Mosby's® Advanced Pharmacy Technician Exam Review

James J. Mizner
Panacea Solutions Consulting
Reston, Virginia

ELSEVIER

Elsevier
3251 Riverport Lane
St. Louis, Missouri 63043

Mosby's® Advanced Pharmacy Technician Exam Review   ISBN: 978-0-323-93539-5

Notice

Publishing Director: Kristin Wilhelm
Senior Content Strategist: Luke Held
Content Development Manager: Danielle Frazier
Senior Content Development Specialist: Maria Broeker
Publishing Services Manager: Deepthi Unni
Project Manager: Thoufiq Mohammed
Senior Book Designer: Amy Buxton

Printed in India

Last digit is the print number: 9 8 7 6 5 4 3 2 1

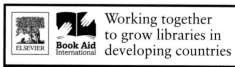

Mosby's® Advanced Pharmacy Technician Exam Review is dedicated to my wife, Mary, and son, Andrew. They have been extremely supportive of me throughout my life and are a constant source of inspiration.

A special thanks to Kristin Wilhelm, Luke Held, Thoufiq Mohammed, and Maria Broeker, who provided their expertise in producing this resource for pharmacy technicians. Finally, thanks to the technical reviewer for assistance in ensuring the accuracy of this review book.

Reviewer

Meera K Brown, PharmD, MBA
Senior Manager, Pharmacy Growth
CVS Health
Austin, Texas

The role of the pharmacy technician has evolved from the days when the early pharmacy technicians accepted prescriptions from walk-in patients, accepted patient refills from the patient over the telephone, and handed the patient their prescription when it was being picked up. The role of the pharmacy technician has always been to assist the pharmacist with dispensing patient prescriptions. Today we find pharmacy technicians entering prescriptions/medication orders into the pharmacy's computer system, pouring and counting out medications, and compounding both sterile and nonsterile preparations. In some pharmacies, the pharmacy technician assists the pharmacist by collecting a patient's medication history, participates in medication therapy management, immunizes patients depending on state regulations, participates in point-of-care testing, and bills out prescriptions and durable medical equipment to various insurance providers.

For the pharmacy technician to perform these advanced pharmacy technician roles, the pharmacy technician is required to undergo specific training, gain valuable experience, and demonstrate knowledge in these specific areas. Upon completion of the training and obtaining practical experience, the pharmacy technician becomes eligible to become a Certified Compounded Sterile Preparation Technician (CSPT), earn the Advanced Certified Pharmacy Technician (CPhT-Adv) credential, or earn a certificate in a variety of pharmacy technician roles. The benefits associated with these credentials and certificates and are listed below:

- CSPT
  - Validates a certified pharmacy technician's (CPhT's) knowledge and skill in compounding sterile preparations and guaranteeing medication safety
- CPhT-Adv
  - Demonstrates knowledge and proficiency in a variety of advanced pharmacy technician roles
- Hazardous Drug Management Certificate
  - Demonstrates responsibility in reducing risk through knowledge of USP <800> standards and requirements for safely managing hazardous drugs.
- Regulatory Compliance Certificate
  - Establishes knowledge of pharmacy laws, regulations, legal requirements, and practice standards
- Controlled Substance Diversion Prevention Certificate
  - Demonstrates knowledge of Drug Enforcement Administration requirements and controlled substance diversion prevention strategies
- Medication History Certificate
  - Denotes knowledge to collect accurate medication histories, review prescriptions to confirm dosing accuracy, and complete specified administrative functions
- Medication Therapy Management Certificate
  - Demonstrates competency in medication use and administration, prescribing accuracy, providing safe medication care, and participating in the medication therapy management process
- Immunization Administration Certificate
  - Shows understanding of immunization schedules, the proper management and storage of immunizations and vaccines, proper usage of personal protective equipment, and safely immunizing patients
- Point-of-Care Testing Certificate
  - Demonstrates competency in performing point-of-care tests, including carefully screening patients, administering tests, collecting specimens, and reading and recording test results; knowledge of Clinical Laboratory Improvement Amendments-waived point-of-care tests; and comprehension of the safe and accurate processes involved with point-of-care testing
- Billing and Reimbursement Certificate
  - Shows knowledge of insurance programs and their eligibility requirements, claim processing and adjudication, prior authorization, and Centers for Medicare and Medicaid Services audits and contract compliance
- Technician Product Verification Certificate
  - Demonstrates ability to complete final verification duties and checking other pharmacy technicians in dispensing medications

Mosby's® Advanced Pharmacy Technician Exam Review has been written to assist active Pharmacy Technician Certification Board (PTCB) CPhTs to prepare for the CSPT examination and the PTCB certificate programs examinations for Hazardous Drug Management, Regulatory Compliance, Controlled Substance Diversion Prevention, Medication History, Medication Therapy Management, Immunization Administration, Point-of-Care Testing, Billing and Reimbursement, and Technician Product Verification.

Each chapter addresses a specific credential or certificate by focusing on the various domains and topics associated with each domain by the PTCB. The medications identified in CSPT have been identified by the PTCB as those medications that a CSPT should know. Medications are covered for the Technician Product Verification Certificate. The vaccines identified in the Medication History and Immunization Administration are common child, adolescent, and adult vaccines, and their schedules are as identified by the Centers for Disease Control and Prevention. Each chapter contains multiple-choice review questions and a sample examination containing the same number of questions as found on the PTCB examination. Each question contains four distractors and rationale identifying why the answer is correct or incorrect. *Mosby's® Advanced Pharmacy Technician Exam Review* contains an online test bank for each examination whereby instructors and students can create their own test to demonstrate their understanding of the content. Information regarding the requirements to earn each credential or certificate are identified below.

Credential	Eligibility requirements	Domains	Test questions	Time to take the test
Certified Compounded Sterile Preparation Technician (CSPT)	Must be an active PTCB CPhT Educational requirements: Pathway 1: Completion of, or enrollment in, a PTCB-recognized education/training program for the CSPT program AND 1 year of full-time continuous compounded sterile preparation (CSP) work experience OR Pathway 2: Three years of full-time continuous CSP work experience	Medications and Components (17%) Facilities and Equipment (22%) Sterile Compounding Procedures (53%) Handling, Packaging, Storage, and Disposal (8%)	75 questions: 60 scored questions and 15 unscored questions	1 hour and 50 minutes
Advanced Certified Pharmacy Technician	At least 3 years of work experience as a pharmacy technician within the past 8 years AND At least four PTCB Assessment-Based Certificate Programs or three Certificate Programs and the CSPT® Certification			
Hazardous Drug Management Certificate	Must hold an active PTCB CPhT Certification and complete a PTCB-Recognized Hazardous Drug Management Education/Training Program	Engineering Controls (22%) Facility Cleaning (16%) Personal Protective Equipment (13%) Transport and Receiving (11%) Dispensing Final Dosage Forms (16%) Administrative (22%)	55 multiple-choice questions	1 hour and 20 minutes
	Must hold an active PTCB CPhT Certification and complete a PTCB-Recognized Regulatory Compliance Education/Training Program	Laws, Regulations, and Guidelines (37%) Legal Requirements and Practice Standards (37%) Patient Safety and Quality Assurance Strategies (26%)	70 multiple-choice questions	1 hour and 20 minutes
Controlled Substance Diversion Prevention Certificate	Must hold an active PTCB CPhT Certification and complete a PTCB-recognized controlled substances diversion prevention education/training program	Controlled Substance Diversion (9%) Controlled Substance Diversion Prevention Program (30%) Drug Enforcement Administration Requirements (38%) Surveillance and Investigation (23%)	70 multiple-choice questions	1 hour and 20 minutes
Medication History Certificate	Must hold an active PTCB CPhT Certification and fulfill one of the following eligibility pathways: Pathway 1: Completion of a PTCB-Recognized Medication History Education/Training Program and at least 6 months of experience conducting medication histories and/or similar experiences of patient-focused communication OR Pathway 2: At least 12 months of full-time experience conducting medication histories and/or similar experiences of patient-focused communication	Concepts/Terminology of Medication History (45%) Patient Safety and Quality Assurance Strategies (55%)	70 multiple-choice questions	1 hour and 20 minutes

Credential	Eligibility requirements	Domains	Test questions	Time to take the test
Medication Therapy Management Certificate	Must hold an active PTCB CPhT Certification and complete a PTCB-Recognized Medication Therapy Management Education/Training Program	Medications and Medical Concepts (40%) Patient Safety and Quality Assurance Strategies (36%) Medication Therapy Management Administration and Management (24%)	65 multiple-choice questions	1 hour and 20 minutes
Immunization Administration Certificate	Must hold an active PTCB CPhT Certification and complete a PTCB-Recognized Immunization Administration Education/Training Program	Concepts/ Terminology of Vaccine Administration (30%) Vaccine Safety and Administration (50%) Documentation, Product Handling, and Adverse Reaction Management for Vaccines (20%)	60 multiple-choice questions	1 hour and 20 minutes
Point-of-Care Testing Certificate	Must hold an active PTCB CPhT Certification and complete a PTCB-Recognized Point-of-Care Testing Education/Training Program	Safety and Precautions (16%) Diseases and Specimens (34%) Clinical Laboratory Improvement Amendments- waived Tests (30%) Test Results, QC, and Recording (20%)	60 multiple-choice questions	1 hour and 20 minutes
Billing and Reimbursement Certificate	Must hold an active PTCB CPhT Certification and fulfill one of the following eligibility pathways: Pathway 1: Completion of PTCB-Recognized Education/ Training Program for the Billing and Reimbursement Certificate and at least 6 months of experience as a pharmacy technician, at least 50% of which must be devoted to pharmacy billing and reimbursement activities OR Pathway 2: At least 12 months of full-time employment with pharmacy technician experience, at least 50% of which must be devoted to pharmacy billing and reimbursement activities	Programs and Eligibility (20%) Claims Processing and Adjudication (48%) Prior Authorization (20%) Audits and Compliance (12%)	70 multiple-choice questions	1 hour and 20 minute
Technician Product Verification Certificate	Must hold an active PTCB CPhT Certification and fulfill one of the following eligibility pathways: Pathway 1: Completion of a PTCB-Recognized Technician Product Verification Education/Training Program OR Pathway 2: Completion of a state board-approved validation program	Identifying the correct product name, strength, and dosage form Calculating the amount of product to dispense based on prescribed dosage and frequency Evaluating the integrity of product characteristics	120 questions	1 hour and 45 minutes

CPhT, Certified Pharmacy Technician; *PTCB*, Pharmacy Technician Certification Board; *QC*, quality control.

Pharmacy technicians should utilize *Mosby's® Advanced Pharmacy Technician Exam Review* as a guide to determine which credential or certificate they may need additional assistance in preparing for examination. Good luck on your examination and your career as an Advanced Pharmacy Technician.

James J. Mizner, MBA, BS, RPh

The Role of the Advanced Pharmacy Technician Today

The practice of pharmacy has evolved over the years, and so has the role of the pharmacy technician. Once known as a drug clerk who accepted a new prescription from the patient and handed the patient's filled prescription back to them in a community retail pharmacy, the role of the pharmacy technician has evolved. Besides assisting the pharmacist in a variety of activities such as inputting a patient's prescription information into the pharmacy information system and pouring and counting a patient's medication, today's pharmacy technician has the opportunity to be involved in a variety of a pharmacy activities to include compounding sterile preparations, conducting a patient's medication history, assisting in immunizing patients, participating in point-of-care testing, and billing for prescriptions.

The Pharmacy Technician Certification Board (PTCB) was formed in 1995 and issued the PTCB Certified Pharmacy Technician (CPhT) Certification to those qualified individuals who met specific eligibility requirements. Since that time, the PTCB has created another credential, the Advance Certified Pharmacy Technician (CPhT-Adv). Individuals who have been awarded the CPhT-Adv are recognized for their pharmacy knowledge and experience. To earn the CPhT an individual must possess at least 3 years of work experience as a pharmacy technician within the past 8 years and complete at least four PTCB Assessment-Based Certificate Programs or three Certificate Programs and the Compounded Sterile Preparation Technician® (CSPT®) Certification. PTCB Assessment-Based Certificate Programs include Hazardous Drug Management Certificate, Regulatory Compliance Certificate, Controlled Substance Diversion Prevention Certificate, Medication History Certificate, Medication Therapy Management Certificate, Immunization Administration Certificate, Point-of-Care Testing Certificate, Billing and Reimbursement Certificate, Technician Product Verification Certificate, and Nonsterile Compounding and Supply Chain and Inventory Management Certificate. The certified CSPT and each certificate have specific educational requirements and work experience associated with the certification/certificate.

Certification/certificate	The pharmacy technician demonstrates knowledge and competency of
Certified Pharmacy Technician (CPhT)	• Medications • Federal requirements • Patient safety and quality assurance • Order entry and processing
Advanced Certified Pharmacy Technician (CPhT-Adv)	• An experienced pharmacy technician committed to ensuring medication safety
Certified Compounded Sterile Preparation Technician® (CSPT®) Certification (CSPT)	• Medications and components • Facilities and equipment • Sterile compounding procedures • Handling, packaging, storage, and disposal of compounded sterile preparations
Hazardous Drug Management Certificate	• Features and characteristics of facilities and engineering controls • Processes and procedures for cleaning facilities where hazardous drugs are handled • Personal protective equipment requirements • Procedures for transporting, receiving, and handling hazardous medications • Dispensing final dosage forms • Federal regulations pertaining to the disposal of hazardous drug
Regulatory Compliance Certificate	• Laws, regulations, and guidelines, such as the Federal Controlled Substances Act • Legal requirements, such as Risk Evaluation and Mitigation Strategies • Practice standards and principles for pharmacy laws and ethics • Patient safety and quality assurance strategies
Controlled Substance Diversion Prevention Certificate	• Consequences of diversion • Signs of impaired health care workers • Areas of vulnerability in procurement, preparation and dispensing, prescribing, administration, and waste/removal processes • Types and functions of security control measures, devices, and software to detect and prevent diversion • Drug Enforcement Administration requirements for registration, record keeping, and conducting physical inventories • Identifying suspicious data patterns, product tampering, and fraudulent prescriptions
Medication History Certificate	• Gathering medication histories with accuracy • Identifying potential errors or necessary clarifications with acute precision • Alleviating pharmacists' time completing various administrative tasks
Medication Therapy Management Certificate	• Medication uses and administration • Prescribing accuracy • Delivering safe patient care • Administration of medication therapy management

Immunization Administration Certificate	• Understanding immunization schedules • Proper management and storage of immunization supplies and vaccine doses in your pharmacy • Safe delivery of immunizations directly to patients • Personal protective equipment and other supplies to protect health care workers and patients
Point-of-Care Testing Certificate	• Conducting point-of-care tests, including carefully screening patients, administering tests, collecting specimens, and reading and recording test results • Knowledge of Clinical Laboratory Improvement Amendments-waived point-of-care tests • Understanding of the safe and accurate processes involved with point-of-care testing
Billing and Reimbursement Certificate	• Insurance programs and eligibility requirements • Claim processing and adjudication • Prior authorizations • Centers for Medicare and Medicaid Services audits and contract compliance
Technician Product Verification Certificate	• Completing final verification duties • Checking other technicians or automated systems for accuracy in dispensing medications • Managing detail-oriented work and administrative tasks

Today's pharmacy technicians are becoming increasingly engaged in a variety of advanced responsibilities such as compounding sterile preparations, assisting in the immunization of patients, performing medication reconciliations, and in some states performing tech-check-tech activities in the pharmacy. By having pharmacy technicians assuming these responsibilities, pharmacists become more involved in direct patient care, which improves patient outcomes. According to William Schimmel, Pharmacy Technician Certification Board Executive Director and CEO, "Assessment-based certificate programs are an important step for pharmacy technicians who seek recognition for their education and training, and their dedication to patient safety."[1] Employers recognize the benefit of using pharmacy technicians in these various advanced pharmacy roles, as it is an intelligent use of their pharmacy resources. Career ladders for pharmacy technicians have incorporated some of these advanced credentials, resulting in new career opportunities and career advancement. In many situations, career advancement results in an increase in employee earnings and career satisfaction.

[1] PTCB developing advanced CPhT credential. https://www.ptcb.org/news/ptcb-developing-advanced-cpht-credential. Accessed July 17, 2023.

Contents

Compounded Sterile Preparation Technician (CSPT)

Eligibility requirements

- Must be an active Pharmacy Technician Certification Board (PTCB) Certified Pharmacy Technician in good standing and satisfy PTCB's education and/or work criteria
- Completion of, or enrollment in, a PTCB-Recognized Education/Training Program for the Compounded Sterile Preparation Technician (CSPT) Program and 1 year of full-time continuous compounded sterile preparation work experience

Or

- Three years of full-time continuous compounded sterile preparation work experience

Compounded sterile preparation technician domains

1.0 Medications and components (17%)

1.1 Generic names, brand names, indications, side effects, and therapeutic classifications of medications used in sterile compounding

1.2 Types of high-alert/narrow-therapeutic-index medications used in sterile compounding (e.g., insulin, heparin, concentrated electrolytes, chemotherapy)

1.3 Dosage (e.g., strength, dosage forms) and administration (e.g., routes, instructions) of compounded sterile preparations

1.4 Drug-specific factors affecting stability of compounded sterile preparations (e.g., containers, light, concentration, closure, temperature, agitation)

1.5 Type, purpose, and use of technical and clinical references for sterile compounding (e.g., package inserts, Safety Data Sheets)

1.6 Factors (e.g., temperature, microbial limits of sterility, storage time, complexity of preparation, location of preparation) that influence the assignment of beyond-use dates for compounded sterile preparations

1.7 Physical and chemical compatibility criteria for components (e.g., medications, ingredients, base solutions, filters, tubing, closures)

2.0 Facilities and equipment (22%)

2.1 Types and uses of primary engineering controls (e.g., laminar airflow workbenches and systems, biological safety cabinets, compounding aseptic isolators, compounding aseptic containment isolators)

2.2 Types of secondary engineering controls (e.g., anteroom, buffer area, segregated compounding areas, containment segregated compounding areas)

2.3 Features of secondary engineering controls (e.g., air pressure differentials, high-efficiency particulate air filtration, International Organization of Standardization (ISO) classification, air changes per hour)

2.4 Temperature, pressure, and humidity parameters and/or tolerances for facilities and controlled environments

2.5 Procedures and requirements for conducting different types of environmental monitoring

2.6 Action levels and parameters for assessing environmental monitoring results (e.g., surface sampling, viable air sampling, nonviable air sampling)

2.7 Common factors contributing to out-of-specification environmental monitoring results

2.8 Operational standards (e.g., food and drink restrictions, facility access) for maintaining the safety and sterility of sterile compounding environments

3.0 Sterile compounding procedures (53%)

3.1 Types, purpose, and procedures for conducting required personnel training and competency assessments (e.g., gloved fingertip sampling, media fill) and the minimum frequency with which they must occur

3.2 Equations and calculations used to prepare compounded sterile preparations (infusion times, percent solutions, dilutions, allegations, dispensing quantities, days' supply, ratios and proportions, quantities, doses, concentrations, conversions)

3.3 Equations and calculations used to prepare compounded sterile preparations (e.g., infusion times, percent solutions, dilutions, allegations, dispensing quantities, days' supply, ratios and proportions, quantities, doses, concentrations, conversions)

3.4   Hand hygiene procedures

3.5   Types of garb and personal protective equipment

3.6   Procedures for donning, doffing, and disposal of garb and personal protective equipment for nonhazardous and/or hazardous drugs

3.7   Properties and usage indications for deactivating, decontaminating, cleaning, and disinfecting agents

3.8   Procedures and requirements for cleaning and disinfecting compounding equipment, primary engineering controls, and secondary engineering controls for nonhazardous compounded sterile preparations

3.9   Procedures and requirements for deactivating, decontaminating, cleaning, and disinfecting compounding equipment, primary engineering controls, and secondary engineering controls for hazardous compounded sterile preparations

3.10   Principles of aseptic manipulation and procedures for operating within horizontal and vertical air flow equipment (e.g., first air, zone of turbulence)

3.11   Types of and requirements for cleaning and disinfecting critical sites of components (e.g., vials, ampoules, ports)

3.12   Safety procedures for handling sharps

3.13   Documentation and record-keeping requirements for sterile compounding (e.g., master formulation record, compounding record)

3.14   Procedures to accurately weigh and measure components; principles of volumetric and gravimetric accuracy

3.15   Procedures for compounding parenteral nutrition

3.16   Procedures for preparing specialized compounded sterile preparations (e.g., epidurals, intrathecals, cassettes, ophthalmics, irrigations)

3.17   Procedures for compounding hazardous drugs (e.g., negative pressure technique, using closed-system drug-transfer devices)

3.18   Procedures for compounding sterile preparations from nonsterile components (e.g., presterilization, terminal sterilization, filtration, aseptic preparation)

3.19   Potential signs of defective compounded sterile preparations (e.g., discoloration, particulates, leaks, turbidity)

3.20   Potential signs of defective compounded sterile preparations (e.g., discoloration, particulates, leaks, turbidity)

3.21   Procedures for interpreting results of sterility, potency, and endotoxin testing

4.0   Handling, packaging, storage and disposal (8%)

4.1   Handling, labeling, packaging, storage, and disposal requirements for nonhazardous medications, components, sharps, and finished compounded sterile preparations

4.2   Handling, labeling, packaging, storage, and disposal requirements for hazardous medications, components, sharps, and finished compounded sterile preparations

4.3   Types of and requirements for supplies used in packaging and repackaging (e.g., bags, syringes, glass, polyvinyl chloride, latex free, Di[2-ethylhexl] phthalate-free)

Medications and components

Sterile compounding medications						
Generic name	Brand name	Classification	Indication	Side effects	Strength	Route of administration
acetaminophen injection	Ofirmev	Centrally acting nonopioid analgesic	Analgesic; antipyretic	Nausea, rash, headache	10 mg/mL	IV
acetazolamide sodium injection	[a]	Carbonic anhydrase inhibitor	Glaucoma, CHF, edema, pseudotumor cerebri, urinary alkalinization	Fatigue, malaise, taste changes	500 mg	IV
acetic acid irrigant	[a]	Irrigating solution	Prevent infection for wounds	Systemic acidosis, hematuria, pain	0.25%	Intravesical
acetylcysteine injection	[a]	Expectorant, mucolytic	Acetaminophen overdose, mucolytic	Anaphylaxis, nausea/vomiting, urticaria	10%, 20%	NG, IV, nebulizer
acyclovir sodium injection	[a]	Antiviral	Herpes/varicella/zoster	Nausea/vomiting, headache, malaise	50 mg/mL	IV
adalimumab	Humira	DMARD, TNF inhibitor	Rheumatoid arthritis, psoriatic arthritis, psoriasis, Crohn disease	Injection site reaction, URI, headache	INJ (pen): 40 mg per 0.4 mL, 40 mg per 0.8 mL, 80 mg per 0.8 mL; INJ (pre-filled syringe): 10 mg per 0.1 mL, 20 mg per 0.2 mL, 40 mg per 0.4 mL, 40 mg per 0.8 mL, 80 mg per 0.8 mL, 20 mg/0.4 mL, 40 mg/0.8 mL	SC

Sterile compounding medications—cont'd						
Generic name	Brand name	Classification	Indication	Side effects	Strength	Route of administration
adenosine injection	Adenocard, Adenoscan	Antiarrhythmics	PSVT conversion, tachycardia	Flushing, dyspnea, chest discomfort	INJ (pre-filled syringe): 6 mg per 2 mL, 12 mg per 4 mL; INJ (vial): 6 mg per 2 mL, 12 mg per 4 mL, 60 mg per 20 mL, 90 mg per 30 mL 3 mg/mL	IV
albumin human injection	Albuked, Albuminar, Albuminex, Albuminex, Albutein, Flexbumin, Kedbumin	Protein	Hypovolemia, hypoalbuminemia, burns	Rapid heart rate, low blood pressure, fever, chills	INJ (5%): 2.5 g per 50 mL, 12.5 g per 250 mL, 25 g per 500 mL; INJ (25%): 5 g per 20 mL, 12.5 g per 50 mL, 25 g per 100 mL 5%, 25%	IV
allopurinol injection	Aloprim	Xanthine oxidase inhibitor	Hyperuricemia	Injection site reaction, elevated alkaline phosphate, eosinophilia	500 mg/vial	IV
alprostadil	a	Vasodilator	Patent ductus arteriosus	Bradycardia, hypotension, tachycardia	500 mcg/vial	IV
alteplase recombinant injection	Activase	Thrombolytic	Acute myocardial infarction, acute ischemic stroke, acute massive pulmonary embolism	Bleeding, thromboembolism, cholesterol embolism	50 mg/mL, 100 mg/mL	IV
amikacin sulfate injection	a	Aminoglycoside	Bacterial infections	Elevated BUN, tinnitus, injection site reaction	250 mg/mL	IM/IV
amino acid injection	Aminosyn II, Travasol, FreAmine	Amino acid	Nutritional support	Local inflammatory reactions	10%, 15%	IV
aminophylline injection	a	Methylxanthine	Asthma, COPD, acute bronchospasm	Insomnia, headache, nausea/vomiting	25 mg/mL	IV
amiodarone HCL injection	Nexterone	Class III antiarrhythmic	Ventricular arrhythmias, ACLS	Malaise/fatigue, ataxia, tremor	50 mg/mL	IV
amphotericin B deoxycholate injection	a	Antifungal	Systemic fungal infections, fungal endocarditis, candidal cystitis	Acute infusion reaction, fever, rigors	50 mg/mL	IV
amphotericin B lipid complex	Abelcet	Antifungal	Systemic fungal infections, fungal endocarditis, aspergillosis	Elevated CR, fever, rigors	5 mg/mL	IV
amphotericin B liposome	AmBisome	Antifungal	Systemic fungal infections, febrile neutropenia, cryptococcal meningitis, aspergillosis, fungal endocarditis	Hypokalemia, hypomagnesma, elevated BUN/CR	50 mg/mL	IV

(Continued)

Sterile compounding medications—cont'd						
Generic name	**Brand name**	**Classification**	**Indication**	**Side effects**	**Strength**	**Route of adminis-tration**
ampicillin injection	a	Penicillin	Bacterial infections, bacterial meningitis, endocarditis, typhoid fever, systemic anthrax	Eosinophilia, glossitis, stomatitis	125 mg, 250 mg, 500 mg, 1 g, 2 g, 10 g/vial	IV
ampicillin sodium/ sulbactam sodium injection	Unasyn	Penicillin	Bacterial infections, PID, sinusitis, infection prophylaxis	Injection site pain, thrombophlebitis, eosinophilia	10 g–5 g, 2 g–1 g, 1 g–0.5 g	IM, IV
antithymocyte globulin (rabbit) injection	Atgam	Immunoglobulin, immunosuppressant	Kidney transplant rejection, aplastic anemia	Fever/rigors, leukopenia, thrombocytopenia	50 mg/mL	IV
argatroban injection	a	Anticoagulant	Anticoagulation	Chest pain, hypotension, hypersensitivity reaction	1 mg/mL, 100 mg/mL	IV
asparaginase injection	Erwinaze	Oncologic	All forms of cancer	Hypersensitivity reaction, hyperglycemia, glucose intolerance	10,000 IU/vial	IM, IV
atracurium besylate injection	a	Neuromuscular blocker	Neuromuscular blockade	Skin flushing, blood pressure changes	10 mg/mL	IV
atropine sulfate injection	a	ACLS/PALS/ NALS	ACLS, anesthesia adjunct, neuromuscular blockade, reversal adjunct	Xerostomia, blurred vision, tachycardia	0.05 mg/mL, 0.1 mg/mL, 0.4 mg/mL, 10 mg/mL	IM, IV, SC
azathioprine sodium injection	a	Immunosuppressant	Kidney transplant rejection prophylaxis	Anemia, leukopenia, thrombocytopenia		IV
azithromycin injection	a	Macrolide	PID	Dyspepsia, impaired hearing, abdominal pain	500 mg/vial	IV
aztreonam injection	Azactam	Antibacterial	Bacterial infections, UTI, surgical infection prophylaxis, hospital-acquired or ventilator-associated pneumonia	Injection site reaction, phlebitis, elevated ALT, AST, and CR levels	1 g/vial, 2 g/ vial, 1 g/50 mL, 2 g/50 mL	IM, IV
bendamustine HCl injection	Bendeka	Alkylating agent	CLL, non-Hodgkin lymphoma	Myelosuppression, neutropenia, thrombocytopenia	25 mg/mL	IV
betamethasone sodium phosphate/ betamethasone acetate injection	Celestone Soluspan	Corticosteroid	Multiple sclerosis, corticosteroid responsive conditions, fetal lung maturation	Cushinoid appearance, hirsutism, weight gain	6 mg/mL	IM
bevacizumab injection	Avastin	Antiangiogenic agents	Metastatic colorectal cancer, metastatic nonsquamous small cell lung cancer, metastatic renal cell cancer, recurrent ovarian cancer, recurrent or metastatic cervical cancer	Thrombo-cytopenia, alopecia, hypertension	25 mg/mL	Bolus, IV

Sterile compounding medications—cont'd						
Generic name	Brand name	Classification	Indication	Side effects	Strength	Route of administration
bivalirudin injection	Angiomax	Anticoagulant	Anticoagulation	Injection site reaction, hypotension, bleeding	260 mg/vial	IV
bleomycin sulfate injection	a	Antibiotic oncologic	Squamous cell cancer, Hodgkin lymphoma, non-Hodgkin lymphoma	Erythema, skin tenderness, rash	15 units/vial, 30 units/vial	IV, IM, SC
bupivacaine injection (HCl and liposomal)	Exparel	Anesthetic	Local anesthesia	Motor dysfunction, arrhythmia, hypokalemia	133 mg/10 mL, 266 mg/mL	Infiltration
calcium chloride injection	a	Mineral	Hypocalcemia, arrhythmias, hypermagnesemia, calcium channel blocker overdose	Hypercalcemia, hypercalciuria, vasodilation, hypotension	100 mg/mL	IV
calcium gluconate injection	a	Mineral	Hypocalcemia, arrhythmias, hypermagnesemia, calcium channel blocker overdose	Hypercalcemia, hypercalciuria, hypomagnesemia	100 mg/mL	IV
carbamazepine injection	Carnexiv	Anticonvulsant	Partial seizures, generalized tonic-clonic seizures, mixed seizure patterns	Dizziness, drowsiness, unsteadiness	200 mg/20 mL	IV
carboplatin injection	a	Alkylating agent	Ovarian cancer	Thrombo-cytopenia, anemia, leukopenia	10 mg/mL	IV
caspofungin acetate injection	Cancidas	Antifungal	Candidiasis, candidemia, aspergillosis, endocarditis	Infusion reaction, elevated ALT, AST, and alkaline phosphate	50 mg/vial, 70 mg/vial	IV
cefazolin sodium injection	a	Cephalosporin	Bacterial infections, UTIs, pneumonia, endocarditis	Thrombophlebitis, elevated ALT/AST	500 mg/vial, 1 g/vial, 10 g/vial	IM, IV
cefepime HCl injection	a	Cephalosporin	Pneumonia, febrile neutropenia, UTI, skin infections, intraabdominal infections	Injection site reaction, hypo-phosphatemia, rash	1 g/vial, 2 g/vial	IV
cefnidir	a	Cephalosporin	Bacterial infections, chronic bronchitis, community acquired pneumonia, uncomplicated UTI	Anaphylaxis, Stevens-Johnson syndrome, aplastic anemia, neutropenia, leukopenia, thrombocytopenia	300 mg, 125 mg/5 ml, 250 mg/5 mL	Oral
cefotaxime sodium injection	a	Cephalosporin	Bacterial infections, pneumonia, gonococcal infections, sinusitis, endocarditis	Injection site reaction, rash, pruritis	1 g/vial	IM, IV
cefotetan disodium injection	Cefotan	Cephalopsorin	Bacterial infections, UTI, PID, infection prophylaxis	Injection site pain, phlebitis, increased ALT, AST, and BUN CR	1 g/vial	IM, IV

(Continued)

Sterile compounding medications—cont'd						
Generic name	Brand name	Classification	Indication	Side effects	Strength	Route of administration
cefoxitin sodium injection [a]		Cephalosporin	Bacterial infections, uncomplicated gonococcal infections, PID, surgical prophylaxis	Thrombophlebitis, induration, hypotension	1 g/vial, 2 g/vial, 10 g/vial	IM, IV
ceftazidime injection	Fortaz, Tazicef	Cephalosporin	Bacterial infections, pneumonia	Injection site pain, elevated ALT, AST, and BUN CR	6 g/vial	IV, IM
ceftriaxone sodium injection [a]		Cephalosporin	Bacterial infections, bacterial meningitis, pneumonia, gonococcal infections, PID, endocarditis, proctitis, epididymitis	Local injection site reaction, thrombocytosis, elevated ALT/AST	250 mg/vial, 500 mg/vial, 1 g/50 mL, 2 g/50 mL, 1 g/vial, 2 g/vial, 10 g/vial	IV, IM
cefuroxime sodium injection [a]		Cephalosporin	Bacterial infections, bacterial meningitis, pneumonia, gonococcal infections, infection prophylaxis	Anemia, renal impairment, elevated ALT/AST	750 mg/vial, 1.5 g vial	IM, IV
chloramphenicol sodium succinate injection [a]		Antibacterial	Bacterial infections, bacterial meningitis, rickettsial infections, systemic anthrax	Peripheral neuropathy, headache, nausea/vomiting	100 mg/mL	IV
chlorpromazine HCl injection [a]		Antipsychotic	Psychosis, nausea, and vomiting	Xerostomia, drowsiness, hypotension	25 mg/mL	IM
ciprofloxacin injection	Cipro	Fluoroquinolones	Bacterial infection, UTI, intraabdominal infection, systemic anthrax exposure	Dyspepsia, photosensitivity, myalgia	200 mg/100 mL, 400 mg/20 mL	IV
cisplatin injection [a]		Alkylating agent	Metastatic ovarian cancer, metastatic testicular cancer, bladder cancer	Elevated BUN and CR, leukopenia, thrombocytopenia	1 mg/mL	IV
clindamycin phosphate injection	Cleocin	Antibacterial	PID, pneumonia, endocarditis, infection prophylaxis, anthrax exposure	Thrombophlebitis, jaundice, hypotension	75 mg/mL, 150 mg/ml	IM, IV
cyclophosphamide injection [a]		DMARDs, alkylating agent	Hodgkin lymphoma, non-Hodgkin lymphoma, multiple myeloma, CML, AML, B-cell precursor ALL, large B-cell lymphoma	Alopecia, neutropenia, leukopenia, thrombocytopenia	500 mg/vial, 1 g/vial, 2 g/vial	IV
cyclosporine injection	Sandimmune	Immunosuppressant	Prophylaxis for heart, liver, and kidney transplants	Nephrotoxicity, hepatotoxicity, leukopenia	50 mg/mL	IV
cytarabine injection (conventional and liposomal) [a]		Antimetabolite agent	Lymphomatous meningitis	Dehydration, peripheral edema, arthralgia	20 mg/mL, 100 mg/mL	Intrathecally
dacarbazine injection [a]		Alkylating agent	Metastatic melanoma, Hodgkin lymphoma	Injection site reaction, anorexia, nausea/vomiting	100 mg/vial, 200 mg/vial	IV

Generic name	Brand name	Classification	Indication	Side effects	Strength	Route of adminis-tration
dactinomycin injection	Cosmegen	Antibiotic oncologic agent	Wilms tumor, Ewing sarcoma, gestational trophoblastic neoplasia, osteosarcoma	Anemia, neutropenia, thrombocytopenia	0.5 mg/mL	IV
daptomycin injection	Cubicin	Antibacterial	Skin/skin structure infections, staphylococcal bacteremia, endocarditis	Insomnia, elevated CK levels, chest pain	350 mg/vial, 500 mg/vial	IV
daunorubicin HCl injection	a	Topoisomerase II inhibitor	ALL, AML	Myelosuppression, cardiotoxicity, alopecia	5 mg/mL	IV
deferoxamine mesylate injection	Desferal	Iron homeostasis	Chronic iron overload, iron intoxication	Injection site reaction, red urine, flushing	500 mg/vial, 2 g/vial	IM, IV
dexamethasone sodium phosphate injection	a	Corticosteroid	Adrenal insufficiency, corticosteroid responsive conditions, cerebral edema, nausea, vomiting, shock, altitude sickness	Cushingoid appearance, hirsutism, weight gain	4 mg/mL, 10 mg/mL	IM, IV
dexmedetomidine HCl injection	Precedex	Sedative	ICU sedation, procedural sedation	Hypotension, bradycardia, nausea	100 mcg/mL	IV
dextrose injection	a	IV fluid	Fluid replenishment and calories	Infection at site of injection, thrombophlebitis, hypervolemia	5%, 10%, 20%	IV
diazepam injection	a	Benzodiazepine	Procedural sedation, status epilepticus	Drowsiness, fatigue, asthenia	5 mg/mL	IM, IV
digoxin injection	Lanoxin	Antiarrhythmic	CHF, atrial fibrillation, PSVT conversion	Dizziness, headache, diarrhea	0.05 mg/mL, 0.25 mg/mL	IM, IV
dihydroergotamine mesylate injection	D.H.E.45	Ergot alkaloid	Migraine and cluster headache	Dizziness, paresthesia, flushing	1 mg/mL	IM, IV, SC
diltiazem HCl injection	a	Calcium channel blocker	Atrial fibrillation, atrial flutter, PSVT conversion	Peripheral edema, headache, nausea	5 mg/mL	IV
dimercaprol injection	BAL in Oil	Heavy metal	Arsenic, gold, lead, or mercury poisoning	Injection site pain, hypertension, tachycardia	100 mg/mL	IM
diphenhydramine HCl injection	a	Antihistamine	Allergy symptoms, allergic reaction	Drowsiness, dizziness, impaired coordination	50 mg/mL	IM, IV
dobutamine HCl injection	a	Inotrope processor	Cardiac decompensation, cardiac output maintenance	Hypertension, tachycardia, premature ventricular contractions	12.5 mg/mL, 5% 200 mg/100 mL, 5% 400 mg/100 mL	IV
docetaxel injection	Taxotere	Mitosis inhibitor	Breast cancer, non–small lung cancer, prostate cancer, gastric cancer, squamous cell head/neck cancer	Neutropenia, leukopenia, anemia	10 mg/mL, 20 mg/mL	IV

Sterile compounding medications—cont'd

(Continued)

Sterile compounding medications—cont'd						
Generic name	Brand name	Classification	Indication	Side effects	Strength	Route of administration
dopamine HCl injection [a]		Inotrope/pressors	Shock, heart failure, bradycardia	Tachycardia, headache, nausea	40 mg/mL	IV
doxorubicin HCl injection (*conventional and liposomal*) [a]		Antibiotic oncologic	ALL, AML, solid tumors	Leukopenia, thrombocytopenia, nausea	2 mg/mL	IV
doxycycline hyclate injection [a]		Tetracycline	Bacterial infections, pneumonia, PID, anthrax exposure, Rocky Mountain spotted fever	Headache, nausea, dyspepsia	100 mg/vial	IV
enalaprilat injection [a]		Angiotensin-converting enzyme inhibitor	HTN	Hypotension, dizziness, elevated BUN, CR, ALT, and AST	1.25 mg/mL	IV
enoxaparin sodium injection	Lovenox	Anticoagulant	DVT prophylaxis, DVT/PE treatment, NQWMI, STEMI	Injection site reaction, anemia, hemorrhage	30 mg/0.3 mL, 40 mg/0.4 mL, 60 mg/0.6 mL, 80 mg/0.8 mL, 100 mg/mL, 120 mg/0.8 mL, 150 mg/mL, 300 mg/mL	SC
ephedrine sulfate injection	Akovaz, Corphedra	Inotropes/pressors	Anesthesia-related hypotension	Headache, restlessness, palpitations	50 mg/mL	IV
epinephrine injection	Adrenalin, Auvi-Q, EpiPen, Symjepi	Inotropes/pressors	Anaphylaxis, asthma exacerbation	Palpitations, tachycardia, nausea/vomiting	0.15 mg/autoinjector, 0.3 mg/autoinjector, 1 mg/mL	IM, SC
epoetin alfa recombinant (erythropoietin) injection	Epogen, Procrit, Retacrit	CSF	Anemia, surgery-associated transfusion reduction	Hypertension, headache, arthralgia	2000 units/mL, 3000 units/mL, 4000 units/mL, 10,000 units/mL, 20,000 units/mL	IV, SC
epoprostenol sodium injection	Flolan, Veletri	Pulmonary arterial hypertension	Pulmonary arterial hypertension	Influenza-like symptoms, tachycardia, hypotension	0.5 mg/vial, 1.5 mg/vial	IV
eptifibatide injection	Integrilin	Antiplatelet	Acute coronary syndrome, PCI	Bleeding, hypotension, thrombocytopenia	0.75 mg/mL, 2 mg/mL	IV
ertapenem sodium injection	Invanz	Carbapenem	Intraabdominal infections, skin/skin structure infections, pneumonia, gynecologic infections, colorectal surgery infection prophylaxis	Infusion site reaction, elevated LFTs, diarrhea	1 g/vial	IM, IV
estradiol cypionate injection	Depo-Estradiol	Estrogen	Vasomotor symptoms, hypogonadal hypoestrogenism	Application site reaction, influenza-like symptoms, dyspepsia	5 mg/mL	IM
etoposide injection [a]		Mitosis inhibitor	Testicular cancer, small cell lung cancer	Neutropenia, thrombocytopenia, hypersensitivity reaction	20 mg/mL	IV

Sterile compounding medications—cont'd						
Generic name	Brand name	Classification	Indication	Side effects	Strength	Route of administration
famotidine injection	a	H$_2$ blocker	Duodenal ulcer, gastric ulcer, GERD, Zollinger-Ellison ulcer	Headache, dizziness, constipation	10 mg/mL	IV
fat emulsion intravenous	Clinolipid, Liposyn	Dietary supplement	Parenteral nutrition	Headache, dizziness, nausea/vomiting	10%, 20%	IV
fentanyl citrate injection	a	Opioid	Analgesia, anesthesia adjunct, postoperative pain, pain	Somnolence, confusion, nausea/vomiting	50 mcg/mL	IM, IV
filgrastim injection	Neupogen, Zarxio, Nivestym	CSF	Neutropenia, PBPC mobilization	Bone pain, musculoskeletal pain, fever	300 mcg/mL, 480 mcg/mL	IV, SC
fluconazole injection	a	Antifungal	Candidiasis, meningitis, BMT fungal prophylaxis	Elevated ALT/AST, nausea, headache	200 mg/100 mL—0.9%, 400 mg/200 mL—0.9%	IV
fludarabine phosphate injection	a	Antimetabolite agent	Refractory CLL, B-cell precursor ALL, large cell B lymphoma	Neutropenia, thrombocytopenia, anemia	25 mg/mL	IV
flumazenil injection	Romazicon	Benzodiazepine antagonist	Benzodiazepine overdose, benzodiazepine sedation reversal	Diaphoresis, bradycardia, tachycardia	0.1 mg/mL	IV
fluorouracil injection	Adrucil	Antimetabolite agent	Breast cancer, colorectal cancer, gastric cancer, pancreatic cancer	Myelosuppression, confusion, nausea/vomiting	50 mg/mL	IV
fluphenazine injection	a	Antipsychotic	Psychosis	Anorexia, dyspepsia, peripheral edema	2.5 mg/mL	IM
folic acid injection	a	Vitamin	Folate-deficient megaloblastic anemia	Anorexia, abdominal pains, disrupted sleep patterns	5 mg/mL	IM, IV, SC
fomepizole injection	Antizol	Environmental/industrial chemical	Ethylene glycol toxicity, methanol toxicity	Transiently elevated ALT/AST, metallic taste, drowsiness	1 g/mL	IV
fondaparinux sodium injection	Arixtra	Anticoagulant	DVT prophylaxis	Injection site bleeding, pruritis, elevated ALT/AST	2.5 mg/0.5 mL, 5 mg/0.4 mL, 7.5 mg/0.6 mL, 10 mg/0.8 mL	SC
foscarnet sodium injection	Foscavir	Antiviral agent	CMV retinitis, acyclovir r-resistant monocutaneous HSV infection, acyclovir-resistant varicella infection, acyclovir-resistant herpes zoster	Anemia, renal impairment, hypokalemia	24 mg/mL	IV
fosphenytoin sodium injection	Cerebyx, Sesquient	Hydantoin	Status epilepticus, seizure disorder	Pruritis, nystagmus, ataxia	100 mg PE/2 mL, 500 mg PE/10 mL	IM, IV
furosemide injection	a	Loop diuretic	Edema, pulmonary edema, HTN, hypercalcemia	Urinary frequency, muscle cramps, elevated ALT/AST	10 mg/mL	IM, IV

(Continued)

Sterile compounding medications—cont'd						
Generic name	Brand name	Classification	Indication	Side effects	Strength	Route of administration
gadoterate meglumine injection	Dotarem	Diagnostic	MRI test	Headache, sleepiness, nausea/vomiting	0.05 mmol/mL	IV
ganciclovir sodium injection	Cytovene	Antiviral	CMV prophylaxis, CMV retinitis	Leukopenia, thrombocytopenia, elevated ALT, AST, and CR	500 mg/vial	IV
gemcitabine HCl injection	Infugem	Antimetabolite	Ovarian cancer, breast cancer, non–small lung cancer, pancreatic cancer	Elevated LFTs, elevated BUN and CR, neutropenia	200 mg/vial, 1 g/vial	IV
gentamicin sulfate injection	a	Aminoglycoside	Bacterial infections, endocarditis, uncomplicated gonococcal infections, PID, pneumonia, surgical infection prophylaxis, respiratory infections in cystic fibrosis patients	Injection site reaction, elevated BUN, tinnitus, hearing loss	10 mg/mL, 40 mg/mL	IM, IV
glucagon injection	GlucaGen	Hypoglycemic anaphylaxis	Hypoglycemia, diagnostics, beta-blocker overdose, calcium channel blocker overdose	Hyperglycemia, tachycardia, hypertension	1 mg/mL	IM, IV, SC
haloperidol decanoate injection	Haldol Decanoate	Antipsychotic	Psychosis	Extrapyramidal symptoms, tardive dyskinesia, akathisia	50 mg/mL, 100 mg/mL	IM
haloperidol lactate injection	a	Antipsychotic	Psychosis, agitation	Extrapyramidal symptoms, tardive dyskinesia, akathisia	5 mg/mL	IM, IV
heparin sodium injection	a	Anticoagulant	Thromboembolism, PCI, acute coronary syndrome	Local injection site reaction, bleeding, thrombocytopenia, prolonged clotting time	1000 units/mL, 5000 units/mL, 10,000 units/mL, 20,000 units/mL	IV, SC
hydralazine HCl injection	a	Vasodilator	Hypertensive crisis	Tachycardia, angina, palpitations	20 mg/mL	IV
hydrocortisone sodium succinate injection	Solu-Cortef	Corticosteroid	Corticosteroid-responsive condition, acute adrenal insufficiency, status asthmaticus, adjunct therapy for septic shock	Cushingoid appearance, hirsutism, weight gain	100 mg/vial, 250 mg/vial, 500 mg/vial, 1000 mg/vial	IM, IV
hydromorphone HCl injection	Dilaudid	Opioid	Pain	Somnolence, dizziness, dysphoria/euphoria	(pre-filled syringe): 0.5 mg per 0.5 mL, 1 mg per mL, 2 mg per mL, 4 mg per mL; INJ (vial): 1 mg per mL, 2 mg per mL, 4 mg per mL	IM, IV, SC

Sterile compounding medications—cont'd						
Generic name	Brand name	Classification	Indication	Side effects	Strength	Route of administration
hydroxocobalamin injection	Cyanokit	Environmental/industrial chemical	Cyanide poisoning	Red urine, erythema, BP transiently elevated	5 g kit	IV
ibuprofen injection	Caldolor	NSAID	Mild to moderate pain, fever	Dyspepsia, nausea, elevated ALT/AST	4 mg/mL	IV
ifosfamide injection	Ifex	Alkylating agent	Germ cell testicular cancer	Alopecia, hematuria, leukopenia, thrombocytopenia	1 g/vial, 3 g/vial	IV
imipenem/cilastatin sodium injection	Primaxin	Carbapenem	Bacterial infections, UTI, pneumonia, anthrax exposure	Increased eosinophils, increased LFTs, increased CR	250 mg/250 mg vial, 500 mg/500 mg vial	IV
infliximab injection	Remicade, Inflectra, Avsola, Renflexis	TNF inhibitor	Crohn disease, ulcerative colitis, rheumatoid arthritis, psoriatic arthritis, ankylosing spondylitis, psoriasis	Infusion reaction, URI, dyspepsia	100 mg/vial	IV
insulin aspart	NovoLog, Flasp	Insulin	Diabetes mellitus type 1, diabetus mellitus type 2	Injection site reaction, hypoglycemia, injection site lipodystrophy	100 units/mL	SC/IV
insulin degludec	Tresiba	Insulin	Diabetes mellitus type 1, diabetes mellitus type 2	Injection site reaction, hypoglycemia, URI	100 units/mL, 200 units/mL	SC
insulin detemir	Levemir	Insulin	Diabetes mellitus type 1, diabetes mellitus type 2	Injection site reaction, hypoglycemia, injection site lipodystrophy	100 units/mL	SC
insulin glargine	Basaglar, Lantus, Toujeo, Semglee	Insulin	Diabetes mellitus type 1, diabetes mellitus type 2	Injection site reaction, hypoglycemia, injection site lipodystrophy	100 units/mL	SC
insulin glulisine	Apidra	Insulin	Diabetes mellitus type 1	Injection site reaction, hypoglycemia, injection site lipodystrophy	100 units/mL	IV, SC
nPH	Humulin N, Novolin N	Insulin	Diabetes mellitus type 1, diabetes mellitus type 2	Injection site reaction, hypoglycemia, injection site lipodystrophy	100 units/mL	SC
nPH and regular	Humulin 50/50, Humulin 70/30, Novolin 70/30	Insulin	Diabetes mellitus type 1, diabetes mellitus type 2	Injection site reaction, hypoglycemia, injection site lipodystrophy	100 units/mL	SC

(Continued)

Sterile compounding medications—cont'd						
Generic name	Brand name	Classification	Indication	Side effects	Strength	Route of adminis-tration
insulin lispro	Admelog, Humalog, Lyumjev	Insulin	Diabetes mellitus type 1, diabetes mellitus type 2	Injection site reaction, hypoglycemia, injection site lipodystrophy	100 units/mL	SC
insulin regular	Humulin R, Novolin R, Myxredin	Insulin	Diabetes mellitus type 1, diabetes mellitus type 2	Injection site reaction, hypoglycemia, injection site lipodystrophy	100 units/mL, 500 units/mL	SC
interferon alfa-2b	Intron A	Interferon	Condyloma acuminate, hairy cell leukemia, hepatitis B infection, melanoma, non-Hodgkin lymphoma	Influenza-like symptoms, anorexia, pruritis/rash	10 million units per mL, 18 million units per 3 mL, 18 million units per mL, 50 million units per mL	IM, SC
iohexol injection	Omnipaque	Diagnostic	Myelography, angiography, aortography	Headache, backache, neckache, nausea/vomiting	180 mg/Iodine/mL, 240 mg iodine/mL, 300 mg iodine/mL	Intrathecal, intravascular
irinotecan injection (HCl and liposomal)	Onivyde	Topoisomerase inhibitor	Metastatic colorectal cancer	Anemia, neutropenia, leukopenia	20 mg/mL	IV
iron dextran injection	INFeD	Iron homeostasis	Iron deficiency anemia, iron replacement	Flushing, taste changes, nausea/vomiting	50 mg/mL	IV, IM
isoniazid injection	[a]	Tuberculosis agent	Tuberculosis	Paresthesia, elevated ALT/AST, pyridoxine deficiency	100 mg/mL	IM
isoproterenol HCl injection	Isuprel	Antiarrhythmic	ACLS (bradycardia), heart block, Adams-Stokes attacks, shock, bronchospasm during anesthesia	Nervousness, blurred vision, skin flushing	0.2 mg/mL	IV
ketamine HCl injection	Ketalar	General anesthetic	General anesthesia induction, general anesthesia maintenance	Sialorrhea, elevated blood pressure, elevated heart rate	10 mg/mL, 50 mg/mL, 100 mg/mL	IV, IM
ketorolac tromethamine injection	[a]	NSAID	Moderate-severe acute pain	Injection site pain, dyspepsia, elevated ALT/AST	15 mg/mL, 30 mg/mL	IV, IM
labetalol HCl injection	[a]	Beta-blocker	Hypertensive emergency	Orthostatic hypotension, paresthesia, elevated BUN/CR	5 mg/mL	IV
leucovorin calcium injection	[a]	Oncologic	Colorectal cancer, leucovorin rescue, folate antagonist overdose, folate-deficient megaloblastic anemia	Urticaria, anaphylactoid reaction, nausea/vomiting	10 mg/mL, 20 mg/mL	IV, IM
leuprolide acetate injection	Eligard, Camcevi, Lupron Depot	Hormonal oncologics	Advance prostate cancer	Hot flashes/diaphoresis, transient tumor flare, depression	1 mg/0.2 mL	SC

Sterile compounding medications—cont'd						
Generic name	Brand name	Classification	Indication	Side effects	Strength	Route of administration
levofloxacin injection	[a]	Fluoroquinolone	Pneumonia, prostatitis, pyelonephritis, skin/skin structure infections, UTI, anthrax exposure	Dyspepsia, tendonitis, insomnia	25 mg/mL, 250 mg/50 mL, 500 mg/100 mL, 750 mg/150 mL	IV
levothyroxine sodium injection	[a]	Thyroid	Myxedema coma	Palpitations, increased appetite, tachycardia	100 mcg/vial, 200 mcg/vial, 500 mcg/vial	IV
lidocaine HCl injection	[a]	Antiarrhythmic, local anesthesia	Ventricular arrhythmias, Ventricular Fibrillation/ Ventricular Tachycardia, local anesthesia, status epilepticus	Injection site pain, light headedness, hypotension	INJ (0.2%): 200 mg per 100 mL; INJ (0.4%): 400 mg per 100 mL; INJ (0.8%): 800 mg per 100 mL; INJ (1%): 10 mg per mL; INJ (1.5%): 15 mg per mL; INJ (2%): 20 mg per mL; INJ (4%): 40 mg per mL; INJ (5% hyperbaric): 50 mg per mL	IV
lidocaine HCl/ epinephrine injection	[a]	Combination local anesthetic-vasoconstrictor	Local anesthesia for dental procedures	Lightheadedness, nervousness, tinnitus	INJ (0.2%): 200 mg per 100 mL; INJ (0.4%): 400 mg per 100 mL; INJ (0.8%): 800 mg per 100 mL; INJ (1%): 10 mg per mL; INJ (1.5%): 15 mg per mL; INJ (2%): 20 mg per mL; INJ (4%): 40 mg per mL; INJ (5% hyperbaric): 50 mg per mL	Oral infiltration
lorazepam injection	Ativan	Benzodiazepine	Anxiety, status epilepticus, nausea/vomiting, preoperative sedation, neuroleptic malignant syndrome	Local injection site reaction, sedation, hypoventilation	2 mg/mL, 4 mg/mL	IV, IM
magnesium sulfate injection	[a]	Mineral	Hypomagnesium, seizures (preeclampsia or eclampsia associated), tocolysis, ventricular arrhythmias, torsades de pointes	Depressed reflexes, hypotension, impaired cardiac function	50%	IV
mannitol injection	Osmitrol	Osmotic diuretic	Oliguria prevention, cerebral edema, elevated IOP or ICP, forced diuresis	Thrombophlebitis, fluid imbalance, electrolyte disorders	25%	IV
medroxy-progesterone acetate injection	Depo-Provera CI, Depo-subQ provera 104	Progestin	Contraception	Cushingoid appearance, hirsutism, sodium and fluid retention	150 mg/mL	IM

(Continued)

Sterile compounding medications—cont'd						
Generic name	Brand name	Classification	Indication	Side effects	Strength	Route of adminis-tration
meperidine HCl injection	Demerol	Opioid	Moderate to severe pain, preoperative sedation, obstetric analgesia	Diaphoresis, dysphoria/euphoria, bradycardia	50 mg/mL	IM, SC
meropenem injection	Merrem	Carbapenem	Skin/skin structures, febrile neutropenia, intraabdominal infections, pneumonia, anthrax exposure	Injection site inflammation, paresthesia, nausea/vomiting	500 mg /vial, 1000 mg/vial	IV
methadone HCl injection	a	Opioid	Opioid dependence, moderate to severe chronic pain	Diaphoresis, lightheadedness, sedation	10 mg/mL	IV, IM, SC
methotrexate injection	Otrexup, Rasuvo, RediTrex	Antimetabolite	Rheumatoid arthritis, psoriasis	Elevated LFTs, anemia, thrombocytopenia	25 mg/mL, 1 g/vial	SC
methylene blue injection	ProvayBlue	Environmental/industrial chemical	Methemoglobinemia	Urine and fecal discoloration, syncope, diaphoresis	10 mg/mL	IV
methylpred-nisolone acetate injection	Depo-Medrol	Corticosteroid	Corticosteroid responsive condition, congenital adrenal hyperplasia, multiple sclerosis	Cushingoid appearance, hirsutism, sodium and fluid retention	40 mg/mL, 80 mg/mL	IM
metoclopramide HCl injection	a	Prokinetic	GERD, diabetic gastroparesis, nausea/vomiting, radiologic examination	Extrapyramidal symptoms, hyperaldo-steronism, hypertension, bradycardia	5 mg/mL, 10 mg/2 mL	IV, IM
metoprolol tartrate injection	a	Beta-blocker	Acute MI	Bradycardia, dyspnea, fatigue	1 mg/mL	IV
metronidazole injection	a	Nitroimidazole	Trichomoniasis, infection prophylaxis	Thrombophlebitis, dark red-brown urine, nausea/vomiting	500 mg/100 mL	IV
midazolam HCl injection	a	Benzodiazepine	Sedation, anesthesia	Injection site pain, sedation, hypotension	1 mg/mL, 5 mg/mL	IM, IV
milrinone lactate injection	a	Inotropes/pressors	CHF, postresuscitation stabilization	Ventricular arrhythmia, ventricular ectopy, ventricular tachycardia	1 mg/mL, 200 mcg/mL-D	IV
morphine injection (sulfate and liposomal)	a	Opioid	Moderate to severe acute pain, moderate to severe chronic pain, unstable angina, acute MI, pulmonary edema	Diaphoresis, dysphoria/euphoria, constipation	4 mg/mL	IV, IM, SC
moxifloxacin HCl injection	a	Fluoroquinolone	Intraabdominal infections, pneumonia, bacterial skin/skin structure infections, plaque, chronic bronchitis, sinusitis, anthrax exposure	Injection site reaction, insomnia, tendinitis	400 mg/250 mL	IV

Sterile compounding medications—cont'd						
Generic name	Brand name	Classification	Indication	Side effects	Strength	Route of administration
mVI	MVI	Vitamin	Vitamin deficiency	Erythema, diplopia, anxiety, urticaria	10 mL dose	IV
mycophenolate mofetil HCl injection	CellCept	Immunosuppressant	Kidney, heart, and liver transplant prophylaxis	Hypotension, peripheral edema, dyspnea	500 mg/Vial	IV
nafcillin sodium injection	[a]	Penicillin	Bacterial infections, bacterial meningitis, endocarditis, osteomyelitis	Injection site pain/irritation, thrombophlebitis, elevated ALT/AST	1 g/vial, 2/vial, 10 g/vial	IV
naloxone HCl injection	[a]	Opioid antagonist	Opioid overdose, opioid reversal	Tachycardia, hypertension/ hypotension, diaphoresis	10 mg/0.4/mL	IV, IM
natalizumab injection	Tysabri	Monoclonal antibody	Multiple sclerosis, Crohn disease	Infusion reaction, depression, arthralgia	300 mg/15 mL	IV
neostigmine methylsulfate injection	Bloxiverz	Cholinesterase inhibitor	Nondepolarizing neuromuscular blockade reversal	Diaphoresis, dyspnea, dizziness	0.5 mg/mL, 1 mg/mL	IV
nitroglycerin injection	[a]	Nitrate	Acute angina, HTN, CHF	Paresthesia, dizziness, flushing	5 mg/mL	IV
nitroprusside sodium injection	Nipride RTU, Nitropress	Nitrate	Hypertensive emergency, hypotension, CHF	Tachycardia/ bradycardia, diaphoresis, dizziness	25 mg/mL	IV
norepinephrine bitartrate injection	Levophed	Inotropes/pressor	Hypotension, cardiac arrest	Bradycardia, dyspnea, anxiety	1 mg/mL	IV
octreotide acetate injection	Sandostatin, Sandostatin LAR Depot, Bynfezia	Growth hormone antagonists	Acromegaly, carcinoid tumor symptoms, VIPoma symptoms, carcinoid crisis, esophageal varices	Injection site pain, hyperglycemia, hypothyroidism	50 mcg/mL, 100 mcg/mL, 200 mcg/mL, 500 mcg/mL, 1000 mcg/mL	IV, SC
ondansetron HCl injection	[a]	Serotonin H-T3 antagonist	Nausea/vomiting	Hypoxia, agitation, Stevens-Johnson syndrome	2 mg/mL	IV, IM
oxacillin sodium injection	[a]	Penicillin	Bacterial infections, endocarditis	Thrombophlebitis, stomatitis, black hairy tongue	1 g/vial, 2 g/vial, 10 g/vial	IV, IM
oxaliplatin injection	Eloxatin	Alkylating agent	Colon cancer	Leukopenia, neutropenia, thrombocytopenia	50 mg/vial, 100 mg/vial, 5 mg/mL	IV
oxytocin injection	Pitocin	Oxytocin binder receptor	Labor induction, postpartum hemorrhage	Uterine hypertonicity, postpartum hemorrhage, arrhythmias	10 units/mL	IV, IM
paclitaxel injection (conventional and protein bound)	[a]	Mitosis inhibitor	Ovarian cancer, breast cancer, non–small cell lung cancer, Kaposi sarcoma	Neutropenia, leukopenia, anemia, injection site reaction, elevated ALT/AST	6 mg/mL	IV
pancuronium bromide injection	[a]	Neuromuscular blocker	Neuromuscular blockade induction and maintenance	Elevated heart rate, elevated blood pressure, increased cardiac output	1 mg/mL	IV

(Continued)

Sterile compounding medications—cont'd						
Generic name	Brand name	Classification	Indication	Side effects	Strength	Route of adminis-tration
pantoprazole sodium injection	Protonix	Proton pump inhibitor	GERD, hypersecretory conditions, upper GI bleeding	Thrombophlebitis, elevated ALT/AST, arthralgia	40 mg/vial	IV
pegaspargase injection	Oncaspar	Oncologic	ALL	Anaphylaxis, hyperglycemia, thrombosis	750 units/mL	IV, IM
peginterferon alfa-2a	Pegasys	Interferon	Hepatitis B infection	Injection site reaction, thrombo-cytopenia, elevated LFTs	180 mcg/0.5 mL	SC
peginterferon beta 1a	Plegridy	Interferon	Adjuvant melanoma treatment	Injection site reaction, increased LFTs, proteinuria	INJ (auto-injector starter pack, SC): 63 mcg and 94 mcg; INJ (auto-injector, SC): 125 mcg; INJ (pre-filled syringe starter pack, SC): 63 mcg per 0.5 mL and 94 mcg per 0.5 mL; INJ (pre-filled syringe, SC): 125 mcg per 0.5 mL; INJ (pre-filled syringe, IM): 125 mcg per 0.5 mL	SC
penicillin G benzathine	Bicillin L-A	Penicillin	Syphilis, pharyngitis, tonsillitis, rheumatic fever	Injection site reaction, elevated BUN/CR, sterile abscess	600,000 units/mL	IM
penicillin G potassium	Pfizerpen	Penicillin	Bacterial infections, meningococcal meningitis, meningococcal septicemia, neurosyphilis, endocarditis, anthrax exposure, pneumonia	Injection site reaction, thrombophlebitis, stomatitis	5,000,000 units, 20,000,000 units	IV, IM
penicillin G procaine	[a]	Penicillin	Group A strep infections, neurosyphilis, fusobacterium infections, anthrax exposure	Injection site reaction, sterile abscess, anaphylaxis	600,000 units/mL	IM
pentobarbital sodium injection	Nembutal	Barbiturate	Procedural sedation, barbiturate coma	Somnolence, hyperkinesias, bradycardia	50 mg/mL	IV, IM
pentostatin injection	Nipent	Antimetabolite	Hairy cell leukemia	Leukopenia, thrombocytopenia, diaphoresis	10 mg	IV
phenobarbital sodium injection	[a]	Barbiturate	Seizure disorder, status epilepticus, sedation	Thrombophlebitis, drowsiness, lethargy	65 mg/mL, 130 mg/mL	IV, IM
phenylephrine HCl injection		Inotrope/pressors	Shock, hypotension, spinal anesthesia, PSVT conversion	CNS stimulation, arrhythmia, hypertension	10 mg/mL	IV, IM, SC

Sterile compounding medications—cont'd						
Generic name	Brand name	Classification	Indication	Side effects	Strength	Route of adminis-tration
phenytoin sodium injection [a]		Hydantoin	Status epilepticus, seizure disorder, seizure prophylaxis	Phlebitis, nystagmus, hyperglycemia	50 mg/mL	IV
phytonadione (vitamin K) injection [a]		Anticoagulant	Hypopro-thrombinemia,	Injection site hematoma, injection site pain, flushing, taste changes	1 mg/0.5 mL, 10 mg/mL	IV
piperacillin sodium/ tazobactam sodium injection	Zosyn	Penicillin	Intraabdominal infections, gynecologic infections, skin/skin structure infections, pneumonia	Electrolyte abnormalities, elevated LFT, leukopenia, neutropenia, thrombocytopenia	2 g/0.25 g, 3 g/0.375 g, 4 g/0.5 g, 36 g/4.5 g	IV
potassium acetate injection [a]		Electrolyte	Hypokalemia	Tingling or burning sensation in hands and feet, mental confusion, weakness	4 mEq/mL	IV
potassium chloride injection [a]		Electrolyte	Hypokalemia	Hyperkalemia, arrhythmias, hypersensitivity reaction, anaphylaxis	2 mEq/mL, 20 mEq/100 mL	IV
potassium phosphate injection [a]		Electrolyte	Hypophosphatemia	Paresthesia, arrhythmias, hypotension	3 millimoles/mL	IV
procainamide HCl injection [a]		Antiarrhythmic	Ventricular arrhythmias	Hypotension, bradycardia, flushing	100 mg/mL, 500 mg/mL	IV
prochlorperazine edisylate injection [a]		Antipsychotic	Schizophrenia, nausea/vomiting,	Hyperglycemia, hypoglycemia, akathisia	5 mg/mL	IM
progesterone injection [a]		Progestin	Amenorrhea, abnormal uterine bleeding	Pain and swelling at the injection site, increased body or facial hair, breast tenderness	50 mg/mL	IM
promethazine HCl injection	Phenergan	Antihistamine	Allergic conditions, nausea/vomiting, sedation	Extravasation/ tissue damage, extrapyramidal symptoms, bradycardia/ tachycardia	25 mg/mL, 50 mg/mL	IV, IM
propofol injection	Diprivan	Anesthetic	Anesthesia	Injection site reaction, hypotension, respiratory acidosis	10 mg/mL	IV
propranolol HCl injection [a]		Beta-blocker	Supraventricular arrhythmia	Bradycardia, hypotension, insomnia	1 mg/mL	IV
protamine sulfate injection [a]		Anticoagulant reversal drug	Heparin reversal, LMWH reversal	Hypotension, bradycardia, dyspnea	10 mg/mL	IV
quinupristin/ dalfopristin injection	Synercid	Streptogramin	Vancomycin resistant enterococci infections, skin/skin structure infections	Injection site reaction, hyperbilirubinemia	350 mg/150 mg	IV

(Continued)

Sterile compounding medications—cont'd						
Generic name	Brand name	Classification	Indication	Side effects	Strength	Route of administration
reteplase recombinant injection	Retavase	Thrombolytic	STEMI	Severe bleeding, arrhythmias, anaphylaxis	10.4 units/vial	IV
rifampin injection	a	Rifamycin	Tuberculosis, endocarditis, anthrax exposure	Elevated ALT/AST, dyspnea, thrombocytopenia, leukemia, anemia	600 mg/mL	IV
risperidone injection	Risperdal Consta, Perseris	Antipsychotic	Schizophrenia, bipolar disease, Tourette syndrome	Somnolence, extrapyramidal symptoms, tachycardia, dyspepsia	1 mg/mL	IM
rituximab injection	Rituxan, Riabni, Ruxience, Truxima	DMARDs	Non-Hodgkin lymphoma, rheumatoid arthritis	Infusion reaction, leukopenia, neutropenia, thrombocytopenia	10 mg/mL	IV
rocuronium bromide injection	a	Neuromuscular blocker	Neuromuscular blockade	Transient hypotension, hypertension, tachycardia	10 mg/mL	IV
sodium acetate injection	a	Electrolyte	Hyponatremia	Sodium overload, excessive hydration, hypokalemia	2 mEq/mL	IV
sodium chloride injection	a	Electrolyte	Fluid and electrolyte replacement	Hypernatremia, fluid retention, hypertension, electrolyte abnormalities	0.45%, 0.9%	IV
sodium ferric gluconate complex injection	Ferrlecit	Mineral	Iron deficiency	Injection site reaction, erythrocyte abnormalities, hypotension	12.5 mg/mL	IV
sodium lactate injection	a	Electrolyte	Metabolic acidosis	Dilution of blood electrolyte concentration, overhydration, pulmonary edema	5 mEq/mL	IV
sodium nitrate/sodium thiosulfate injection	Nithiodote	Industrial/environmental chemical	Cyanide poisoning	Arrhythmias, syncope, hypotension	30 mg–250 mg/mL	IV
sodium phosphate injection	a	Electrolyte	Hypophosphatemia	Phosphate intoxication, hypocalemic tetany	3 mmole/mL	IV
succinylcholine chloride injection	Anectine	Neuromuscular blocker	Neuromuscular blockade	Elevated IOP, hypotension, bradycardia/tachycardia	20 mg/mL	IV, IM
sulfamethoxazole/trimethoprim injection	a	Sulfonamide	UTI, typhoid fever, toxoplasmosis	Infusion reaction, photosensitivity, hepatotoxicity	80–16 mg/mL	IV
tacrolimus injection	Prograf	Immunosuppressant	Heart, liver, and kidney transplant	Increased CR, elevated LFTs, hyperglycemia, hyperkalemia	5 mg/mL	IV

Sterile compounding medications—cont'd						
Generic name	Brand name	Classification	Indication	Side effects	Strength	Route of adminis-tration
tenecteplase recombinant injection	TNKase	Thrombolytic	STEMI	Bleeding, arrhythmia, stroke	50 mg/vial	IV
testosterone injection	[a]	Androgen	Hypogonadism	Injection site reaction, elevated ALT/AST, hyperlipidemia	100 mg/mL, 200 mg/mL	IM
theophylline injection	[a]	Methylxanthine	Acute bronchospasms	Arrhythmias, seizures, hypotension	25 mg/mL	IV
tobramycin injection	[a]	Aminoglycoside	Bacterial infections, pneumonia, respiratory infections in cystic fibrosis patients, endocarditis	Elevated BUN/CR, ototoxicity, nephrotoxicity	40 mg/mL, 1.2 g vial	IV, IM
trace elements combinations injection	Multitrace-5 Concentrate	Supplement	Supplement	The quantities of each element are extremely small and toxicities are unlikely to occur	Zinc 5 mg, copper 1 mg, manganese 0.5 mg, chromium 10 mcg, selenium 60 mcg/mL	IV
tranexamic acid injection	Cyklokapron	Fibrinolysis inhibitor	Bleeding prophylaxis	Hypotension, anaphylaxis, thromboembolism	100 mg/mL	IV
trastuzumab injection	Herceptin, Herzuma, Kanjinti, Ogivri, Ontruzant, Trazimera	Antiangiogenic	Breast cancer, gastric cancer	Infusion reaction, neutropenia, anemia, leukopenia	150 mg/vial	IV
tuberculin purified protein derivative injection	Tubersol	Vaccine	Diagnostic for tuberculosis	Injection site pain, injection site pruritis, injection site erythema	5 units/0.1 mL	Intradermal
valproate sodium injection	Depacon	Glutamate/NMDA receptor inhibitor	Absence and partial seizures	Thrombocyto-penia, dyspepsia, elevated ALT/AST	100 mg/mL	IV
vancomycin HCl injection	[a]	Glycopeptides	Severe bacterial conditions, *Clostridium difficile* infection, pneumonia, endocarditis, anthrax exposure	Red-man syndrome, hypotension, elevated BUN/CR	500 mg/vial, 750 mg/vial, 1 g/vial, 5 g/vial, 10 g/vial	IV
vasopressin injection	Vasostrict	Inotropes/pressors	Vasodilatory shock	Diaphoresis, hyponatremia, ischemic injury	20 units/mL	IV
vecuronium bromide injection	[a]	Neuromuscular blocker	Neuromuscular blockade	Muscle weakness, respiratory depression, apnea	10 mg/vial, 20 mg/vial	IV
verapamil HCl injection	[a]	Calcium channel blocker	PSVT conversion, atrial fibrillation/flutter	Hypotension, congestive heart failure, atrioventricular block, bradycardia, hepatotoxicity	2.5 mg/mL	IV

(Continued)

Sterile compounding medications

Generic name	Brand name	Classification	Indication	Side effects	Strength	Route of adminis-tration
vinblastine sulfate injection	[a]	Mitosis inhibitor	Hodgkin lymphoma, testicular cancer	Injection site reaction, leukopenia, neutropenia, thrombophlebitis	1 mg/mL	IV
vincristine sulfate injection (and liposome)	[a]	Mitosis inhibitor	ALL, Hodgkin lymphoma, non-Hodgkin lymphoma, solid tumors	Peripheral neuropathy, hyper-uricemia, blood pressure changes	1 mg/mL	IV
vinorelbine tartrate injection	Navelbine	Mitosis inhibitor	Non–small cell lung cancer	Leukopenia, granulocytopenia, elevated LFTs	10 mg/mL	IV
voriconazole injection	Vfend	Antifungal	Severe fungal infections, aspergillosis, candidemia, candidiasis	Elevated ALT/AST, elevated alkaline phosphate, tachycardia	40 mg/mL, 200 mg/vial	IV

[a]Brand name discontinued in the United States.

Italicized drugs are included on IInstitute for Safe Medication Practices List of High-Alert Medications in Acute Care, Community and Ambulatory Healthcare, and Long-Term Care (LTC) Settings. *CHF*, congestive heart failure; *NG*, nasogastric; *SC*, subcutaneous; *DMARD*, disease-modifying antirheumatic drug; *URI*, upper respiratory infection; *PSVT*, paroxysmal supraventricular tachycardia; *ACLS*, advanced cardiac life support; *IM*, intramuscular; *ACLS/PALS/NALS*, advanced care life support/pediatric advanced life support/neonatal advanced life support; *ALT*, alanine aminotransferase; *AST*, aspartate aminotransferase; *PID*, pelvic inflammatory disease; *BUN*, blood urea nitrogen; *CR*, creatine; *CML*, chronic myelogenous leukemia; *AML*, acute myelogenous leukemia; *ALL*, acute lymphoblastic leukemia; *CK*, creatine kinase; *DVT*, deep vein thrombosis; *PE*, pulmonary embolism; *NQWMI*, non Q-wave myocardial infarction; *STEMI*, ST elevation myocardial infarction; *PCI*, percutaneous coronary intervention; *LFT*, liver function test; *GERD*, gastroesophageal reflux disease; *PBPC*, peripheral blood progenitor cell; *BMT*, bone marrow transplantation; *CLL*, chronic lymphocytic leukemia; *CMV*, cytomegalovirus; *HSV*, herpes simplex virus; *HTN*, hypertension; *IOP*, intraocular pressure; *ICP*, intracranial pressure; *LMWH*, low-molecular-weight heparin; *NMDA*, N-methyl-D-aspartate; *MVI*, multivitamins parenteral; *NPH, insulin isophane; NSAID*, nonsteroidal antiinflammatory drug; *TNF*, tumor necrosis factor; *CSF*, colony-stimulating factor; *COPD*, chronic obstructive pulmonary disease; *UTI*, urinary tract infection; *ICU*, intensive care unit; *MI*, myocardial infarction; *GI*, gastrointestinal; *BP*, blood pressure; *CNS*, central nervous system.

Large-volume IV solutions

Injection	Common name	Concen-tration (%)	Therapeutic use
Dextrose	D5W	5	Hydration, calories
	D10W	10	Insulin shock, calories
	D20W	20	Insulin shock, calories
	D50W	50	Insulin shock, calories
Sodium chloride	Normal saline	0.9	Extracellular fluid replacement
	½ Normal saline	0.45	Dehydration
Ringer's solution NaCl KCl CaCl₂	Ringer's solution	0.86 0.03 0.033	Fluid and electrolyte replacement
Lactated Ringer's solution NaCl KCl CaCl₂ Na lactate	Hartman's solution	0.6 0.03 0.02 0.3	Fluid and electrolyte replacement

Types of injectable water

- **Purified water USP:** not intended for parenteral administration; used in the reconstitution of oral products
- **Sterile water for injection USP:** has been sterilized but has no antimicrobial agents; can be used in parenteral solutions
- **Bacteriostatic water for injection USP:** sterile water with antimicrobial agents that can be used for injection
- **Sterile water for irrigation USP:** has been sterilized but contains no antimicrobial agents; used as an irrigating solution

High-alert and narrow therapeutic index medications

High-alert drug classifications in acute care settings

- Adrenergic agonists, IV (e.g., epinephrine, phenylephrine, norepinephrine)
- Adrenergic antagonists, IV (e.g., propranolol, metoprolol, labetalol)
- Anesthetic agents, general, inhaled and IV (e.g., propofol, ketamine)
- Antiarrhythmics, IV (e.g., lidocaine, amiodarone)
- Antithrombotic agents, including:

- Anticoagulants (e.g., warfarin, low-molecular-weight heparin, IV unfractionated heparin)
- Factor Xa inhibitors (e.g., fondaparinux, apixaban, rivaroxaban)
- Direct thrombin inhibitors (e.g., argatroban, bivalirudin, dabigatran etexilate)
- Thrombolytics (e.g., alteplase, reteplase, tenecteplase)
- Glycoprotein IIb/IIIa inhibitors (e.g., eptifibatide)
- Cardioplegic solutions
- Chemotherapeutic agents, parenteral and oral
- Dextrose, hypertonic, 20% or greater
- Dialysis solutions, peritoneal and hemodialysis
- Epidural or intrathecal medications
- Hypoglycemics, oral
- Inotropic medications, IV (e.g., digoxin, milrinone)
- Insulin, subcutaneous and IV
- Liposomal forms of drugs (e.g., liposomal amphotericin B) and conventional counterparts (e.g., amphotericin B desoxycholate)
- Moderate sedation agents, IV (e.g., dexmedetomidine, midazolam)
- Moderate sedation agents, oral, for children (e.g., chloral hydrate)
- Narcotics/opioids
  - Includes IV, transdermal, and oral (including liquid concentrates, immediate and sustained-released formulations)
- Neuromuscular blocking agents (e.g., succinylcholine, rocuronium, vecuronium)
- Parenteral nutrition preparations
- Radiocontrast agents, IV
- Sterile water for injection, inhalation, and irrigation (excluding pour bottles) in containers of 100 mL or more
- Sodium chloride for injection, hypertonic, greater than 0.9% concentration

Narrow-therapeutic-index medications

Narrow-therapeutic-index (NTI) drugs are defined as those drugs where small differences in dose or blood concentration may lead to dose- and blood concentration–dependent serious therapeutic failures or adverse drug reactions. Serious events are those that are persistent, irreversible, slowly reversible, or life-threatening, possibly resulting in hospitalization, disability, or even death.

- Examples of injectable NTI drugs:
  - amiodarone
  - argatroban
  - amphotericin B
  - cisplatin
  - cyclosporine
  - digoxin
  - fluorouracil
  - fosphenytoin
  - gentamicin
  - haloperidol
  - heparin
  - interferon alfa-2b
  - levothyroxine
  - methotrexate
  - olanzapine

- paclitaxel
- Phenytoin
- procainamide
- sotalol
- sirolimus
- tacrolimus
- tobramycin

Factors affecting compounded sterile preparations

Light

- Light may cause some medication such as amphotericin B and cisplatin to break down and lose their therapeutic effect.

Temperature

- IV solutions must be stored at the correct temperature to maintain the stability of the compound.
- In many situations, heat causes many admixtures to break down.
- Not all admixtures should be refrigerated because a precipitate may form.

pH

- If the IV solution and medication being added possess conflicting pH values, either the medication may break down or a precipitate may form. In many cases normal saline solution is used in compounding a sterile compound.

Containers

- Some medications are incompatible with the plastic, such as polyvinyl chloride plastics, which may be found in its container or IV administration kits.
- Plasticizers may leach out of the plastic bag and bind with the active ingredient in the administration.

Concentration

- Depending on the concentration of the drug in an IV fluid, it may become incompatible with other drugs. This is a common occurrence when using electrolytes.

Agitation

- Some IV medications may require that they are properly mixed before the medication or additive is mixed, which reduces the possibility of another drug being added will come in contact with the other drug.

Clinical reference materials

- A medication's package insert contains information to determine the correct beyond-use date (BUD), how to reconstitute a powder, and the appropriate solution to reconstitute a powder.

- *Handbook on Injectable Drugs* (Trissel) provides a standardized source of primary research on the stability, compatibility, and incompatibilities of injectable drugs.
- *The King Guide to Parenteral Admixtures* provides stability and compatibility data using different infusion fluids and lists drug compatibility and stability in small-volume and large-volume parenteral solutions.
- *Extended Stability for Parenteral Drugs* provides information to safely extend dating of parenteral drugs beyond the usual 24-hour limit—minimizing waste, lowering medication costs, and enabling optimal patient administration schedules at alternate infusion sites.
- *Safety Data Sheets (SDS)* is a document that contains information on the potential hazards (health, fire, reactivity, and environmental) and how to work safely with the chemical product. Information contained on an SDS includes all hazards associated with the chemical, first aid measures, accidental release measures, handling and storage, exposure control/personal protection, physical/chemical properties, stability and reactivity, and toxicological measures.

Compounded sterile preparation categories

- Category 1 CSPs are compounded under the least controlled environmental conditions and therefore are assigned a BUD of 12 hours or less at controlled room temperature or 24 hours or less when refrigerated.
- Category 2 CSPs require more environmental controls and testing than Category 1 CSPs and may be assigned a BUD of greater than 12 hours at controlled room temperature or more than 24 hours if refrigerated.

Urgent-use compounded sterile preparations (formerly known as immediate-use compounded sterile preparations)

- It is only intended if there is a need for emergency or immediate patient administration of a CSP.
- Examples of emergencies include cardiopulmonary resuscitation, emergency room treatment, preparation of diagnostic agents, and critical therapy where using Category 1 CSPs would result in additional patient risk due to delay in therapy.
- Storage for anticipated use is not permitted.
- Hazardous drug (HD) products are not allowed.
- Exempt from normal compounding guidelines only if all of the following are true:
  - Compounding is continuous and does not exceed 1 hour.
  - Aseptic technique is used throughout preparation.

- Administration begins no more than 1 hour following the start of the preparation.
- Administration of CSP must begin immediately upon completion.

Beyond-use dates

- BUD is used to determine the expiration date of a CSP.
- Each CSP label must state the date, or the hour and date, beyond which the preparation must not be used and must be discarded.
- BUD is either the date, or hour and date, after which a CSP must not be used.
- BUD is determined from the date and time the preparation of the CSP was compounded.
- BUD applies to all CSPs.
- Expiration date is the time during which a product can be expected to meet the requirements of the United States Pharmacopeia-National Formulary monograph, if one exists, or maintain expected quality provided it is kept under the specified storage conditions
- Expiration dates apply to all conventionally manufactured products
- BUDs are based upon:
  - Conditions of the environment in which the CSP is prepared
  - Aseptic processing and sterilization method
  - Starting components (e.g., sterile or nonsterile ingredients)
  - Whether or not sterility testing is performed
  - Storage conditions (e.g., packaging and temperature)

Category 1 compounded sterile preparation beyond-use date

A shorter BUD must be assigned when the stability of the CSP or its components is less than the hours or days stated in the previous table. The BUD must not exceed the shortest remaining expiration date or BUD of any of the starting components, regardless of the source. The table establishes the longest permitted BUDs for Category 1 CSPs. Category 1 CSPs may be prepared in an segregated compounding area (SCA) or clean room suite.

	Controlled room temperature (20°C–25°C)	Refrigerator (2°C–8°C)
Beyond-use date	≤12 h	≤24 h

Category 2 compounded sterile preparations beyond-use date

The tables establishes the longest permitted BUDs for Category 2 CSPs. Category 2 CSPs must be prepared in a clean room suite.

Compounding method	Sterility testing performed and passed	Controlled room temperature (20°C–25°C)	Refrigerator (2°C–8°C)	Freezer (−25°C–10°C)
Aseptically processed CSPs	No	Prepared from one or more nonsterile starting component(s): 1 day	Prepared from one or more nonsterile starting component(s): 4 days	Prepared from one or more nonsterile starting component(s): 45 days
Aseptically processed CSPs	No	Prepared from only sterile starting components: 4 days	Prepared from only sterile starting components: 10 days	Prepared from only sterile starting components: 45 days
Aseptically processed CSPs	Yes	30 days	45 days	60 days
Terminally sterilized CSPs	No	14 days	28 days	45 days
Terminally sterilized CSPs	Yes	45 days	60 days	90 days

CSP, Compounded sterile preparation.

In-use time

- The time before which a conventionally manufactured product or CSP must be used after it has been opened or needle punctured

- Cannot exceed the expiration date of the conventionally manufactured product or BUD of the CSP

In-use times		
Container type	In-use time, ISO 5 or better	In-use time, worse than ISO 5
Ampoule	Use immediately after opening	Use immediately after opening
Pharmacy bulk package	As specified by manufacturer	Cannot be used
Single-dose container	6 h	Use for single patient within manufacturer-specified time or by end of case/procedure, whichever comes first
Multidose container	28 days unless otherwise specified by manufacturer	28 days unless otherwise specified by manufacturer
CSP type		
Compounded single-dose container	6 h	Use for single-patient only, disregard remainder
Compounded multidose container	28 days unless otherwise specified by manufacturer	Not permitted

CSP, Compounded sterile preparation.

Microbial limits of sterility

USP <797> has established air standards based on 0.5-mcm particle size. These standards have been implemented to avoid contamination in the following work areas.

ISO Class	US FS 209E	Particle count/m³	Particle count/ft³	Area in pharmacy	Required testing for compliance
ISO Class 5	Class 100	3520	100	IV hood	Checked every 6 months
ISO Class 6	Class 1,000	35,200	1,000	Ante-area	Checked every 6 months
ISO Class 7	Class 10,000	352,000	10,000	Clean room (buffer and ante-area)	Checked every 12 months
ISO Class 8	Class 100,000	3,520,000	100,000	Nonhazardous room	Checked every 12 months

US FS 209E, US Federal Standard 209E; ISO, International Standard for Organization.

Location of preparation

According to USP <797>, CSPs are prepared in a primary engineering control (PEC), such as a laminar airflow workbench (LAFW) biological safety cabinet (BSC), compounding aseptic isolator (CAI), or compounding aseptic containment isolator (CACI).

Physical and chemical stability

Compatibility

- "Compatibility" describes how effectively a sterile product combines with another sterile product.

- Not all sterile products are compatible with each other.

Incompatibility

- "Incompatibility" describes the negative effects of combining a sterile product with another sterile product, surface material.
- Effects of incompatibilities may result in the formation of a precipitate or a gas, a decrease in the potency of the medication, or the action of the drug may not occur.

Physical incompatibility

- Signs of physical incompatibilities include cloudiness, an increase or decrease in the temperature of the solution due to mixing, a change in color of the solution, or a separation of the solution.
- Results from a physical incompatibility:
  - A precipitate is formed when the solute does not dissolve in solvent.
  - Adsorption takes place when a CSP in a gas or liquid form collects on the surface of a solid or liquid.
  - Absorption happens when a material or container soaks up all or part of a liquid CSP.
  - Color change arises when the original color of one or more products in the mixture changes.
  - Separation occurs when one of the ingredients separates out of the mixture, such as in compounding a total parenteral nutrition (TPN). Creaming, aggregation, and coalescence are examples of separation.

Chemical incompatibility

- Occurs when two chemicals are combined, resulting in a chemical reaction.
- Examples of chemical incompatibilities:
  - Hydrolysis occurs a product combines with water resulting in two new products.

- Oxidation/reduction occurs when two products interact, resulting in one product gaining an electron and the other product losing an electron.
- Photolysis occurs when a product breaks down due to exposure to light.

Minimizing incompatibilities

- Check incompatibility references when the additive drug will create a very high or very low pH in the solution. The pH may cause the drug to form a precipitate.
- Check incompatibility reference when an additive drug contains calcium, magnesium, or phosphate salt; salt forms may cause the drug to precipitate.
- Check incompatibility reference when an additive drug contains acetate or lactate salt, which may increase the buffer capacity.
- Minimize the number of drugs that will be added in a solution at one time.
- Use solutions promptly after compounding.

Medication ingredients

- When two or more ingredients are mixed together, they may form a new chemical entity. As a result of this mixing, the therapeutic effect of the drug may change.

Base solutions

- Some medications may require a specific solution or diluent to be used when compounding them. Selecting the wrong solution may result in the drug breaking down too quickly or in a precipitate being formed. Some medications are packaged with the correct diluent to be used when reconstituting the medication.

Filters

- A filter such as a final filter may reduce the concentration of the drug if it becomes trapped inside the filter. For example, if nitroglycerin is being injected and in-line filter is being used the final concentration may be reduced by 90%.

Tubing

- Certain medications are incompatible with the plastics being used in select administration sets. An example is polyvinyl chloride plastics. In this situation a medication binds to the plastic material, which makes it unavailable to produce its therapeutic effect. This problem can be prevented by adding albumin to the solution, resulting in the albumin binding to the plastic surface and allowing the medication to exert its therapeutic action. Plasticizers may seep out of the plastic bag or the administration kit, bind with the drug, and possibly inactivate it.

Facilities and equipment

Primary engineering controls

- A device or room that provides an ISO Class 5 environment for compounding sterile preparations
- Requires use of high-efficiency particulate air (HEPA) filter that is ≥99.99% efficient in removing particles as small as 0.3 mcm

Laminar airflow workbenches

Class I

- A BSC that protects personnel and the environment but does not protect the product/preparation
- Has a minimum velocity of 75 linear feet/minute of unfiltered room air and is passed through a HEPA/ULPA (ultra-low particulate air) filter
- Must be turned on for at least 10 minutes prior to compounding

Class II (Types A1, A2, B1, and B2) biological safety cabinets

Class II BSCs are a partial barrier system that relies on the movement of air to provide personnel, environmental, and product/preparation protection. Protection is provided by a combination of inward and downward airflow, and there is a minimization of side-to-side contamination. BSCs must be turned on for at least 10 minutes prior to compounding.

- **Type A1 hoods:** Recirculates a portion of the air (after it first passes through a HEPA filter) within the hood and exhausts a portion of this air back into the parenteral room. Type A1 BSCs are not suitable for use with volatile toxic chemicals and radionucleotides.
- **Type A2:** They maintain a minimum inflow velocity of 100 feet/minute; have HEPA-filtered, downflow air that is a portion mixed downflow and inflow air from a common exhaust. If a Type A2 is used for minute quantities of volatile toxic chemicals and trace amounts of radionucleotides, they must be exhausted through properly functioning exhaust canopies.
- **Type B1 hoods:** They maintain a minimum inflow velocity of 100 feet/minute, and they expel most of the contaminated air through a duct to the outside atmosphere and pass through a HEPA filter. If a Type B1 is used for minute quantities of volatile toxic chemicals and trace

amounts of radionucleotides, they must be done in the directly exhausted portion of the cabinet.
- **Type B2 (total exhaust) hoods:** They maintain a minimum inflow velocity of 100 feet/minute. They remove all of the contaminated air to the outside atmosphere after it passes through a HEPA filter. This air is not recirculated within the hood or returned to the parenteral room atmosphere. Type B2 cabinets may be used with volatile toxic chemicals and radionucleotides.
- Class III cabinets are designed for work with highly infectious microbiological agents and other hazardous operations. It provides the maximum protection for the environment and the worker. Both the supply and exhaust air are HEPA/ULPA filtered.

Laminar airflow systems

- Vertical laminar workbench (Fig. 1.1)
  - Used in compounding chemotherapeutic and non-chemotherapeutic agents
  - Provides negative air pressure
  - Filtered air enters at the top of the workbench and moves downward
  - Must be turned on for at least 30 minutes before compounding
- Horizontal laminar workbench
  - Used in compounding nonchemotherapeutic medications
  - Provides positive air pressure

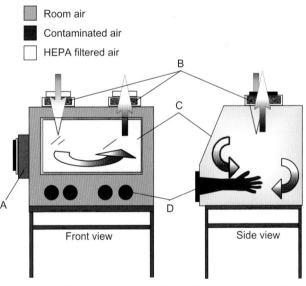

Fig. 1.1 Schematic representation of a Class III biological safety cabinet. This cabinet is completely sealed from the environment. Any materials entering or leaving the cabinet are passed through a chemical dunk tank or autoclave (A) in order to sterilize them and prevent environmental contamination. Air entering or leaving these cabinets is passed through HEPA filters (B). Access to the workspace is by means of rubber gloves (D) and the workspace is visualized through a sealed window (C). rom Pepper IL, Charles, P, Gerba TJ: Environmental Microbiology, ed 3 Elsevier, 2015

- Room air is channeled through a HEPA filter and the filtered air moves outward toward the preparer
- Preparer must work 6 inches from the side and the front of the workbench
- Must be turned on for at least 30 minutes before compounding

Restricted access barrier systems (formerly known as compounding aseptic isolators and compounding aseptic containment isolators)

- Restricted access barrier systems (RABSs) are designed to maintain an aseptic compounding area.
- They provide worker protection from exposure to undesirable levels of airborne drugs.
- They are used in compounding nonhazardous and hazardous medications.
- Must be within at least ISO 7 area to prepare Category 2 CSPs or within a segregated area to prepare Category 1 CSPs.
- Compounding isolators may be within an ISO 8 area to prepare Category 2 CSPs.
- They utilize an airtight glove/glove port design that allows the pharmacy personnel to perform hands-on tasks.
- All transport ports must be closed; the recovery time to achieve ISO 5 air must be documented after opening.
- Materials and supplies for aseptic compounding must enter through a special air-lock box.

Primary engineering controls

PEC device	Used to prepare nonhazardous CSPs	Used to prepare hazardous CSPs
Conventional	Laminar airflow workbench	Class II biological safety cabinet
Isolators	Restricted access barrier systems	Restricted access barrier systems

CSP, Compounded sterile preparation; *PEC*, primary engineering control.

Types of secondary engineering controls

- **Ante-area:** Transition area between the general area and the room containing the containment primary engineering control (C-PEC). Hand hygiene, garbing, staging of components, order entry, and other particle-generating activities are performed in the ante-area. For sterile compounding, the ante-area shall meet ISO Class 7 and also provides assurance that pressure relationships between rooms are constantly maintained.
- **Buffer area:** Part of the HD compounding area under negative pressure where the C-PEC is physically located. Activities that occur in this area are limited to the preparation and staging of components and supplies used when compounding HDs.

- **Containment segregated compounding area (C-SCA):** A type of containment secondary engineering control (C-SEC) with nominal airflow (12 air changes per hour [ACPH]) and room pressurization requirements (negative pressure between 0.01 and 0.03 inches of water column) as they pertain to HD compounding. The C-SCA is limited for use with a BSC or an RABS.
- **SCA:** A designated space; either a demarcated area or room.

Features of secondary engineering controls

Air pressure differentials

- Positive pressure room is an area in which the air pressure is higher than nearby areas, resulting in the air flowing out of the room. Positive pressure is required from the buffer area to the ante-area for non-HDs.
- Negative pressure room is an area in which the air pressure is lower than the nearby areas resulting in air flowing into the room. Negative pressure is required from the buffer area to the ante-area for HDs. A compounding aseptic containment isolator is located in a negative pressure room.
- Differential airflow shall be a minimum of 40 feet/minute between buffer area and ante-area when compounding Category 1 and Category 2 compounds.

HEPA filtration standards			
Class	**Risk levels**	**Safety level**	**Filtering system**
Class I	Low- to moderate-risk biologicals	Biosafety level I	HEPA filters exhaust air
Class II	Low- to moderate-risk biologicals	Biosafety level II	HEPA filters exhaust air to room or to a facility exhaust system
Class III	High-risk biologicals	Biosafety level III	Containment of hazardous materials

HEPA, High-efficiency particulate air.

ISO class particle classification

ISO class particle classification	
ISO Class	**Particle count (per m³)[a]**
3	35.2
4	352
5	3,520

ISO class particle classification	
ISO Class	**Particle count (per m³)[a]**
6	35,200
7	352,000
8	3,520,000

[a]The particles are 0.5 mcm or larger (3520 particles per cubic meter is equivalent to 100 particles per cubit foot).

Air changes per hour

- **Ante-area:** must maintain a minimum of 20 ACPH
- **Buffer area:** must maintain a minimum of 30 ACPH

Temperature, pressure, and humidity parameters

- Any controlled temperature area used for compounding sterile preparations or for storage of sterile products or CSPs must be monitored at least once daily and results documented in a log.
- The facilities should maintain a comfortable room temperature (20°C [68°F] or cooler).
- A pressure gauge must be installed to monitor the differential airflow between buffer area and the ante-area and between the ante-area and general environment.
- Results of pressure differential and/or velocity of air displacement must be reviewed and documented each shift (at least daily) or by a continuous device with alarms.
- Humidity should be less than 60% because high humidity supports microbial growth.

Environmental monitoring

Environmental monitoring examines the conditions of the PECs, buffer areas, ante-areas, and SCAs. Each element of the monitoring program must be included in a sampling plan with sample locations, methods of collection, sampling frequency, and other specifics depending on the type of monitoring being performed. The environmental monitoring sampling frequency must occur at a minimum as listed here, with possible additional times based on the type of testing:

- At the commissioning and certification of new facilities and equipment
- Every 6 months during routine recertification of equipment and facilities
- After any facility or equipment maintenance, including construction or remodeling of adjacent departments or work on shared air handlers
- At any point when problems are identified with products, preparations, or employee technique or if a CSP is suspected to be the source of a patient infection

Growth medium

- A general microbiological medium such as Soybean-Casein Digest Medium should be used to support growth of bacteria.
- Malt extract agar or some other media that supports the growth of fungi should be used in high-risk level compounding environments.
- Surface sampling medium should be supplemented with additives to neutralize the effects of disinfecting agents, such as tryptic soy agar (TSA) with lecithin and polysorbate 80.

Viable air sampling

- Air samples are obtained from ISO Class 5, 7, and 8 environments.
- Each facility must have an air sampling plan.
- Samples are obtained:
  - when equipment or facilities are built
  - after equipment or facilities are serviced
  - every 6 months as a requirement for recertification
  - when concerns are raised about the end-product
- Sampling plan should include:
  - the location of the plan
  - method of collection
  - frequency of sampling
  - volume of air sampled
  - time of day the sample was taken
- Reevaluation of work practices and cleaning procedures should occur if the colony forming unit (CFU) count exceeds the suggested action levels.

Recommended action levels for personnel testing (adapted from USP Chapter 797)	PEC	Buffer area	Ante-area
Viable airborne particle testing action levels for contamination (CFUs per cubic meter [1000 L] of air per plate)	>1	10	100

CFU, Colony forming unit; PEC, primary engineering controls.

Incubation period

- TSA should be incubated at 30°C–35°C for 48–72 hours.
- Malt agar should be incubated at 26°C–30°C for 5–7 days.

Viable air sampling

- Sampling measures the performance of the engineering controls used to create the various levels of air cleanliness in ISO Class 5, 7, and 8 environments.
- Sampling is performed to assure that contamination levels are within acceptable limits for both primary and secondary environmental controls. Sampling must be performed no less than every 6 months.
- Total particle counts must be performed no less than every 6 months and must not exceed the following requirements:

- ISO Class 5: not more than 3520 particles 0.5 mcm and larger size per cubic meter of air for any LAFW, BSC, or RBAS
- ISO Class 7: not more than 352,000 particles 0.5 mcm and larger size per cubic meter of air for any buffer area
- ISO Class 8: not more than 3,520,000 particles 0.5 mcm and larger size per cubic meter of air for any ante-area

Particle counting

- Particle counting involves obtaining samples of nonairborne particles in:
  - ISO Class 5, which includes air found in LAFWs, BSCs, and RBA
  - ISO Class 7 for air found in any buffer area
  - ISO Class 8 for air found in any ante-areas
- Particle counting is to occur when there is activity in the ISO Class 5, 7, and 8 areas.
- Results of particle counts must be maintained.

- Particle counts must be performed:
  - At least every 6 months
  - When the PEC has been relocated
  - When the environment has been altered

Temperature

- Cold temperature (2°C–8°C).
- Freezing temperature (–25°C to 10°C)
- Temperatures in controlled area monitored and documented at least daily

Temperature limits

- Proper room temperature is 20°C or cooler.
- Storage of some products must be in controlled room temperature area (20°C–25°C).
- Deviation of controlled room temperature may be up to 5°C warmer or colder.

Environmental monitoring requirements according to USP <797>		
Parameter	Monitored by	Frequency
Temperature	Compounding personnel or facilities management staff	Documented daily (at a minimum)
Pressure differential or velocity across line of demarcation	Compounding personnel	Documented each shift (preferably) or daily (at a minimum)
Viable particles	Qualified certifier	At least every 6 months
Surface sampling	Compounding or laboratory personnel	Periodically, as defined by compounding and infection control personnel, at least every 6 months or after significant changes in procedures or cleaning practices

Environmental monitoring requirements according to USP <797>		
Parameter	Monitored by	Frequency
Electronic device sample of viable particles	Compounding personnel or qualified certifier	At least every 6 months

USP, United States pharmacopeia.

Operational standards

- Access to buffer area is restricted to qualified personnel.
- Carton supplies are decontaminated by using a spray disinfectant.
- Frequently used supplies are decontaminated and stored on shelving in the ante-area.
- Carts used in bringing supplies from the storeroom cannot be rolled past the demarcation line in the anteroom.
- Carts used in the buffer area cannot be rolled outward beyond the demarcation line unless cleaned and disinfected before returning.
- Regularly used compounding supplies must be disinfected and brought into the buffer area using a cart.
- Nonessential supplies that shed particles should not be taken into the buffer area.
- Essential paper-related supplies must be disinfected before being brought into the buffer area.
- Traffic in and out of the buffer area must be minimized.
- Individuals entering the buffer area should not wear outer garments (coats), cosmetics, jewelry, or piercings that can interfere with the effectiveness of personal protective equipment (PPE).
- Appropriate PPEs should be worn into the anteroom.
- Hands and forearms should be washed with soap and water for at least 30 seconds.
- An air dryer or disposable nonshedding towel should be used in drying hands and forearms.
- Upon entering the buffer area, antiseptic hand cleansing must be performed before sterile gloves are donned.
- No food, drink, or chewing gum is permitted in buffer or ante-area.
- At the beginning of the compounding session and whenever anything is spilled, the area is cleaned with USP-purified water followed by a disinfecting agent with a non-residue-generating agent using a nonlint wipe.
- Only one individual is permitted to enter the buffer area to turn the blower on, which must be on for 30 minutes prior to compounding. During sterile compounding the PECs shall be operating continuously.
- Traffic in the area of the direct compounding area (DCA) is minimized and controlled.
- Supplies used in the DCA are decontaminated using sterile 70% Isopropyl alcohol (IPA).
- All supply items are arranged orderly in the DCA to avoid clutter.
- Supplies in the DCA, where critical sites are exposed to unidirectional HEPA-filtered air, are disinfected with 70% IPA.
- Gloves are disinfected with 70% isopropyl alcohol.
- All rubber stoppers of vials and necks of ampoules are disinfected with 70% IPA, and the preparer must wait 10 seconds prior to compounding.

- All injectable drugs and other CSPs must be prepared in a "clean room" using a laminar flow hood.
- Laminar air flow hoods are recertified after at least 6 months or when the laminar airflow hood is moved.
- No objects should be between the first air from a HEPA filter and the critical site.
- HEPA filters must be changed when they become wet.
- Inspection records must be kept on file within the pharmacy department.

Sterile compounding procedures

Personal training and competency assessments

Personnel training

- All personnel who prepare CSPs shall be trained by expert personnel.
- Training must be completed and documented prior to compounding personnel preparing CSPs.
- Compounding personnel must complete didactic training, pass written competence assessments, and undergo skill assessment using observational audit tools and media-fill testing.
- Media-fill testing of aseptic work skills must be performed initially before beginning to prepare CSPs for Category 1, Category 2 CSPs.
  - For personnel compounding Category 1 and Category 2 CSPs, the aseptic manipulation competency must occur initially and at least every 6 months thereafter.
- Compounding personnel who fail written tests or observational audits or whose media-fill test vials have one or more units showing visible microbial contamination must be reinstructed and reevaluated by expert compounding personnel to ensure correction of all aseptic work practice deficiencies.
- Compounding personnel shall pass all evaluations prior to resuming compounding of sterile preparations.
- Compounding personnel must demonstrate proficiency of proper hand hygiene, garbing, and consistent cleaning procedures in addition to didactic evaluation and aseptic media fill.
- Cleaning and disinfecting procedures performed by other support personnel shall be thoroughly trained in proper hand hygiene and garbing, cleaning, and disinfection procedures by a qualified aseptic compounding expert.
- Support personnel should routinely undergo performance evaluation of proper hand hygiene, garbing, and all applicable cleaning and disinfecting procedures conducted by a qualified aseptic compounding expert.

Competency assessments

All sterile compounding personnel should be able to demonstrate at least the following in a hands-on, witnessed assessment, initially and at least every 12 months thereafter:

- Hand hygiene
- Garbing
- Cleaning and disinfection

- Calculations, measuring, and mixing
- Aseptic technique
- Achieving and/or maintaining sterility and apyrogenicity
- Use of equipment
- Documentation of the compounding process (e.g., master formulation and compounding records
- Principles of HEPA-filtered unidirectional airflow within the ISO 5 area
- Proper use of PECs
- Principles of movement of materials and personnel within the compounding area

Aseptic work practice assessment and evaluation

- Pharmacy personnel must pass a didactic, practical skills assessment and media-fill testing.

Garbing and gloving competency evaluation

- Personnel must demonstrate proficiency of proper hand hygiene, garbing, and applicable cleaning and disinfecting procedures.
- Evaluation includes the preparer:
- Presents in a clean appropriate attire
- Wears no cosmetics or jewelry
- Does not bring food or beverages into the ante-area or buffer area
- Is aware of the demarcation separating the clean and dirty sides and observes the required activities
- Dons shoe covers properly and places the designated shoe on the clean side of the demarcation
- Dons beard covering if necessary
- Dons head covering to ensure all hair is covered
- Dons face mask to cover bridge of nose down to include the chin
- Performs hand hygiene procedure by wetting hands and forearms and washing using soap and warm water for at least 30 seconds
- Dries hands and forearms using a lint-free towel or hand dryer
- Selects appropriate-sized gown, examines it, and dons it to ensure full closure
- Disinfects hands again using a waterless alcohol-based surgical hand scrub and allows hands to dry thoroughly prior to donning sterile gloves
- Dons appropriate-sized gloves that are tight with no excess glove material at the fingertips
- Examines gloves for any defects, holes, or tears
- Disinfect gloves with 70% IPA prior to work in the DCA
- Removes PPEs on the clean side of the ante-area
- Removes gloves and performs hand hygiene
- Removes gown and discards it; hangs it on a hook if it is to be worn again on the same workday
- Removes and discards mask, head cover, and beard cover (if used)
- Removes shoe covers one at a time, ensuring that the uncovered foot is placed on the dirty side of the demarcation line, and performs hand hygiene again

Gloved fingertip sampling

- Prior to individuals being permitted to compound, they must undergo a competency evaluation a minimum of three times before working in a clean room.

- Monitoring of all compounding personnel glove fingertips should be performed for all CSP risk-level compounding.
- Sampling evaluates the competency of personnel performing hand hygiene and garbing procedures.
- All personnel must demonstrate competency in proper hand hygiene and garbing procedures.
- Individuals must don PPE and sterile gloves and press each finger and thumb into agar culture.
- Individuals must place their gloved finger or thumb into agar.
- Another staff member must incubate the sample at 30°C–35° C for 48–72 hours; the sample must read zero colony-forming units.
- After passing the initial evaluation, the individual must undergo a sampling at least once a year.
- In this assessment gloves are not to be disinfected with sterile 70% IPA prior to sampling.
- The CFU action level for gloved hands should be based on the total number on CFU on both gloves.
- Results are reported as number of CFU per employee hand.
- Reevaluation of work practices and cleaning procedures should occur if the CFU count exceeds the suggested action levels.

Personnel evaluation and testing	
Competency	Frequency
Core skills	Initially and at least every 1 2 months
Garbing	Every 6 months for personnel compounding Category 1,2, and 3 CSPs.
Aseptic manipulation (media fill, gloved fingertip/thumb sampling and surface sampling)	Every 6 months for personnel compounding Category 1, 2 and 3 CSPs.
CSP, Compounded sterile preparation.	

Cleaning and disinfecting competency evaluation

- Evaluations show the effectiveness of the disinfecting processes being used by the facility in the clean room.
- Cleansing and disinfecting evaluation involves:
  - Removing all items from the area to be cleaned
  - Cleaning surfaces by removing loose residue and remains from spills
  - Using sterile 70% IPA to wipe down the surfaces and allow to air dry
- Using a sterile nutrient agar contact plate for flat surfaces or swabs for equipment and other nonflat surfaces, sampling must be performed in all ISO classified areas on a periodic basis.
- Reevaluation of work practices and cleaning procedures should occur if the CFU count exceeds the suggested action levels.

Subsequent testing must be performed in the same location as previously done.

Surface sampling

- Surface sampling is performed at the end of compounding or at regular intervals as specified by the policies of the facility.
- Use contact plates for regular or flat surfaces, and swabs are used for irregular surfaces.
- Contact plate collection utilizes rolling an agar plate across the sampling area.
- Swab collection is performed by wiping a swab across the sampling area and placing on agar.

Surface collection methods

- Immediately after sampling a surface with the contact plate, the sample shall be thoroughly wiped with a non-shedding wipe soaked in sterile 70% IPA.
- Results should be reported as CFU per unit of surface area.
- If levels measured during surface sampling exceed the levels in identified below for each ISO classification, then the cause must be investigated and corrected.

Air and surface sampling	
	<797> Guidelines
ISO certification/viable airborne particle testing	Every 6 months
Viable airborne particle testing	Monthly
Surface sampling	Monthly

Action levels for surface sampling				
ISO class	Work surface samples (plates)	Work surface samples (swabs)	Non–work surface (plates)	Non–work surface (swabs)
5	>3	>3	a	a
7	>5	>5	>10	>10
8	>25	>25	>50	>50
aAll ISO 5 surfaces are considered work surfaces.				

Pharmacy calculations in sterile compounding

Concentrations

- Percent Weight-in-Volume (%w/v)
  - The number of grams of solute dissolved in 100 milliliters of solvent (e.g. 1% w/v contains 1 gram of solute dissolved in 100 milliliters of solvent.
- Percent Volume-in-Volume (%v/v)
  - The number of milliliters of solute dissolved in 100 milliliters of solvent (e.g. 5% v/v contains 5 milliliters of solution dissolved in 100 mL of solvent).

- Percent Weight-in-Weight (%w/w)
  - The number of grams of solute dissolved in 100 grams of solvent (e.g. 10% w/w contains 10 grams of solute dissolved in 100 grams of solvent).
- Ratio strength
  - Method of expressing strength in the form of a ratio
    - 5% can be written 5:100 which means there are 5 parts per 100 parts
    - For example, 1:1000 ratio strength can be interpreted:
      - Solids in liquids=1 gram of solute in 1000 mL of solution
      - Liquids in liquids=1 milliliter of solute in 1000 mL of solution
      - Solids in solids=1 gram of solute in 1000 grams of mixture

Dosage

- Actual body weight is defined as the number of quantity (micrograms, milligrams, grams) per kilogram or pound of body weight.
- Ideal body weight (IBW) is used in calculating dosages for obese patients.
  - Adult males: $IBW_{kg} = 50 + (2.3 \times$ height in inches over 5 feet)
  - Adult women: $IBW_{kg} = 45.5 + (2.3 \times$ height in inches over 5 feet)
  - Children under 5 feet tall: $IBW_{kg} = (height^2_{cm} \times 1.65)/1000$
  - Children over 5 feet tall:
    - Males $IBW_{kg} = 39 + (2.27 \times height_{in}$ over 5 feet)
    - Females $IBW_{kg} = 42.2 + (2.27 \times height_{in}$ over 5 feet)
- Body surface area (BSA) (weight in pounds and height in inches):
  - $BSA (m^2) = \sqrt{(Height(in) \cdot Weight(lb)/3131}$
- BSA (weight in kilograms and height in centimeters):
  - $BSA (m^2) = \sqrt{(Height(cm) \cdot Weight(kg)/3600}$
- BSA dose for adults:
  - $BSA \times$ adult dose
- BSA dose for children:
  - $(BSA \times$ adult dose$)/1.7$

Powder volume

- Final volume = volume of diluent + volume of powder

Drip (flow) rates

Pharmacy technicians must be aware of calculations associated with IV fluids. Pharmacy technicians must be able to determine the flow rates of IV infusions, calculate the volume of fluids administered over a period, and control the total volume of fluids administered to a patient over a period of time.

A variety of IV sets are available for infusing IV fluids. They are identified by the number of drops of a fluid per milliliter. Common IV sets include 10 drops/mL, 15 drops/mL, and 60 drops/mL (minidrip set).

Time of infusion: volume of fluid (or amount of drug)/rate of infusion

Rate of infusion: Volume of fluid (or amount of drug)/time of infusion

Infusion rate: drops/minute = (number of mL/h) × (number of drops/mL) divide by 60 min/h

The number of drops per milliliter may vary.

Personal health and hygiene requirements

- USP <797> states that compounding personnel with rashes, sunburn, weeping sores, conjunctivitis, active respiratory infection, and cosmetics are prohibited from preparing CSPs.

Hand hygiene procedures

Hand hygiene (Fig. 1.2) must be performed prior to and after gowning and includes:

- Washing hands under the fingernails, on the wrists, and up to the elbow for 30 seconds with a facility-approved agent
- Drying hands and arms with nonshedding disposable towels or an electronic hand dryer
- Sanitizing hands with application of a waterless, alcohol-based hand rub with persistent activity prior to donning sterile gloves

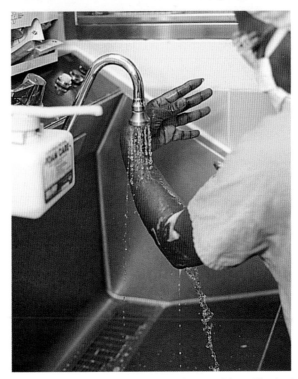

Fig. 1.2 Hands and forearms are thoroughly rinsed in an upright position, beginning with the fingertips down to the elbows. (From Davis K, Guerra T. *Mosby's Pharmacy Technician Principles and Practice*, 6th ed. Elsevier: 2022.)

Personal protective equipment

- Any individual compounding a Category 1, 2, or 3 CSP must wear PPEs as outlined in institutional standard operating procedure (SOP).
- Minimum garbing requirements for compounding Category 1 and 2 CSPs include
  - Low-lint garment with sleeves that fit snugly around the wrists and an enclosed neck (e.g., gowns) should be worn.
  - Low-lint covers for shoes should be worn.
  - Low-lint cover for head that covers the hair and ears, and if applicable, cover for facial hair should be worn.
  - Low-lint face mask should be worn.
  - Sterile powder-free gloves should be worn.
  - If using an RABS (i.e., a compounding aseptic isolators or compounding aseptic containment isolators), disposable gloves should be worn inside the gloves attached to the RABS sleeves. Sterile gloves must be worn over the gloves attached to the RABS sleeve.
  - Garb must be replaced if it becomes visibly soiled.
  - Gowns may be reused within the same shift.
- If an HD is being compounded, appropriate PPE must be worn and disposed of according to USP <800>.
- Gloves must be sterile and powder free.

Usage of personal protective equipment				
PPE	Receiving damaged or broken containers	Compounding (sterile and nonsterile)	Cleanup	Collection and disposal of waste/spills
Gloves	X	X	X	X
Gown	X	X	X	X
Hair, face, beard, and shoe covers	X	X	X	X
Eye and face protection	X			X
Respiratory protection	X			X
PPE, Personal protective equipment.				

Donning and disposing of PPEs

- For preparing Category 1 CSPs, all garbing (Fig. 1.3) must occur within the SCA.
- Compounding Category 2 CSPs, all garb must be donned before entering the buffer area.

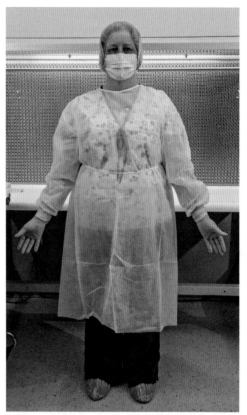

Fig. 1.3 Personal protective equipment. Start at feet first. (From Davis K, Guerra T. *Mosby's Pharmacy Technician Principles and Practice*, 6th ed. Elsevier: 2022.)

- The proper sequence of donning PPEs, performed in the ante-area, is as follows:
  - Don shoe covers, hair and beard covers, and a mask.
  - Perform hand hygiene.
  - Don gown, fastened securely at the neck and wrists.
  - Sanitize hands using an alcohol-based hand rub and allow hands to dry.
  - Enter the buffer area (if facility layout dictates, this step may occur after the following two steps).
  - Don sterile powder-free gloves.
  - Sanitize the gloves with application of 70% sterile IPA and allow gloves to dry.
- The proper sequence in removing PPEs is:
  - gloves
  - goggles/face shield
  - gown
  - mask/respirator
  - hand hygiene

Properties and usages of deactivating, decontamination, cleaning, and disinfecting agents

Common disinfectants used in health care facilities for inanimate objects		Isopropyl alcohol	Accelerated hydrogen peroxide	Quaternary ammonium	Phenolics	Chlorine (e.g., sodium hypochlorite)	Iodophors (e.g., povidone-iodine)
Concentration used		60%–95%	0.5%	0.4%–1.6% aq	0.4%–1.6% aq	100–500 ppm	30–50 ppm
Microbial inactivator	Bacteria	+	+	+	+	+	+
Microbial inactivator	Lipophilic viruses	+	+	+	+	+	+
Microbial inactivator	Hydrophilic viruses	±	+	±	±	+	±
Microbial inactivator	*Mycobacterium tuberculosis*	+	+	±	+	+	±
Microbial inactivator	Mucolytic agents	+	+	+	+	+	±
Microbial inactivator	Bacterial spores	–	–	–	–	+	–
Chemical and physical properties	Corrosive	±	–	–	–	±	±
Chemical and physical properties	Nonevaporating residue	–	–	+	+	–	+
Chemical and physical properties	Inactivated by organic matter	+	±	+	±	+	+
Chemical and physical properties	Skin irritant	±	–	+	+	+	–
Chemical and physical properties	Eye irritant	–	–	+	+	+	–
Chemical and physical properties	Respiratory irritant	–	–	–	–	+	–
Chemical and physical properties	Systemic toxicity	+	–	+	+	+	±

aq; Aqueous; *ppm*, parts per million.

Procedures and requirements for cleaning and disinfecting compounding equipment

- Areas to be cleaned and disinfected include all ISO Class 5 compounding areas, buffer areas, ante-areas, and SCA.
- Disinfectants used are dependent on microbial activity, inactivation by organic matter, type of residue, and shelf-life of the disinfectant.
- Work surfaces in ISO Class 7 (buffer area) and ISO Class 8 (ante-area) shall be cleaned and disinfected at least once daily.
- Floors in the buffer or clean area, ante-area, and segregate compounding area are cleaned by mopping with a cleaning and disinfecting area once daily.
- All cleaning materials should be of nonshedding material.
- Supplies and equipment removed from shipping cartons should be wiped with sterile 70% IPA.

Cleaning a horizontal laminar flow workbench

- Remove all items from within the laminar flow workbench (Fig. 1.4).
- Using a lint-free wipe and sterile water, clean all surfaces within the laminar flow hood.

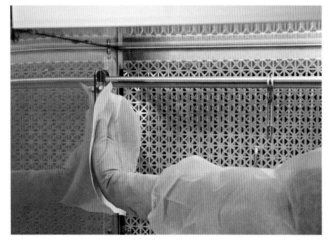

Fig. 1.4 Wipe the top of the hood first. Clean in a side-to-side motion from left to right, working from back to front. (From Davis K, Guerra T. *Mosby's Pharmacy Technician Principles and Practice*, 6th ed. Elsevier: 2022.)

- Look at all surfaces for any signs of crystallized solutions; if any are found, clean them with sterile water.
- Using sterile 70% alcohol, moisten a 4-by-4-inch gauze or lint-free cloth.
- Wipe the top of the hood first. Clean this surface with a side-to-side motion from left to right, working from back to front.
- Wipe the horizontal IV pole and all hooks or brackets.
- Wipe from top to bottom on each side of the hood, working from back to front using overlapping strokes.
- Wipe the rear wall of the hood using a side-to-side motion from left to right, beginning at the top and working down to the bottom.
- Wipe the flat work surface using a side-to-side motion from left to right, working from the back to the front of the laminar flow hood.
- Before compounding, allow the 70% alcohol to remain on the disinfected areas for a minimum of 30 seconds.

Cleaning a vertical laminar flow workbench

- Remove all items from within the laminar flow workbench.
- Using a lint-free wipe and sterile water, clean all surfaces within the laminar flow hood.
- Look at all surfaces for any signs of crystallized solutions; if any are found, clean them with sterile water.
- Using sterile 70% alcohol, moisten a 4-by-4-inch gauze or lint-free cloth.
- Wipe the horizontal IV pole and all hooks or brackets.
- Wipe from top to bottom on each side of the hood, working from back to front using overlapping strokes.
- Wipe the rear wall of the hood using a side-to-side motion from left to right, beginning at the top and working down to the bottom.
- Wipe the flat work surface using a side-to-side motion from left to right, working from the back to the front of the laminar flow hood.
- Before compounding allow the 70% alcohol to remain on the disinfected areas for a minimum of 30 seconds.

Cleaning a biological safety cabinet

- Remove all items from within the BSC.
- Using a lint-free wipe and sterile water, clean all surfaces within the BSC.
- Look at all surfaces for any signs of crystallized solutions; if any are found, clean them with sterile water.
- Using sterile 70% alcohol, moisten a 4-by-4-inch gauze or lint-free cloth.
- Wipe the horizontal IV pole and all hooks or brackets.
- Wipe from top to bottom on each side of the BSC using overlapping strokes.
- Wipe the rear wall of the BSC and inside the front shield using a side-to-side motion from left to right, beginning from the top and working to the bottom.
- Wipe the flat work surface using a side-to-side motion from left to right, working from the back to the front of the BSC.
- Before compounding allow the 70% alcohol to remain on the disinfected areas for a minimum of 30 seconds.

Minimum frequency of cleaning and disinfecting compounding areas for ISO Class 5	
Site	**Minimum frequency**
ISO Class 5 (primary engineering control, e.g., LAFW, BSC, RABS)	At the frequency of each shift, before each batch, not longer than 30 min following the previous surface disinfection when ongoing compounding activities are occurring, after spills, when surface contamination is known or suspected
Counters and easily cleanable work surfaces	Daily
Floors	Daily
Walls	Monthly
Ceilings	Monthly
Storage shelving	Monthly

BSC, Biological safety cabinet; *ISO*, International Organization for Standardizaion; *LAFW*, laminar airflow workbench; *RABS*, restricted access barrier system.

Principles of aseptic manipulation within a horizontal or vertical laminar airflow workbench

Critical air

- Enters the prefilters in front of the hood; travels through the HEPA filter where all air contaminants, including bacteria, are removed; and then flows horizontally across the work surface. Purified air circulates from the back to the front in parallel lines.

First air

- In the DCA, there is exposure to HEPA-filtered air or first air when preparing sterile compounds. The critical sites should be exposed to first air to avoid contamination from particles present in the air. Needles, syringe plungers, and vial tops should always be exposed to first air.

Zones of turbulence

- In a horizontal LAFW one should not perform critical procedures or place objects downstream of an object, within the zone of turbulence, which is approximately three times the diameter of the object.

Critical sites

- Any location where contamination might come into contact with a CSP is a critical site.
- These sites are never touched or swabbed with alcohol prior to needle entry.
- Examples of critical sites include the needle, needle hub, and syringe plunger.
- Examples of critical sites that may be exposed to the air include the tip of the needle, an opened ampoule of medication, and the injection port.

Critical area

- A critical area is a place where CSPs, containers, and closures are exposed to the environment.
- In an ISO Class 5 environment (laminar workbenches, BSCs, and compounding isolators) has no more than 3520 particles per cubic meter of air.

Cleaning critical sites of vials, ampoules, and injection ports

- Clean the critical site of an ampoule, vial, or an injection port with an alcohol swab of 70% IPA. Take a fresh alcohol swab and gently wipe the entire surface of the ampoule to clean it. If it seems wet or slippery afterward, let it dry for 1–2 minutes before handling it.

Straight draw

- This procedure must be performed in a clean air environment.
- Wipe rubber top of vial with 70% IPA and allow to dry.
- Make sure the needle is firmly attached to the syringe.
- Prime the plunger by pulling it back and forth; then pull plunger back to slightly less than the amount of solution to be withdrawn.
- Remove needle cap. Insert the bevel of the needle with a 30-degree angle into the center of the rubber stopper.
- Upon entering the rubber stopper, adjust needle such that it is entering at a 90-degree angle.
- Remove bubbles from the syringe.
- Invert vial and needle without shadowing, withdraw the needle, and carefully recap the end or inject into the injection port of the IV bag.

Reconstituting a powder

- Wipe the rubber top of the vial with 70% sterile IPA and allow to dry.
- Make sure the needle is firmly attached to the syringe.
- Insert the needle into the vial of the diluent and withdraw the correct amount of diluent to reconstitute the powder.
- Pull back the plunger to clear the neck of the syringe.
- Remove the needle and replace it with a vented needle.
- Insert vented needle into the vial of powder and slowly add the diluent to powder in the vial.
- Shake and swirl the vial to completely dissolve the powder.
- Clean the rubber stopper with 70% IPA if it has become contaminated.
- Using a new syringe with a regular needle, withdraw the desired amount of the drug.
- Remove any air bubbles from the syringe.
- Recap the needle and insert the needle into the injection port of the IV bag.

Removing air bubbles

- Draw back on the plunger, allowing fluid into the syringe.
- Turn the large air bubbles around the syringe to pick up smaller air bubbles. If smaller air bubbles continue to exist, tap the syringe to displace them.
- Hold the syringe upright and pull the plunger back to clear the hub.
- Slowly push the plunger to remove any remaining air.

Using transfer needles

- Wipe the IV injection port and the rubber top of the vial with an alcohol swab.
- Insert the longer of the two needles into the IV bag injection port.
- Place the shorter of the two needles into the vial.
- Squeeze the IV bag, gently forcing the IV fluid to fill the vial.
- Shake the vial gently, causing the powder to dissolve in the solution.
- Hold the IV bag such that the air rises to the top of the IV bag.
- Squeeze the bag, causing the air to move into the vial, which will force the fluid down into the IV bag.
- Ensure that all fluid from the vial has moved into the IV bag before removing the transfer syringe.
- Remove the transfer needle from the IV bag injection port.
- Remove the transfer needle from the vial and dispose of it in a sharps container.

Withdrawing fluid from an ampoule

- This procedure should be done in an ISO Class 5 PEC.
- Remove air bubbles from the body of the ampoule.
- Swab the neck of the ampoule and IV injection port and allow to dry.
- Hold the ampoule at a 20-degree angle toward the side of laminar flow hood.

- Using your thumbs, apply pressure to the neck of the ampoule using a hands-away motion.
- Attach a filter needle or filter straw to the syringe.
- Withdraw the solution from the ampoule.
- Empty the filter needle or filter straw into the syringe, cleaning the hub of the syringe.
- Change the filter needle or filter straw to a regular needle.
- Remove any air bubbles.
- Insert the needle into the IV injection port and inject the fluid slowly.

Handling sharps containers

- The FDA recommends that used needles and other sharps be immediately placed in FDA-cleared sharps disposal containers.
- Sharps disposal containers should be:
  - Made of a heavy-duty plastic
  - Able to close with a tight-fitting, puncture-resistant lid, without sharps being able to come out
  - Upright and stable during use
  - Leak resistant
  - Properly labeled to warn of hazardous waste inside the container
- Sharps containers should never be overfilled; they should only be filled to three-quarters full of the sizes of the container.
- Pharmacy personnel should never force materials into the opening or reach inside of a sharps container.
- Disposal of sharps containers should be done according to community guidelines, which may include drop box or supervised collection sites, household hazardous waste sites, mail-back programs, or residential special waste pickup services.

Record-keeping requirements

- Written documentation is required to demonstrate full compliance with <797>.
- Documentation includes
  - Personnel training, competency assessments, and qualification records including corrective actions for any failures
  - Certification reports, including corrective actions for any failures
  - Environmental air and surface monitoring procedures and results
  - Equipment records (e.g., calibration, verification, and maintenance reports)
  - Receipt of components
  - SOPs; Master Formulation Records (if required) and compounding records (if required)
  - Release of inspection and testing records
  - Information related to complaints and adverse events including corrective actions taken
  - Results of investigations and corrective actions
- The Master Formulation Record (MFR) is a list of ingredients, preparation methods, safety requirements, BUD,

and references for the compounder. It contains the steps involved in compounding the product. It must contain the following information: name, strength, and dosage form of the CSP.
  - Identifies amounts of all ingredients
  - Type and size of container closure system
  - Complete instructions for preparing the CSP, including equipment, supplies, a description of the compounding steps and any special precautions
  - Physical description of the final CSP
  - BUD and storage requirements
  - Reference source to support the stability of the CSP
  - Quality control procedures (e.g., pH testing, filter integrity testing)
  - Other information as needed to describe the compounding process and ensure repeatability (e.g., adjusting pH and tonicity; sterilization method, such as steam, dry heat, irradiation, or filter)
- Compounding record (CR) contains a record of all finished compounds. A compounding record must be maintained for a minimum of 3 years from the date medication was prepared and at the pharmacy. Information found on a compounding record includes:
  - name, strength and dosage form of the CSP
  - date and time of preparation
  - assigned internal identification number (e.g., prescription, order)
  - a method to identify the individuals involved in the compounding process and individuals identifying the final CSP
  - name of each component
  - vendor, lot number, and expiration date for each component for CSPs for more than one patient and for CSPs prepared from nonsterile ingredients
  - weight or volume of each component
  - strength of each component
  - total quantity compounded
  - final yield
  - assigned BUD and storage requirements
  - results of quality control procedures (e.g., visual inspection, filter integrity testing, pH testing)
- All records specific to compounding a particular CSP must be kept for at least 3 years or as required by state law, whichever is greater.
- Facility design and initial qualification records must be kept as facility is in operation.
- All other records such as personnel training records, equipment maintenance, and environmental monitoring should be maintained for 3 years or per state law, whichever is greater.

Weighing and measuring components

Volumetric analysis

- The volumetric method is limited by human error.
- In a situation where the pharmacy utilizes the pullback method, an error can occur by pulling the plunger back incorrectly and injecting the incorrect volume into the IV bag. The pullback method should not be used in

preparing CSPs. There is nothing to prevent a wrong dose from accidentally being injected into a bag only to have the technician pull the empty syringe back to the correct volume.

- Using either a step-check process or photo-assisted volumetrics is significantly better than the pullback method but has its own shortcomings. A pharmacy technician may pull the wrong dose and the pharmacist may verify it.

Gravimetric analysis

- The specific gravity of a solution is used to quantitatively determine the amount of drug in the solution.
- In the case of an IV preparation, the gravimetric method can be used to determine the accuracy of a dose drawn into a syringe, removed from a vial, injected into an IV bag, and so on.
- If the preparer knows the weight of an object—syringe, IV bag, a vial of medication, etc.—before and after adding or removing a substance, then one knows exactly how much drug was added or removed.

Compounding parenteral nutrition procedures

Peripheral parenteral nutrition

- IV nutrition administered through veins of the peripheral areas of the body that provides part of an individual's daily nutritional requirements.

Total peripheral nutrition

- IV nutrition that provides all an individual's daily nutritional requirements

Adult daily body nutrient and fluid requirements

- Dextrose: 30 to 45 kcal/kg per day
- Protein: 1.0 to 2.0 g/kg per day
- IV fat emulsion: administered as 1, 2, or 3 kcal/mL; should account for 1%–4% of daily calories
- Fluids: 30 to 40 mL/kg per day

Components of a total parenteral nutrition

- Dextrose is a source of calories and is available as a 70% or 50% solution.
- Amino acids are required for protein synthesis and are available as 10% solution. They provide a source of nitrogen, which is necessary in utilizing proteins in the body. There are two types of amino acids—essential amino acids and nonessential amino acids. Essential amino acids are not produced by the body, and nonessential amino acids are produced by the body.

- Fat provides the necessary fatty acids for the body and are available as 10%, 20%, and 30%.
- Sterile water is necessary.
- Additives include both electrolytes and minerals.
  - Calcium: assists in many body functions required for proper bone formation, nerve function, muscle contraction, heart function, and blood clotting
  - Chloride: controls water balance inside and outside of the cells, maintains appropriate pH of body fluids, blood volume, and blood pressure
  - Magnesium: required for the muscular and nervous system
  - Phosphate: essential for bone growth, muscle function, and fighting infection
  - Potassium: regulates water balance in cells and assists in maintaining nerve and muscle function
  - Sodium: establishes total body water volume

Calcium and phosphate concerns

- A precipitate may form if the calcium and phosphate are not added in the proper sequence and the amounts are incorrect or at the incorrect temperature.
- Phosphate should be added first to a TPN admixture.

Preparing total parenteral nutrition

- Aseptic technique is required because TPN is infused into the right atrium of the heart.
- TPN compounders have been developed, which include a multichannel pump for the amino acids, dextrose, fats, and other additives, that are connected to a personal computer. The computer assists in the calculations and drives the pump. Microcompounding pumps are used for the electrolytes and other additives.
- TPN and peripheral parenteral nutrition are premixed from the manufacturer, but electrolytes, vitamins, and medications may be added to the nutrients at the pharmacy.

Preparing total parenteral nutrition solutions (requires aseptic technique)

- **Method 1:** Amino acids and dextrose are mixed first. Fat emulsion is added next, followed by the additives.
- **Method 2:** Amino acids are added to the fat emulsion. Dextrose is added next, followed by the additives.
- **Method 3:** Dextrose, amino acids, and fat emulsion are added simultaneously while swirling and mixing. Additives are incorporated last.
- Examples of TPN additives include:
  - potassium chloride (KCl)
  - potassium phosphate (KPO_3)
  - calcium gluconate (Ca gluconate)
  - magnesium sulfate ($MgSO_4$)
  - sodium phosphate ($NaPO_4$)
  - sodium chloride (NaCl)
  - multivitamin
  - multiple trace elements
  - zinc (Zn)

Specialized compounded sterile preparations

Epidurals

- Used in surgery and childbirth where the dosage form is injected intrathecally to control pain
- May contain a narcotic and anesthetic or just an anesthetic
- Dosage form must be preservative free

Dialysis solutions

- Dialysis is the separation of particles in a liquid on the basis of differences in their ability to pass through a membrane.
- During dialysis a drug travels from a higher concentration to a lower concentration.
- Peritoneal dialysis is a form of dialysis where the dialysis solution flows into the peritoneal cavity and the organs are protected by a peritoneal membrane that removes toxic substances from the blood. When this solution accumulates waste and toxins, it is exchanged.
- Hemodialysis is a form of dialysis where toxic substances are removed from the blood.

Ophthalmics

- Sterile, particle-free solution or suspension administered to the eye
- May be either water based or isotonic, sodium chloride based
- May contain buffers, preservatives, antioxidants, and other additives
- Aseptic technique must be used during compounding
- Must be compounded in either a LAFW or a compounding aseptic isolator
- Must be sterilized using either an autoclave or a bacterial filter
- Tonicity of ophthalmic medications must be between 0.6% and 2%
- pH of ophthalmic medications should be approximately 7.4
- Thickening agents used to increase the viscosity of the solution, which increases the effectiveness of the ophthalmic agent
- Packaged in soft plastic container with a fixed built-in dropper

Otic medications

- Compounded in a sterile environment using an aseptic technique
- Not considered a sterile medication because they are applied externally

Nasal preparations

- Preparations are water-based solutions that are indicated for rhinitis.

- They may contain buffers and preservatives.
- FDA requires that nasal preparations must be sterile before being dispensed.
- Compounding occurs in a LAFW or a compounding aseptic isolator.
- A bacterial filter and a sterile container are used during compounding.
- Upon compounding the preparation, an autoclave may be used to sterilize the medication.

Irrigations

- Used to bathe or wash wounds, incisions, or body tissues
- Not injected directly into a vein but rather applied outside the circulatory system
- Examples of irrigation solutions:
  - Acetic acid irrigation USP is indicated for irrigating the bladder or rinsing away blood or surgical debris.
  - Ringer's Irrigation USP is used to irrigate body surfaces and must be labeled as "Not for Injection."
  - Sodium chloride irrigation USP is used in washing wounds.
  - Sterile water USP must be labeled "Not for Injection."

Negative pressure technique

- It is intended to prevent exposure of health care personnel to the drugs being compounding.
- The negative pressure technique involves:
  - Swabbing the vial septum with sterile 70% IPA and allowing to dry
  - Performing manipulations in the DCAs and in such a manner in which critical sites remain in unobstructed HEPA-filtered air
  - Using a syringe that is 25% larger than the total dose
  - Attaching the needle and syringe carefully to avoid touch contamination of the critical site
  - Drawing up the amount of air that is equal to the total dose to be drawn up
  - Inserting the needle into the septum
  - Pulling back on the plunger slightly to create a negative pressure within the vial without touching the barrel
  - Inverting the vial and withdrawing no more than 15%–25% of the dose into syringe, until resistance is observed
  - Allowing the syringe plunger to return to original position
  - Repeating process until entire volume is withdrawn

Closed-system drug-transfer devices

- The National Institute for Occupational Safety and Health (NIOSH) defines a closed-system drug-transfer device as a system that "mechanically prohibits the transfer of environmental contaminants into the system and the escape of HD or vapor outside the system."
- After connecting a vial to the closed-system drug-transfer devices, the device balances the pressure difference between the container with the drug and the syringe.

- The presence of differences in pressure may result in an aerosol escaping into the environment and exposing individuals to HDs.

Compounding sterile preparations from nonsterile components

Sterilization methods

- Filtration
  - The passage of a fluid or solution through a sterilizing grade membrane produces a sterile waste product.
  - All CSPs shall be pyrogen free and have a nominal pore size of 0.2–0.22 mcm.
  - Filters must be chemically and physically stable.
- Steam
  - Applying a lethal process such as autoclaving or steam under pressure to a sealed container can be used for quality assurance purposes.
  - All materials should be exposed to steam at 121°C at 15 pounds/inch for 20–60 minutes.
  - Prior to sterilization all plastic, glass, and metal devices are to be wrapped in low-particle paper or fabric or sealed in envelopes to prevent poststerilization microbial penetration.
- Dry heat
  - Performed as a batch process in a specialized oven for sterilization
  - Heat-filtered air distributed throughout the oven through the use of a blower
  - Requires higher temperature for a longer period of time than steam

Signs of defective compounded sterile preparations

- Solubility
  - Solute does not dissolve in solvent resulting in a precipitate.
  - Drug must be soluble in the base solution.
  - Reconstitution requires the proper diluent is used.
- Adsorption
  - Adsorption occurs when a CSP in gas or liquid form accumulates on the surface of the solid or liquid.
  - Adsorption problems can be resolved by adjusting the amount of drug injected into the solution. For example, insulin may be adsorbed on the surface of the IV container, resulting in a lower concentration in the solution.
- Absorption
  - Occurs when a material or container soaks up of the CSP. As an example, absorption occurs when nitroglycerin is placed in a plastic container, which explains why nitroglycerin is packaged in a glass container.
  - Color changes occur when the original color of one or more components changes.
  - Aggregation occurs when triglycerides clump together in an emulsion.

- Cracking occurs when there is a separation of oil and water in an emulsion.
- Creaming results when an accumulation of a triglyceride forms at the top of an emulsion.
- Separation may occur when one of the ingredients separates out in a mixture, which may happen when in a 3:1 TPN.

Sterility, potency, and endotoxin testing

- CSPs prepared in batches of more than 25 units, with the exception of inhalation or ophthalmic preparations, must be tested to ensure that they do not contain excessive bacterial endotoxins.

Sterility testing requirements

- Sterility testing is not required for Category 1 CSPs.
- Category 2 CSPs assigned a BUD require a sterility testing.
- The maximum batch size for all CSPs requiring sterility testing is limited to 250 units.
- If 1–39 CSPs are compounded in a single batch, the sterility testing must be performed on 10% of the number of CSP s prepared, rounded up to the next whole number.
- Pyrogen testing is used to identify the presence of fever-producing microorganisms due to microbial contamination.
  - *Limulus* amebocyte lysate test
  - Rabbit test

Handling, packaging, storage, and disposal

Nonhazardous medications

Labeling of nonhazardous IV medications
- Name of pharmacy
- Patient's name
- Date the medication was filled
- Ingredients with quantity of each in IV
- Total quantity of IV
- Directions for usage
- Infusion rate
- Any special notes
- BUD
- Must be initialed by the technician who prepared it
- Licensed pharmacist's initial

Storage
- Medications must be in a secure area away from unauthorized personnel and visitors.
- Outdated and unused medications are to be returned to the compounding area for disposition according to SOPs.
- Refrigerators are to be kept at 2°C–8°C.
- Daily monitoring and documentation of drug storage refrigerators are required.

- Monthly inspections must be performed for all storage areas.

Transporting

- Staff must be properly trained in transporting sterile compounds.
- Transportation methods for CSPs should be evaluated to ensure the stability and integrity of the CSP is maintained.
- Not all methods of transportation are appropriate for all CSPs. For instance, pneumatic tube delivery may require additional padding around containers to ensure that heat and light exposure and impact are minimized. Other medications may degrade if shaken.

Hazardous medications

A HD is any drug identified as hazardous or potentially hazardous on the basis of at least one of these six criteria: carcinogenicity, teratogenicity, reproductive toxicity in humans, organ toxicity, genotoxicity, or new drugs that mimic existing HDs in structure or toxicity.

Hazardous drugs classification

- Nonantineoplastic drugs
- Antineoplastic drugs
- Drugs with reproductive risks for men or women

Examples of hazardous drugs

- NIOSH maintains a list of antineoplastic and other HDs used in health care.
- Examples of HDs include
  - azathioprine
  - cisplatin
  - cyclophosphamide
  - cyclosporine
  - docetaxel
  - estradiol
  - ethinyl estradiol
  - etoposide
  - fluorouracil
  - ganciclovir
  - isotretinoin
  - methotrexate
  - paclitaxel
  - tamoxifen
  - zidovudine
- Some dosage forms of HDs may not pose a risk as a result of exposure.

Potential areas of unintentional exposure risk from hazardous drugs	
Activity	**Potential exposure**
Receiving HDs	■ Contacting residue on drug containers, individual dosage units, outer containers, work surfaces, or floors

Potential areas of unintentional exposure risk from hazardous drugs	
Activity	**Potential exposure**
Dispensing HDs	■ Counting or repackaging tablets and/or capsules
Compounding and other manipulations	■ Crushing or splitting tablets, opening capsules ■ Pouring liquids from one container to another ■ Weighing or mixing components ■ Constituting or reconstituting HDs ■ Withdrawing or diluting injectable HDs from parenteral containers ■ Expelling air or diluting injectable HDs from syringes ■ Contacting residue on PPE or other garments ■ Deactivating, decontaminating, cleaning, and disinfecting areas contaminated or suspected to be contaminated with HDs ■ Maintenance activities for potentially contaminated equipment
Administration of HDs	■ Generating aerosols during administration by various routes, such as injection, irrigation, and topical application ■ Performing certain specialized procedures such as intraoperative intraperitoneal injection ■ Priming an IV administration set
Patient care activities	■ Handling body fluids or body fluid–contaminated clothing, dressings, and linens
Spills	■ Spill generation, management, and disposal
Transport	■ Moving HDs within a health care facility
Waste	■ Collection and disposal of hazardous waste and trace contaminated waste

HD, Hazardous drug; *PPE*, personal protective equipment.

Personal protective equipment

- Must be worn for any handling of HDs
- Chemotherapy gloves
  - American Society of Testing and Materials–tested chemotherapy gloves may be worn when transporting intact supplies or compounded HDs or receiving or stocking HDs.
  - The gloves must be worn for handling all HDs.
  - They must be powder free.
  - For sterile compounding the outer pair must be sterile.
  - They should be changed every 30 minutes.
  - Hands should be washed with soap and water after removal of gloves.
- Gowns
  - Must be disposable
  - Must be resistant to permeability by HDs
  - Must close in the back and have long sleeves
  - Must have closed cuffs that are elastic or knot
  - Must have no seams or closures that could allow HDs to pass through

- Should be changed based on manufacturer information (If manufacturer information is not available, a gown should be changed every 2–3 hours or immediately after a spill or splash.)
- Covers
  - Head and hair covers (including beard covers)
  - Sleeve covers optional
  - Eye and face protection
    - Must be worn when working outside C-PEC (for example, cleaning a spill)
    - Goggles (face shields, full-piece respirators)
  - Shoe covers
    - Second pair must be donned before entering C-SEC.
    - Second pair must be removed when exiting C-SEC.

- Respiratory protection
  - Surgical masks should not be used when respiratory protection is required.
  - N95 respirator is acceptable for most activities (workers should be fit tested and trained).
  - A full-piece, chemical cartridge or powered air-purifying respirator should be worn with:
    - HD spills larger than be contained by spill kit
    - Tasks such as deactivating, decontaminating, or cleaning under work surface of C-PEC
    - Known or suspected airborne exposure to vapor or powder

Personal protective equipment requirements when handling hazardous drugs summary				
PPE	Receiving damaged or broken hazardous drugs	Compounding (sterile and nonsterile) hazardous drugs	Cleanup (routine) hazardous drugs	Collection and disposal of waste/spills
Gloves	X	X	X	X
Gowns	X	X	X	X
Hair, face, beard, and shoe covers	X	X	X	X
Eye and face protection	X			X
Respiratory protection	X			X
PPE, Personal protective equipment.				

Hazard Communication Standard

- A facility must create SOPs that address the labeling, transporting, storing, and disposing of HDs.
- The Hazard Communication ensures chemical safety in the workplace by providing information regarding the identities and hazards associated with chemicals in the workplace and providing the information to the employees.
- Manufacturers are required to evaluate the hazards associated with the chemicals they produce and prepare labels and SDSs to convey the hazard information.
- SDSs are required for each hazardous chemical used and must be easily accessible exposed personnel. Personnel must be properly trained to handle all chemicals.
- SDS must contain the following sixteen sections:
  - Section 1: Identification
  - Section 2: Hazard(s) identification
  - Section 3: Composition/information on ingredients
  - Section 4: First-aid measures
  - Section 5: Firefighting measures
  - Section 6: Accidental release measures
  - Section 7: Handling and storage
  - Section 8: Exposure controls/personal protection
  - Section 9: Physical and chemical properties
  - Section 10: Stability and reactivity
  - Section 11: Toxicological information

  - Section 12: Ecological information (nonmandatory)
  - Section 13: Disposal considerations (nonmandatory)
  - Section 14: Transport information (nonmandatory)
  - Section 15: Regulatory information (nonmandatory)
  - Section 16: Other information
- The Hazard Communication Standard provides specific criteria for classification of health and physical hazards, as well as classification of mixtures.
  - All containers of hazardous chemicals must be labeled, which includes a harmonized signal word, pictogram, and hazard statement for each hazard class and category. Labeling must include precautionary statement.
  - Personnel who may be exposed to hazardous chemicals must be provided with training and information before they begin working work with hazardous chemicals and whenever the hazard changes.
  - All personnel of reproductive capability must confirm in writing that they understand the risks of handling HDs.

Personnel training

- All training must be done based on job functions, and personnel must be trained before they independently handle HDs.
- Personnel competency must be reassessed at least every 12 months.

- Personnel must be trained prior to introduction of a new HD or new equipment or before significant changes to process of SOP.
- All training and assessment must be documented.

Training requirements

- Overview of entity's list of HDs and their risks
- Review of facility's SOPs pertaining to HDs
- Proper use of PPE
- Proper use of equipment and devices
- Correct response to known or suspected HD exposure
- Spill management
- Proper disposal of HDs and trace-contaminated materials

Facilities and engineering controls

- Certain areas required to have negative pressure
- Recommended use of UPS for ventilation system in the event of power loss
- Designated areas must be available for:
  - Receipt and unpacking of HDs
  - Storage of HDs
  - Nonsterile HD compounding
  - Sterile HD compounding

Receiving hazardous drugs

- SOPs must be established for receiving HDs.
  - Chemotherapy gloves must be worn.
- HDs should be received from supplier in impervious plastic to allow for safety.
- Antineoplastic HDs and all HD APIs must be unpacked in a neutral or negative pressure area compared with its surrounding areas.
- HDs cannot be unpacked in the sterile compounding area(s).
- HDs cannot be unpacked in positive pressure area.
- After unpacking, HDs must be delivered immediately to the storage area.
- Spill kit must be accessible. Spill kits contain:
  - Absorbent chemotherapy pads and towels
  - Disposable chemotherapy-resistant gowns (with back covers)
  - Chemotherapy-resistant shoe covers
  - Chemotherapy gloves
  - Chemical splash goggles
  - NIOSH-approved respirator masks
  - Disposable dustpan
  - Plastic scraper
  - Puncture-proof container for glass
  - Large, heavy-duty, sealable waste disposal bags
  - Hazardous waste label, if bags are unlabeled

Receiving damaged containers	
If container appears damaged	■ Seal container without opening and contact supplier. ■ For returns to supplier, seal in impervious container and label outside of container "Hazardous." ■ For items not returned, dispose as hazardous waste.

Receiving damaged containers —cont'd	
If damaged container must be opened	■ Seal container in plastic or impervious container. ■ Transport to C-PEC and place on chemotherapy mat. ■ Open package, remove undamaged items. ■ Wipe undamaged items with disposable wipe. ■ Follow process for returned/nonreturned items. ■ Deactivate, decontaminate, and clean C-PEC; dispose mat and cleaning items as hazardous waste.

C-PEC, Containment primary engineering control.

Labeling hazardous drugs

- All containers of hazardous material must be labeled as such, identifying the material and appropriate hazard warnings.
- HD labels must indicate the following: "Caution Hazardous Drug Observe Special Handling, Administration, and Disposal Requirements."
- HDs identified by the entity as requiring special HD-handling precautions must be clearly labeled at all times during their transport.
- Personnel must ensure that the labeling processes for compounded preparations do not introduce contamination into the non-HD handling areas.

Storage

- Access to areas where HDs are handled must be restricted to authorized personnel only.
- Storage areas must be located away from employee break areas, patients, and visitors.
- Storage area must be ventilated and in a negative pressure room with a minimum of 12 ACPH to dilute and remove any airborne contaminants
- Designated area must be available for:
  - Receipt and unpacking of HDs
  - Storage of HDs
  - Nonsterile HD compounding
  - Sterile HD compounding
- Storage of HDs should be secure enough to prevent spillage or breakage.
- Storage of HDs should not be on the floor.
- Storage must meet appropriate safety precautions.
- Sterile and nonsterile HDs may be stored together.
- Nonantineoplastic, reproductive risk only, and final dosage forms of HDs may be stored with other inventory if permitted by facility.
- Upon receipt of HDs, there must be a visual inspection of the packaging, looking for possible damage to the medication or external container. Facility must have a plan if it is damaged.
- Areas designated for the handling of the HDs must be separate from areas for non-HDs.
- Unpacking of HDs must be done in a room with negative or neutral pressure with at least 12 ACPH.
- Unpacking of HDs cannot occur in sterile compounding areas.
- HDs requiring refrigeration must be placed in a designated refrigerator in the HD storage room, buffer room, or containment C-SCA. Room must have negative pressure.

- It is recommended that exhaust be placed adjacent to the refrigerator's compressor.
- HDs should be stored at eye level; they should not be stored on the floor.
- HDs must be appropriately labeled to ensure proper handling.

Packaging, transport, and disposal

- A facility must have written SOPs to describe appropriate shipping containers and insulating materials, based on information from product specifications, vendors, and mode of transport.
- All packaging containers and materials must maintain physical integrity, stability, and sterility (if needed) of the HD during transport.
- Packaging materials must protect the HD from damage, leakage, contamination, and degradation, while protecting health care workers who transport them.
- Pneumatic tube systems cannot be used in transporting HDs.

Spills

- SOPs must be in place in the event of a spill.
- All personnel who may be required to clean HDs spills must be trained in spill management, the use of PPE, and respirators.
- Qualified personnel must be available at all times when HDs are being handled.
- Spill kits must be readily available in all areas where HDs are routinely handled.
- All incidents involving spills must be documented.

Medical surveillance

- All workers who handle HDs as a regular part of their job should be enrolled.
- Initial baseline of health status and medical history (to include history of exposure to HDs).
- Periodic surveillance required using baseline data as reference point.
- Follow-up plan should be developed for workers who have had health changes suggesting toxicity or have experienced acute exposure.
- Exit examination when employment ends.

Follow-up plan

- In the event of an exposure:
  - Examination must be tailored to the type of exposure, such as a spill or needlestick.
  - Compare controls against recommended standards.
  - Verify and document that engineering controls are in proper working condition.
  - Develop plan of action to prevent additional exposure.
  - Provide and document medical follow-up survey.

Procedures for compounding hazardous materials

- A facility must maintain a list of all HDs and must include any items on the current list published by NIOSH.

- NIOSH maintains criteria to identify HDs:
  - For drugs marketed after most current NIOSH list published
  - For investigational drugs
  - If information is not available, the medication must be treated as a hazardous substance
- List must be reviewed every 12 months.
- Three basic levels of engineering controls are required for containment:
  - C-PEC such as Class I or II BSC or RABS
  - C-SEC
    - Externally vented, physically separated from other preparation areas
    - Minimum 12 ACPH
    - Negative pressure between 0.01 and 0.03 inches
  - Supplementary engineering controls such as closed-system drug-transfer devices
    - Must not be used as a substitute for a C-PEC
    - Should be used whenever allowed dosage form
    - Cannot be used with drugs that are incompatible
- For nonsterile compounding regulations, regulations under <795> must be followed in addition to those under <800>.
- For sterile compounding regulations, regulations under <797> must be followed in addition to those under <800>.
- Non-HDs cannot be made in a C-PEC used for HDs, unless placed in a protective wrapper and labeled to require PPE handling precautions.
- C-PEC must be ISO 5 or better.
- May be ISO 7 or better in both the buffer and anterooms.
- BUDs limited to those specified in <797>.
- BUDs will be based on CSP category sterility testing and storage temperature.
- For a C-SCA:
  - Fixed walls, negative pressure, minimum 12 ACPH
  - Externally vented
  - Sink at least 1 m from C-PEC
  - BUD to not exceed <797> guidelines for CSPs made in a SCA

Disposal

Hazardous wastes are wastes that cause or contribute to an increase in mortality or an increase in irreversible or incapacitating reversible illness.

Hazardous Waste Characteristics

- Ignitability: Ignitable wastes can create fires under certain conditions, are spontaneously combustible, or have a flash point less than 60°C (140 °F). Examples include waste oils and used solvents.
- Corrosivity: Corrosive wastes are acids or bases (pH ≤2, or ≥12.5) and/or are capable of corroding metal containers; an example is acetic acid.
- Reactivity: Reactive wastes are unstable under "normal" conditions. They can cause explosions; undergo violent reactions; generate toxic fumes, gases, or vapors or explosive mixtures when heated, compressed, or mixed with water. An example of reactive waste is nitroglycerin.
- Toxicity: Toxic wastes (such as mercury or lead) are harmful or fatal when ingested or absorbed.

USP <800> Requirements

- All personnel who perform routine custodial waste removal and cleaning activities in HD-handling areas must be trained in appropriate procedures to protect themselves and the environment to prevent HD contamination.
- The disposal of all HD waste, including, but not limited to, unused HDs and trace-contaminated PPE and other materials, must comply with all applicable federal, state, and local regulations.
- Various types of waste can be the result of preparing and administering HDs. They include partially filled vials, undispensed products, unused IVs, needles and syringes, gloves, gowns, underpads, and contaminated materials from spill cleanups.
- Place trace wastes (those that contain less than 3% by weight of the original quantity of HDs)—such as needles, empty vials and syringes, gloves, gowns, and tubing—in yellow chemotherapy waste containers.
  - Place soft trace items (those that are contaminated with trace amounts of HDs) in yellow chemotherapy bags for disposal by incineration at a regulated medical waste facility.
  - Place soft trace items (those that are contaminated with trace amounts of HDs) in yellow chemotherapy bags for disposal by incineration at a regulated medical waste facility.
- Do not place HD-contaminated sharps in red sharps containers that are used for infectious wastes, since these are often autoclaved or microwaved.
- Dispose of P-listed arsenic trioxide and its containers and any bulk amounts of U-listed drugs in hazardous waste containers at a RCRA-permitted incinerator.
- Dispose of other bulk HDs (that is, expired or unused vials, ampoules, syringes, bags, and bottles of HDs or solutions of any other items with more than trace contamination) in a manner similar to that required for RCRA-defined hazardous wastes.

The Occupational Safety and Health Administration technical manual recommendations

- Label needle containers and breakable items of hazardous waste as HD waste only.
- Properly labeled, sealed, and covered disposal containers should be handled by trained and protected personnel.
- Thick, leak-proof plastic bags, colored differently from other hospital trash bags, should be used for routine collection of discarded gloves, gowns, and other disposable material and labeled as HD-related wastes.
- The hazardous waste bag should be kept inside a covered waste container clearly labeled "Hazardous Drug Waste Only." At least one such receptacle should be located in every area where the drugs are prepared. The bag should be sealed when filled and the covered waste container taped.

CHAPTER REVIEW QUESTIONS

1. Which is the generic name for Humira?
   a. Adalimumab
   b. Enoxaparin
   c. Rituximab
   d. Tacrolimus

2. Which is the brand name for docetaxel?
   a. Cubicin
   b. Retavase
   c. Sandimmune
   d. Taxotere

3. What is the brand name for insulin glargine?
   a. Apidra
   b. Lantus
   c. NovoLog
   d. Tresiba

4. Which medication is indicated for a fungal infection?
   a. Amiodarone
   b. Amphotericin B liposome
   c. Argatroban
   d. Paclitaxel

5. Which medication is classified as a mitosis inhibitor?
   a. Acyclovir
   b. Azathioprine
   c. Carboplatin
   d. Docetaxel

6. Which of the following medications has a NTI?
   a. Amiodarone
   b. Ampicillin
   c. Azithromycin
   d. Calcium gluconate

7. How many risk levels are associated with compounded sterile products?
   a. 2
   b. 3
   c. 4
   d. 6

8. Which medication is administered subcutaneously?
   a. Alteplase
   b. Bivalirudin
   c. Cefazolin
   d. Enoxaparin

9. What is the minimum inflow velocity for a Type A 2 BSC?
   a. 50 feet/minute
   b. 75 feet/minute
   c. 100 feet/minute
   d. 150 feet/minute

10. Which ISO classification must the anteroom be?
    a. ISO Class 5
    b. ISO Class 6
    c. ISO Class 7
    d. ISO Class 8

11. How often must an ISO Class 5 be tested for sterility according to USP <800>?
    a. Every 3 months
    b. Every 6 months
    c. Every 9 months
    d. Every 12 months

12. **Which of the following is an example of a secondary engineering control?**
    a. Buffer area
    b. Class II biological cabinet
    c. Environmental monitoring
    d. Viable air sampling

13. A patient has been diagnosed with candidiasis. Which of the following medications would be a appropriate treatment?
    a. Chlorpromazine
    b. Fluconazole

   c. Fluorouracil
   d. Heparin
14. Which large-volume IV solution is used to provide extracellular fluid replacement to the body?
   a. D5W
   b. Hartman's solution
   c. Normal saline solution
   d. Ringer's solution
15. Which form of water is *not* sterile and cannot be used in aseptic compounding of sterile products?
   a. Bacteriostatic water for injection USP
   b. Purified water USP
   c. Sterile water for irrigation USP
   d. Water for injection USP
16. Which medication is an example of a high-alert parenteral medication used in an acute care setting?
   a. Amiodarone
   b. Glyburide
   c. Rivaroxaban
   d. Warfarin
17. What is the in-use time for a multidose container in an ISO 5 or better environment?
   a. 6 hours
   b. 12 hours
   c. 14 days
   d. 28 days
18. What is the maximum number of particles per cubic meter for a Class 7 environment?
   a. 3520
   b. 35,200
   c. 352,000
   d. 3,520,000
19. According to USP <797> how often does the temperature need to be monitored and documented?
   a. Daily
   b. Weekly
   c. Biweekly
   d. Monthly
20. According to USP <797> how often must a qualified certifier monitor viable particles?
   a. Bimonthly
   b. Monthly
   c. Every 3 months
   d. Every 6 months
21. How often must a pharmacy technician be evaluated for gloved fingertip sampling?
   a. Every 3 months
   b. Every 6 months
   c. Every 9 months
   d. Every 12 months
22. A pharmacy technician is compounding a Category 2 CSP that was aseptically processed and underwent sterility testing and passed. Which BUD should be assigned to the compounded preparation if stored in the refrigerator (2°C–8°C)?
   a. 14 days
   b. 28 days
   c. 30 days
   d. 45 days
23. What is the in-use time for a single-dose container in an ISO 5 environment?
   a. Immediately
   b. Refer to manufacturer's labeling

   c. 6 hours
   d. 28 days
24. Which additive may increase the buffer capacity of a CSP?
   a. Acetate
   b. Calcium
   c. Magnesium
   d. Phosphate
25. How long must a Class II biological cabinet be on before compounding?
   a. 10 minutes
   b. 15 minutes
   c. 20 minutes
   d. 30 minutes
26. Which of the following environments would you find the IV hood?
   a. ISO Class 5
   b. ISO Class 6
   c. ISO Class 7
   d. ISO Class 8
27. How often must the clean room be tested to comply with USP <797> air standards?
   a. Every 3 months
   b. Every 6 months
   c. Every 9 months
   d. Every 12 months
28. What is the minimum air differential between the buffer area and ante-area when compounding Category 1 and Category 2 sterile products?
   a. 40 feet/minute
   b. 60 feet/minute
   c. 80 feet/minute
   d. 100 feet/minute
29. What is the minimum number of ACPH in the ante-area?
   a. 20
   b. 25
   c. 30
   d. 35
30. How often must viable air samples be collected from ISO Class 5, 7, and 8 environments?
   a. Monthly
   b. Every 3 months
   c. Every 6 months
   d. Every 12 months
31. What is the minimum frequency that pressure differential must be documented by the compounding personnel?
   a. Daily
   b. Weekly
   c. Bimonthly
   d. Monthly
32. What is the time of infusion if 500 mL are being infused at a rate 125 mL/hour?
   a. 0.25 hours
   b. 2 hours
   c. 4 hours
   d. 8 hours
33. What is the minimum amount of time pharmacy technicians should spend on washing their hands, under the fingernails, on the wrists, and up to the elbows?
   a. 15 seconds
   b. 30 seconds
   c. 1 minute
   d. 2 minutes

34. Which piece of PPE should be removed first?
    a. Gloves
    b. Goggles/face shield
    c. Gown
    d. Mask/respirator
35. Which area of a horizontal laminar flow workbench should be cleaned first?
    a. Flat work surface of the laminar flow workbench
    b. Rear wall of the laminar flow workbench
    c. Side of the laminar flow workbench
    d. Top of the laminar flow workbench
36. Which is the first thing pharmacy technicians should do if they observe that air bubbles have appeared in a syringe?
    a. Draw back on the plunger, allowing fluid into the syringe.
    b. Hold the syringe upright and pull the plunger back to clear the hub.
    c. Slowly push the plunger to remove any remaining air.
    d. Turn the large air bubbles around the syringe to pick up smaller air bubbles. If smaller air bubbles continue to exist, tap the syringe to displace them.
37. How long must a compounding record be maintained for a prepared medication?
    a. Minimum of 2 years from the date the medication was prepared
    b. Minimum of 3 years from the date the medication was prepared
    c. Minimum of 4 years from the date the medication was prepared
    d. Minimum of 5 years from the date the medication was prepared
38. What function does sodium have when added to a total parenteral nutrition IV?
    a. Sodium is necessary for proper bone formation.
    b. Sodium controls water inside and outside of the cells.
    c. Sodium is required for fighting infection.
    d. Sodium establishes total body water volume.
39. What pH should an ophthalmic solution be?
    a. 4.8
    b. 6.2
    c. 7.4
    d. 9.2
40. A sign of a defective CSP is absorption. Which form of absorption occurs when there is a separation of oil and water in an emulsion?
    a. Aggregation
    b. Cracking
    c. Creaming
    d. Separation
41. CSPs must be tested to ensure that they do not contain excessive bacterial endotoxins. What is the minimum number of units to be tested if the batch size is 80 bags?
    a. 4 bags
    b. 8 bags
    c. 10 bags
    d. 12 bags
42. When transporting, compounding, receiving, or stocking HDs, what type of chemotherapy gloves must be worn?
    a. American Society of Health System Pharmacists-tested chemotherapy gloves
    b. American Society of Testing and Materials–tested chemotherapy gloves
    c. NIOSH-tested chemotherapy gloves
    d. Occupational Safety and Health Administration–tested chemotherapy gloves
43. When collecting and disposing of waste/spills, which PPEs must be worn?
    a. Gloves, gowns, and hair, face, beard and shoe covers
    b. Gloves, gowns, and hair, face, beard, shoe covers and eye/face protection
    c. Gloves, gowns, and hair, face, beard, shoe covers and respiratory protection
    d. Gloves, gowns, and hair, face, beard, shoe covers and eye/face protection and respiratory protection
44. Which of the following must appear on an HD label?
    a. "Caution Hazardous Drug"
    b. "Caution Hazardous Drug: Observe all FDA Regulations"
    c. "Caution Hazardous Drug: Observe all Federal, State, and Local Laws and Regulations"
    d. "Caution Hazardous Drug: Observe Special Handling, Administration, and Disposal Requirements"
45. Which of the hazardous wastes is an example of being corrosive?
    a. Acetic acid
    b. Lead
    c. Mercury
    d. Nitroglycerin
46. Which of the following is a component of a spill kit?
    a. Adsorbent chemotherapy pad and towel
    b. Disposable gown with back covers
    c. Latex gloves
    d. NIOSH-approved respirator mask
47. Which is an example an unintentional exposure risk associated with dispensing a hazardous medication?
    a. Counting or repackaging tablets and/or capsules
    b. Expelling air or diluting injectable HDs from syringes
    c. Reconstituting an HD
    d. Weighing or mixing components
48. Which of the following is an example of an HD?
    a. Ampicillin
    b. Insulin glargine
    c. Levothyroxine
    d. Methotrexate
49. Which medication is indicated for deep vein thrombosis?
    a. Enoxaparin
    b. Epoetin alpha recombinant
    c. Famotidine
    d. Fluorouracil
50. Which medication is classified as an antipsychotic?
    a. Amiodarone
    b. Amphotericin B
    c. Carboplatin
    d. Chlorpromazine

REFERENCES

USPC-797 Pharmaceutical Compounding. 8/1/21. https://www.uspnf.com/sites/default/files/usp_pdf/EN/USPNF/usp-nf-commentary/797-commentary-20221101.pdf

2

Hazardous Drug Management Certificate

Engineering controls

Facilities and engineering controls for receiving and storing hazardous

Hazardous drugs must be handled under conditions that promote patient safety, worker safety, and environmental protection. Signs designating the hazard must be prominently displayed before the entrance to the hazardous drug (HD) handling areas. Access to areas where HDs are handled must be restricted to authorized personnel to protect persons not involved in HD handling. HD handling areas must be located away from breakrooms and refreshment areas for personnel, patients, or visitors to reduce risk of exposure.

Designated areas must be available for:

- Receipt and unpacking
- Storage of HDs
- Nonsterile HD compounding
- Sterile HD compounding

Certain areas are required to have negative pressure from surrounding areas to contain HDs and minimize risk of exposure. Consideration should be given to uninterrupted power sources for the ventilation systems to maintain negative pressure in the event of power loss.

Antineoplastic HDs and all HD active pharmaceutical ingredients (APIs) must be unpacked (i.e., removal from external shipping containers) in an area that is neutral/normal or negative pressure relative to the surrounding areas. HDs must not be unpacked from their external shipping containers in sterile compounding areas or in positive pressure areas.

HDs must be stored in a manner that prevents spillage or breakage if the container falls. Do not store HDs on the floor. In areas prone to specific types of natural disasters (e.g., earthquakes) the manner of storage must meet applicable safety precautions, such as secure shelves with raised front lips.

Antineoplastic HDs requiring manipulation other than counting or repackaging of final dosage forms and any HD API must be stored separately from non-HDs in a manner that prevents contamination and personnel exposure. These HDs must be stored in an externally ventilated, negative pressure room with at least 12 air changes per hour (ACPH). Non-antineoplastic, reproductive risk only, and final dosage forms of antineoplastic HDs may be stored with other inventory if permitted by entity policy.

Sterile and nonsterile HDs may be stored together, but HDs used for nonsterile compounding should not be stored in areas designated for sterile compounding to minimize traffic into the sterile compounding area.

Refrigerated antineoplastic HDs must be stored in a dedicated refrigerator in a negative pressure area with at least 12 ACPH (e.g., storage room, buffer room, or containment segregated compounding area [C-SCA]). If a refrigerator is placed in a negative pressure buffer room, an exhaust located adjacent to the refrigerator's compressor and behind the refrigerator should be considered.

Facilities and engineering controls features for manipulating sterile hazardous drugs

Engineering controls are required to protect the preparation from cross-contamination and microbial contamination (if preparation is intended to be sterile) during all phases of the compounding process. Engineering controls for containment are divided into three categories representing primary, secondary, and supplementary levels of control.

- A containment primary engineering control (C-PEC):
  - Is a ventilated device designed to minimize worker and environmental HD exposure when directly handling HDs
  - Is where sterile and nonsterile HDs must be compounded
  - Must operate continuously if it supplies some or all of the negative pressure in the containment secondary engineering control (C-SEC) or if it is used for sterile compounding
  - Should be covered according to manufacturer's recommendations

- The C-SEC is the room in which the C-PEC is placed.
  - The C-SEC used for sterile and nonsterile compounding must:
    - Be externally vented
    - Be physically separated (i.e., a different room from other preparation areas)
    - Have an appropriate air exchange (e.g., ACPH)
    - Have a negative pressure between 0.01 and 0.03 inches of water column relative to all adjacent areas
    - Have a minimum of 12 ACPH
    - Handwashing sink placed at least 1 m from C-PEC, which may be either inside the C-SCA or directly outside the C-SCA
- Supplemental engineering controls (e.g., closed-system drug-transfer device [CSTD]) are adjunct controls to offer additional levels of protection.
  - CSTD must not be used as a substitute for a C-PEC when compounding.
  - CSTDs should be used when compounding HDs when the dosage form permits it.
  - CSTDs must be used when administering antineoplastic HD when the dosage form permits it.

The C-PEC must operate continuously if it supplies some or all of the negative pressure in the C-SEC or if it is used for sterile compounding. If there is any loss of power to the C-PEC, all activities occurring in the C-PEC must cease immediately. Once power is restored to the C-PEC, decontamination, cleaning, and disinfecting should occur for all sterile compounding surfaces. Compounding may resume after manufacture-specified recovery time has lapsed. A sink must be available for handwashing. An eyewash station and/or other emergency or safety precautions that meet applicable laws and regulations must be readily available. Water sources and drains must be located at least 1 m away from the C-PEC.

For facilities that compound both nonsterile and sterile HDs, the respective C-PECs must be placed in separate rooms, unless the facility is able to maintain an ISO 7 classification throughout the nonsterile compounding. In situations where the C-PECs used for sterile and nonsterile compounding are placed in the same room, they must be placed at least 1 m apart and particle-generating activity must not be performed when sterile compounding is occurring. In addition to USP <800>, sterile compounding must follow standards in <797>.

All C-PECs used for manipulation of sterile HDs must be externally vented. Sterile HD compounding must be performed in a C-PEC that provides an ISO Class 5 or better air quality, such as a Class II or III biological safety cabinets (BSC) or compounding aseptic containment isolator (CACI). Examples of Class II BSCs include types A2, B1, and B2.

A laminar airflow workbench or compounding aseptic isolator must not be used for the compounding of an antineoplastic HD. A BSC or CACI used for the preparation of HDs must not be used for the preparation of a non-HD unless the non-HD preparation is placed into a protective outer wrapper during removal from the C-PEC and is labeled to require personal protective equipment (PPE) handling precautions.

The C-PEC must be located in a C-SEC, which may either be an ISO Class 7 buffer room with an ISO Class 7 anteroom or an unclassified C-SCA. If the C-PEC is placed in a C-SCA, the beyond-use date (BUD) of all compounded sterile preparations (CSPs) must follow USP <797> requirements for CSPs prepared in a segregated compounding area.

Configuration	C-PEC	C-SEC
ISO Class 7 buffer room with an ISO Class 7 anteroom	Externally vented Examples include Class II BSC or CACI	Externally vented 30 ACPH Negative pressure between 0.01 and 0.03 inches of water column relative to adjacent areas
C-SCA	Externally vented Examples include Class II BSC or CACI	Externally vented 12 ACPH Negative pressure between 0.01 and 0.03 inches of water column relative to adjacent area

ACPH, Air changes per hour; *BSC*, biological safety cabinet; *CACI*, compounding aseptic containment isolator; *C-PEC*, containment primary engineering control; *C-SEC*, containment secondary engineering control.

ISO Class 7 buffer room

The C-PEC is placed in an ISO Class 7 buffer room that has fixed walls, high-efficiency particulate air (HEPA)-filtered supply air, a negative pressure between 0.01 and 0.03 inches of water column relative to all adjacent areas and a minimum of 30 ACPH. The buffer room must be externally vented. Other buffer room requirements include:

- Minimum of 30 ACPH of HEPA-filtered supply air
- Maintain a positive pressure of at least 0.02 inches of water column relative to all adjacent unclassified areas
- Maintain an air quality of ISO Class 7 or better

ISO Class 7 anteroom

An ISO Class 7 anteroom with fixed walls is necessary to provide inward air movement of equal cleanliness classified air into the negative pressure buffer room to contain any airborne HD. A handwashing sink must be placed in the anteroom at least 1 m from the entrance to the HD buffer room.

If a negative pressure HD buffer room is entered though the positive pressure non-HD buffer room, the following are also required:

- A line of demarcation must be defined within the negative pressure buffer room for donning and doffing PPE.
- A method to transport HDs, HD CSPs, and HD waste into and out of the negative pressure buffer room to minimize the spread of HD contamination. This may be accomplished by use of a pass-through chamber.

HD CSPs prepared in an ISO Class 7 buffer room with an ISO Class 7 anteroom may use the BUDs described in USP <797>. A category 1 CSP prepared in segregated compounding area or cleanroom suite has a BUD of ≤12 hours at a controlled room temperature 20°C–25°C or ≤24 hours in a refrigerator of 2°C–8°C. Depending on compounding method, the sterility testing performed and passed and the storage conditions will determine the BUD for a Category 2 CSP.

Compounding method	Sterility testing performed and passed	Controlled room temperature (20°C–25°C)	Refrigerator (2°C–8°C)	Freezer (−25°C to −10°C)
Aseptically Processed CSPs	No	Prepared from one or more nonsterile starting component (s): 1 day	Prepared from one or more nonsterile starting component(s): 4 days	Prepared from one or more nonsterile starting component(s): 45 days
	No	Prepared from only sterile starting components: 4 days	Prepared from only sterile starting components: 10 days	Prepared from only sterile starting components: 45 days
	Yes	30 days	45 days	60 days
Terminally sterilized CSPs	No	14 days	28 days	45 days
	Yes	45 days	60 days	90 days

CSP, Compounded sterile preparation.

Only Category 1 HD CSPs may be prepared in a C-SCA. HD CSPs prepared in the C-SCA must not exceed the BUDs described in <797> for CSPs prepared in a segregated compounding area.

Containment supplemental engineering controls, such as CSTDs, provide adjunct controls to offer an additional level of protection during compounding or administration. Some CSTDs have been shown to limit the potential of generating aerosols during compounding. However, there is no certainty that all CSTDs will perform adequately. Until a published universal performance standard for evaluation of CSTD containment is available, users should carefully evaluate the performance claims associated with available CSTDs based on independent, peer-reviewed studies and demonstrated contamination reduction.

Biological safety cabinets

- Class I: A BSC that protects personnel and the environment but does not protect the product/preparation
  - A minimum velocity of 75 linear feet/minute of unfiltered room air is drawn through the front opening and across the work surface, providing personnel protection.

- The air is passed through a HEPA/ULPA (ultra-low particulate air) filter providing environmental protection.
- Class II: Class II (Types A1, A2, B1, and B2) biological safety cabinets
  - These partial barrier systems rely on the movement of air to provide personnel, environmental, and product/preparation protection.
  - Personnel and product/preparation protection are provided by the combination of inward and downward airflow captured by the front grille of the cabinet.
  - Side-to-side cross-contamination of products/preparations is minimized by the internal downward flow of HEPA/ULPA filtered air.
  - Environmental protection is provided when the cabinet exhaust air exhaust air is passed through a HEPA/ULPA filter.
  - Type A1 (formerly, Type A)
    - Maintain a minimum inflow velocity of 75 feet/minute
    - Have HEPA-filtered, downflow air
    - May exhaust HEPA-filtered air back into the laboratory
    - May have positive pressure contaminated ducts and plenums that are not surrounded by negative pressure plenums
    - Not suitable for use with volatile toxic chemicals and volatile radionuclides
  - Type A2 (formerly, Type B3)
    - Maintain a minimum inflow velocity of 100 feet/minute
    - Possess HEPA-filtered, downflow air
    - May exhaust HEPA-filtered air back into the laboratory through an exhaust canopy
    - Has all contaminated ducts and plenums under negative pressure
    - If used for volatile toxic chemicals or radionucleotides, must be exhausted through exhaust canopies
  - Type B1: These Class II BSCs
    - Maintain a minimum inflow velocity of 100 feet/minute
    - Have HEPA-filtered, downflow air composed largely of uncontaminated, recirculated inflow air
    - Exhaust most of the contaminated downflow air through a dedicated duct through HEPA filters
    - Have all contaminated ducts and plenums under negative pressure
    - If involving minute quantities of volatile toxic chemicals and trace amounts of radionuclides, the work must be done in the directly exhausted portion of the cabinet
  - Type B2 (total exhaust)
    - Maintain a minimum inflow velocity of 100 feet/minute
    - Have HEPA-filtered, downflow air drawn from the laboratory or the outside
    - Exhaust all inflow and downflow air to the atmosphere after filtration through a HEPA filter
    - Have all contaminated ducts and plenums under negative pressure
    - May be used with volatile toxic chemicals and radionuclides

- Class III (Class III BSC)
  - Is used for work with highly infectious microbiological agents
  - Provides maximum protection for the environment and the worker
  - Consists of gas-tight enclosure
  - Has HEPA/ULPA-filtered supply and exhaust air
  - Exhaust air to pass through two HEPA/ULPA filters in series before discharge to the outdoors

Facilities and engineering controls features for manipulating nonsterile hazardous drugs

- Nonsterile hazardous compounding must follow USP <795>.
- A C-PEC is not required if manipulations are limited to handling of final dosage forms such as counting or repackaging tablets or capsules.
- C-PECs used for manipulating nonsterile HDs must be either externally vented or have redundant-HEPA filters in series.
- Nonsterile HD compounding must be performed in a C-PEC that provides personnel and environmental protection such as Class I BSC or containment ventilated enclosure, a Class II BSC, or a CACI.
- A C-PEC used only for nonsterile compounding does not require unidirectional airflow.

Engineering Controls	
C-PEC	C-SEC requirements
Externally vented (preferred) or redundant-HEPA filtered in series	Externally vented
Examples include CVE, Class I or II BSC, CACI	12 ACPH
	Negative pressure between 0.01 and 0.03 inches of water column relative to adjacent areas

ACPH, Air changes per hour; *BSC*, biological safety cabinet; *CACI*, compounding aseptic containment isolator; *C-PEC*, containment primary engineering control; *C-SEC*, containment secondary engineering control; *CVE*, containment ventilated enclosure.

Facility cleaning

Deactivating, decontaminating, cleaning, and disinfecting areas

- Written procedures must be in place for decontamination, deactivation, and cleaning and for sterile compounding area disinfection.
- Cleaning of nonsterile compounding areas must comply with <795>, and cleaning of sterile compounding areas must comply with <797>.
- Detailed procedures for cleaning must be in place to include agents used, dilutions (if used), frequency, and documentation requirements.

- All individuals involved in deactivation, decontamination, cleaning, and disinfection activities must be trained in the appropriate procedures.
- Cleaning must be conducted in properly ventilated areas.
- Individuals must wear appropriate PPE resistant to the cleaning agents used, to include two pairs of chemotherapy gloves and impermeable disposable gowns.
  - Eye protection and face shields must be used if splashing may occur.
  - Respiratory protection must be used if necessary.

Deactivation

- After deactivating an HD contaminant, it must be removed by decontaminating the surface.
- Chemical agents used in deactivation include sodium hypochlorite and peroxide formulations.
  - If sodium hypochlorite is used, it should be neutralized with sodium thiosulfate followed by either sterile alcohol, sterile water, a germicidal detergent, or a sporicidal agent.

Decontamination

- Process must be noted for inactivating, neutralizing, or removing HD residue from nondisposable surfaces and transferring it to absorbent, disposable materials such as wipes, pads, or towels.
- Decontaminants consist of Environmental Protection Agency (EPA)-approved oxidizing agents, which include alcohol, water, sodium hypochlorite, and peroxide.
- HD contamination in the C-PEC may be reduced by wiping down HD containers.
- The work surface of the C-PEC must be decontaminated between compounding different HDs.
- Decontamination must be done at least daily (when used), any time a spill occurs, before and after certification, any time voluntary interruption occurs, and if the ventilation tool is moved.
- Contamination may occur under the work tray of the C-PEC. When deactivating, decontaminating and cleaning the area under the work tray of a C-PEC must occur monthly. Respiratory equipment may be required.

Cleaning

- Cleaning is a process resulting in the removal of contaminants (e.g., soil, microbial contamination, HD residue) from objects and surfaces.
- Cleaning agents include water, detergents, surfactants, solvents, and/or other chemicals.
- Cleaning should not occur while compounding is taking place.

Disinfection

- Disinfection is the process of inhibiting or destroying microorganisms.
- Surfaces must be cleaned before disinfecting takes place.
- Sterile alcohol is used as a disinfectant.

Accidental exposure of hazardous drugs

- Exposure (e.g., breathing vapors, dusts, or aerosols; absorbing it through skin contact; swallowing it; or accidental injection) of HDs to health care can be extremely severe depending upon the following:
  - A drug's toxicity must be considered.
  - A drug's potency must be considered.
  - Route of exposure must be considered.
  - A drug's physical and chemical properties to include its vapor pressure, physical state (solid, liquid, or gas), and molecular weight of the drug. Medications in liquid or powder form may be inhaled as aerosols, droplets, or dusts. HD may be absorbed through skin, especially if the skin is chapped or abraded or has cuts or scrapes.
  - Drug formulation refers to the form the drug takes for administration—such as a powder, liquid, capsule, or prefilled syringe. The type of formulation will help determine the required precautions to be taken to avoid exposure.
  - Workplace activity refers to how health care employees use and handle the drug in the workplace. In a pharmacy, pharmacists and pharmacy technicians receive, compound, and dispense hazardous medications.

Preventing employee exposure

The National Institute for Occupational Safety and Health (NIOSH) recommends the following to prevent health care worker exposure to HDs:

- Assess the hazards in the workplace.
  - Evaluate the workplace to identify and assess hazards before anyone begins work with HDs. As part of this evaluation, assess the following:
    - Total working environment
    - Equipment (i.e., ventilated cabinets, CSTDs, glove bags, needleless systems, and PPE)
    - Physical layout of work areas
    - Types of drugs being handled
    - Volume, frequency, and form of drugs handled (tablets, coated versus uncoated, powder versus liquid)
    - Equipment maintenance
    - Decontamination and cleaning
    - Waste handling
    - Potential exposures during work, including HDs, blood-borne pathogens, and chemicals used to deactivate HDs or clean drug-contaminated surfaces
    - Routine operations
    - Spill response
    - Waste segregation, containment, and disposal
  - Regularly review the current inventory of HDs, equipment, and practices, seeking input from affected workers.
  - Conduct regular training reviews with all potentially exposed workers in workplaces where HDs are used.
- Handle drugs safely.
  - Implement a program for safely handling HDs at work and review this program annually on the basis of the workplace evaluation.

- Establish procedures and provide training for handling HDs safely, cleaning up spills, and using all equipment and PPE properly.
- Establish work practices related to both drug manipulation techniques and to general hygiene practices—such as not permitting eating or drinking in areas where drugs are handled (the pharmacy or clinic).
- Use and maintain equipment properly.
  - Develop workplace procedures for using and maintaining all equipment that functions to reduce exposure—such as ventilated cabinets, CSDTs, needleless systems, and PPE.

Addressing accidental exposure to hazardous medications

A postexposure examination should be conducted and is dependent upon the nature of the exposure. An assessment to the degree of the exposure is made and is included in the incident report. After exposure has occurred, the following is recommended:

- Have the individual remove contaminated clothes.
- Refer to the hazardous medication's safety data sheet (SDS) and decontaminate according to instructions.
- Have individual visit the employee health professional to document and confirm complete decontamination.
- Have individual undergo physical examination at the site of exposure. In addition, the examination may focus on target organs for drug(s) involved.
- Obtain blood sample for baseline counts and archiving (spin and freeze) after major exposures.
- Schedule appropriate follow-up visits based on drug half-life.
- Patient should be counseled and encouraged to report symptoms, and a medical follow-up should be recommended.

Addressing hazardous drug spills

- Assess the size and scope of the spill.
- Post signs to limit access to spill area.
- Obtain spill kit and respirator.
- A spill kit contains absorbent chemotherapy pads and towels, disposable cvhemotherapy gowns with back covers, chemotherapy resistant shoe covers, chemotherapy gloves, chemical splash goggles, respirator mask (NIOSH approved), disposable dust pan, puncture proof for glass, large heavy-duty sealable waste disposable bag and hazardous waste label (if not attached to the bag).
- Don appropriate PPEs to include gloves and respirator.
- After being totally garbed, contain the spill using the spill kit.
- Carefully remove any broken glass fragments and place them in a puncture-resistant container.
- Absorb liquids with spill pads.
- Absorb powder with damp disposable pads or soft toweling.
- Spill cleanup should proceed progressively from areas of lesser to greater contamination.
- Completely remove and place all contaminated material in the disposal bags.

- Rinse the area with water and then clean with detergent, sodium hypochlorite solution, and neutralizer or other validated decontamination solution.
- Rinse the area several times and place all materials used for containment and cleanup in disposal bags.
- Seal bags and place them in the appropriate final container for disposal as Resource Conservation and Recovery Act (RCRA) hazardous waste.
- Carefully remove all PPE using the inner gloves. Place all disposable PPE into disposal bags. Seal bags and place them into the hazardous waste container (not trace-contaminated waste).
- Remove inner glovers, contain them in a small, sealable band, and place them into a small, sealable container for disposal as hazardous waste.
- Wash hands with soap and water.
- After the spill has initially been decontaminated, have the area cleaned by housekeeping or environmental services.

Personal protective equipment

Personal protective equipment requirements when handling hazardous drugs

- PPE protects the health care worker from exposure to HD aerosols and residues.
- Refer to the NIOSH list of antineoplastic drugs and other HDs for additional guidance on wearing PPEs when performing various tasks within a health care setting.
- Disposable PPEs should never be reused.
- Reusable PPEs must be decontaminated and cleaned after use.

Gloves

- Gloves must meet the American Society for Testing and Material standard D6978-05 and are required for compounding sterile and non-sterile HDs, administration of HDs, and the cleanup of HD spills.
- Gloves must be powder-free since powder may absorb the hazardous material.
- Chemotherapy gloves should be worn for handling all HDs, including non-antineoplastics, and for reproductive risk–only HDs.
- Double gloves should be worn during any handling of HD shipping cartons or drug vials and handling of HD waste or waste from patients recently treated with HDs.

Gowns

- Gowns must be disposable.
- Selection of gowns must be based on the HDs handles.
- Gowns must close in the back (no open front), be long sleeved, have closed cuffs (elastic or knit)
- Gowns must be changed according to manufacturer's information for permeation of the gown. If no permeation information is provided, the gown should be changed every 2–3 hours or immediately after a spill or splash.

- Gowns should not be worn in areas outside of HD handling to avoid spreading HD contamination or exposing other workers
- Cloth laboratory coats, surgical scrubs, isolation gowns, or other absorbent materials are *not* appropriate protective outerwear when handling HDs because they permit the permeation of HDs and can hold spilled drugs against the skin, thereby increasing exposure.

Head, hair, shoe, and sleeve covers

- Head and hair covers (including beard and moustache), shoe covers, and sleeve covers provide protection from contact with HD residue.
- A second pair of shoe covers must be donned prior to entering the C-SEC and removed when exiting the C-SEC.
- Shoe covering should not be worn to other areas to prevent spreading HD contamination.
- Disposable sleeve covers may be used to protect areas of the arm that may come in contact with HDs.
- Sleeve covers made of polyethylene-coated polypropylene provide better protection than uncoated materials.

Eye and face protection

- Appropriate eye and face protection must be worn when there is a risk for spills or splashes of HDs or HD waste materials when working outside of a C-PEC.
- A full-facepiece respirator provides eye and face protection.
- Goggles must be used when eye protection is warranted.
- Faced shields with goggles provide protection against splashes to the face and eyes.

- Eye glasses or safety glasses with side shields do not protect the eyes from splashes.
- Face shields alone do not offer full eye and face protection.

Respiratory protection

- Individuals unpacking HDs that are not contained in plastic should wear an elastomeric half-mask with a multigas cartridge and P100-filter until it can be determined that no breakage or spillage occurred during transport.
- When respiratory protection from HD exposure is required, a surgical mask must not be worn because it does not provide respiratory protection from drug exposure.
  - A surgical N95 respirator provides the respiratory protection of an N95 respirator and provides a barrier to splashes, droplets, and sprays around the nose and mouth.
  - A NIOSH-certified N95 respirator provides sufficient protection against airborne particles but do not offer protection against gases and vapors and little protection against direct liquid splashes.
  - An appropriate full-facepiece, chemical cartridge-type respirator or powered air-purifying respirator should be worn when there is a risk of respiratory exposure to HDs, including when:
    - Attending to HD spills larger than what can be contained with a spill kit
    - Deactivating, decontaminating, and cleaning underneath the work surface of a C-PEC
    - Knowing or suspecting airborne exposure to powders or vapors

Engineering controls, administrative controls and personal protective equipment for working with hazardous drugs in health care settings						
Formulation	Activity	Double Chemotherapy Gloves	Protective Gown	Eye/Face Protection	Respiratory Protection	Engineering Control
All types of hazardous drugs	Receiving, unpacking, and placing in storage	No (single glove can be used, unless spills occur)	Yes, when spills and leaks occur	No	Yes, when spills and leaks occur	No
Tablets or capsules	Cutting, crushing, or manipulating tablets or capsules; handling uncoated tablets	Yes	Yes	No	Yes, if not done in a control device	Yes
Oral liquid drug or feeding tube	Compounding	Yes	Yes	Yes, if not done in a control device	Yes, if not done in a control device	Yes
Topical drug	Compounding	Yes	Yes	Yes, if not done in a control device	Yes, if not done in a control device	Yes, C-PEC
Subcutaneous/ intramuscular injection from a vial	Preparation (withdrawing from vial)	Yes	Yes	Yes, if not done in a control device	Yes, if not done in a control device	Yes, C-PEC
Withdrawing and/or mixing intravenous or intramuscular solution from a vial or ampoule	Compounding	Yes	Yes	No	No	yes, C-PEC; use of CSTD recommended

(Continued)

Formulation	Activity	Double Chemotherapy Gloves	Protective Gown	Eye/Face Protection	Respiratory Protection	Engineering Control
Solution for irrigation	Compounding	Yes	Yes	Yes, if not done in a control device	Yes, if not done in a control device	Yes, C-PEC; use of CSTD recommended
Powder/solution for inhalation/ aerosol treatment	Compounding	Yes	Yes	Yes, if not done in a control device	Yes, if not done in a control device	Yes, C-PEC
Drug-contaminated waste	Disposal and cleaning	Yes	Yes	Yes, if liquid that could splash	Yes, if inhalation potential	N/A
Spills	Cleaning	Yes	Yes	Yes	Yes	N/A

Engineering controls, administrative controls and personal protective equipment for working with hazardous drugs in health care settings—cont'd

C-PEC, Containment primary engineering control; *CSTD*, closed-system drug-transfer device; *N/A*, not applicable.

Process for disposing personal protective equipment

- All PPE worn when handling HDs should be considered contaminated with trace quantities of HDs.
- PPEs must be placed in an appropriate waste container and disposed of according to local, state, and federal regulations prior to leaving the secondary engineering control.
- Chemotherapy gloves and sleeve covers worn during compounding must be removed and discarded immediately into an approved waste container for trace contaminated wasted inside the C-PEC or in a sealable bag for discarding outside the C-PEC.

Transport and receiving

Procedures and environmental requirements for receiving and transporting hazardous medications

Receiving

- An institution's standard operating procedure (SOP) must outline the procedures to be followed when receiving HDs.
- HDs listed as antineoplastic HDs on the current NIOSH HD list and all HD APIs must be unpacked in areas that are neutral/normal or negative pressure relative to the surrounding areas.
- PPEs, including chemotherapy gloves, must be worn when unpacking HDs, and a spill kit must be accessible in the receiving area.
- A visual examination of the carton for outward signs of damage or breakage, which include visible stains from leakage and sounds of broken glass, must be conducted by the individual responsible for HDs.

Transporting

- HDs identified as requiring special HD handling precautions must be clearly labeled at all times.

- Packaging containers for HDs and materials must maintain physical integrity, stability, and sterility during transport.
- Health care workers responsible for transporting HDs must undergo training to include spill control.
- The transported HDs must be properly labeled, stored, and handled in accordance with applicable federal, state, and local regulations.
- Labels and accessory labeling for the HDs include storage instructions, disposal instructions, and HD category information.
- Pneumatic tubes should never be used to transport any liquid HDs or any antineoplastic HDs because of the potential for breakage and contamination.

Procedures for handling damaged shipping containers containing hazardous drugs

- If the shipping container appears damaged:
  - Seal the container without opening and contact the supplier.
  - If the unopened package is to be returned to the supplier, enclose the package in an impervious container and label the outer container "Hazardous."
  - If the supplier will not accept the return, dispose of it as hazardous waste.
- If a damaged shipping container must be opened:
  - Damaged containers should be considered a spill and reported to the designated individual according to SOPs.
  - Seal the container in plastic or an impervious container.
  - Transport it to a C-PEC and place on a plastic-backed preparation mat.
  - Open the package and remove undamaged items.
  - Wipe the outside of the undamaged items with a disposable wipe.
  - Enclose the damaged item(s) in an impervious container and label the outer container "Hazardous."
  - Segregate HDs waiting to be returned to the supplier in a designated negative pressure area.
  - If the supplier declines return, dispose of as hazardous waste.

- Deactivate, decontaminate, and clean the C-PEC and discard the mat and cleaning disposables as hazardous waste.

Dispensing final dosage forms

National Institute for Occupational Safety and Health criteria

- An HD is any drug identified as hazardous or potentially hazardous on the basis of at least one of these six criteria:
  - Carcinogenicity, which is the ability to cause cancer in humans, animals, or both
  - Teratogenicity, which is the ability to cause defects in fetal development or fetal malformation
  - Reproductive toxicity, which causes fertility impairment in humans
  - Organ toxicity at low doses in humans or animal models
  - Genotoxicity, which is the ability to cause a change or mutation in genetic material
  - New drugs that mimic existing HDs in structure or toxicity

Hazardous drug classifications

- Group 1: antineoplastic drugs that may pose a reproductive threat
- Non-antineoplastic drugs
- Drugs that pose a reproductive risk for men or women

In 2020, NIOSH updated its List of Hazardous Drugs in Healthcare Settings. It classified HDs into two categories, which are:

- Drugs that contain the manufacturer's special handling information in the package insert and/or meet the NIOSH definition of an HD and are classified by the National Toxicology Program as "known to be a human carcinogen" and/or classified by the International Agency for Research on Cancer as "carcinogenic" or "probably carcinogenic." Examples of this category include azathioprine, bleomycin, cisplatin, cyclophosphamide, conjugated estrogens, fluorouracil, ganciclovir, hydroxyurea, paclitaxel, tamoxifen, thalidomide, vinblastine, and vincristine.
- Drugs that meet the NIOSH definition of an HD but are not drugs that have the manufacturer's special handling information or are classified by the National Toxicology Program as "known to be a human carcinogen" or classified by the International Agency for Research on Cancer as "carcinogenic" or "probably carcinogenic." Examples of this category include abacavir, anastrozole. clomiphene, clonazepam, colchicine, divalproex, estradiol, fluconazole, methimazole, oxytocin, and warfarin.

Containment supplemental engineering controls, protective medical devices, and techniques for administering hazardous drugs to patients

Engineering controls, administrative controls, and personal protective equipment for administering with hazardous drugs in health care settings						
Formulation	Activity	Double chemotherapy gloves	Protective gown	Eye/face protection	Respiratory protection	Engineering control
Intact tablet or capsule	Administration from unit-dose package	No (single glove can be used)	No	No	No	N/A
Prefilled syringe or injector	Administration	No (single glove can be used)	No	No	No	N/A
Tablets or capsules	Administration	No (single glove can be used)	No	Yes, if vomit or potential to spit up	No	N/A
Oral liquid drug or feeding tube	Administration	Yes	Yes	Yes, if vomit or potential to spit up	No	N/A
Topical drug	Administration	Yes	Yes	Yes, if liquid that could splash	Yes, if inhalation potential	N/A
Subcutaneous/ intramuscular injection from a vial	Administration from prepared syringe	Yes	Yes	Yes, if liquid that could splash	No	N/A
Withdrawing and/or mixing intravenous or intramuscular solution from a vial or ampoule	Administration of prepared solution	Yes	Yes	Yes, if liquid that could splash	No	N/A; CSTD required per USP 800 if the dosage form allows

(Continued)

Engineering controls, administrative controls, and personal protective equipment for administering with hazardous drugs in health care settings—cont'd

Formulation	Activity	Double chemotherapy gloves	Protective gown	Eye/face protection	Respiratory protection	Engineering control
Solution for irrigation	Administration (bladder, HIPEC, limb perfusion)	Yes	Yes	Yes	Yes	N/A
Powder/solution for inhalation/ aerosol treatment	Aerosol administration	Yes	Yes	Yes	Yes	Yes, when applicable
	Administration	Yes	Yes	Yes, if liquid that could splash	Yes, if inhalation potential	N/A

CSTD, Closed-system drug-transfer device; *HIPEC*, hyperthermal intraperitoneal chemotherapy; not applicable; *USP*, United States pharmacopeia.

Administrative

Federal regulations pertaining to the disposal of hazardous drugs

- The RCRA was passed to track hazardous waste from its generation to its disposal. It applies to pharmaceuticals and chemicals disposed of by pharmacies, hospitals, and clinics.
- Hazardous waste is defined as waste that causes or contributes to an increase in mortality or an increase in irreversible or incapacitating reversible illness.
- Hazardous waste also refers to waste that may cause a danger to human health when improperly treated, stored, transported, disposed of, or mismanaged.
- The EPA is responsible for enforcing the regulations contained in the RCRA.

Characteristics of hazardous waste

- Ignitability
  - Refers to flammable liquids with a flash point <140 °F or 60°C
  - Solids that can ignite by friction or absorption of moisture and certain compressed gases
  - Ignitable substances containing mixtures of alcohol and water
- Corrosivity
  - Refers to strong acids (pH < 2) and bases (pH > 12.5)
  - Examples: glacial acetic acid potassium permanganate and sodium hydroxide
- Reactivity
  - May be unstable under normal conditions, may react with water, may give off toxic gases and may be capable of detonation or explosion under normal conditions or when heated.
  - Example: nitroglycerin
- Toxicity
  - Refers to a substance that is harmful when ingested or absorbed through the skin
  - Examples: chromium, lindane, mercury and selenium

A waste is determined to be a hazardous waste if it is specifically listed on one of four lists (the F, K, P, and U lists). If a medication possess one of substance's characteristic and is identified on either the P or U list, it is considered as hazardous waste. Examples of medications found on the P list include warfarin > 0.3%, nicotine, physostigmine, epinephrine, and nitroglycerin. Mitomycin, chlorambucil, cyclophosphamide, daunomycin, lindane, melphalan, reserpine, selenium sulfide, uracil mustard, and warfarin < 0.3% are identified on the U list. Substances identified on the P or U list require special handling, containment, and disposal. Examples of hazardous waste products include:

- Used medications, unused medications. expired medications and patient medications
- Partial doses remaining in syringes, vials, ampoules, IV bags, and other liquid packaging that is not completely administered
- Chemotherapy agents
- Liquids, creams, transdermal patches, tablets, capsules
- Supplies used in cleaning up hazardous spills

"Empty containers" are exempted from these hazardous waste regulations under the RCRA. The RCRA defines empty containers "as those that have held U-listed or characteristic wastes and from which all wastes have been removed that can be removed using the practices commonly employed to remove materials from that type of container and no more than 3% by weight of the total capacity of the container remains in the container." The disposal of "RCRA-empty" containers, needles, syringes, trace-contaminated gowns, gloves, pads, and empty IV sets may be collected and incinerated at a regulated medical waste incinerator.

Under the RCRA, if a syringe with a needle holding a listed chemotherapeutic agent drug cannot be used, it should be managed as a dual waste. In this situation, a black needle box labeled for both hazardous and biohazardous wastes should be used for containment.

After hazardous waste has been identified, it must be collected, stored, and transported according to the requirements established by both the EPA and Department of Transportation. Hazardous waste must be packaged in leakproof and spill-proof containers, which are composed of nonreactive plastic and are properly labeled. Needles, scalpels, and waste contaminated with blood or other body fluids must not be mixed with hazardous waste.

Medical surveillance programs and surface wipe sampling

- Medical surveillance is an element of a comprehensive exposure control program that takes into consideration engineering controls, safe work processes, and use of PPE.
- Any health care worker who handles HDs should be enrolled in a medical surveillance program.
- The goal of medical surveillance is to reduce the incidence of adverse health effects in employees who have been exposed to HDs.
- A medical surveillance program involves assessing and documenting a health care worker's symptoms, physical findings, and laboratory values associated with an HD and deciding whether there is a deviation from the expected norms.

According to USP <800>, a medical surveillance program should

- Develop an orderly method to identify workers who are potentially exposed to HDs as a result of their job responsibilities.
- Employ an entity-based or contracted employee health service to perform the medical surveillance and protect the employees' confidential personal medical information.
- Conduct employees' initial baseline assessments and collect their medical history. Information collected should include a medical (including reproductive) history and work history to assess exposure to HDs, physical examination, and laboratory testing. Methods used to measure exposure history include a review of:
  - Records of HDs handled, with quantities and dosage forms
  - Estimated number of HDs handled per week
  - Estimates of hours spent handling HDs per week and/or per month
  - Performance of a physical assessment and laboratory studies related to target organs of commonly used HDs, such as a baseline complete blood count (Monitoring the blood or urine levels of specific HDs is not recommended in medical surveillance procedures; however, they may be beneficial in the follow-up of acute spills of an HD.)
- Maintain medical records of surveillance following Occupational Safety and Health Administration regulations regarding access to employee exposure and medical records.
- Monitor workers' health through regular surveillance based upon data gathered by utilizing updated health and exposure history, physical assessment, and laboratory measures.
- Monitoring of the data may be utilized to identify prevention failure resulting in adverse health effects.
- Develop a follow-up plan for health care workers who have demonstrated health changes indicating toxicity or have experienced an acute exposure.
- Complete an exit examination when a worker's employment at the health care facility ends, to document the information on the employee's medical, reproductive, and exposure histories.

The occurrence of exposure-related health changes should prompt urgent reevaluation of primary preventive measures to include administrative and engineering controls and PPEs. The organization should take the following actions:

- Perform a postexposure examination tailored to the type of exposure whether it is a spill or needlesticks from syringes containing an HD. The physical examination should focus on the involved area as well as other organ systems commonly affected.
- Compare performance of controls with recommended standards.
- Verify and document that all engineering controls are in proper operating condition.
- Verify and document that the health care worker followed all existing institutional policies to include all PPE policies.
- Develop and document a plan of action to prevent future exposure of health care workers.
- Guarantee confidential communication between the health care worker and the employee health unit(s).
- Provide and document a follow-up medical survey to demonstrate that the plan implemented is effective.
- Ensure that any exposed worker receives confidential notification of any adverse health effect. Offer alternative duty or temporary reassignment.
- Provide ongoing medical surveillance of all workers at risk for exposure to HDs to determine whether the plan implemented is effective.

Environmental wipe sampling for HD surface residue should be performed routinely (e.g., initially as a benchmark and at least every 6 months, or more often as needed, to verify containment). Surface wipe sampling should include:

- Interior of the C-PEC and equipment contained in it
- Pass-through chambers
- Surfaces in staging or work areas near the C-PEC
- Areas adjacent to C-PECs (e.g., floors directly under C-PEC, staging, and dispensing area)
- Areas immediately outside the HD buffer room or the C-SCA
- Patient administration areas

Best Standard Operating Procedures

- The health care facility must maintain SOPs for the safe handling of HDs.
- SOPS must be reviewed at least every 12 months and the review documented. Staff should be notified of SOP revisions involving HDs.
- The SOPs for handling of HDs should include a Hazard Communication Program.
- The Hazard Communication Program must include
  - All containers of hazardous chemicals must be labeled, tagged, or marked with the name of the material and appropriate hazard warnings.
  - All health care organizations must have an SDS for each hazardous chemical they use and it must be readily available to the user.
  - Personnel who may be exposed to hazardous chemicals when working must be provided information and training before the initial assignment to work with a hazardous chemical and also whenever the hazard changes.

- Personnel of reproductive capability must confirm in writing that they understand the risks of handling hazardous.
- Designation of HD areas:
  - A sign must be conspicuously posted prior to entering any area where HDs are handled.
  - Access to areas where HDs are being handled must be restricted to authorized personnel.
  - HD handling areas must be located away from breakrooms for personnel, patients, and visitors to minimize the risk of exposure.
  - Designated area must be available for receiving and unpacking HDs, storing HDs, compounding nonsterile HDs, and compounding sterile HDs.
- SOPs must be established for receiving HDs and should require:
  - Chemotherapy gloves must be worn.
  - Antineoplastic HDs and all HD APIs must be unpacked in a neutral or negative pressure area compared with its surrounding areas.
  - HDs should *not* be unpacked from their external shipping containers in sterile compounding areas or in positive pressure areas.
  - Unpacked HDs are required to be delivered immediately to the storage area.
  - Spill kit must be readily accessible.

Best practices for storage of hazardous drugs

- All health care workers who work with or around HDs must receive appropriate training to perform their jobs adhering to established precautions and required PPEs.
- HDs should be handled with caution using appropriate chemotherapy gloves during receiving, distribution, stocking, and inventorying.
- Access to HD areas must be restricted to authorized personnel only.
- Drug packages, bins, shelves, and storage areas for HDs should display unique labels identifying those drugs as requiring special handling precautions. These labels should be applied to all HD containers, as well as the shelves and bins where these containers are stored. Warning labels and signs must be in English and in other languages if non-English readers are employed to work in these areas.
- HD storage areas should be designed to prevent containers from falling to the floor.
- USP <800> requires the HD be segregated from other drug inventory.
- USP <800> mandates that storage areas should at least 12 ACPH.
- The health care facility should identify all drugs covered by HD policies.
- Health care workers should be aware of all spill and emergency contact procedures for HDs.
- Storage areas must be located away from employee break areas and patients and visitors

Best practices for compounding hazardous drugs

- A ventilated cabinet designed to reduce worker exposures while compounding HDs should be used.
- All staff who use ventilated cabinets should be trained to employ work appropriate practices established for the equipment.
- Implement initial and periodic assessments of technique in the safety program and verify technique during drug administration.
- Wear protective gloves and gowns if you are involved in preparation activities such as opening drug packaging, handling vials or finished products, labeling HD containers, or disposing of waste.
- Wear PPE (including double gloves and protective gowns) while reconstituting and admixing drugs.
- Make sure that gloves are labeled as chemotherapy gloves and make sure such information is available on the box (American Society for Testing and Material in press) or from the manufacturer.
- Use double gloving for all activities involving HDs. Make sure that the outer glove extends over the cuff of the gown.
- Inspect gloves for physical defects before use.
- Wash hands with soap and water before donning protective gloves and immediately after removal.
- Change gloves every 30 minutes or when torn, punctured, or contaminated. Discard them immediately in a yellow chemotherapy waste container.
- Dispose of protective gowns after each use.
- Use disposable sleeve covers to protect the wrist area and remove the covers after the task is complete.
- When drug preparation is complete, seal the final product in a plastic bag or other sealable container for transport before taking it out of the ventilated cabinet.
- Seal and wipe all waste containers inside the ventilated cabinet before removing them from the cabinet.
- Remove all outer gloves and sleeve covers and bag them for disposal while you are inside the ventilated cabinet.
- Wash hands with soap and water immediately after removing gloves.
- Have pharmacy personnel prime the IV tubing and syringes inside the ventilated cabinet or prime them in line with nondrug solutions—never in the patient's room.

Best practices involving engineering controls (e.g., containment primary engineering controls, containment secondary engineering controls, and closed-system drug-transfer devices)

- Mix, prepare, and otherwise manipulate, count, crush, compound powders, or pour liquid HDs inside a ventilated cabinet designed to prevent HDs from being released into the work environment.

- Do not use supplemental engineering or process controls (such as needleless systems, glove bags, and CSDTs) as a substitution for ventilated cabinets, even though such controls may reduce the potential for exposure when preparing and administering HDs.
- Select a ventilated cabinet depending on the need for aseptic processing.
- When asepsis is not required, a Class I BSC or an isolator intended for containment applications (a "containment isolator") may be sufficient.
- When aseptic technique is required, use one of the following ventilated cabinets:
  - Class II BSC (Type B2 is preferred, but Types A2 and B1 are allowed under certain conditions.)
  - Class III BSC
  - Isolators intended for asepsis and containment
- Use a HEPA filter for the exhaust from these controls.
- Install the outside exhaust so that the exhausted air is not pulled back into the building.
- Place fans downstream of the HEPA filter so that contaminated ducts are maintained under negative pressure.
- Have a written safety plan for all routine maintenance activities performed on equipment that could be contaminated with HDs.
- Properly install and maintain and routinely clean any Class II BSC. Field certify its performance (1) after installation, relocation, maintenance repairs to internal components and HEPA filter replacement and (2) every 6 months thereafter.
- Prominently display a current field-certification label on the ventilated cabinet.

Best practices involving hand hygiene and personal protective equipment

- Minimize contamination through proper handwashing. Proper handwashing involves these steps:
  - All personal electronic devices, such as cell phones, iPods, and any associated devices must be removed before handwashing.
  - Remove all visible jewelry and cosmetics before handwashing begins.
  - Turn on water. Wash hands, nails, wrists, and forearms up to the elbows for at least 30 seconds with a brush and/or sponge, warm water, and an antibacterial soap.
  - Rinse thoroughly with the hands and forearms in an upward position beginning with the fingers down town to the elbows.
  - Dry the hands and arms with a nonshedding or lint-free cloth or with an electric hand dryer.
  - After the hands and arms are completely dry, throw away damp towels and use a new towel to turn off the water.
  - Sanitize the hands by applying a waterless, alcohol-based hand rub and allow it to dry completely before putting on sterile gloves.
- USP <800> requires gowns, head, hair, shoe covers, and two pairs of chemotherapy gloves are required for compounding sterile and nonsterile HDs. Two pairs of chemotherapy gloves are required for administering

injectable antineoplastic HDs. Gowns shown to withstand penetrability by HDs are required when administering injectable antineoplastic HDs. Appropriate PPEs must be worn when handling HDs during
- their receipt
- storage
- transport
- compounding
- administering
- deactivating/decontaminating, cleaning, and disinfecting
- spill control
- waste disposal

Best practices during deactivation, decontamination, cleaning, and disinfection

- Perform cleaning and decontamination work in areas that are sufficiently ventilated to prevent buildup of hazardous airborne drug concentrations.
- Clean work surfaces with an appropriate deactivation agent (if available) and cleaning agent before and after each activity and at the end of the work shift.
- Establish periodic cleaning routines for all work surfaces and equipment that may become contaminated.
- Wear safety glasses with side shields and protective gloves for cleaning and decontaminating work.
- Wear face shields if splashing may occur.
- Wear protective double gloves when performing decontamination and cleaning processes.

Best practices for dispensing hazardous drugs

- Clean equipment should be dedicated for use with HDs and should be decontaminated after every use.
- Antineoplastic tablet and capsule dosage forms must not be placed in automated counting or packaging machines, since they may create powdered contaminants.

Best practices for transporting hazardous drugs

- HDs must be transported in containers that minimize the possibility of breakage or leakage.
- Pneumatic tube must not be used to transport any liquid HDs or any antineoplastic HDs due to the potential for breakage and contamination.
- When HDs are transported to areas outside the facility, the pharmacy must refer to Section 14: Transport Information of the Safety Data Sheet.
- Labeling for transporting HDs must include storage and disposal instructions.

Best practices for administering hazardous drugs

- Handle all HDs safely when administering them.
- Wear PPE (including double gloves, goggles, and protective gowns) for all activities associated with drug administration to include opening the outer bag, assembling the delivery system, delivering the drug to the patient, and disposing of all equipment used to administer drugs.

- Utilize protective medical devices (such as needleless and closed systems) and employ appropriate techniques (such as priming of IV tubing by pharmacy personnel inside a ventilated cabinet or priming in line with non-drug solutions) when administering HDs.
- Never remove tubing from an IV bag containing an HD.

Best practices for environmental monitoring of hazardous drugs

- Environmental wipe sampling for HD surface residue should be performed routinely at least every 6 months, or more often as needed.
- Surface wipe sampling includes
  - Interior of the C-PEC and equipment contained in it
  - Pass-through chambers
  - Surfaces in staging or work areas near the C-PEC
  - Areas adjacent to C-PECs (e.g., floors directly under C-PEC, staging, and dispensing area)
  - Areas immediately outside the HD buffer room or the C-SCA

Best practices for disposal of hazardous drugs

- Various types of waste can be the result of preparing and administering HDs. They include partially filled vials, undispensed products, unused IVs, needles and syringes, gloves, gowns, underpads, and contaminated materials from spill cleanups.
- Place trace wastes (those that contain less than 3% by weight of the original quantity of HDs)—such as needles, empty vials and syringes, gloves, gowns, and tubing—in yellow chemotherapy waste containers.
  - Place soft trace items (those that are contaminated with trace amounts of HDs) in yellow chemotherapy bags for disposal by incineration at a regulated medical waste facility.
  - Place soft trace items (those that are contaminated with trace amounts of HDs) in yellow chemotherapy bags for disposal by incineration at a regulated medical waste facility.
- Do not place HD-contaminated sharps in red sharps containers that are used for infectious wastes, since these are often autoclaved or microwaved.
- Dispose of P-listed arsenic trioxide and its containers and any bulk amounts of U-listed drugs in hazardous waste containers at a RCRA-permitted incinerator.
- Dispose of other bulk HDs (that is, expired or unused vials, ampoules, syringes, bags, and bottles of HDs or solutions of any other items with more than trace contamination) in a manner similar to that required for RCRA-defined hazardous wastes.

Best practices for spill control of hazardous drugs

- SOPs must be developed to prevent spills and to direct the clean up of HD spills. These procedures must address the size and scope of the spill and indicate who is responsible for spill management and the type of PPE required.

- All health care workers required to clean up an HD spill must receive proper training in spill management and the use of PPE and NIOSH-certified respirators.
- Spills must be contained and cleaned immediately only by properly trained personnel wearing appropriate PPE.
- A spill kit must be readily available in any area where HDs are handled, compounded, or administered. SOPs must address the location of spill kits and cleanup materials as well as the capacity of the spill kit.
- A spill kit contains the following:
  - Absorbent chemotherapy pads and towels
  - Disposable chemotherapy gowns with back closures
  - Chemotherapy-resistant shoe covers
  - Chemotherapy gloves
  - Chemical splash goggles
  - Respirator masks (NIOSH approved)
  - Disposable dust pan
  - Plastic scraper
  - Puncture-proof container for glass
  - Large, heavy-duty sealable waste disposable bags
  - Hazardous waste label (if not attached to the bag)
- Warning signs should be posted to control access to the area
- Employees who are possibly exposed during the spill or spill cleanup or who have direct skin or eye contact with HDs are required to receive immediate evaluation.

American Society of Health System Pharmacists recommended general spill procedure

- Assess the size and scope of the spill. Call for trained help, if necessary.
- Obtain spill kit and respirator, if needed. Spills that cannot be contained by two spill kits may require outside assistance.
- Don PPE including double gloves and respirator.
- Once fully garbed, contain spill using spill kit.
- Carefully remove any broken glass fragments and place them in a puncture-resistant container.
- Absorb liquids with spill pads or toweling.
- Absorb powder with damp disposable pads or soft toweling.
- Spill cleanup should proceed progressively from areas of lesser to greater contamination.
- Completely remove and place all contaminated material in the HD waste disposal bags.
- Rinse the area with water and then clean with detergent, sodium hypochlorite solution, and neutralizer (if the area may be bleached; if not, use detergent and rinse 3 times).
- Rinse the area several times and place all materials used for containment and cleanup in disposal bags. Seal bags and place them in the appropriate final container for disposal as hazardous waste.
- Carefully remove all PPE using the inner gloves. Place all disposable PPE into disposal bags. Seal bags and place them into the appropriate final container.
- Remove inner gloves, contain in a small, sealable bag, and then place into the appropriate final container for disposal as hazardous waste.
- Wash hands thoroughly with soap and water.

- Once a spill has been initially cleaned, have the area recleaned by housekeeping, janitorial staff, or environmental services per facility policy.

American Society of Health System Pharmacists recommended procedures for spills in a containment primary engineering control

- Spills occurring in a C-PEC should be cleaned up immediately.
- Obtain a spill kit if the volume of the spill exceeds 30 mL or the contents of one drug vial or ampoule.
- Additional HD gloves should be worn to remove broken glass in a C-PEC. Care should be taken not to damage the fixed-glove assembly in a CACI.
- Place glass fragments in the puncture-resistant HD waste container.
- Thoroughly clean and decontaminate the C-PEC. Clean and decontaminate the drain spillage trough located in the C-PEC if so equipped.
- If the spill results in liquid being introduced onto the HEPA filter, or if powdered aerosol contaminates the "clean side" of the HEPA filter, use of the C-PEC should be suspended until the equipment has been decontaminated and the HEPA filter replaced.
- Contaminated reusable items, for example, glassware and scoops, should be cleaned with mild detergent and water after use. Items contaminated with HDs should be washed twice with detergent by a trained employee wearing PPE as described in the PPE section.

Hazardous drug training

USP <800> require HD training must address the following topics:

- The institutional HD list and risks associated with HDs
- Institutional SOPs for HDs
- Proper use of PPE
- Proper use of equipment and devices (e.g., engineering controls)
- Actions to take in response to known or suspected HD exposure
- HD disposal procedures and trace-contaminated materials
- HD spill management procedures

In addition to USP <800>, health care workers who are required to wear respirators must be fitted and trained to meet all Occupational Safety and Health Administration respirator requirements to include:

- The properties of the HDs located in the work area
- The techniques and safe handling practices that have been implemented in the work area to protect employees from exposure to HDs, such as identification of drugs that should be handled as hazardous, appropriate work practices, safety equipment, and PPE to be used, and emergency procedures for spills or employee exposure

- The details of the hazard communication program developed by the employer, including an explanation of the labeling and HD identification system used by the employer, the SDSs, and how employees can obtain and use the appropriate hazard information
- Proper use of safety equipment such as BSCs, compounding aseptic containment isolators, and CSDTs
- Proper donning and removal of PPE
- Drug preparation, administration, disposal, and spill management procedures that minimize worker and environmental exposure.

Training must be provided, and competence must be demonstrated prior to assuming HD responsibilities. Personnel must be trained prior to the introduction of a new HD or new equipment and prior to a new or significant change in process or SOP. All training and competency assessment must be documented. Individuals must be reassessed at least annually.

CHAPTER REVIEW QUESTIONS

1. What is the minimum number of ACPH a refrigerated antineoplastic HD be stored?
   a. 8
   b. 10
   c. 12
   d. 14
2. An antineoplastic HD may be unpacked from its shipping container in which of the following areas?
   a. Neutral/normal pressure
   b. Positive pressure areas
   c. Sterile compounding area
   d. All of the above
3. Which classification of BSCs must have a minimum inflow velocity of 75 feet/minute?
   a. Class II Type A1
   b. Class II Type A2
   c. Class II Type B1
   d. Class II Type B 2
4. Which term refers to the process of inhibiting or destroying microorganisms?
   a. Cleaning
   b. Deactivation
   c. Decontamination
   d. Disinfecting
5. How often must a C-PEC be deactivated, decontaminated, and cleaned?
   a. Daily
   b. Weekly
   c. Monthly
   d. Every 6 months
6. If no manufacturer's information regarding a gown's permeability is provided, how often should a gown be changed?
   a. Every hour or immediately after a spill or splash
   b. Every 2–3 hours or immediately after a spill or splash
   c. Every 3–4 hours or immediately after a spill or splash
   d. Every 4–7 hours or immediately after a spill or splash

7. Which term refers to the process of inactivating, neutralizing, or removing of HD contaminants from nondisposable surfaces and transferring it to absorbent, disposable materials such as wipes, pads, or towels?
   a. Cleaning
   b. Deactivation
   c. Decontamination
   d. Disinfecting

8. Which organization recommends evaluating the workplace to identifying and assessing the hazards prior to anyone working with HDs?
   a. Centers for Disease Control
   b. Drug Enforcement Administration
   c. FDA
   d. NIOSH

9. All of the following are recommended after an individual has been accidentally exposed to a HD *except* which one?
   a. Complete an incident report.
   b. Conduct a postexposure examination.
   c. Isolate the employee.
   d. Refer to SDSs.

10. Which is the first thing that should be done when a HD spill has occurred?
    a. Assess the size and scope of the spill.
    b. Don appropriate PPEs to include double gloves and respirator.
    c. Obtain spill kit and respirator.
    d. Contain the spill using the spill kit.

11. Which is a *true* statement regarding wearing gloves when handling HDs?
    a. Gloves are only required when compounding sterile and nonsterile drugs.
    b. Gloves must contain powder since they will absorb the hazardous material.
    c. Chemotherapy gloves should be worn for handling all HDs, including non-antineoplastics and for reproductive risk–only HDs.
    d. Triple gloves should be worn during any handling of HD shipping cartons or drug vials and handling of HD waste or waste from patients recently treated with HDs.

12. Which activity does *not* require a pharmacy technician to wear eye/face protection?
    a. Compounding an oral liquid drug
    b. Compounding a topical drug
    c. Cutting, crushing, or manipulating tablets or capsules
    d. Withdrawing a subcutaneous injection from a vial

13. Which of the following medications is an example of medication containing manufacturers' special handling information?
    a. Anastrozole
    b. Clomiphene
    c. Cyclophosamide
    d. Fluconazole

14. Which of the following is an example of a criteria for a drug to be identified as hazardous or potentially hazardous?
    a. Corrosivity
    b. Ignitability

c. Reactivity
d. Teratogenicity

15. A waste is determined to be a hazardous waste if it is specifically listed on one of four lists. Which of the following is an example of a list?
    a. J list
    b. K list
    c. L list
    d. M list

16. A pharmacy technician was compounding an HD. After compounding the drug, which color container should they use to dispose of their gloves?
    a. Black
    b. Red
    c. Yellow
    d. Any of the above

17. Which is a classification of HDs?
    a. Antineoplastic drugs
    b. Non-antineoplastic drugs
    c. Drugs that pose a reproductive risk for men or women
    d. All of the above

18. How often must environmental sampling be performed?
    a. At least monthly
    b. At least every 3 months
    c. At least every 6 months
    d. At least once a year

19. How often must SOPs for the safe handling of HDs be conducted?
    a. Every 6 months
    b. Every 12 months
    c. Every 18 months
    d. Every 24 months

20. Which chapter of the USP addresses the storage of HDs?
    a. USP <795>
    b. USP <797>
    c. USP <800>
    d. USP <825>

21. What is the first thing to be done after an individual has been accidentally exposed to an HD?
    a. Have individual undergo physical examination at the site of exposure.
    b. Have individual visit the employee health professional to document and confirm complete decontamination.
    c. Refer to the hazardous medication's SDS and decontaminate.
    d. Remove the individual's contaminated clothes.

22. Which term refers to the ability to cause cancer in humans, animals, or both?
    a. Carcinogenicity
    b. Genotoxicity
    c. Reproductive toxicity
    d. Teratogenicity

23. Which individual should be enrolled in a medical surveillance program
    a. A nurse who administers an HD to a patient
    b. A pharmacist who prepares a sterile HD
    c. A pharmacy technician who unpacks a delivery of HDs
    d. All the above

24. Which organization is responsible for enforcing the RCRA?
    a. Drug Enforcement Administration
    b. FDA
    c. EPA
    d. All of the above
25. How many pairs of chemotherapy gloves are required to be worn when compounding both sterile and nonsterile hazardous medications?
    a. One pair
    b. Two pairs
    c. Three pairs
    d. Four pairs

RESOURCES

https://go.usp.org/l/323321/2020-03-09/3125jw
https://www.cdc.gov/niosh/topics/hazdrug/riskmanagement.html
https://www.osha.gov/hazardous-drugs/controlling-occex#hazcom_written
https://www.cdc.gov/niosh/docs/2004-165/pdfs/2004-165.pdf?id=10.26616/NIOSHPUB2004165
ASHP Guidelines on Handling Hazardous Drugs: https://www.ashp.org/-/media/assets/policy-guidelines/docs/guidelines/handling-hazardous-drugs.ashx

3

Regulatory Compliance Certificate

- Must hold an active Pharmacy Technician Certification Board–Certified Pharmacy Technician Certification.
- Must complete a Pharmacy Technician Certification Board–Recognized Regulatory Compliance Education/Training Program.

Regulatory compliance domains

Laws, regulations, and guidelines (37%)
- Roles of various regulatory bodies
- Use of United States Pharmacopeia (USP) Standards pertaining to Regulatory Compliance (e.g., appropriate application and interpretation of USP Chapters)
- Federal requirements for pharmacy (e.g., nondiscrimination; fraud, waste, and abuse; Office of Inspector General exclusion list; Health Insurance Portability and Accountability Act; Substance Abuse and Mental Health Services Administration; Nuclear Regulatory Commission)
- Environmental Protection Agency's hazardous waste management in the pharmacy
- Federal Controlled Substances Act
- Federal Food, Drug, and Cosmetic Act
- Drug Quality and Security Act—Title I Compounding Quality Act, Title II Drug Supply Chain Security Act
- Accreditation standards (e.g., types of accreditations, elements of accreditation, reasons for accreditation)

Legal requirements and practice standards (37%)
- Regulatory and accreditation-related terminology (e.g., statute, law, regulation, standard, code, certification, certificate, licensure, registration)
- Basic principles that serve as the foundation for pharmacy laws and pharmacy ethics (e.g., evolution of the Federal Food, Drug, and Cosmetic Act, other key legislation that has shaped pharmacy practice)
- Federal requirements (e.g., Drug Enforcement Administration, FDA) for controlled substances (i.e., receiving, storing, ordering, labeling, dispensing, reverse distribution, take back programs, and loss or theft of controlled substances)

- Federal requirements for handling and disposal of nonhazardous, hazardous, and pharmaceutical substances and waste
- Federal requirements for restricted drug programs and related medication processing (e.g., pseudoephedrine, Risk Evaluation and Mitigation Strategies)
- Laws and/or regulations regarding compliance and auditing functions
- Federal requirements pertaining to the medication dispensing process
- Federal requirements pertaining to personnel competency
- Federal requirements pertaining to compounding sterile preparations
- Federal requirements pertaining to nonsterile compounding
- Licensing and reporting requirements for personnel and facility

Patient safety and quality assurance strategies (26%)
- Elements of compliance programs (e.g., Just Culture, continuous quality improvement, quality assurance, patient safety organization)
- Methods or techniques to systematically improve accuracy (e.g., barcode scanning, failure mode and effects analysis, root cause analysis)
- Cause and impact of medication dispensing errors (e.g., abnormal doses, early refill, incorrect quantity, incorrect strength, incorrect patient, incorrect drug, incorrect route of administration, incorrect directions, wrong timing, missing dose, misinterpretation of drug concentration)
- Cause and impact of other types of quality-related events (e.g., incomplete counseling, patient language barrier, adverse events)
- Medication storage requirements (e.g., refrigeration, freezing)
- Rules, policies, and regulations related to the disposal of pharmaceutical drugs (e.g., prescription drug take back programs; proper medication destruction)
- Reporting of medication errors and quality-related events (e.g., internal reporting, MedWatch, Vaccine Adverse Event Reporting System, Board of Pharmacy)
- Institute for Safe Medication Practices best practices (e.g., List of High-Alert Medications; Targeted Medication Safety Best Practices for Hospitals; Safe Preparation of Compounded Sterile Preparations; look-alike/sound-alike medications)

Laws, regulations, and guidelines

Roles of various regulatory bodies

Food and Drug Administration

- Food and Drug Administration (FDA) is responsible for protecting the public health by guaranteeing the safety, efficacy, and security of human and veterinary drugs, biological products, medical devices, our nation's food supply, cosmetics, products that emit radiation and tobacco. The FDA has released regulations involving:
  - Drug development
  - Drug labeling involves:
    - Drug monographs, which provide comprehensive information regarding a medication's actions. Information contained in a drug monograph includes indications and usage; dosage and administration; dosage forms and strengths; contraindications; warnings and precautions; adverse reactions; drug interactions; usage in specific populations; drug abuse and dependence; overdosage; description; clinical pharmacology; references; how it is supplied, stored, and handled; and patient counseling information.
    - Boxed Warning "black box warning" label draws attention to serious attention to serious or life-threatening risks.
    - Patient package inserts (PPIs) provide FDA-approved information regarding the medication and its usage.
    - Medication guides are paper handouts that come with many prescription medicines and assist patients in avoiding serious adverse events.
    - Instructions for use is a document developed by the manufacturer, approved by the FDA, and dispensed with specific products that have complicated dosing instructions to help the patient use the product properly.
- Supervising risk evaluation and mitigation strategy (REMS), which is a drug safety program that the FDA requires for particular medications with serious safety concerns to help ensure the benefits of the medication outweigh its risks
- Overseeing drug recall process
  - Class I recall is issued with a dangerous or defective product that could cause serious health problems or death.
  - Class II recall is issued when a product might cause a temporary health problem or pose slight threat of a serious nature.
  - Class III recall is issued when a product is unlikely to cause any adverse health reactions but that violates FDA labeling or manufacturing laws.

Drug Enforcement Administration

The Drug Enforcement Administration (DEA) is responsible for:

- Regulating the manufacture and distribution of controlled pharmaceuticals and listed chemicals

- The oversight of dispensing and administering controlled substances
- Enforcing the Controlled Substance Act, Combat Methamphetamine Epidemic Act of 2005 (CMEA), and the Ryan Haight Online Pharmacy Consumer Protection Act of 2008
- Classifying medications based upon their potential for abuse
- Enforcing the registration requirements for prescribers in prescribing controlled substances and pharmacies for dispensing controlled substances
- The oversight of ordering controlled substances for pharmacies
- Enforcing inventory requirements of controlled substances for pharmacies
- Enforcing valid prescription requirements for controlled substances
- Enforcing pharmacy dispensing requirements for controlled substances
- Overseeing pharmacy security requirements
- The oversight for transferring or disposing of controlled substance

Environmental Protection Agency

Under the Resource Conservation Act, the Environmental Protection Agency (EPA) is responsible regulating the handling of hazardous waste, which is defined as waste with properties that make it dangerous or capable of having a harmful effect on human health or the environment. Hazardous waste characteristics includes ignitability, corrosivity, reactivity, and toxicity. The EPA established a comprehensive regulatory program to ensure that hazardous waste is managed safely from "cradle to grave," meaning from the time it is created, while it is transported, treated, and stored, and until it is disposed of.

Many types of medications are regulated as hazardous waste and they include:

- Used, unused or expired medications, including patient's leftover medications
- Liquids, creams, transdermal patches, and solid preparations such as tablets, pills, capsules, and powders
- Partial doses in syringes, vials, ampoules, and IV bags that were not administered
- Chemotherapeutic agents
- Spill cleanup materials

Centers for Medicare and Medicaid Services

The Centers for Medicare and Medicaid Services (CMS) is responsible for administering Medicare, Medicaid, the Children's Health Insurance Program, and the Health Insurance Portability and Accountability Act (HIPAA) standards. Medicare is a federal program to provide health care for adult patients over the age of 65, persons with disabilities, and patients with end-stage renal disease. Medicare consists of:

- Medicare Part A, which covers inpatient hospital care, skilled nursing facilities, hospice, and home health care
- Medicare Part B, which provides for physician services, outpatient care, and some physical/occupational therapy

- Medicare Part C (Medicare Advantage), which permits patients enrolled in Medicare Part A and B to obtain coverage through an HMO or PPO that provides additional services
- Medicare Part D, which provides for prescription medications, biologicals, insulin, vaccines, and select medical supplies (Medicare Part D does not pay for all medications.)

Use of USP Standards pertaining to Regulatory Compliance (e.g., appropriate application and interpretation of USP chapters)

- USP <795> Pharmaceutical Compounding—Nonsterile Preparations
- USP <797> Pharmaceutical Compounding—Sterile Preparations
- USP <800> Hazardous Drugs—Handling in Healthcare Settings
- USP <825> Radiopharmaceuticals—Preparation, Compounding, Dispensing, and Repackaging
- USP <1160> Pharmaceutical Calculations in Pharmacy Practice
- USP <1163> Quality Assurance in Pharmaceutical Compounding
- USP <1176> Prescription Balances and Volumetric Apparatus Use in Compounding

Federal requirements for pharmacy

Nondiscrimination

- Affordable Care Act (ACA) requires health care entities receiving federal financial assistance (e.g., Medicaid and Medicare) to engage in practices designed to prevent discrimination on the basis of age, race, color, nationality, or gender, including gender identity.
- The ACA requires pharmacies to take reasonable steps to provide access to individuals with limited English skills or who possess a disability.
- Best practices for pharmacies to prevent discrimination include:
  - Providing aids and services, free of charge, when necessary, so that people with disabilities have an equal opportunity to communicate effectively with the pharmacy staff to include written information in other formats such as large print, audio, and available electronic formats
  - Providing language services such as an interpreter or information written in their languages

Fraud, waste, and abuse

- Fraud is knowingly and willfully executing, or attempting to execute, a scheme or artifice to defraud any health care benefit program or to obtain, by means of false or fraudulent pretenses, representations, or promises, any of the money or property owned by, or under the custody or control of, any health care benefit program. Fraud

requires intent to obtain payment and the knowledge the actions are wrong. An examples of fraud would involve billing for nonexistent prescriptions.
- Waste involves practices that, directly or indirectly, result in unnecessary costs to the Medicare program, such as overusing services. Waste is generally not considered to be caused by criminally negligent actions but rather by the misuse of resources. An example of waste would involve a physician prescribing for more medications than necessary to treat a specific medication.
- Abuse encompasses actions that may, directly or indirectly, result in unnecessary costs to the Medicare program. Abuse includes paying for items or services when there is no legal entitlement to that payment, and the provider has not knowingly or intentionally misrepresented facts to obtain payment. Waste and abuse may involve obtaining an improper payment or creating an unnecessary cost to the Medicare program but do not require the same intent and knowledge. An example of waste would be unknowingly billing for brand-name drugs when generics are dispensed.
- An individual must report suspected instances of fraud, waste, and abuse occurring in a pharmacy.
- Once fraud, waste, or abuse is detected in your pharmacy, it should be corrected immediately.
- Signs of potential fraud, waste, and abuse:
  - Is the provider filling numerous identical prescriptions for this beneficiary, possibly from different doctors?
  - Is the prescription appropriate based on the beneficiary's other prescriptions?
  - Are the provider's prescriptions appropriate for the member's health condition (medically necessary)?
  - Does the provider write prescriptions for diverse drugs or primarily for controlled substances?
  - Is the provider prescribing a higher quantity than medically necessary for the condition?
  - Does the physician's prescriptions contain their active and valid National Provider Identifier on it?
  - Are drugs being diverted (drugs meant for nursing homes, hospice, and other entities being sent elsewhere)?
  - Are the dispensed drugs expired, fake, diluted, or illegal?
  - Are generic drugs provided when the prescription requires dispensing brand drugs?
  - Are pharmacy benefits managers billed for prescriptions that are unfilled or never picked up?
  - Are proper provisions made if the entire prescription is not filled (no additional dispensing fees for split prescriptions)?
  - Do you see prescriptions being altered (changing quantities or "dispense as written")?

Office of Inspector General List of Excluded Individuals/Entities

- List of Excluded Individuals/Entities provides information to the health care industry, patients, and the public regarding individuals and entities currently excluded from participation in Medicare, Medicaid, and all other federal health care programs. Individuals and entities who have been reinstated are removed from the List of Excluded Individuals/Entities.

Health Insurance Portability and Accountability Act of 1996

The purpose of their Health Insurance Portability and Accountability Act (HIPAA) is:

- To improve portability and continuity of health coverage in the group and individual markets
- To combat waste, fraud, and abuse in health insurance and health care delivery
- To promote the use of medical savings accounts
- To improve access to long-term care (LTC) services and coverage
- To simplify the administration of health insurance

All pharmacy personnel shall respect and protect patient confidentiality by safeguarding access to all patient information. Patient information shall be shared only with authorized health professionals and others authorized within the hospital or health system as needed for the care of patient.

Health Insurance Portability and Accountability Act's administrative simplification provisions

- HIPAA Privacy Rule—covers patients health information
- HIPAA Security Rule—administrative, technical, and physical safeguards are required to protect patient's health information
- HIPAA Electronic Health Care Transactions and Code Sets Standards—require every provider that does business electronically to use the same health care transactions, code sets, and identifiers

Health Insurance Portability and Accountability Act Privacy Rule

Covered entities must:

- Have a set of privacy practices that are appropriate for its health care services
- Notify patients of their privacy rights and how information can be used or disclosed
- Train employees to understand the privacy practices
- Appoint a privacy official who is responsible for ensuring the privacy practices are adopted and followed
- Safeguard patient's records

Protected health information

Protected health information is individually identifiable health information that is transmitted or maintained over electronic media such as the Internet. Protected health information includes:

- Any information related to past, present, or future physical and mental health
- Past, present, or future payments for health services received
- Specific care the patient received, is receiving, or is willing to receive
- Any information that can identify the patient as the individual receiving the care, such as patient name or address

(including street addresses, city, county, and zip code); names of relatives or employers; Social Security number; date of birth, admission, discharge, or death; telephone and fax numbers; email or addresses, medical records or account numbers or health plan beneficiary numbers; certificate or license numbers; photographs; biometric indicators

Health Insurance Portability and Accountability Act Security Rule

- Encryption required
- Security measures include:
  - Access control, passwords, and log files to keep intruders out
  - Backups to replace items after damage (It is necessary after a minor or major security incident.)
  - Security policies that inform employees about protecting electronically stored information; examples include changing passwords after a given period of time or having employees sign confidentiality agreements to prevent from disclosing their usernames and passwords

Health Insurance Portability and Accountability Act Electronic Health Care Transactions and Code Sets Standard

- Permits providers and health care plans to exchange electronic data using a standard format and standard code sets
- Standard transactions
  - Consist of a name and number
  - Apply to electronic data that are sent back and forth between providers, health plans, and employers; standards contain both a number and a name

Standard code sets

- Provide codes for diseases, injuries, impairments, and other health-related problems
- Provide codes for procedures to prevent, diagnose, treat, or manage diseases, injuries, or impairment such as pharmacist services
- Code for medications as is found in a medication's National Drug Code (NDC)

Substance Abuse and Mental Health Services Administration

- Is an agency within the US Department of Health and Human Services
- Goal is to reduce the impact of substance abuse and mental illness in communities
- Collects mental health and substance abuse data
- Provides tools, training, and technical assistance to practitioners
- Produces and distributes public education materials
- Develops workplace drug testing guidelines
- Establishes regulations for opioid treatment programs
- Oversees programs for:
  - HIV/AIDS
  - Now Is the Time
  - Children's Mental Health Initiative

- Trauma
- Criminal and Juvenile Justice
- Primary and Behavioral Health Care Integration
- Screening, Brief Intervention, Referral to Treatment
- Suicide Prevention
- Substance Abuse Prevention
- Consumer and Family Support
- Protection and Advocacy for Individuals With Mental Illness

Nuclear Regulatory Commission

Nuclear pharmacy is a specialized pharmaceutical care service that has been defined as a patient-oriented service that embodies the scientific knowledge and professional judgement required to improve and promote health through assurance of the safe and efficacious use of radioactive drugs for diagnosis and therapy. The states regulate the practices of medicine and pharmacy and administer programs associated with radiation-producing x-ray machines and accelerators. The Nuclear Regulatory Commission (NRC) oversees medical uses of nuclear material through licensing, inspection, and enforcement programs.

The NRC has established standards in:

- Procurement
- Compounding
- Quality assurance (QA)
- Dispensing
- Distribution
- Health and safety
- Provision of information and consultation
- Monitoring patient outcomes
- Research and development

The NRC controls the use and disposal of radioactive materials and the safety of employees and the public. Any pharmacy that deals with radioactive compounding must possess:

- A license from the NRC
- A traditional pharmacy license issued by the state board of pharmacy
- A nuclear pharmacist in charge
- A list of personnel who have met specialized requirements for training and experience to handle radioactive materials
- Detailed floor plans that have been approved by the NRC
- Maintenance of records for the receipt, storage, compounding, disposal of, and transport of radioactive materials
- Compounding records
- Compounding areas surveyed daily
- Records demonstrating regular monitoring of external radiation exposure and contamination
- Records indicating the storage area is surveyed weekly
- Personnel exposure limits records
- Radiopharmaceutical labeling
- Postradioactive caution signs
- Documentation of radioactive spills
- Radiopharmaceutical error documentation

Environmental Protection Agency's hazardous waste management in the pharmacy

- Hazardous wastes are classified as either "P-list" or "U-list." Examples of P-list medications include chemotherapeutic agents, warfarin, nicotine, and physostigmine. An example of a U-list" medication is cyclophosphamide.
- The EPA and the Department of Transportation have issued specific conditions regarding the storage and transportation of hazardous waste.
- Hazardous drug (HD) waste must be placed in thick, leakproof bags of a different color from ordinary trash bags and labeled as "Hazardous Drug Waste."
- HD waste bags should be placed in a covered waste container and labeled as such.
- Bags containing hazardous waste should be sealed and tightly taped when full.
- The EPA requires hazardous waste be stored in a secure area until it is properly disposed of.

Federal Controlled Substances Act

Controlled substance schedules

Under the Controlled Substance Act of 1970, five drug schedules were created. A controlled substance is assigned a drug schedule based upon whether it has a currently accepted medical use in treatment in the United States and its relative potential and likelihood of causing dependence.

- Schedule I Controlled Substances
  - Have a high potential of abuse
  - No currently accepted medical use in the United States
  - Lack of accepted safety for use of the drug under medical supervision
  - Examples: heroin, lysergic acid diethylamide (LSD), marijuana (cannabis), 3,4-methylenedioxymethamphetamine ("Ecstasy"), peyote, hashish, and "crack" cocaine
- Schedule II Controlled Substances
  - Have a high potential for abuse, which may lead to severe psychological or physical dependence
  - Have a currently accepted medical use in the United States with severe restrictions
  - Examples: morphine, codeine, opium, hydrocodone with acetaminophen, fentanyl, hydromorphone (Dilaudid), methadone, meperidine (Demerol), oxycodone (OxyContin), oxycodone with acetaminophen (Percocet), dextroamphetamine (Dexedrine), dextroamphetamine/amphetamine (Adderall), methylphenidate (Ritalin, Concerta), lisdexamfetamine (Vyvanse), and cocaine nasal (Goprelto)
- Schedule III Controlled Substances
  - Have a potential for abuse less than substance in Schedules I or II
  - Have a currently accepted medical use in the United States
  - Possibility of abuse leading to moderate or low physical dependence or high psychological dependence
  - Examples: acetaminophen with codeine, buprenorphine, ketamine, and benzphetamine

- Schedule IV Controlled Substances
  - Have a low potential for abuse relative to substances in Schedule III
  - Have a currently accepted medical use with severe restrictions
  - Possibility of abuse leading to limited physical dependence or psychological dependence compared with substances in Schedule III
  - Examples: acetaminophen with alprazolam (Xanax), clonazepam (Klonopin), clorazepate (Tranxene T-Tab), diazepam (Valium), eszopiclone (Lunesta), lorazepam (Ativan), temazepam (Restoril), tramadol, triazolam (Halcion), and zolpidem (Ambien)
- Schedule V Controlled Substances
  - Have a low potential for abuse relative to substances listed in Schedule IV
  - Have a currently accepted medical use in treatment in the United States
  - Possibility of abuse leading to limited physical dependence or psychological dependence compared with Schedule IV substances
  - Are often classified as antitussives and antidiarrheals
  - Cough preparations not containing more than 200 mg of codeine per 100 mL or per 100 g
  - Examples: codeine/guaifenesin (Cheratussin AC), diphenoxylate/atropine (Lomotil), pregabalin (Lyrica)

Drug Enforcement Administration registration requirements

- Every pharmacy dispensing a controlled substance must be registered with the DEA and must have a state license. The DEA Form 224 must be completed and should be completed online but may be submitted using a paper version of the DEA Form 224 (Application for New Registration Under Controlled Substance Act of 1970) by writing to the DEA. Upon receipt of the completed DEA Form 224, a DEA Form 223 (Certificate of Registration) is issued to the pharmacy and must be kept on site at the pharmacy and available for inspection. A renewal of the pharmacy's registration must be completed every 3 years using a DEA Form 224a (Application for Renewal of Registration Under the Controlled Substance Act of 1970).
- A pharmacy may authorize one or more individuals to obtain and complete DEA Form 222 (US Official Order Form for Schedule I and II Controlled Substances) for the pharmacy by allowing them a power of attorney. The power of attorney must be signed by the registrant of the pharmacy and the individual to whom the power of attorney is being issued and by two witnesses. The power of attorney may be withdrawn at any time by the individual who signed the most current DEA registration or reregistration and two witnesses. The power of attorney must be kept with completed DEA Form 222.

Validating a Drug Enforcement Administration number

A practitioner's DEA may be verified by the pharmacy using the following link: https://apps.deadiversion.usdoj.gov/webforms2/spring/validationLogin?execution=e1s1. A DEA number can be validated manually by remembering the following:

- New DEA registration numbers issued before 1985 to physicians, dentists, veterinarians and other health care prescribers began with the letter A.
- New DEA registration numbers issued after 1985 began with either the letters B or F.
- A DEA number beginning with the letter M indicates the practitioner is a midlevel practitioner (physician assistant or nurse practitioner).
- Prescribers employed by a drug addiction treatment facility will have the letter X as the first letter of their DEA number.
- The letter G is assigned to prescribers under the Department of Defense.
- The second letter of the DEA registration number begins with the first letter of practitioner's last name.
- The first two letters are followed by a sequence of seven numbers. To determine if the DEA number is valid:
  - Add the first, third, and fifth numbers together.
  - Next add the second, fourth, and sixth numbers together. Multiply this sum by two.
  - Add the first and second set of numbers together. The number located in the one's column should be same as seventh number in the DEA number.
    - Example: What should the seventh number in Dr. Andrew Shed's DEA number be if his DEA number begins with BS452589?
      Add 4 + 2 + 8, which totals 14.
      Add 5 + 5 + 9, which totals 19; multiply 19 by 2 and the product is 38.
      Add 14 + 38, which totals 52. The last number should be a 2.
      A valid DEA number for Dr. Andrew Shed would be BS4525892.

Using a hospital's Drug Enforcement Administration number

Practitioners, such as interns, residents, staff physicians, or midlevel practitioners, may prescribe controlled substances using the hospital's DEA registration number under the following conditions:

- Dispensing, administering, or prescribing is a part of their professional practice.
- The practitioner is licensed by the state.
- The hospital has confirmed the practitioner is licensed to administer, dispense, or prescribe controlled substances within the state.
- The hospital approves the practitioner to administer, dispense, or prescribe under its controlled substance registration and designates an internal code number to the practitioner.

Drug Enforcement Administration physical inventories

- An "inventory" is a complete and accurate list of all stocks and forms of controlled substances in the possession of the pharmacy as determined by an actual physical count for Schedule II Controlled Substances. The pharmacy may make an estimated count of all Schedule III,

IV, or V substances for bottles containing less than 1000 tablets or capsules. An exact count must be made if the bottle contains more than 1000 tablets or capsules. All inventory counts of controlled substances must be retained at the pharmacy for a minimum of 2 years. Inventory records of Schedule II Controlled Substances must be kept separate from other pharmacy records, and Schedule III, IV, and V records must be kept separate from other pharmacy records and be easily retrieved.

Initial inventory

- When issued a DEA registration, the pharmacy must take an exact count of all controlled substances in the pharmacy during an initial inventory. Inventory information should include
  - The date of the inventory
  - Whether the inventory was taken at the beginning or close of business
  - The name of each controlled substance inventoried
  - The finished form of each of the substances (e.g., 100-mg tablet)
  - The number of dosage units or volume in the manufacturer's container
  - The number of manufacturer's container of each finished form (e.g., five 100-tablet bottles)
  - Total count of the substance
- The initial inventory does not need to be submitted to the DEA but needs to be maintained by the pharmacy.
- Best practices indicate that an initial inventory record contains the name, address, pharmacy address, and signature of the individual taking the inventory.

Biennial inventory

- Is taken at least every 2 years.
- The inventory contains the same information taken during an initial inventory:
  - The date of the inventory
  - Whether the inventory was taken at the beginning or close of business
  - The name of each controlled substance inventoried
  - The finished form of each of the substances (e.g., 100-mg tablet)
  - The number of dosage units or volume in the manufacturer's container
  - The number of manufacturer's container of each finished form (e.g., five 100-tablet bottles)
  - Total count of the substance
- Biennial inventory does not need to be submitted to the DEA but does need to be maintained by the pharmacy.

Newly scheduled controlled substance inventory

- When a noncontrolled substance has been reclassified as a controlled substance, the medication must be inventoried if in stock on its effective date as a controlled substance.

Inventory for damaged substances

- If a controlled substance is damaged, defective, or adulterated and is being held for quality control (QC) purposes, an inventory must be conducted. Inventory information to be maintained includes:
  - Name of substance

- Quantity of the substance to the nearest metric unit weight or total number units of the drug
- Reason for the medication to be maintained

Perpetual inventory

- A perpetual inventory indicates the actual quantity of a specific medication on hand at a specific time.

Federal Food, Drug, and Cosmetic Act (1938)

- FDA was created under the Federal Food, Drug, and Cosmetic Act (FDCA) of 1938
- Requires that all new drug applications be filed with the FDA
- Clearly defined adulteration and misbranding of drugs and food products
- Requires drug manufacturers to include package inserts

Adulteration

- Consisting "in whole or in part of any filthy, putrid, or decomposed substance"
- "Prepared, packed, or held under unsanitary conditions"
- Prepared in containers "composed, in whole or in part, of any poisonous or deleterious substance"
- Containing unsafe color additives
- Claimed to be or represented as drugs recognized "in an official compendium" but differing in strength, quality, or purity of the drugs

Misbranding

- Labeling that is "false or misleading in any particular way"
- Packaging that does not bear a label containing the name and place of business of the manufacturer, packer, or distributor or an accurate quantity of contents or is not conspicuously and clearly labeled with information required by the act
- Failure to carry a label indicating "Warning—May be habit forming" if the product is habit forming
- Failure to "bear the established name of the drug and in case it carries more than two or more active ingredients, the quantities of the ingredients, the amount of alcohol and also including—whether active or not—the established name and quantity of certain other substances described in the act"
- Failure to label "adequate directions for use" or "adequate warnings against use in certain pathological conditions"
- Products that are "dangerous to health when used in the dosage or manner or duration prescribed, recommended or suggested in the labeling"

Manufacturer drug labeling

- All drug manufacturer labeling must meet FDA requirements. Please note that manufacturer drug labeling is different than prescription drug labeling (community pharmacy), medication order labeling (hospital), and unit dose labeling. Labeling requirements include:
  - Name and place of business of manufacturer, packer, or distributor

- NDC number
- Adequate directions for use
- No misleading statements
- Statement of ingredients
- Prominence of required label statements
- Spanish language version of certain required statements
- Expiration date
- Manufacturer lot or control numbers
- Declaration of presence of FD&C Yellow No. 5 or FD&C Yellow No. 6 in certain drugs for human use
- Declaration of presence of phenylalanine as a component of aspartame in over-the-counter (OTC) and prescription drugs for human use
- Prescription drugs containing sulfites; required warning statements

Over-the-counter package labeling

The FDA requires the following on all OTC packages:

- Drug's name and place of business of manufacturer, packer, or distributor of drugs and devices
- NDC number
- Active ingredient
- Established name of a drug
- Inactive ingredient
- Content requirements
- "Purpose" or "Purposes" followed by the general pharmacologic category(ies) or the principal intended action(s) of the drug or, when the drug consists of more than one ingredient, the general pharmacologic categories or the principal intended actions of each active ingredient
- "Use" or "Uses," followed by the indication(s)
- "Warning" or "Warnings" and "Do not use," followed by all contraindications for use with the product. These include:
  - "Ask a doctor before use if you have" (a particular condition)
  - "Ask a doctor or pharmacist before use if you are" (taking specific medications)
  - "When using this product" followed by the side effects that the consumer may experience
  - "Stop use and ask a doctor if" followed by any signs of toxicity or other reactions that would necessitate immediately discontinuing use of the product, including a pregnancy and breastfeeding warning
  - "Keep out of reach of children" warning, and an accidental overdose or ingestion warning
  - "Directions" followed by the directions for use
  - "Inactive ingredients" followed by a listing of the established name of each inactive ingredient
  - "Questions?" or "Questions or comments?" followed by the telephone number of the manufacturer to answer questions about the product

Drug Quality and Security Act

Title I Compounding Quality Act

- Enhanced compounding drug oversight
- Created a new entity known as an "outsourcing facility," which is larger than a traditional compounding pharmacy

and supplies compounds to hospitals and other health care facilities

- Exempts compounds from the drug approval provisions of the FDCA
- Provides guidelines for labeling, and does not require that a compounding facility meet the current Good Manufacturing Practices
- Established penalties various activities related to compounded medication to include selling compounded medications marked "not for resale"
- Sets up a system for easier communication between the FDA and state pharmacy boards on drug compounding
- Prevents compounding pharmacies from making copies of any commercial drugs or any drugs the FDA has removed from the market for safety or efficacy purpose

Title II Drug Supply Chain Security Act

The Drug Supply Chain Security Act outlines critical steps to build an electronic, interoperable system to identify and trace certain prescription drugs as they are distributed in the United States. The goals of the system will:

- Allow verification of the authenticity of the drug product identifier down to the package level
- Improve detection and notification of illegitimate products in the drug supply chain
- Make possible more well-organized recalls of drug products

Key provisions of the Drug Supply Chain Security Act

- Manufacturers and repackagers will be required to put a unique product identifier on certain prescription drug packages, such as a barcode that can be easily read electronically.
- Manufacturers, wholesaler drug distributors, repackagers, and dispensers in the drug supply chain must provide information about a drug and who handled it each time it is sold in the US market.
- Manufacturers, wholesaler drug distributors, repackagers, and dispensers will be required to develop systems and processes to be able to verify the product identifier on certain prescription drug packages.
- Manufacturers, wholesaler drug distributors, repackagers, and dispensers will be required to isolate and promptly investigate a drug that has been identified as suspect (counterfeit, unapproved, or potentially dangerous).
- Manufacturers, wholesaler drug distributors, repackagers, and dispensers to establish systems and processes must notify the FDA if an illegitimate drug is found.
- Wholesale drug distributors must report their licensing status and contact information to the FDA that will be available on a database.
- Third-party logistics providers, those who provide storage and logistical operations related to drug distribution, must obtain a state or federal license.

Accreditation Standards

Accreditation is the external recognition of an institution's adherence to a set of standards to obtain a certain status.

Types of accreditation

- Utilization Review Accreditation Commission
  - The Utilization Review Accreditation Commission (URAC) Standards address risk management, consumer protection and empowerment, operations and infrastructure, performance monitoring and improvement, pharmacy dispensing, pharmacy product handing and security, patient service and communication, and reporting performance measures to URAC.
  - Accreditation is available in the following areas:
    - Specialty Pharmacy Accreditation
    - Mail Order Service Pharmacy Accreditation
    - Pharmacy Services Accreditation
    - Rare Disease Designation
    - Specialty Pharmacy Services Accreditation
    - Specialty Pharmacy Accreditation for Small Business
    - Mail Service Pharmacy Accreditation for Small Business
    - Infusion Pharmacy Accreditation
    - Medicare Home Infusion Therapy Supplier Accreditation
    - Pharmacy Benefit Management Accreditation
    - Opioid Stewardship Designation
- Accreditation Commission for Health Care
  - Accreditation is available in the following settings:
    - Acute Inspection Service
    - Compounding Pharmacy Accreditation
    - Durable Medical Equipment, Prosthetics, Orthotics, and Supplies
- Center for Pharmacy Practice Accreditation
  - Accredits outpatient pharmacy practices in community, hospitals, health systems, and clinics
  - Address practice management, patient care services, and quality improvement
- Joint Commission
  - Accredits and certifies hospitals and health care organizations that provide ambulatory and office-based surgery, behavioral health, home health care, laboratory, and nursing care center services
  - Accreditation evaluates the pharmacy's
    - Controlled substance security and diversion mitigation
    - High-risk medication processes
      - Sterile compounding and USP 797 compliance
      - Chemotherapy safety
      - Pediatric medication processes
    - HD management and USP readiness
    - Alignment with Joint Commission requirements for Complex Medication Orders
    - Medication-related technologies including computerized order entry, barcode medication administration, smart pump technology, and in-pharmacy technology
    - Specialty pharmacy and home infusion pharmacy under the home care accreditation
  - Has been granted "deemed" status for participation in Medicare (This status states that the institution has met the Medicare Conditions of Participation and is eligible for Medicare funding. The institution does not need to meet the requirements for annual Medicare surveys by state inspectors.)
  - Provides certification for disease-specific and advanced disease-specific care, palliative care and home care staffing
  - Establishes national patient safety goals and universal protocols for those accredited or certified
  - Addresses health care associated infections, infection control, and patient safety concerns to include medication errors

Elements of accreditation

- Elements of pharmacy accreditation include:
  - Policies and procedures
  - Training and documentation
  - Clinical patient management program
  - Marketing materials
  - Call center
  - Quality management program and evaluation tool

Reasons for accreditation

- Demonstrates to stakeholders that the pharmacy meets high standards that permit patients to receive specific treatments
- Increases public health by expanding the level of patient care services
- Enables high quality of all services provided to patients, as well as safe and effective dispensing services
- Requires pharmacy to utilize patient data to improve care, medication, and care delivery
- Provides the pharmacy the opportunity to obtain recognition by adhering to agency standards
- Meet payor requirements for financial reimbursement

Legal requirements and practice standards

Regulatory and accreditation-related terminology

- A statute is a written law passed by a legislature on the state or federal level. Statutes set forth general propositions of law that courts apply to specific situations. A statute may forbid a certain act, direct a certain act, make a declaration, or set forth governmental mechanisms to aid society. A statute is also known as an act.
- A law is a system of rules that are created and are enforceable by social or governmental institutions to regulate behavior.
- A regulation is a rule and administrative code issued by governmental agencies at all levels, municipal, county, state and federal. For example, state boards of pharmacy issue regulations, which affect the practice of pharmacy within the state.
- A standard is established by authority, custom, or general consent as a model, example, or point of reference. For

example, the US Pharmacopoeia has established standards for nonsterile compounding USP <795>, sterile compounding USP <797>, and HDs USP <800>.

- A code is a collection of laws, rules, or regulations that are systematically arranged.
- A certification is a legal document certifying that an individual meets certain objective standards usually provided by a neutral professional organization. For example, pharmacy technicians may be certified by the Pharmacy Technician Certification Board (PTCB) or National Healthcareer Association (NHA).
- A certificate is a document attesting a level of achievement in a course of study or training.
- Licensure is the granting of a license to practice a profession. For example, pharmacists are licensed to practice pharmacy.
- Registration is the action or process of registering or of being registered. An example of registration would be requiring pharmacy technicians to be registered with the state board of pharmacy.
- Reciprocation is a mutual agreement between two US states whereby each agrees to grant a license to practice pharmacy to any individual licensee by the other state.

Basic principles that serve as the foundation for pharmacy laws and pharmacy ethics

Pure Food and Drug Act of 1906

- Regulated the development, compounding, distribution, storage, and dispensing of drugs
- Prohibited the interstate transportation of adulterated and misbranded drugs and food

Durham-Humphrey Amendment to Federal Food, Drug, and Cosmetic Act of 1951

- Distinguished legend and nonlegend drugs
- Required legend drugs to bear the federal legend "Federal law prohibits dispensing without a prescription"
- Required all prescriptions to have adequate directions for use
- OTC label required to have a listing of all ingredients

Kefauver-Harris Amendment to Federal Food, Drug, and Cosmetic Act of 1962

- Required all drugs be safe and effective
- All pharmaceutical manufacturers to file an Investigational New Drug Application (INDA) prior to starting clinical trials on human beings
- Drug manufacturers follow good manufacturing practices

Drug Listing Act of 1972

- Each medication is assigned an 11-digit number known as a National Drug Code (NDC).
- The NDC consists three sets of numbers whereby the first five numbers indicate the drug manufacturer, the next four numbers indicate the drug entity, and the last two numbers indicate the medication packaging.

Prescription Drug Marketing Act of 1987

- Prohibits the reimportation of a drug into the United States other than the drug manufacturer
- Forbids the sale or distribution of samples to anyone other than those licensed to prescribe medications
- Requires veterinarian medication to bear the following labeling "Caution: Federal law restricts this drug to use by or on the order of a licensed veterinarian"

Anabolic Steroid Control Act of 1990

- Reclassified anabolic steroids as Schedule III Controlled Substance

Dietary Supplement Health and Education Act of 1994

- Classified herbal supplements as a food product not a drug product
- Prohibited manufacturers from making claims that the supplement treats or cures a specific condition

Medicare Modernization Act of 2003

- Provided a voluntary prescription drug benefit to Medicare beneficiaries
- Added preventive medical benefits to Medicare beneficiaries
- Changed the way Medicare pays for outpatient Part B medications
- Permitted Medicare Part D beneficiaries to enroll in either regional or national insurance plans
- Created health saving accounts
- Provided medication therapy management for Medicare beneficiaries
- Permitted pharmacists to be reimbursed for medication counseling and medication therapy management

FDA Modernization Act of 2003

- Changed federal legend to "Rx" only

Patient Protection and Affordable Care Act (2010)

- Mandated universal health care coverage for US citizens
- Established health insurance exchanges
- Provided catastrophic coverage for high-cost illnesses
- Prohibited insurers from refusing coverage to individuals with preexisting conditions

Pharmacy ethics

Ethics are defined as a study of standards and moral judgment; it is a moral philosophy that is influenced by a particular group, society, philosophy, religion, or profession. According to *Remington: The Science and Practice of Pharmacy*, 23rd edition, 2020 ethics and laws are related in that both share the social purpose of encouraging the right conduct. Whereas laws are enacted by the government to achieve a goal, ethics are embraced by a profession without the involvement of government.

American Pharmacists Association Code of Ethics for Pharmacists

Preamble

Pharmacists are health professionals who assist individuals in making the best use of medications. This Code, prepared and supported by pharmacists, is intended to state publicly the principles that form the fundamental basis of the roles and responsibilities of pharmacists. These principles, based on moral obligations and virtues, are established to guide pharmacists in relationships with patients, health professionals, and society.

Principles

1. A pharmacist respects the covenantal relationship between the patient and pharmacist.
2. A pharmacist promotes the good of every patient in a caring, compassionate and confidential manner.
3. A pharmacist respects the autonomy and dignity of each patient.
4. A pharmacist acts with honesty and integrity in professional relationships.
5. A pharmacist maintains professional competence.
6. A pharmacist respects the values and abilities of colleagues and other health professionals.
7. A pharmacist serves individual, community and societal needs.
8. A pharmacist seeks justice in the distribution of health resources.[1]

American Association of Pharmacy Technicians Code of Ethics

Preamble

Pharmacy technicians are health care professionals who assist pharmacists in providing the best possible care for patients. The principles of this code, which apply to pharmacy technicians working in any and all settings, are based on the application and support of the moral obligations that guide the pharmacy profession in relationships with patients, health care professionals, and society.

Principles

A. A pharmacy technician's first consideration is to ensure the health and safety of the patient and to use knowledge and skills to the best of his/her ability in serving others.
B. A pharmacy technician supports and promotes honesty and integrity in the profession, which includes a duty to observe the law, maintain the highest moral and ethical conduct at all times, and uphold the ethical principles of the profession.
C. A pharmacy technician assists and supports the pharmacist in the safe, efficacious, and cost-effective distribution of health services and health care resources.
D. A pharmacy technician respects and values the abilities of pharmacists, colleagues, and other health care professionals.
E. A pharmacy technician maintains competency in his/her practice and continually enhances his/her professional knowledge and expertise.
F. A pharmacy technician respects and supports the patient's individuality, dignity, and confidentiality.
G. A pharmacy technician respects the confidentiality of a patient's records and discloses pertinent information only with proper authorization.
H. A pharmacy technician never assists in the dispensing, promoting, or distribution of medications or medical devices that are not of good quality or do not meet the standards required by law.
I. A pharmacy technician does not engage in any activity that will discredit the profession, and will expose, without fear or favor, illegal or unethical conduct in the profession.
J. A pharmacy technician associates with and engages in the support of organizations that promote the profession of pharmacy through the utilization and enhancement of pharmacy technicians.[2]

Federal requirements (e.g., Drug Enforcement Administration, FDA) for controlled substances

Receiving controlled substances

- All receipts (invoice or packing slip) for controlled substances must indicate the date the medications were received and contain the signature of the individual receiving it.
- Receipts must indicate:
  - Name of substance
  - Each finished form
  - Number of units of finished form
- Receipts must be maintained separately from other records but readily retrievable

Storing controlled substances

- Schedule II, III, IV, and V Controlled Substances maybe store in a locked cabinet or disperse among noncontrolled medications.

Ordering controlled substances

DEA Form 222

Schedule I and II Controlled Substances may be ordered by using a DEA Form 222. Effective October 31, 2021, the DEA Form 222 will be to is single sheet format instead of a triplicate form. A DEA Form 222 is required for each distribution or transfer of a Schedule I or Schedule II Controlled Substance. The pharmacy will request the DEA provide a limited number of DEA Form 222 to the pharmacy based upon the pharmacy's business activity. A DEA Form 222 contains an order form number; the name, address, and registration number of the pharmacy; and the schedules the pharmacy is authorized to dispense.

When completing a DEA Form 222, the purchaser must:

- Use a typewriter, computer printer, pen or indelible pencil
- Only enter one item on each number line
- Indicate the number of lines completed at the bottom of the form in its respective box

- Enter the name and address for whom the controlled substances are being ordered must be on the DEA form
- Make a copy of the DEA form and submit the original to the supplier
- Be signed and dated by the individual who is authorized a registration application or have power of attorney

In addition, the purchaser must:

- Upon receipt of the ordered medications indicate the number of containers for each medication and the date they were received
- Maintain a copy of the completed DEA form for a minimum of 2 years
- Keep any defective DEA forms for a minimum of 2 years
- Retain all DEA Forms 222 separate from other pharmacy records

Electronic copies of DEA Form 222 do not need to be stored on a different server.

A supplier of controlled substances may decline to honor a DEA Form 222 if the order is not complete, legible, or properly prepared, executed, or endorsed. If the Form 222 shows any alteration, erasure, or change of any description, it should not be accepted. If for any reason the order cannot be filled, then the original DEA Form 222 must be returned to the purchaser with a reason for its return. A defective DEA Form 222 can be amended but a new DEA Form 222 must be issued in its place. In situations where a DEA Form 222 has been lost, the pharmacy must complete a new DEA Form 222 and provide a statement that the DEA Form 222 has been lost. If a pharmacy determines that a DEA Form 222 has been stolen, it must be promptly reported to the local DEA Diversion Field Office and the serial number(s) of the stolen form(s) provided.

Drug Enforcement Administration Controlled Substance Ordering System

The Controlled Substance Ordering System (CSOS) is another method by which Schedule II Controlled Substances can be ordered. The CSOS allows secure electronic ordering of controlled substances without using a paper DEA Form 222. Using the CSOS, a pharmacy is able to order Schedule II medications from controlled substance manufacturers, distributors, and pharmacies. Advantages of the CSOS include

- Does not have a maximum number of line items per order
- CSOS certificates including the same identification information as is found on a paper DEA Form 222, resulting in timely and accurate authentication by the supplier
- Allows just-in-time ordering resulting in smaller pharmacy inventories
- Reduces the number of ordering errors resulting in more accurate orders
- Lowers transaction costs for the pharmacy due to order accuracy and decreases paperwork

A certificate will be canceled if the certificate holder is no longer permitted to sign Schedule II orders.
Electronic orders for controlled substances will not be filled if:

- The required data fields have not been filled in properly.
- The order is not signed using a digital certificate issued by DEA.
- The digital certificate used has ended or been canceled prior to signature.

- The purchaser's public key will not authorize the digital certificate.
- The order is invalid for any reason.

A supplier must notify the purchaser and provide an explanation for not filling the order. Neither the purchaser nor supplier cannot correct an electronic order for controlled substances, but a new order must be provided by the purchaser.

Labeling controlled substances

Prescription labels must contain the following information:

- Date of filling
- Pharmacy name and address
- Serial (prescription) number
- Patient name
- Prescribing practitioner name
- Directions for use
- Cautionary statements
- "CAUTION: Federal law prohibits the transfer of this drug to any person other than the patient for whom it was prescribed"

Dispensing controlled substances
Schedule II Controlled Substances

- Schedule II prescriptions may be sent electronically from the prescriber's office, or they can be handwritten or computer generated but must be signed in ink by the physician with no allowable refills.
- A partial filling of a Schedule II medication is allowed if the remaining quantity is available to the patient within 72 hours.
- A new prescription must be issued by the prescriber if additional quantities are to be provided after 72 hours.
- The pharmacist should notify the physician if the balance cannot be provided to the patient.

Emergency filling of Schedule II drug prescriptions

An emergency oral prescription for a Schedule II medication can be issued to a pharmacy under the following conditions:

- Pharmacist must make a good faith attempt to identify the physician.
- Prescription is limited to a quantity to treat the patient during this emergency period.
- Pharmacist must reduce order to writing.
- Physician must write a prescription for this emergency quantity, and the pharmacy must receive it within 7 days of the oral order.
- If the pharmacy does not receive the written prescription, the DEA must be notified immediately.

Issuance of multiple prescriptions for Schedule II medications

A prescriber of controlled substances may issue multiple prescriptions authorizing the patient to receive a total of up to a 90-day supply of a Schedule II Controlled Substance if the following conditions are met:

- Each prescription must be issued on a separate prescription blank.

- Each separate prescription must be issued for a legitimate medical purpose by an individual practitioner acting in the usual course of professional practice.
- The individual practitioner must provide written instructions on each prescription (other than the first prescription if the prescribing practitioner intends for that prescription to be filled immediately) indicating the earliest date on which a pharmacy may fill each prescription.
- The individual practitioner concludes that providing the patient with multiple prescriptions in this manner does not create an undue risk of diversion or abuse.
- The issuance of multiple prescriptions is permitted under applicable state laws.

Schedule III–V Controlled Substances

- Schedule III–V prescriptions may be sent electronically from the prescriber's office or they can be handwritten or computer generated by a physician's office, but they must be signed by the physician in ink.
- The physician's office may telephone a Schedule III–V prescription in to the pharmacy or may fax one, depending on state law.
- Partial fillings are permitted if refills are indicated on the original prescription, refills do not exceed the total quantity prescribed by the physician, and no partial filling occurs after 6 months of the original date of the prescription.
- A prescriber may permit a maximum of five refills for a Schedule III-V prescriptions and m,ust be filled within six months of being issued.

Exempt narcotics (select Schedule V medications)

- Select cough and antidiarrheal prescription items can be purchased by an individual if permitted by state law.
- The quantity dispensed must be in the original manufacturer's container and must not exceed the quantity established by law.
- The purchaser must be at least 18 years of age and must complete the exempt narcotic book with the following information: date purchased, name of purchaser, address of purchaser, name of product and quantity purchased, price of transaction, and pharmacist's signature.
- There is a limit of one container in a 48-hour period.

Facsimile prescriptions

- A faxed prescription for a Schedule II drug is permissible, but the pharmacy must have the original prescription prior to dispensing the medication.
- A faxed prescription for a Schedule III, IV, or V drug may serve as the original prescription. The following situations are exceptions:
  - A narcotic Schedule II substance that is to be compounded for direct administration to a patient by parenteral, IV, intramuscular, subcutaneous, or intraspinal infusion is an exception.
  - A Schedule II substance for a resident of a LTC facility is an exception.
  - A practitioner prescribing a Schedule II narcotic substance for a patient in hospice care, as certified by Medicare under Title XVIII or licensed by the state, may transmit a prescription to the dispensing pharmacy by fax regardless of whether the patient resides in a hospice facility or other care setting. The practitioner's agent may also transmit the prescription to the pharmacy. The practitioner will note on the prescription that it is for a hospice patient

Reverse distribution

- A pharmacy may transfer controlled substances to a DEA-registered reverse distributor who handles the disposal of controlled substances.
- A reverse distributor must issue an official order form (DEA Form 222) or the electronic equivalent to the pharmacy when a pharmacy transfers Schedule II Controlled Substances to a reverse distributor.
- A pharmacy must maintain a record of Schedule III–V Controlled Substances transferred to a reverse distributor. The record must contain the drug name, dosage form, drug strength, quantity, and date transferred.
- A reverse distributor must submit a DEA Form 41 to the DEA when the controlled substances have been destroyed.

Take back programs of controlled substances

- The National Prescription Drug Take Back Day aims to provide a safe, convenient, and responsible means of disposing of prescription drugs, while also educating the general public about the potential for abuse of medications.
- Some facilities are registered with the DEA to collect unused or expired medications. Locations accepting controlled substance can be identified by accessing the following website https://apps.deadiversion.usdoj.gov/pubdispsearch/spring/main?execution=e1s1.

Loss or theft of controlled substances
Drug Enforcement Administration Form 106

The DEA Diversion Drug Theft Loss system has been replaced by the Theft Loss Reporting system. The Theft Loss Reporting system provides the means for a registrant to submit a Form 106 and/or a Form 107. The Theft Loss Reporting system automatically determines which form(s) need to be produced and submitted depending on the type of registrant and the data entered. The Diversion Drug Theft Loss system is used to electronically submit a DEA Form 106 (Report of Theft or Loss of Controlled Substances) and DEA Form 107 (Report of Theft or Loss of Listed Chemicals).

The DEA Form 106 (Report of Theft or Loss of Controlled Substances) is used in conveying the theft or loss of controlled substances, mail-back packages, and/or inner liners. A pharmacy must notify the area DEA in writing within 1 day of discovering the theft or significant loss of controlled substances by submitting a DEA Form 106 electronically. Information to be submitted on a DEA Form 106 includes:

- DEA registration number
- Name of business
- Address
- City, state, and zip code
- Point of contact
- Date of theft or loss
- Number of thefts and losses within the past 24 months
- Principal business of registrant
- Type of theft or loss (break-in/burglary, employee theft, hijacking of transport vehicle, packaging discrepancy, robbery, customer theft, loss in transit, or disaster)

- Theft reported to police to include responding officer's name and police report number
- Corrective measures take to prevent future thefts or losses
- Listing and quantity of controlled substances lost or stolen

  The DEA Form 106 must be maintained for 2 years.

Loss or theft of chemicals
Drug Enforcement Administration Form 107

The DEA Form 107 (Report of Theft or Loss of Listed Chemicals) is used to report any theft or loss of listed chemicals. The DEA has issued two lists of chemical, which are classified as List I and List II. List I and II chemicals are precursors in the manufacture of controlled substances. Examples of List I chemicals include ephedrine, ergocristine, ergotamine, and phenylpropanolamine. Acetone, benzyl chloride, ethyl ether, and potassium permanganate are examples of List II chemicals. DEA Form 107 should only be used for reporting any theft or loss of listed chemicals. When completing a DEA Form 107, the following information is required:

- The pharmacy's DEA number and your last name or the business name you used to register for DEA number are required.
- CMEA registrants are compelled to provide the certificate ID number and the business name used to certify with the DEA.
- Background information regarding the loss or theft incident is required, to include the date and place, the type (night break-in, armed robbery, etc.), and the estimated value of the substances stolen.
- NDC or chemical and quantity of the controlled substance being reported as a theft or loss is required. Quantity should be reported in milligrams, kilograms, milliliters, tablets, or capsules.
- DEA Form 107 is submitted electronically to the DEA. A copy of the DEA-107 must be maintained by the pharmacy for a minimum of 2 years.

Federal requirements for handling and disposing of hazardous drugs
Handling of hazardous drugs

- Wear personal protective equipment when manipulating HDs.
- Utilize appropriate primary and secondary equipment controls.
- Clearly label all HDs.
- Use liquid formulations, when possible, to avoid crushing tablets or opening capsules.
- Avoid cutting, crushing, or otherwise manipulating pills or capsules since powder may be produced and contaminate the work area.
- Automated counting machines should not be used with HDs since powder may be produced and contaminate the work area.

Disposal of hazardous drugs

- Use thick, leak-proof plastic bags, colored differently from other facility trash bags, for disposal of discarded gloves, gowns, and other related disposable material and labeled as "Hazardous Drug-Related Wastes."
- Keep the waste bag inside a covered waste container clearly labeled "Hazardous Drug Waste Only." Do not move waste from one area to another. Seal the bag when filled and tape the covered waste container.
- Label needle and sharps containers in the pharmacy unit as "Hazardous Drug Waste Only."
- Dispose of HD-related wastes according to federal (e.g., EPA), state, and local regulations for hazardous waste.
- Use either an incinerator or a licensed sanitary landfill for toxic wastes as appropriate to dispose of this waste.

Federal requirements for restricted drug programs and related medication processing
Restricted drug programs
Pseudoephedrine

The CMEA established conditions to be followed in selling of Scheduled Listed Chemical Product (SLCP). An SLCP is any product that contains ephedrine, pseudoephedrine, or phenylpropanolamine and is marketed as a nonprescription (OTC) medication in the United States.

Requirements of the Combat Methamphetamine Epidemic Act of 2005

- SLCPs are to be placed behind the counter or in locked cabinets.
- Purchaser's identity must be checked.
- A log (paper or electronic) must be maintained of all purchasers of SLCPs. The log requires
  - Purchaser's name and complete address
  - Purchaser's signature
  - Product sold
  - Quantity sold
  - Date and time
- The purchaser must provide approved federal or state photo identification. Approved federal government identification includes:
  - US passport
  - US Armed Forces military identification card
  - Foreign passport with a temporary I-551 stamp
- Individuals 18 years of age or older may provide the following:
  - Driver's license or identification card with a photograph
  - School identification card with a photograph
  - Voter's registration card
  - US military card
  - Military dependent's identification card
  - Native American tribal documents
- The logbook must be maintained for 2 years.

Other Scheduled Listed Chemical Product requirements

- Pharmacy must train all employees selling SLCPs on CMEA requirements and indicate training has occurred.
- A maximum of 3.6 g of the chemical can be sold in 1 day.
- Product packaging is limited to blister packs with no more than two dosage units per blister.
- The maximum amount that can be purchased in 30 days is 9 g, of which no more than 7.5 g can be imported by private or commercial carrier or US Postal service.
- Annual self-certification of all sellers of SLCPs must take place, which indicates the seller is stating that:
  - All employees have received SLCP training.
  - Training records are maintained.
  - Sales of SLCPs do not exceed 3.6 g per day to purchaser.
  - SLCPs are stored behind the counter or in a locked cabinet.
  - Maintaining a written or electronic logbook.

Isotretinoin

Isotretinoin is a very powerful medication indicated in treating acne. Isotretinoin has been found to cause severe birth defects, induce spontaneous abortions, and produce adverse psychiatric effects, including depression, psychosis, suicidal ideation, suicide attempts, and suicide. The Isotretinoin Safety and Risk Management Act was enacted, resulting in the following:

- Requiring all patients receiving isotretinoin prescriptions, practitioners prescribing isotretinoin, and pharmacists dispensing isotretinoin to be enrolled in a mandatory registry
- Mandating all practitioners and pharmacists to receive education regarding the risks associated with isotretinoin, including birth defects and mental health risks
- Requiring isotretinoin to be only prescribed only for severe recalcitrant nodular acne
- Mandating monthly education of patients, both male and female, regarding the need to avoid pregnancy, as well as completion of a survey to warn the patient of the adverse side effects (Patient visits include one-on-one counselling, and patients or parents must sign an informed consent form.)
- Requiring certification of medical offices and clinics as treatment centers
- Prohibiting Internet, telephone, or mail order prescriptions of isotretinoin prescriptions from being filled
- Limiting isotretinoin prescriptions to only a 30-day supply with no refills
- Requiring all female patients undergo monthly pregnancy testing and providing documentation of a negative pregnancy test result before a prescription is renewed
- Requiring blood testing during treatment and 30 days after treatment
- Evaluating all treatment centers on a yearly basis to ensure compliance with the program
- Requiring prescribers to provide mandatory quarterly reporting of all adverse reactions and mandatory reporting within 15 days of all patient deaths associated with the drug

Clozapine

- The Clozaril National Registry was developed in response to an FDA mandate to ensure the safety of patients treated with clozapine (Clozaril), which has potentially dangerous side effects if not strictly monitored.
- The program must provide dedicated 800 numbers for internal clients, consumers, and health care professionals to call for information, education, and patient enrolment.
- The Clozaril Administration Registry Enrolment (CARE) is a secured Internet application that facilitates the reporting of white blood cell values and absolute neutrophil counts of patients taking brand clozapine (Clozaril) to the Clozaril National Registry.
- CARE is designed to safeguard patient information, protect patients' privacy, and assist physicians and pharmacists with effective monitoring functionalities.
- Clozaril is only available through a strict monitoring and distribution system to detect the early onset of agranulocytosis. With proper white blood cell and absolute neutrophil counts monitoring and reporting, Clozaril-induced agranulocytosis can be reversible if detected early.
- Prescribers and pharmacies must be registered before they can treat patients with Clozaril. CARE is designed and developed to streamline this process.
- Approved generic manufacturers of clozapine must have established similar programs to comply with the FDA mandate.

Thalidomide

- Thalidomide is indicated for multiple myeloma.
- Thalidomide must not be taken by women who are pregnant or who could become pregnant while taking this medication. A single dose of thalidomide taken during pregnancy can cause severe birth defects (physical problems present in the baby at birth) or death of the unborn baby.
- System for Thalidomide Education and Prescribing Safety (STEPS) is a program approved by the FDA to ensure pregnant women do not take thalidomide and that women do not become pregnant while taking thalidomide. All patients who are prescribed thalidomide, including men and women who cannot become pregnant, must register with STEPS. They can only receive a thalidomide prescription from a doctor who is registered with STEPS. The prescription can only be filled at a pharmacy that is registered with STEPS to receive this medication.
- Patients must see their doctors every month during their treatment to discuss their condition and any side effects they may be experiencing. During the patient's visit, the doctor may provide a prescription for up to a 28-day supply of medication with no refills. The patient must have this prescription filled within 7 days.
- Patients are prohibited from donating blood while being prescribed thalidomide.
- If a woman is taking thalidomide and can become pregnant, she will need to meet certain requirements during her treatment. A woman will need to meet these requirements even if she has a history of not being able to become pregnant. A woman may be excused

from meeting these requirements only if she has not had a period for 24 months in a row or if she has had a hysterectomy.

- A woman must use two acceptable forms of birth control for 4 weeks before beginning to take thalidomide, during treatment, and for 4 weeks after treatment. The patient's doctor will inform her about which forms of birth control are acceptable. A woman must always use two forms of birth control unless she can guarantee that she will not have any sexual contact with a man for 4 weeks before, during, and for 4 weeks after treatment.
- A woman must have a negative pregnancy test result within the 24 hours before beginning treatment with thalidomide. In addition, she will also need to be tested for pregnancy in a laboratory weekly during the first 4 weeks of the treatment and then once every 4 weeks if she has regular menstrual cycles or once every 2 weeks if she has irregular menstrual cycles.
- A woman should stop taking thalidomide and contact her physician immediately if she thinks she is pregnant; has a late, irregular, or missed menstrual period; experiences any change in menstrual bleeding; or has sex without using two forms of birth control. If a woman becomes pregnant during treatment, the physician is required to call the FDA and the manufacturer.
- If a man is prescribed thalidomide, he must be aware that thalidomide is present in his semen and must either use a latex condom or completely avoid any sexual contact with a woman who is pregnant or may become pregnant while taking this medication and for 4 weeks after treatment. Although a man may have had a vasectomy, this is still required. The man must notify his physician immediately if he has had unprotected sex with a woman who can become pregnant or if he thinks for any reason that his partner is pregnant. A man should not donate semen or sperm while taking thalidomide.

Risk Evaluation and Mitigation Strategies

REMSs are required risk management plans that utilize risk minimization strategies. REMSs ensure that the benefits of certain prescription drugs outweigh their risks as authorized by the Food and Drug Administration Amendments Act of 2007.

Risk evaluation and mitigation strategy key points

- FDA can require a REMS if the agency determines that safety measures are needed beyond the professional labeling to ensure that a drug's benefits outweigh its risks.
- Drug sponsors are responsible for developing REMS programs, and it is the FDA's responsibility to review and approve REMS programs.
- FDA can require a REMS before or after a drug is approved.
- REMS can be required for a single drug or a class of drugs.
- Each REMS has specific safety measures unique to the safety risks associated with a particular drug or class of drugs (i.e., no two REMS are exactly alike).

- Health care professionals and distributors may need to follow specific safety procedures prior to prescribing, shipping, or dispensing the drug.
- A REMS for a New Drug Application or Biologic License Application may also contain any of the following elements:
  - Medication guide or PPI
  - Communication plan
  - Elements to assure safe use
  - Implementation system

Medication guides

Medication guides are paper handouts that come with many prescription medicines. The guides address issues that are specific to a specific drug or drug classes. They contain FDA-approved information that can help patients avoid serious adverse events. The FDA requires that medication guides be issued with specific prescribed drugs and biological products when the agency determines that:

- Certain information is necessary to prevent serious adverse effects,
- Patient decision making should be informed by information about a known serious side effect with a product, or
- Patient adherence to directions for the use of a product are essential to its effectiveness.

A medication guide must be provided to the patient or the patient's agent:

- When the patient or the patient's agent requests a medication guide
- When a drug is dispensed in an outpatient setting (e.g., retail pharmacy, hospital ambulatory care pharmacy), and the product will then be used by the patient without direct supervision by a health care professional
- The first time a drug is dispensed to a health care professional for administration to a patient in an outpatient setting, such as in a clinic or dialysis or infusion center
- The first time a drug is dispensed in an outpatient setting of any kind, after a medication guide is changed (e.g., after addition of a new indication, new safety information)
- When a drug is subject to a REMS that includes specific requirements for reviewing or providing a medication guide as part of an element to assure safe use (possibly in conjunction with distribution), the medication guide must be provided in accordance with the terms of the REMS

Examples of medications requiring a medication guide be provided to the patient include:		
Aripiprazole (Abilify)	Canagliflozin (Prozac)	Fluoxetine (Prozac)
Isotretinoin (Absorica)	Warfarin (Jantoven)	Mirtazapine (Remeron)
Rabeprazole (Aciphex)	Metformin/sita-gliptin (Janumet)	Ramelteon (Rozerem)
Risedronate (Actonel)	Sitagliptin (Januvia)	Salmeterol (Serevent Diskus)
Metformin/pioglita-zone (Actoplus Met)	Lopinavir/ritonavir (Kaletra)	Quetiapine (Seroquel XR)

Examples of medications requiring a medication guide be provided to the patient include:—cont'd		
Dextroamphetamine/ amphetamine (Adderall XR)	Lamotrigine (Lamictal)	Atomoxetine (Strattera)
Fluticasone/salme- terol (Advair HFA or Diskus)	Lurasidone (Latuda)	Carbamazepine (Tegretol)
Zolpidem (Ambien)	Escitalopram (Lexapro)	Topiramate (Topamax)
Metformin/rosiglita- zone (Avandamet)	Pregabalin (Lyrica)	Linagliptin (Tradjenta)
Ibandronate (Boniva)	Dronedarone (Multaq)	Emtricitabine and tenofovir (Truvada)
Exenatide (Byetta)	Primidone (Mysoline)	Venlafaxine (Effexor XR)
Celecoxib (Celebrex)	Naproxen (Naprosyn)	Vilazodone (Viibryd)
Ciprofloxacin (Cipro)	Gabapentin (Neurontin)	Bupropion (Wellbutrin XL)
Methylphenidate (Concerta)	Esomeprazole (Nexium)	Rivaroxaban (Xarelto)
Duloxetine hydro- chloride (Cymbalta)	Saxagliptin (Onglyza)	Tofacitinib (Xeljanz)
Divalproex (Depakote ER)	Amiodarone (Pacerone)	Sertraline (Zoloft)
Dexlansoprazole (Dexilant)	Paroxetine (Paxil)	
Dexmethylphenidate (Focalin XR)	Dabigatran (Pradaxa)	
Alendronate (Fosamax)	Lansoprazole (Prevacid)	

A complete listing of medications requiring medication guides can be found at http://www.fda.gov/Drugs/DrugSafety/ucm085729.htm.

Communication plan

- A communication plan educates, informs, and raises awareness of risk to health care providers.

Elements to assure safe use

Elements to assure safe use (EASU) are required medical interventions or other actions health care professionals need to execute prior to prescribing or dispensing the drug to the patient. Some actions may also be required for the patient to continue treatment. A REMS may require any or all the following:

- Pharmacies, practitioners, or health care settings that dispense the drug be specially certified
- Drug be dispensed only in certain health care settings (e.g., infusion settings, hospitals)
- Drug be dispensed with evidence of safe-use conditions such as laboratory test results
- Each patient using the drug be subject to monitoring
- Each patient using the drug be enrolled in a registry

Assessment results may be used to modify the REMS, or even eliminate it, if the assessment shows changes are needed or that the REMS has met its goals.

Patient package inserts

A PPI is an informational leaflet written for the lay public describing the benefits and risks of medications. Information found on a package insert includes the following:

- Description
- Clinical pharmacology
- Indications and usage
- Contraindications
- Warnings
- Precautions
- Adverse reactions
- Drug abuse and dependence
- Overdosage
- Dosage and administration
- How supplied
- Date of the most recent revision of the labeling

A pharmacy is required to provide PPIs to all patients receiving metered-dose inhalers, oral contraceptives, estrogen, and progesterone. PPIs should be given to any patient receiving a new medication.

Laws and/or regulations regarding compliance and auditing functions

- The DEA is responsible for enforcing Controlled Substance Act
  - Administrative inspection
    - Requires notice of inspection, informed consent (Form 82), and administrative warrant
    - The following records are reviewed:
      - Initial inventory
      - Biennial inventory
      - Closing inventory
      - Receiving records (DEA Form 222 and CSOS)
      - Distribution records
      - Theft and loss records (DEA Form 106)
      - Drug destruction (DEA Form 41), reverse distributor, and return to manufacturer documentation
      - Dispensing records
  - Common findings in administrative inspections
    - Failure to maintain complete and accurate records
    - Failure to maintain control substance records
    - Failure to perform adequate inventory records
    - Prescriptions missing patient addresses and dates
    - Prescription forms lacking security features
    - Theft/loss not reported in timely manner
    - Improperly completed DEA Form 222
    - Missing power of attorney
    - No background checks
    - Ignoring "red flags when dispensing controlled substances
    - Failure to run prescription drug monitoring program (PDMP) reports
  - Common "red flags"

- Excessive filling compared with similar situated pharmacies
- Unusual combination of controlled substances
- Patients obtaining controlled substances from multiple practitioners
- Customers paying in cash
- Filling prescriptions without obtaining a PDMP report
- Early refills
  - May result in monetary penalties
- Criminal inspection
  - Requires search warrant
  - May result in surrender, immediate suspension/revocation of license, prosecution, and arrest

Federal requirements pertaining to the medication dispensing process

- FDCA of 1938
  - Requires medication guides be dispensed with specific medications
- Durham-Humphrey Amendment to FDCA of 1951
  - Permitted new prescriptions and refills to be called into the pharmacy from a physician's office
- Comprehensive Drug Abuse Prevention and Control Act (Controlled Substance Act)
  - Created controlled substance drug schedules and the maximum number or refills permitted for each schedule
  - Created prescription requirements for controlled substances to include being dated as of and signed on the day when issued and bearing the full name and address of the patient, drug name, strength, dosage form, quantity prescribed, directions for use, and name, address, and registration number of the practitioner
  - Established requirements for paper prescription files
    - Option 1
      - A file for Schedule II Controlled Substances dispensed
      - A file for Schedules III, IV, and V Controlled Substances dispensed
    - Option 2
    - A file for all Schedule II Controlled Substances dispensed
    - A file for all other drugs dispensed (noncontrolled and those in Schedules III, IV, and V) (If this method is used, a prescription for a Schedule III, IV, or V drug must be made readily retrievable by use of a red "C" stamp not less than 1 inch high.)
  - Permits the transmission of electronic prescriptions for controlled substances
  - Established requirements for electronic prescription files:
    - If a prescription is created, signed, transmitted, and received electronically, all records related to that prescription must be retained electronically.
- Occupational Safety and Health Act of 1970
  - Requires safety data sheets be provided to purchasers of hazardous chemical
  - Established universal precautions

- Poison Prevention Packaging Act of 1970
  - Required child resistant containers for most prescription and OTC medications
  - Identified medications that do not need to be dispensed in a child-resistant container
  - Established exceptions whereby a prescription drug did not need to be dispensed in a child-resistant container, which included
    - Single-time dispensing of product in noncompliant container as ordered by the prescriber
    - Single-time or blanket dispensing of product in noncompliant container as requested by patient or customer in a signed statement
    - One noncompliant size of an OTC product for elderly or disabled patients provided that the package contains the warning "This Package for Households Without Young Children" or "Package Not Child Resistant"
    - Drugs dispensed to institutionalized patients provided the medications are administered by institution employees
    - Medications not requiring child-resistant containers to include nitroglycerin, methylprednisolone tablets with no more than 85 mg per package, prednisone tablets with no more than 105 mg per package, sodium fluoride tablets, inhalation aerosols, and oral contraceptives
- Omnibus Budget Reconciliation Act of 1990
  - Required pharmacists to perform a retrospective drug utilization review for every prescription
  - Compelled pharmacists to offer prescription counseling for all Medicaid patients
  - Required pharmacists to maintain patient profiles that contain the patient's name, address, telephone number, date of birth, gender, and medication history
- Combat Methamphetamine Epidemic Act of 2005
  - Created a category of medications referred to as SLCPs, which includes ephedrine, pseudoephedrine, and phenylpropanolamine
  - Established sales restrictions, storage, and record-keeping requirements
  - Limited the quantity of SLCP that can be sold daily to 3.6 g of the chemical base

Federal requirements pertaining to personnel competency

- USP <795>
  - Personnel compounding compounded nonsterile preparations (CNSPs) to complete a training program prior to compounding a CNSP and on a yearly basis thereafter
  - Must demonstrate a knowledge competency at least every 12 months in the following:
    - Hand hygiene
    - Garbing
    - Cleaning and sanitizing
    - Handling and transporting components and CNSPs
    - Measuring and mixing
    - Proper use of equipment and devices selected to compound CNSPs

- Documentation of the compounding process to include master formulation and compounding records
- USP <797>
  - Competency must be demonstrated, and written/electronic testing must be conducted initially and at least every 12 months in the following areas:
    - Hand hygiene
    - Garbing
      - Consists of a visual observation and gloved fingertip and thumb sampling of both hands
      - Must be conducted initially and at least every 6 months thereafter for Category 1 and Category 2 compounding sterile preparations (CSPs)
      - Must be conducted initially and every 3 months for Category CSPs
    - Cleaning and disinfection
    - Calculations, measuring, and mixing
    - Aseptic technique
      - Consists of media-fill testing followed by a gloved fingertip and thumb sampling on both hands and surface sampling of the direct compounding area
      - Must be conducted initially and at least every 6 months for Category 1 and 2 CSPs
      - Must be conducted initially and every 3 months for Category CSPs
      - Surface sampling to be conducted at the end of the compounding activity
      - Surface sampling of all classified areas and pass-through chambers for Category 1 and 2 CSPs to be done monthly
    - Achieving and/or maintaining sterility and apyrogenicity
    - Use of equipment
    - Documentation of the compounding process to include master formulation and compounding records
    - Principles of high-efficiency particulate air (HEPA)-filtered unidirectional airflow within the International Organization for Standardization (ISO) Class area
    - Proper use of primary engineering controls (PECs)
    - Principles of movement of materials and personnel within the compounding area
    - Must include competency in every procedure relating to their job function
- USP <800>
  - Prior to handling HDs personnel must receive training in the following areas:
    - Overview of the entity's list of HDs and their risk
    - Review of the entity's standard operating procedures (SOPs) related to handling of HDs
    - Proper use of personal protective equipment
    - Proper use of equipment and devices (e.g., engineering controls)
    - Response to known or suspected HD exposure
    - Spill management

- Proper disposal of HDs and trace-contaminated materials
- Additional training
- Personnel competency to be reassessed at least every 12 months
- Combat Methamphetamine Epidemic Act of 2005
  - Requires sellers of SLCP to undergo training regarding CMEA to include the maximum quantity that may be sold daily, verifying proper identification of the purchaser, documentation of the transaction, and appropriate storage of SLCPs in a pharmacy

Federal requirements pertaining to compounding sterile preparations

USP <797>

Compounded sterile preparations affected

- Injections, including infusions
- Irrigations for internal body cavities
- Ophthalmic dosage forms
- Aqueous preparations for pulmonary inhalation
- Baths and soaks for live organs and tissues
- Implants

Categories of immediate-use compounded sterile preparations

- Category 1 CSPs
  - Compounded under the least controlled environmental conditions
  - Assigned a BUD of 12 hours or less at controlled room temperature or 24 hours or less when refrigerated
- Category 2 CSPs
  - Require more environmental controls and testing than Category 1 CSPs
  - May be assigned a BUD of greater than 12 hours at controlled room temperature or more than 24 hours if refrigerated

Personnel training and evaluation

- Personnel compounding only immediate-use CSPs must complete training as required by the facility's SOPs
- Personnel competency must be demonstrated, and written/electronic testing must be completed initially and at least every 12 months in the following areas:
  - Hand hygiene
  - Garbing
  - Cleaning and disinfecting
  - Calculations, measuring, and mixing
  - Aseptic technique
  - Achieving and /or maintaining sterility and apyrogenicity
  - Use of equipment
  - Documentation of the compounding process (master formulation and compounding records)
  - Principles of HEPA-filtered unidirectional airflow within the ISO Class 5 area

- Proper us of PECs
- Principles of movement of materials and personnel withing the compounding area
  - Garbing and hand hygiene competency
    - Consists of a minimum of three separate competency evaluations
    - Consists of a visual observation and gloved fingertip and thumb sampling of both hands
      - Gloved fingertip and thumb sampling procedure
        - Use one sampling device (e.g., plates, paddles, or slides) per hand, containing general microbial growth agar.
        - Label each sampling device with a personnel identifier, right or left hand, and the date and time of sampling.
        - Do not apply sterile 70% isopropyl alcohol (IPA) to gloves immediately before touching sample. Using a separate sampling device for each hand, collect samples from all gloved fingertips and thumbs from both hands by rolling fingertip.
        - Incubate the sampling device at 30°C–35°C for no less than 48 hours and then at 20°C–25°C for no less than 5 additional days.
        - Record the number of colony-forming unit (cfu) per hand (left hand, right hand).
        - Determine whether the cfu action level is exceeded by counting the total number of cfu from both hands.
        - After the initial garbing competency evaluations, compounding personnel must successfully complete the garbing competency at least one time every 6 months for personnel compounding Category 1 and Category 2 CSPs, and at least one time every 3 months for personnel compounding CSPs.
  - Aseptic manipulation competency testing
    - All personnel compounding Category 1, Category 2, and CSP must undergo manipulation competency evaluation consisting of media-fill testing and gloved fingertip and thumb sampling for both hands and surface sampling.
    - Personnel compounding Category 1 and Category 2 CSPs must be evaluated for initially and every 6 months.
    - Failure in media-fill testing occurs when visible turbidity or visual growth is present in one container.
    - Gloved fingertip and thumb sampling must be performed on both hands and inside of an ISO Class 5 PEC immediately following the media fill test. Successful completion of the gloved fingertip and thumb sampling after media-fill testing is defined as ≤3 cfu as a total from both hands.
    - A failure in media-fill, gloved fingertip and thumb sampling or surface samples is an immediate failure in aseptic manipulation.
    - Results of evaluation and corrective actions taken must be documented, which consists of:
      - Name of individua evaluated
      - Evaluation date and time

- Media and components used to include manufacturer's name
- Expiration dates and lot numbers
- Starting temperature of each incubation
- Dates of incubation
- Test results
- Name of observer and individual who read and documented the results

Personal hygiene and garbing

- Prior to compounding a Category 1 or Category 2 CSPs, an individual must:
  - Remove personal outer garments (e.g., bandanas, coats, hats, jackets, sweaters, vests).
  - Remove all cosmetics because they shed flakes and particles.
  - Remove all hand, wrist, and other exposed jewelry, including piercings that could interfere with the effectiveness of garbing.
  - Remove earbuds or headphones.
  - Do not bring electronic devices that are not necessary for compounding or other required tasks into the compounding area.
  - Keep nails clean and neatly trimmed to minimize particle shedding and avoid glove punctures. Nail products (e.g., polish, artificial nails, and extenders) must not be worn.
  - Wipe eyeglasses, if worn.
- Any person entering a compounding area where Category 1 or Category 2 CSPs are prepared must wash hands and forearms up to the elbows with soap and water before initiating compounding activities.
  - Handwashing procedures
    - Remove visible debris from underneath fingernails under warm running water using a disposable nail cleaner.
    - Wash hands and forearms up to the elbows with soap and water for at least 30 seconds.
    - Dry hands and forearms up to the elbows completely with low-lint disposable towels or wipes.
  - Hand sanitizing procedures
    - Apply an alcohol-based hand sanitizer to dry skin following the manufacturer's instructions for the volume of product to use.
    - Apply product to one hand and rub hands covering all surfaces of hands and fingers, until hands are dry.
    - Allow hands to dry thoroughly before donning sterile gloves.
- Garbing
  - Minimum garbing requirements for Category 1 or Category 2 CSPs
    - Low-lint garment with sleeves that fit snugly around the wrists and an enclosed neck (e.g., gowns)
    - Low-lint covers for shoes
    - Low-lint cover for head that covers the hair and ears, and if applicable, cover for facial hair

- Low-lint face mask
- Sterile powder-free gloves
- If using a restricted access barrier system (RABS) (i.e., a compounding aseptic isolator or compounding aseptic containment isolator), disposable gloves to be worn inside the gloves attached to the RABS sleeves, and sterile gloves to be worn over the gloves attached to the RABS sleeve
- Garb to be replaced immediately if it becomes visibly soiled
- Gowns may be reused during the same shift if the gown is maintained inside the segregated compounding area (SCA)
- Gloves to be sterile and powder free

Facilities and engineering controls

ISO classification of particulate matter in room air	
ISO Class	Particle count per cubic meter
3	35.2
4	352
5	3520
6	35,200
7	352,000
8	3,520,000

Design requirements to maintain air quality

- Anterooms
  - Anterooms providing access only to positive pressure buffer rooms must meet at least ISO Class 8 classification.
  - Anterooms providing access to negative pressure buffer rooms must meet at least ISO Class 7 classification.
  - There must be transition areas to ensure that proper air classification and pressure relationships are maintained between classified and unclassified areas.
- Buffer room
  - Must meet at least ISO Class 7 air quality
- Category 1 and Category 2 CSPs must be prepared in an ISO Class 5 or better PEC. If compounding only Category 1 CSPs, the PEC may be placed in an unclassified SCA.

Facility design and environmental controls

- Clean room suite should be maintained at a temperature of 20°C or cooler and a relative humidity of 60% or below.
- Temperature and humidity must be monitored and documented daily.
- Temperature and humidity monitoring devices must be verified for accuracy at least every 12 months or as required by the manufacturer.

Types of secondary engineering controls

- Access to secondary engineering control (SEC) must be restricted to authorized personnel
- Clean room suite
  - The PEC must be located in the buffer room of the clean room suite or the SCA.
  - Classified rooms must be equipped with pressure differential monitoring system.
  - Anteroom must have a line of demarcation separating the clean side from the dirty side, where the clean side is closest to the buffer room.
- SCA
  - It may be located within an unclassified area without anteroom or buffer area.
  - Only Category I CSPs can be compounded in the SCA.

Types of primary engineering controls

Laminar airflow system offers an ISO Class 5 or better environment for sterile compounding. The laminar airflow system provides unidirectional HEPA-filtered airflow that is intended to reduce the risk of contamination of a sterile compounding environment.

- Laminar airflow workbench provides an ISO Class 5 or better environment for sterile compounding. It provides either horizontal or vertical unidirectional HEPA-filter airflow. It is not to be used in compounding antineoplastic or HDs.
- Integrated vertical laminar flow zone is a designated ISO Class 5 area serving as the PEC within an ISO Class 7 or cleaner buffer room. The unidirectional HEPA-filtered zone must be separated from the ISO Class 7 area with a physical barrier to direct the airflow downward over the work area to separate the direct compounding area from potential sources of contamination.
- Class II biological safety cabinet is a ventilated cabinet with an open front and inward and downward unidirectional HEPA-filtered airflow and exhaust. Biological safety cabinets must be turned on for at least 10 minutes prior to compounding. The exhaust airs must be externally vented when preparing antineoplastic and HDs.
- RABS provides HEPA-filtered ISO Class unidirectional air.
  - Compounding aseptic isolator is designed for compounding nonhazardous CSP. It cannot be used in preparing antineoplastic or HDs.
  - Compounding aseptic containment isolator maintains an ISO Class environment for compounding sterile hazardous preparations.
- Pharmaceutical isolator maintains an ISO Class environment and consists of:
  - Controlled workspace
  - Transfer device(s)
  - Access device(s)
  - Integral decontamination system

Minimum requirements for placement of primary engineering controls for compounding non–hazardous drug compounded sterile preparations			
PEC type	Device type	Placement for compounding only Category 1 CSPs	Placement for compounding Category 2 CSPs
LAFS	LAFW	Unclassified SCA	ISO Class 7 positive pressure buffer room with an ISO Class 8 positive pressure anteroom
LAFS	IVLFZ	N/A	ISO Class 7 positive pressure buffer room with an ISO Class 8 positive pressure anteroom
LAFS	BSC	Unclassified SCA	ISO Class 7 positive pressure buffer room with an ISO Class 8 positive pressure anteroom
RABS	CAI or CACI	Unclassified SCA	ISO Class 7 positive pressure buffer room with an ISO Class 8 positive pressure anteroom
Pharmaceutical isolator	Pharmaceutical isolator	Unclassified SCA	ISO Class 8 positive pressure room

BSC, biological safety cabinet; *CACI*, Compounding aseptic containment isolator; *CAI*, Compounding aseptic isolator; *CSP*, compounded sterile preparations; *IVLFZ*, integrated vertical laminar flow zone; *LAFS*, laminar airflow system; *LAFW*, laminar airflow workbench; *N/A*, not available; *PEC*, primary engineering control; *RABS*, restricted access barrier system; *SCA*, segregated compounding area.

ACPH Requirements for nonhazardous sterile compounding areas	
Compounding area	ACPH requirement
Unclassified SCA	No requirement
ISO Class 7 rooms	≥30 ACPH
ISO Class 8 rooms	≥20 ACPH

ACPH, air changes per hour; *SCA*, segregated compounding area.

Certification and recertification

- Certification of the classified areas including the PEC must be performed initially, and recertification must be performed at least every 6 months and must include:
  - Airflow testing
  - HEPA filter integrity testing
  - Total particle counting
  - Dynamic airflow smoke pattern test

Action levels for viable airborne particle air sampling	
ISO Class	Air sampling action levels (cfu/cubic meter [1000 L] of air plate)
5	>1
7	>10

Action levels for viable airborne particle air sampling	
ISO Class	Air sampling action levels (cfu/cubic meter [1000 L] of air plate)
8	>100

cfu, colony-forming units.

Action levels for viable airborne particle air sampling	
ISO Class	Surface sampling action levels (cfu/device)
5	3
7	>5
8	>50

cfu, colony-forming units.

Cleaning, disinfecting, and applying sporicidal disinfectants

Purpose of cleaning, disinfecting and sporicidal disinfectants	
Type of agent	Purpose
Cleaning	An agent used for the removal of residues (e.g., dirt, debris, microbes, and residual drugs or chemicals) from surfaces
Disinfectant	A chemical or physical agent used on an inanimate surfaces and objects to destroy fungi, viruses, and bacteria
Sporicidal	A chemical or physical agent that destroys bacterial and fungal spores when used at a sufficient concentration for a specified contact time; all vegetative microorganisms are expected to be killed

Procedures for cleaning and disinfecting the primary engineering control

- Remove visible particles, debris, or residue with an appropriate solution such as sterile water for injection or sterile water for irrigation using a sterile low-lint wiper.
- Using a sterile low-lint wiper, apply a sterile cleaning agent followed by a sterile disinfecting agent or an EPA-registered one-step disinfectant cleaner to equipment and all interior surfaces of the PEC.
- Guarantee the contact time required by manufacturer is met.
- Apply 70% IPA to equipment and all interior surfaces in the PEC.
- Allow surface to dry completely prior to compounding.

Procedures for applying a sporicidal disinfectant in the primary engineering control

- Remove visible particles, debris, or residue with an appropriate solution such as sterile water for injection or sterile water for irrigation using a sterile low-lint wiper.
- After cleaning and disinfecting the PEC, apply the sterile sporicidal disinfectant using a sterile low-lint wipe to all surfaces and area under the work tray. If an

EPA-registered one-step sporicidal disinfectant is used, separate cleaning and disinfecting steps are not necessary.

- Guarantee the contact time required by manufacturer is met.

- Apply 70% IPA to equipment and all interior surfaces in the PEC.
- Allow surface to dry completely prior to compounding.

Minimum frequency for cleaning and disinfecting surfaces and apply sporicidal disinfectants in classified areas and within the perimeter of the segregated compounding area			
Site	**Cleaning**	**Disinfecting**	**Apply sporicidal disinfectant**
PEC(s) and equipment inside the PEC(s)	Equipment and all interior surfaces of the PEC on days when compounding occurs and when surface contamination is known or suspected	Equipment and all interior surfaces of the PEC daily and when surface contamination is known or suspected. Apply sterile 70% IPA to the horizontal work surface at least every 30 min if the compounding process takes 30 min or less; if the compounding takes more than 30 min, compounding must not be interrupted, and the work surface of the PEC must be disinfected immediately after compounding	Monthly for entities compounding Category 1 and/or Category 2 CSPs
Removable work tray of the PEC, when applicable	Work surface of the tray daily on days when compounding occurs. All surfaces and the area underneath the work tray monthly	Work surface of the tray before compounding on days when compounding occurs. Apply sterile 70% IPA to the horizontal work surface at least every 30 min if the compounding process takes 30 min or less; if the compounding takes more than 30 min, compounding must not be interrupted, and the work surface of the PEC must be disinfected immediately after compounding. All surfaces and the area underneath the work tray monthly	Work surface of the tray monthly. All surfaces and the area underneath the work the work tray monthly
Pass-throughs	Daily on days when compounding occurs	Daily on days when compounding occurs	Monthly for entities compounding Category 1 and/or Category 2 CSPs
Work surface(s) outside the PEC	Daily on days when compounding occurs	Daily on days when compounding occurs	Monthly for entities compounding Category 1 and/or Category 2 CSPs
Floors	Daily on days when compounding occurs	Daily on days when compounding occurs	Monthly for entities compounding Category 1 and/or Category 2 CSPs
Wall(s), door(s), and door frame(s)	Monthly	Monthly	Monthly
Ceilings	Monthly	Monthly	Monthly
Storage shelving and bins	Monthly	Monthly	Monthly
Equipment outside the PEC(s)	Monthly	Monthly	Monthly for entities compounding Category 1 and/or Category 2 CSPs
CSP, compounded sterile preparation; *IPA*, isopropyl alcohol; *PEC*, primary engineering control.			

Introducing items into the secondary engineering control and primary engineering control

- An item must be wiped with a sporicidal disinfectant, EPA-registered disinfectant, or sterile 70% IPA using low-lint wipers by personnel wearing gloves prior to it being introduced into the clean side of the anteroom, or placed into pass-throughs or brought insides the perimeter of the SCA.
- Wiping the item must not make the label unreadable.
- Critical sites (e.g., vial stoppers, ampule necks, and intravenous bag septums) must be wiped with sterile 70% IPA in the PEC to provide both chemical and mechanical actions to remove contaminants.

Equipment, supplies, and components

- All equipment brought into classified areas must be wiped with a sporicidal disinfectant, EPA-registered disinfectant, or sterile 70% IPA using low-lint wipers.
- Records for equipment calibration, verification, and maintenance must be kept.
- Automated compounding devices (ACDs) must have an accuracy assessment performed before each day the ACD is used.
- Supplies in direct contact with CSP must be sterile and depyrogenated.
- All compounding ingredients must meet the criteria in the USP-NF monograph.
- Compounding components must be examined for deterioration upon receipt of the component.
- All components must be stored in closed containers complying with the temperature, humidity, and lighting conditions as indicated on monograph.

Sterilization and depyrogenation

- The sterilization method used must sterilize the CSP without damaging its physical, chemical, or packaging integrity.
- Terminal sterilization such as dry heat, steam, or irradiation is the preferred method of sterilization.
- Steam sterilization should not be used if moisture, pressure, or temperatures utilized would break down the CSP.
- Filtration should not be when compounding a suspension.
- Dry heat depyrogenation should not be used to make glassware, metal, and components pyrogen free.
- Depyrogenation processes typically operate at a range of temperatures, from approximately 170°C to 400°C.
- Sterilization by filtration requires sterilizing filters be sterile and depyrogenated and have a pore size of 0.22-μm or smaller.
- Sterilization by steam heat requires temperatures to be lower than those used for depyrogenation.
- Sterilization by dry heat is used for CSPs that cannot be sterilized by steam. The process requires higher temperatures and longer exposure times than sterilization by steam.

Master formulation records and compounding records

- A master formulation record (MFR) is a detailed record of procedures that describes how the CSP is tube prepared.
- An MFR must be created for Category 1 and Category2 immediate-use CSPs prepared for more than one patient and for CSPs prepared from nonsterile ingredient(s).

Master formulation records must contain the following

- Name, strength, or activity and dosage of the CSP
- Identities and amounts of all ingredients
- Type and size of container closure system(s)
- Compete instructions for preparing CSP, including equipment, supplies, description of the compounding steps, and special precautions
- Physical and description of the final CSP
- BUD and storage requirements
- Reference source to support stability of the CSP
- QC procedures such as pH testing and filter integrity testing
- Other information as needed to describe the compounding process and ensure repeatability such as adjusting pH and tonicity and sterilization method

Compounding records

- The compounding record must be produced to document the compounding process or repackaging process.
- A compounding record must be created for all Category 1, Category 2 immediate-use CSPs prepared for more than one patient and for CSPs prepared from nonsterile ingredient(s).

Compounding records must contain the following

- Name, strength, and dosage form of the CSP
- Date and time of preparation
- Assigned internal identification number such as prescription number, order, or lot number
- Method to confirm the individual involved in the compounding of the preparation and the individual involved with confirming the final CSP
- Name of each component
- Vendor, lot number, and expiration date for each component for the CSP compounded
- Weight or volume of each component
- Strength of each component
- Quantity compounded
- Final yield such as quantity, containers, or number of units
- Assigned BUD and storage requirements
- Results of QC procedures such as visual inspection, filter integrity testing, or pH testing
- MFR reference for the CSP
- Calculations made to determine and verify quantities and or concentrations

Release inspections and testing

- Visual inspection
  - CSP must be visually inspected to ensure the physical appearance is as expected such as having no visible particulate matter or discoloration.
  - A visual inspection of the of the container to ensure there is no leakage from the container or seals.
- Sterility testing
  - Sterility testing is not required for Category 1 CSPs.
  - Category 2 CSPs must undergo sterility testing.

- If 1–39 CSPs are compounded in a single batch, 10% of the units compounded must undergo sterility testing.
  - Maximum batch size is 250.
- Bacterial endotoxins testing
  - Category 1 CSPs do not require bacterial endotoxins testing.
  - Category 2 CSPs compounded from one or more nonsterile components must undergo bacterial endotoxin testing.

Labeling

- All Category 1 and Category 2 CSPs must be labeled with appropriate, legible, identifying information to prevent errors during storage, dispensing, and use.
- Label must contain the following:
  - Assigned internal identification number such as a barcode, prescription, order, or lot number
  - Active ingredient(s) and their amounts, concentrations, or activity(ies)
  - Storage conditions if other than controlled room temperature
  - BUD
  - Route of administration
  - Total amount or volume
  - If it is a single-dose container, a statement stating such when space permits
  - If it is a multiple-dose container, a statement stating so
  - Any special handling instructions
  - Applicable warning statements
- Label must be verified to confirm that meets:
  - Prescription or medication order

- MFR
- Compounding record

Beyond-use dates

- Each CSP label must state the date, or the hour and date, beyond which the preparation must not be used and must be discarded.
- BUD is either the date, or hour and date, after which a CSP must not be used.
- BUD is determined from the date and time the preparation of the CSP was compounded.
- BUD applies to all CSPs.
- Expiration date is the time during which a product can be expected to meet the requirements of the USP-NF monograph, if one exists, or maintain expected quality provided it is kept under the specified storage conditions.
- Expiration dates apply to all conventionally manufactured products.
- BUDs are based upon
  - Conditions of the environment in which the CSP is prepared
  - Aseptic processing and sterilization method
  - Starting components (e.g., sterile or nonsterile ingredients) and whether or not sterility testing is performed
  - Storage conditions (e.g., packaging and temperature)

Best-used-by date for Category 1 compounded sterile preparations	
Storage conditions	
Controlled room temperature (20°C–25°C)	Refrigerator (2°C–8°C)
≤12h	≤24h

Best-used-by date for Category 2 compounded sterile preparations				
Preparation characteristics		**Storage conditions**		
Compounding method	**Sterility test performed and passed**	**Controlled room temperature (20°C–25°C)**	**Refrigerator (2°C–8°C)**	**Freezer (−25°C to −10°C)**
Aseptically processed CSPs	No	Prepare from one or more sterile starting components: 1 day	Prepared from one or more nonsterile starting components: 4 days	Prepared from one or more nonsterile component(s): 4 days
Aseptically processed CSPs	No	Prepared from only sterile starting components: 4 days	Prepare from only sterile starting components: 10 days	Prepare from only sterile starting components: 45 days
Aseptically processed CSPs	Yes	30 days	45 days	60 days
Terminally sterilized CSPs	No	14 days	28 days	45 days
Terminally sterilized CSPs	Yes	45 days	60 days	90 days
CSP, compounded sterile preparation.				

Standard operating procedures

Facilities that prepare CSPs must develop SOPs for the compounding process and other support activities. SOPs must include the types of CSPs that are prepared (i.e., Category 1, Category 2). All compounding personnel must:

- Recognize potential problems, deviations, failures, or errors associated with preparing a CSP (e.g., those related to equipment, facilities, materials, personnel, the compounding process, or testing) that could potentially result in contamination or other adverse impact on CSP quality.
- Report any problems, deviations, failures, or errors to the designated person(s).

SOPs must be reviewed every 12 months and documented.

Quality assurance and quality control

- QA is a system of procedures, activities, and oversight that guarantees the compounding process meets quality standards.
- QC is the sampling, testing. and documentation of results that guarantee that specifications have been met before the release of the CSP.
- An institution's QA and QC programs must be documented in the institution's SOP.
- QA and QC programs must have a system that:
  - Adheres to procedures
  - Prevents and detects errors and other quality problems
  - Evaluates complaints and adverse events
  - Investigates and takes corrective actions

Handling, storage, packaging, shipping, and transport

- Handling and storing
  - Controlled temperature area must be established and monitored.
  - Temperature must be monitored daily manually or by a continuous recording device daily and documented.
  - Temperature monitoring devices must be evaluated at least every 12 months.
- Packaging
  - Packaging must protect CSP from damage, leakage, contamination, degradation, and adsorption.
  - Light-sensitive packaging must be used if CSP is sensitive to light.
  - In select situations, the CSP must be packaged in special containers to protect it from temperature variations.
- Shipping and transporting
  - Transporting CSP must ensure the CSP is undamaged, sterile, and stable .condition
  - CSPs requiring special handling must bear specific handling instructions on the outside of the container.

Documentation

Facilities preparing CSPs must have and maintain written electronic documentation for the following:

- Personnel training, competency assessments, and qualification records including corrective actions for any failures
- Certification reports, including corrective actions for any failure
- Environmental air and surface monitoring procedures and results
- Equipment records (e.g., calibration, verification, and maintenance reports)
- Receipt of components
- SOPs, MFRs (if required), and compounding records (if required)
- Release inspection and testing records
- Information related to complaints and adverse events including corrective actions taken
- Results of investigations and corrective actions

Federal requirements (USP <795>) pertaining to nonsterile compounding

Nonsterile compounding is combining, admixing, diluting, pooling, reconstituting other than as provided in the manufacturer's package insert or otherwise altering a drug or bulk drug substance to create a nonsterile medication. CNSPs includes solid oral preparation, liquid oral preparations, rectal preparations, vaginal preparations, topical preparations, nasal and sinus preparations intended for local application, and otic preparations.

Personnel

- Personnel must be trained in the preparation and handling of CNSPs, must demonstrate competency, and must undergo annual refresher training.
- A designated individual must develop a written training program that describes the required training, the frequency of training, and the process for evaluating the competency of personnel involved in CSNPs.
- Proficiency must be demonstrated in the following areas:
  - Hand hygiene
  - Garbing
  - Cleaning and sanitizing
  - Component selection, handling, and transport
  - Performing calculations
  - Measuring and mixing
  - Use of equipment
  - Documentation (MFRs and compounding records)

Personal hygiene and garbing

- Personnel must:
  - Remove all personal outer garments.
  - Remove all hand, wrist, and other exposed jewelry or piercing.
  - Remove headphones and earphones.
  - Keep nails clean and neatly trimmed.
- Hand hygiene is required before beginning any compounding that includes:
  - Wash hands and forearms up to the elbows with soap and water for at least 30 seconds.
  - Dry hands and forearms to the elbows completely with disposable towels or wipes.
  - Allow hands and forearms to dry thoroughly before donning gloves.

- Gloves are required to be worn for all compounding activities. Shoe covers, head and facial covers, face masks, and gowns may be required to be worn depending on the type of compounding performed.
- Gowns maybe redonned during the same work shift.
- Gloves, shoe covers, hair covers, facial hair covers, face masks, or head may not be reused.

Cleaning and sanitizing

Minimum frequency for cleaning and sanitizing surfaces in nonsterile compounding areas	
Site	**Minimum frequency**
Work surfaces	At the beginning and end of each shift, after spills, and when surface contamination (e.g., from splashes) is known or suspected Between compounding CNSPs with different components
Floors	Daily, after spills, and when surface contamination (e.g., splashes) is known or suspected
Walls	Every 3 months, after spills, and when surface contamination (e.g., splashes) is known or suspected
Ceilings	Every 3 months, after spills, and when surface contamination (e.g., splashes) is known or suspected
Storage shelving	Every 3 months, after spills, and when surface contamination (e.g., splashes) is known or suspected
CNSP, compounded nonsterile preparations.	

Equipment and components

- Equipment surfaces that contact components must not be reactive, additive, absorptive, or adsorptive and must not alter the quality of the CNSPs.
- Any weighing, measuring, or other manipulation of an active pharmaceutical ingredient (API) or added substance that may cause airborne contamination must be done in a containment ventilate enclosure.
- Safety data sheets must be available for all substances and bulk chemicals.
- APIs must be purchased from an FDA-registered facility.
- Purified water must be used to reconstitute nonsterile products.

Minimum frequency for cleaning and sanitizing equipment in nonsterile compounding areas	
Site	**Minimum frequency**
CVE and work surfaces outside the CVE	At the beginning and end of each shift, and after spills and when surface contamination is known or suspected. Clean and sanitize the horizontal work surface of the CVE between compounding of different drugs.
BSC	At the beginning and end of each shift, after spills, and when surface contamination (e.g., from splashes) is known or suspected. Clean and sanitize the horizontal work surface of the BSC between compounding CNSPs with different components. Clean and sanitize under the work surface at least monthly.

Minimum frequency for cleaning and sanitizing equipment in nonsterile compounding areas—cont'd	
Site	**Minimum frequency**
Equipment used in compounding operations	Before first use and thereafter in accordance with the manufacturer's recommendations. If no recommendation is available after each use.
BSC, biological safety cabinet; CVE, containment ventilate enclosure.	

Standard operating procedures/master formulation records/compounding records

- An MFR is a detailed record of procedures that describes how each CNSP is prepared.
- A MFR must be prepared for each unique product and contain the following:
  - Name, strength or activity, and dosage form of the CNSP
  - Identities and amounts of all components; if applicable, relevant characteristics of components (e.g., particle size, salt form, purity grade, solubility)
  - Container closure system(s)
  - Complete instructions for preparing the CNSP including equipment, supplies, and description of compounding steps
  - Physical description of the final CNSP
  - Assigned BUD and storage requirements
  - Reference source to support the assigned BUD and storage requirements
  - If applicable, calculations to determine and verify quantities and/or concentrations of components and strength or activity of the API(s)
  - Labeling requirements (e.g., "Shake Well")
  - QC procedures (e.g., pH testing, visual inspection) and expected results
  - Other information needed to describe the compounding process and ensure repeatability (e.g., adjusting pH, temperature)
- A compounding record documents the compounding of each CNSP and be created for each CNSP. It contains the following information:
  - Name, strength or activity, and dosage form of the CNSP
  - Date and time of preparation of the CNSP
  - Assigned internal identification number (e.g., prescription, order, or lot number)
  - A method to identify the individuals involved in the compounding process and individuals verifying the final CNSP
  - Name, vendor or manufacturer, lot number, and expiration date of each component
  - Weight or measurement of each component
  - Total quantity of the CNSP compounded
  - Assigned BUD and storage requirements
  - If applicable, calculations to determine and verify quantities and/or concentrations of components and strength or activity of the API(s)
  - Physical description of the final CNSP
  - Results of QC procedures (e.g., pH testing and visual inspection)
  - MFR reference for the CNSP

Labeling

The labeling on the CNSP must display the following:

- Assigned internal identification number (e.g., prescription or lot number)
- Chemical and/or generic name(s), or active ingredient(s), and amounts or concentrations
- Dosage form
- Total amount or volume
- Storage conditions
- BUD
- Indication that the preparation is compounded
- Route of administration
- Any special handling instructions
- Any warning statements that are applicable
- Name, address, and contact information of the compounding facility if the CNSP is to be sent outside of the facility or health care system in which it was compounded

Beyond-use dates

- Each CNSP label must state the date beyond which the preparation cannot be used and must be discarded.
- Expirations date identifies the time during which a conventionally manufactured drug product may be expected to maintain its labeled identity, strength, purity, and quality assuming it has been stored properly.
- Temperature, humidity, and light are some of the factors that can affect whether a product will break down over time.
- When an expiration date is identified by month and year, it is intended that the medication will expire on the last day of the month.
- Expiration dates is not appropriate for CNSPs.
- A BUD cannot exceed the expiration date. A BUD indicates the number of days after the CNSP is prepared and beyond which the CNSP cannot be used. The day CNSP is prepared is considered day 1.
- Factors affecting BUD
  - The chemical and physical stability properties of the API and any added substances in the preparation
  - The compatibility of the container-closure system with the finished preparation
  - Degradation of the container-closure system
  - The potential for microbial growth in the CNSP

Maximum beyond-use dates by the type of preparation in the absence of compounded nonsterile preparations–specific stability information		
Type of preparation	BUDs (days)	Storage temperature
Solid dosage forms (e.g., capsules tablets, granules, powders)	180	Controlled room temperature or refrigerator
Preserved aqueous dosage forms (e.g., emulsions, gels, creams, solutions, sprays, or suspensions)	35	Controlled room temperature or refrigerator
Nonpreserved aqueous dosage forms (e.g., emulsions, gels, creams, solutions, sprays, or suspensions)	14	Refrigerator

Maximum beyond-use dates by the type of preparation in the absence of compounded nonsterile preparations–specific stability information —cont'd		
Type of preparation	BUDs (days)	Storage temperature
Nonaqueous dosage forms (e.g., suppositories and ointments)	90	Controlled room temperature or refrigerator

BUD, beyond-use date.

Quality assurance and quality control

- QA is a set of written processes that, at a minimum, verifies, monitors, and reviews the adequacy of the compounding process.
- QC is an observation of techniques and activities that demonstrate that requirements are met.
- Facility must have a written QA and QC program.

Compounded nonsterile preparation handling, packaging, storage, and transport

- SOPs must outline processes or techniques for storing, handling, packaging, and transporting CNSPs.
- Garb, spill kits, and safety data sheets must be readily accessible for those handling CNSPs.
- Hazard labels (if appropriate) should be on all chemical containers.
- Packaging materials must protect CNSPs from damage, leakage, contamination, degradation, and adsorption, while simultaneously protecting transport personnel from exposure.
- A controlled room temperature area must be either monitored manually at least once daily on days that compounding is performed or by a continuous temperature recording device to determine whether the temperature is appropriate for CNSP.
- Temperature readings must be documented and readily retrievable.
- Temperature monitoring must be calibrated or verified for accuracy at least every 12 months.
- Humidity of storage area must be at or below 60%.
- SOPs that describe appropriate shipping containers, insulating materials, and packaging materials based on physical and chemical properties of CNSP.
- SOPs must indicate mode of transportation.

Complaint handling and adverse event reporting

- A designated person must review all complaints to determine whether the complaint indicates a potential quality problem with the CNSP. If so, an investigation must take place. If it is determined that the quality problem exists, corrective action must be taken to include product recalls. A readily retrievable written or electronic record of each complaint must be maintained. The record must contain the name of the complainant, the date the complaint was received, the nature of the complaint, and the response to the complainant.

- A designated individual must review all reports of potential adverse events. If an adverse event identifies as being a quality event, then all affected patients and prescribers must be notified. All adverse events should be reported to the FDA through MedWatch.

Documentation

All CNSPs must have and maintain written or electronic documentation to include the following:

- Personnel training, competency assessment, and qualification records including corrective actions for any failures
- Equipment records (e.g., calibration, verification, and maintenance reports)
- Receipt of components
- SOPs, MFRs, and compounding records
- Release testing, including corrective actions for any failures
- Information related to complaints and adverse events including corrective actions taken

All required compounding records for a particular CNSP (e.g., MFR, compounding record, and testing results) must be readily retrievable for at least 3 years.[3]

Licensing and reporting requirements for personnel and facility	
Licensing requirements	
Pharmacists	**Licensed by state board of pharmacy**
Pharmacy technicians	State boards of pharmacy may require a pharmacy technician to be certified by the PTCB or NHA, be registered with the state board of pharmacy, or licensed by the state board of pharmacy; some states do not have requirements for pharmacy technicians
Community pharmacies	Licensed by the state board of pharmacy Possess an NPI number Possess a DEA number if controlled substances are dispensed Be enrolled as a Medicare/Medicaid provider Possess a business license
Hospital pharmacies	Licensed by the state board of pharmacy Accredited by the Joint Commission Possess an NPI Number Possess a DEA number to dispense controlled substances Be enrolled as Medicare/Medicaid provider Possess a business license

DEA, Drug Enforcement Administration; *NHA*, national healthcareer association; *NPI*, national provider identifier.

Patient safety and quality assurance strategies

Elements of compliance programs

Just Culture

- "Just Culture" refers to a system of shared accountability in which organizations are accountable for the systems they have designed and for responding to the behaviors of their employees in a fair and just manner.

- Employees are accountable for the quality of their choices and for reporting errors and system vulnerabilities.
- The elements of Just Culture include building awareness, implementing policies that support Just Culture, and building Just Culture principles into the practices and processes of daily work.
- The goal of a Just Culture is the development of an organizational culture that promotes and exhibits a quality learning environment as a responsibility to both employees and patients.
- Three behaviors are found in a Just Culture and include human error, at risk, and reckless:
  - Human error is when the mistake was not intended.
  - At-risk behavior is when a person chooses to do something not knowing or not ascertaining the risk.
  - Reckless behavior is substantial, nonjustified, and conscious disregard.

Continuous quality improvement

- Medicare Part D requires participating pharmacies to implement a continuous quality improvement program.
- The purpose of a continuous quality improvement program is to assess errors that occur in the pharmacy during the review, preparation, and dispensing of prescription medications and to allow the pharmacy to take appropriate action to prevent or reduce the likelihood of a recurrence.
- A continuous quality improvement program requires pharmacy team members to ask questions such as "How are we doing?" and "Can we do it better?"
- A continuous quality improvement program ss nonpunitive and seeks to identify weaknesses in process and systems resulting in making the appropriate corrections to improve them.

Steps in continuous quality improvement process

- Step 1. Identify a need/issue/problem and develop a problem statement.
- Step 2. Define the current situation—break down the problem into component parts, identify major problem areas, and develop a target improvement goal.
- Step 3. Analyze the problem—identify the root causes of the problem and use charts and diagrams as needed.
- Step 4. Develop an action plan—outline ways to correct the root causes of the problem, specific actions to be taken, and identify who, what, when, and where.
- Step 5. Look at the results—confirm that the problem and its root causes have decreased, identify if the target has been met, and display results in graphic format before and after the change.
- Step 6. Start over—go back to the first step and use the same process for the next problem.

Quality assurance

- QA is the maintenance of a desired level of quality in a service or product by means to every stage in the process or delivery or production.
- QA focuses on the processes and procedures that improve quality, including training documentation, monitoring, and audits.

- Most states require pharmacies to have a QA program to address prescription (medication) errors.
  - States vary on how a pharmacy needs to respond to the medication error, but most agree that investigation should commence as soon as possible. The investigation should identify the cause of the mistake and preventative steps to be implemented,
- Most states require that all compounding pharmacies maintain a written QA designed to monitor and ensure the integrity, potency, quality, and labeled strength of compounded drug products. Components of a compounding QA include:
  - Written procedures for verification, monitoring, and review of the adequacy of the compounding processes
  - Written standards for qualitative and quantitative integrity, potency, quality, and labeled strength analysis of compounded drug products
  - Written procedure for scheduled action in the event a compounded drug is below minimum standards for integrity, potency, quality, or labeled strength

Patient safety organization

- Patient safety organizations were created under the Patient Safety and Quality Act of 2005.
- Patient safety organizations collect and analyze data voluntarily reported by health care providers to help improve patient safety and health care quality.
- Patient safety organizations provide feedback to health care providers with the intent to promote futures safety events.
- Providers who establish relationships with a patient safety organization receive uniform federal protections (conferring privilege and confidentiality) that are expected to remove fear of legal liability or professional sanctions
- Patient safety organizations must meet specific requirements to become certified as a patient safety organization.

Methods or techniques to systematically improve accuracy

Barcode scanning

- Barcode scanning improves patient safety during prescription dispensing process in pharmacy settings.
- Barcode scanning verifies the drug product and strength selected from storage matches what has been entered into the patient's profile in the pharmacy computer system.
- If implemented properly, barcode scanning will not permit the dispensing process to continue if a match does not occur.

Barcode scanning tips

The Institute of Safe Medication Practices recommends the barcode scanning practices:

- Ensure barcode scanning is used consistently and as intended each time a medication is dispensed, including refills and owed quantities.

- Always scan the barcode printed from the pharmacy computer system and the barcode on the medication product being dispensed.
- Avoid verifying product selection by typing the NDC number from the patient's label or the computer screen, as this undermines the system safeguards.
- If you must type the NDC number because the barcode will not scan, type it from the medication product.
- During order entry, either type the drug name and strength or use the computer system's drug look-up feature. Do not first retrieve the product from storage and scan the barcode as a way of entering the drug; if the wrong product is selected from storage, there will be no opportunity to catch the error later in the dispensing process by scanning the barcode.
- When more than one stock bottle is needed for a specific drug quantity, scan each stock bottle. If more than one container will be dispensed, ensure that each one has a pharmacy-generated label.
- Scan each medication product for verification. For example, dispensing three albuterol inhalers should require three individual computer-generated labels and the scanning of each albuterol inhaler package barcode.
- Invest in barcode scanners that can read at least 90% of barcodes and all symbols used by pharmaceutical manufacturers. Notify the manufacturer and Institute for Safe Medication Practices (ISMP) if product labels do not scan.
- Review system reports on scanning overrides to discover problems in workflow and make necessary changes. This also can help identify issues with specific products (e.g., the barcode is not readable or is bent around the curvature of the bottle, making it difficult to scan).
- Never bypass the barcode scan in the interest of delivering the prescription more quickly.
- If a mismatched scan is identified, investigate the cause.

Failure mode and effects analysis

- Is a proactive process to systematically identify areas of potential failure within a process and gauge what the effects would be—before an error actually takes place
- Can be used before new medications are prescribed, purchased, dispensed, and administered so that preemptive action can be taken to detect, eliminate, or mitigate any potential patient harm

Federal Emergency Management Agency process for introduction of a new medication to the pharmacy's inventory

- Create a detailed diagram of the process and tasks involved with storing and dispensing the new product. Explore how the intended product would be prescribed. How will the prescription be received? Who would prescribe it and for which patients? What clinical patient information will be needed before it is prescribed or dispensed? How would it be procured, stored, and used, from acquisition through dispensing and administration? Who would prepare and dispense it? What information will need to be given to the patient or caregiver?
- Identify how and where systems and processes may fail (failure modes) and what can go wrong while considering how the product would be used.

Examples of drug characteristics and questions to ask in failure mode and effects analysis for new medications	
Drug characteristic	**Probing question**
Drug names	Does the drug name (brand or generic) look or sound like another drug name?
Drug indication(s)	Is the drug's indication similar to another product with a similar drug name?
Storage location	Would it be store near another similarly packaged product?
Drug name on computer screen	Would a similarly spelled drug name be listed in close proximity to the intended product?
Manufacturer container label	Does the container or label look similar to another product?
Manufacturer's barcode	Wil your barcode system read the barcode?

- Determine for each failure mode the likelihood of making an error, as well as the potential consequences of the failures. How often could this failure mode occur? What would happen to the patient if the drug were given at the wrong dose or at the wrong time or by the wrong route? What would happen if a patient received the wrong medication or if the wrong patient received the medication?
- Consider the severity of the outcome and identify any preexisting processes that could help eliminate or detect the error before it reaches the patient. Evaluate each process for its effectiveness based upon what was learned in previous steps.
- Develop actions to prevent the error, detect it before it reaches the patient, or minimize its consequences if failure modes reveal errors with significant consequences.

Root cause analysis

- Is a systematic process to identify the causal factors that contributed to the occurrence of a sentinel event that is an unexpected occurrence involving death or serious physical or psychological injury or risk
- Focuses primarily on systems and processes, not individual performance
- Should be performed whenever a sentinel event or any medication error not defined as a sentinel event occurs

Root cause analysis characteristics

- Identifies system and process changes needed to improve performance and reduce the risk of a similar event or close call from recurring
- Focuses primarily on systems and processes rather than individual performance
- Provides in-depth understanding of the events being investigated by continuously asking "Why did this (or that) happen?" until all root causes have been identified
- Includes organizational leadership participation in problem solving and quality and safety improvement

- Includes participation by individuals most closely involved in the processes and systems under review and who are knowledgeable in human factors and error prevention measures
- Internally consistent—does not contradict itself or leave obvious questions unanswered
- Includes consideration of relevant literature; if a similar error was reported and published, it takes into consideration of recommended strategies

Root causes of medication errors

- Human: An error caused by an individual by not following procedures or missing or ignoring a step or lack of training. For example, a pharmacy technician pulls a bottle of amoxicillin 250 mg from the shelf instead of amoxicillin 500 mg.
- Manufacturing: An error caused during manufacturing in which the medication is not manufactured according to specifications, or the packaging or educational materials provided are incorrect. An example is one whereby patient product insert is not provided by the manufacturer.
- Organizational: The health care organization's policy and procedures lack appropriate directions for the staff to perform their jobs properly, to include training. An example would be the pharmacy is not following the current USP <795> standards for nonsterile compounding, USP <797> standards for sterile compounding, or USP <800> standards for handling HDs.
- Technical: The equipment used in processing or compounding a prescription is not working properly. For example, the pharmacy scale used to weigh ingredients is not calibrated properly or the automatic dispensing equipment is not working properly.

Root cause analysis process

1. Form a team.
2. Determine what happened.
   a. Review documentation.
   b. Assess the physical environment.
   c. Review labeling and packaging.
   d. Interview pharmacy staff.
3. Develop a flow chart of the sequence of the event.
   a. At each step of the event, identify any contributing or root causes.
4. Identify the root cause.
   a. Determine if each factor is a root cause or contributing factor and whether action should be taken.
   b. Take into consideration human factors and communication, human factors and training, human factors and fatigue/scheduling, environment and equipment, rules, policies, and procedures.
5. Write root cause statement.
   a. For each item, write a concise description of the cause-and-effect relationship.
6. Develop action plan and measures.
   a. Form action plan.
   b. Establish measures.
   c. Communicate the results.

Cause and impact of medication dispensing errors

Causes of dispensing errors

- Wrong formulation error occurs when a different dosage form or salt is dispensed without the prescriber's permission. An example would be dispensing metoprolol tartrate instead of metoprolol succinate.
- Wrong drug error occurs when a drug was dispensed that is different than the drug prescribed. An example would be atorvastatin 40 mg was ordered and atomoxetine 40 mg was dispensed.
- Medication education error is one where proper education material is not provided to the patient. An example is the failure of the pharmacist or pharmacy technician to provide a medication guide to the patient.
- Adverse drug error occurs when a drug utilization review warning is missed or ignored. The pharmacy technician overrides a warning for warfarin in a 75-year-old patient and does not inform the pharmacist of the situation.
- Wrong amount/dosage error occurs when the dose given is 5% greater or less than the dose prescribed. An example would be dispensing levothyroxine 0.025 mg instead of levothyroxine 0.125 mg.
- Documentation error occurs when essential information is missing or incorrect. An example of this is when the medication list in the pharmacy information system is not updated with current information.
- Compliance error occurs when a patient fails to adhere to the directions provide by their physician and pharmacist regarding taking their medication. An example would be a patient completing their 30-day therapy in 10 days and the pharmacist failing to address the issue with the patient.
- Monitoring error is a failure to review a prescribed regimen for appropriateness and detection of problems or failure to use appropriate clinical or laboratory data for adequate assessment of patient response to prescribed therapy. An example would be failing to monitor properly medications with narrow therapeutic indexes such as warfarin and levothyroxine.
- Wrong drug preparation error is one where the medication has been incorrectly formulated or manipulated before administration. An example would be using the incorrect diluent when preparing a sterile compound.
- Deteriorated drug error is one where a drug dispensed has expired or for which the physical or chemical dosage-form integrity has been compromised. An example would be dispensing a medication on September 30 when the label on the manufacturer's package indicates the expiration date is July 31 of that year. Another example would be dispensing a medication that has exceeded its beyond-use-date.

Impact of dispensing errors

- Patient receives a subtherapeutic dose and the condition is not treated properly.
- Patient receives a supratherapeutic dose than prescribed and experiences adverse effects.
- Medication dispensed is contraindicated with other prescription medications prescribed or OTC medications the patient is taking.
- Medication dispensed may affect the patient's renal or hepatic function.
- Patient may develop an allergy or anaphylactic reaction to the dispensed medication.

Cause and impact of other types of quality-related events

Incomplete counseling

- The Omnibus Budget Reconciliation Act of 1990 required pharmacists to offer prescription counseling for all Medicaid patients.
- It has been shown that patients who receive prescription counseling are more likely to be compliant with their medication therapy.
- Failing to counsel a patient may cause patient nonadherence resulting in patients not experiencing the full benefits of their medication and possible side effects that could have been prevented.

Patient language barrier

- Differences in education, English proficiency, socioeconomic status, and situational circumstances can affect an individual's health literacy.
- Health literacy refers to the degree to which individuals have the ability to find, understand, and use information and services to inform health-related decisions and actions for themselves and others.
- Health literacy requires a patient to be able to read, listen, communicate, and comprehend to follow a medication regimen.
- Low health literacy skills hinder a patients' ability to build knowledge about their illness and therapy resulting in nonadherence.

Adverse event

- Is an appreciably harmful or unpleasant reaction resulting from a medication

Medication storage requirements

All medications have specific storage conditions determined by the manufacturer, which include the type of container (e.g., a light-resistant container) and temperature. The following definitions indicate the proper temperature at which a drug is to be stored:

- Freezer: Temperature maintained thermostatically between −25°C and −10°C (−13°F and 14°F)
- Cold: Not to exceed 8°C (46°F)
- Cool: Any temperature between 8°C and 15°C (46°F and 59°F)
- Room temperature: Any temperature between 15°C and 30°C (59°F and 86°F)

- Warm: Any temperature between 30°C and 40°C (86°F and 104°F)
- Excessive heat: Any temperature above 40°C (104°F)
- Protect from freezing: Freezing medication leads to a loss of strength, potency, or destructive alterations
- Dry temperature: Conditions not to exceed 40% humidity at controlled room temperature

Many medications must be stored at refrigerated temperatures to ensure their stability. One should refer to the pharmaceutical manufacturer's product information to determine if the product needs to be refrigerated upon receipt, upon reconstitution, or when a diluent is added. If a reconstituted product needs to be refrigerated, the manufacturer will state how long the medication will be stable upon being reconstituted.

Rules, policies, and regulations related to the disposal of pharmaceutical drugs

Prescription drug take back programs

Medication take back programs are the best way to properly dispose of unused or expired prescription and nonprescription (for example, OTC) medicines.

- Permanent collection sites are registered with the DEA to take collect unused or expired medications. These sites may be found in local pharmacies, hospitals, clinic pharmacies, or law enforcement facilities. Collection sites may include drop-off boxes, mail back boxes or in-home disposal methods.
- National Prescription Drug Take Back events are sponsored by the DEA. They involve setting up temporary collection sites in communities.
- Local law enforcement authorities may promote take back events in the community.

Proper medication destruction

- In situations in which a drug take back location is not present in the community, select medications may be flushed down the toilet. Medications that appear on the FDA Flush List for Certain Medicines include buprenorphine, fentanyl, hydrocodone, benzhydrocodone, hydromorphone, meperidine, methadone, morphine, oxycodone, oxymorphone, tapentadol, sodium oxybate, diazepam rectal gel, and methylphenidate transdermal system.
- Nonflush medications may be disposed of in the trash.
  - Refer to a medication's medication guide or package insert to determine if specific disposal instructions are present. If not, adhere to the following steps:
    - Mix medicines (liquid or pills; do not crush tablets or capsules) with an unappealing substance such as dirt, cat litter, or used coffee grounds.
    - Place the mixture in a container such as a sealed plastic bag.
    - Throw away the container in your trash at home.
    - Delete all personal information on the prescription label of empty medicine bottles or medicine packaging, then trash or recycle the empty bottle or packaging.

Reporting of medication errors and quality-related events

Internal reporting

Most states require pharmacies to have a QA program to address prescription (medication) errors. States vary on how a pharmacy needs to respond to the medication error, but most agree that investigation should commence as soon as possible. The investigation should identify the cause of the mistake and preventative steps to be implemented.

MedWatch

MedWatch was established by the FDA as a voluntary program to report adverse events or sentinel events that are observed or suspected in human medical products. These adverse events include serious drug side effects, product use errors, product quality problems, and therapeutic failures. FDA regulated products that include:

- Prescription or OTC medicines
- Biologics (including blood components, blood and plasma derivatives, and gene therapy)
- Medical devices including hearing aids, pacemakers, and breast pumps
- Combination products such as prefilled drug syringe, metered-dose inhalers, and nasal spray
- Special nutritional products such as dietary supplements, infant formulas, and medical foods
- Cosmetics to include moisturizers, makeup, shampoos, hair dyes, and tattoos
- Foods/beverages (including reports of serious allergic reactions)
- Reports are generated from health providers using FDA Form 3500 and consumers/patients use FDA Form 3500B. MedWatch provides safety alerts for human medical products that include drugs, biologics, medical devices, special nutrition, and cosmetics. MedWatch is not used to report vaccine events.

Vaccine Adverse Event Reporting System

- The FDA cosponsors the Vaccine Adverse Event Reporting System with the Centers for Disease Control.
- It is a postmarketing safety surveillance program that collects information about adverse events (possible side effects) that occur after the administration of vaccines licensed for use in the United States.
- Information collected is used to identify any new safety concerns that otherwise may not come to light before licensing.
- Reports may be generated by health care providers, vaccine manufacturers, vaccine recipients, and state immunization programs.
- Health care providers are required to report the following:
  - Any event listed by the vaccine manufacturer as a contraindication to subsequent doses of the vaccine
  - Any event listed in the Reportable Events Table that occurs within the specified time period after vaccination

Board of pharmacy

The practice of pharmacy in a state is overseen by the state board of pharmacy, which is responsible for:

- Determining the qualifications for a pharmacist or pharmacy technician (to include certification, registration, and/or licensing) to practice their profession in the state
- Establishing continuing education requirements for pharmacists and pharmacy technicians
- Disciplining pharmacists and pharmacy technicians for unlawful or inappropriate pharmacy practice behaviors. (The state board of pharmacy may suspend, revoke, or fine a pharmacist or pharmacy technician for their actions.)
- Issuing regulations and standards regarding the pharmacy facility, its security system, personnel, processing prescription drug order, record keeping, and prepackaging of medications
- Overseeing the state's PDMP

Institute for Safe Medication Practices best practices

High-alert medications in acute care settings

High-alert medications are drugs that exhibit an increased risk of causing considerable harm when used in error in an acute care setting. ISMP has identified both specific medications and classes/categories of medication that require specific strategies to reduce risk of errors and minimize harm.

- Specific medications
  - EPINEPHrine, intramuscular, subcutaneous
  - Epoprostenol (e.g., Flolan), IV
  - Insulin U-500
  - Magnesium sulfate injection
  - Methotrexate, oral, nononcologic use
  - Nitroprusside sodium for injection
  - Opium tincture
  - Oxytocin, IV
  - Potassium chloride for injection concentrate
  - Potassium phosphate, injection
  - Promethazine, injection
  - Vasopressin, V and intraosseous
- Classes/categories of medications
  - Adrenergic agonists, IV (e.g., EPINEPHrine, phenylephrine, norepinephrine)
  - Adrenergic antagonists, IV(e.g., propranolol, metoprolol, labetalol)
  - Anesthetic agents, general, inhaled and IV (e.g., propofol, ketamine)
  - Antiarrhythmics, IV (e.g., lidocaine, amiodarone)
  - Antithrombotic agents, including:
    - Anticoagulants (e.g., warfarin, low-molecular-weight heparin, unfractionated heparin)
    - Direct oral anticoagulants and factor Xa inhibitors (e.g., dabigatran, rivaroxaban, apixaban, edoxaban, betrixaban, fondaparinux)
    - Direct thrombin inhibitors (e.g., argatroban, bivalirudin, dabigatran) glycoprotein IIb/IIIa inhibitors (e.g., eptifibatide)
    - Thrombolytics (e.g., alteplase, reteplase, tenecteplase)
  - Cardioplegic solutions

- Chemotherapeutic agents, parenteral and oral
- Dextrose, hypertonic 20% or greater
- Dialysis solutions, peritoneal dialysis and hemodialysis
- Epidural and intrathecal medications
- Inotropic medications, IV (e.g., digoxin, milrinone)
- Insulin, subcutaneous and IV
- Liposomal forms of drugs (e.g., liposomal amphotericin B) and conventional counterparts (e.g., amphotericin B desoxycholate)
- Moderate sedation agents, IV (e.g., dexmedetomidine, midazolam, LORazepam)
- Moderate and minimal sedation agents, oral, for children (e.g., chloral hydrate, midazolam, ketamine [using the parenteral form])
- Opioids, including:
  - IV
  - Oral (including liquid concentrates, immediate- and sustained-release formulations)
  - Transdermal
- Neuromuscular blocking agents (NMBs) (e.g., succinylcholine, rocuronium, vecuronium)
- Parenteral nutrition preparations
- Sodium chloride for injection, hypertonic, greater than 0.9% concentration
- Sterile water for injection, inhalation and irrigation (excluding pour bottles) in containers of 100 mL or more
- Sulfonylurea hypoglycemics, oral (e.g., chlorproPAMIDE, glimepiride, glyBURIDE, glipiZIDE, TOLBUTamide)[4]

High-alert medications in community/ambulatory care settings

High-alert medications are drugs that show an added risk of producing substantial harm when used in error in a community/ambulatory care setting.

- Specific medications
  - CarBAMazepine
  - EPINEPHrine, IM, subcutaneous
  - Insulin U-500 (special emphasis)*
  - LamoTRIgine
  - Methotrexate, oral and parenteral, nononcologic use (special emphasis)
  - Phenytoin
  - Valproic acid
- Classes/categories of medications
  - Antithrombotic agents, oral and parenteral, including:
    - Anticoagulants (e.g., warfarin, low-molecular-weight heparin, unfractionated heparin)
    - Direct oral anticoagulants and factor Xa inhibitors (e.g., dabigatran, rivaroxaban, apixaban, edoxaban)
    - Direct thrombin inhibitors (e.g., dabigatran)
  - Chemotherapeutic agents
    - Oral and parenteral chemotherapy (e.g., capecitabine, cyclophosphamide)

*All oral and parenteral chemotherapy, and all insulins are considered high-alert medications. These specific medications have been singled out for special emphasis to bring attention to the need for distinct strategies to prevent the types of errors that occur with these medications.

- Oral targeted therapy and immunotherapy (e.g., palbociclib [IBRANCE], imatinib [GLEEVEC], bosutinib [BOSULIF])
  - Excludes hormonal therapy
- Immunosuppressant agents, oral and parenteral (e.g., azaTHIOprine, cycloSPORINE, tacrolimus)
- Insulins, all formulations and strengths (e.g., U-100, U-200, U-300, U-500)
- Medications contraindicated during pregnancy (e.g., bosentan, ISOtretinoin)
- Moderate and minimal sedation agents, oral, for children (e.g., chloral hydrate, midazolam, ketamine [using the parenteral form])
- Opioids, all routes of administration (e.g., oral, sublingual, parenteral, transdermal), including liquid concentrates, immediate- and sustained-release formulations, and combination products with another drug
- Pediatric liquid medications that require measurement
- Sulfonylurea hypoglycemics, oral (e.g., chlorproPAMIDE, glimepiride, glyBURIDE, glipiZIDE, TOLBUTamide)[5]

High-alert medications in long-term care settings

High-alert medications are drugs that demonstrate an additional risk of creating considerable harm when used in error in a LTC setting.

- Specific medications
  - Concentrated morphine solution (20 mg/mL), oral (special emphasis)
  - Digoxin, parenteral and oral
  - EPINEPHrine, IM, subcutaneous
  - Insulin U-00
  - Iron dextran, parenteral
  - Methotrexate, oral and parenteral, nononcologic use (special emphasis)
  - Phenytoin
  - Sacubitril and valsartan (ENTRESTO)
- Classes/categories of medications
  - Anti-Parkinson's drugs, including carbidopa, levodopa, and combination products that contain at least one of these ingredients
  - Antithrombotic agents, parenteral and oral, including:
    - Anticoagulants (e.g., warfarin, low-molecular-weight heparin, unfractionated heparin)
    - Direct oral anticoagulants (e.g., dabigatran, rivaroxaban, apixaban, edoxaban, betrixaban)
    - Direct thrombin inhibitors (e.g., dabigatran)
  - Chemotherapeutic agents
    - Oral and parenteral chemotherapy (e.g., capecitabine, cyclophosphamide)
    - Oral targeted therapy and immunotherapy (e.g., palbociclib [IBRANCE], imatinib [GLEEVEC], bosutinib [BOSULIF])
    - Excludes hormonal therapy
  - GABA (gamma-aminobutyric acid) analogs (e.g., gabapentin, pregabalin) used to treat neuropathic pain
  - Immunosuppressants, oral and parenteral (e.g., azaTHIOprine, cycloSPORINE, cyclophosphamide, tacrolimus, abatacept [ORENCIA], adalimumab [HUMIRA])

- Insulins, all formulations and strengths (e.g., U-100, U-200, U-300, U-500
- Opioids, all routes of administration (e.g., oral, sublingual, parenteral, transdermal), including liquid concentrates, immediate- and sustained-release formulations, and combination products with another drug
- Parenteral nutrition preparations
- Sulfonylurea hypoglycemics, oral (e.g., chlorproPAMIDE, glimepiride, glyBURIDE, glipiZIDE, TOLBUTamide)[6]

Targeted medication safety best practices for hospitals

The Institute of Safe Medication Practices has identified specific medication issues that have resulted in patient harm and in some situations, death. These "best practices" include:

- Dispense vinCRIStine and other vinca alkaloids in a mini bag of a compatible solution and not in a syringe.

- Use a weekly dosage regimen default for oral methotrexate in electronic systems when medication orders are entered.

Require a hard stop verification of an appropriate oncologic indication for all daily oral methotrexate orders.

- Double-check all printed medication lists and discharge instructions to ensure that they indicate the correct dosage regimen for oral methotrexate prior to providing them to the patient.
- Ensure that the process for providing discharge instructions for oral methotrexate includes clear written instructions *and* clear verbal instructions that specifically review the dosing schedule, emphasize the danger with taking extra doses, and specify that the medication should not be taken "as needed" for symptom control.
- Require the patient to repeat back the instructions to validate that the patient understands the dosing schedule and toxicities of the medication if taken more frequently than prescribed.

3. Weigh each patient as soon as possible on admission and during each appropriate outpatient or emergency department encounter. Avoid the use of a stated, estimated, or historical weight. Measure and document patient weights in metric units only.
   - Ensure that electronic health record screen views, medication device screens (e.g., infusion pumps), printed patient information documents, and printed order and/or communication forms list or prompt for the patient's weight in metric units only.
   - Document the patient's weight in metric units only in all electronic and written formats.
4. Segregate, sequester, and differentiate all NMBs from other medications, wherever they are stored in the organization.
   - Eliminate the storage of NMBs in areas of the hospital where they are not routinely needed.
   - Limit availability in automated dispensing cabinets (ADCs) to perioperative, labor and delivery, critical care, and emergency department settings; in these areas, store NMBs in a rapid sequence intubation kit, or locked-lidded ADC pockets/drawers.

- Segregate NMBs from all other medications in the pharmacy by placing them in separate lidded containers in the refrigerator or other secure, isolated storage area.
- Place auxiliary labels on all storage bins and/or ADC pockets and drawers that contain NMBs as well as all final medication containers of NMBs (e.g., syringes, IV bags) that state: "Warning: Causes Respiratory Arrest—Patient Must Be Ventilated" or "Warning: Paralyzing Agent—Causes Respiratory Arrest" or "Warning: Causes Respiratory Paralysis—Patient Must Be Ventilated" to clearly communicate that respiratory paralysis will occur and ventilation is required.

5. Administer medication infusions via a programmable infusion pump utilizing dose error-reduction systems. Maintain a compliance rate of greater than 95% for the use of dose error-reduction systems. Monitor compliance with use of smart pump dose error-reduction software on a monthly basis.

6. Ensure all appropriate antidotes, reversal agents, and rescue agents are readily available. Have standardized protocols and/or coupled order sets in place that permit the emergency administration of all appropriate antidotes, reversal agents, and rescue agents used in the facility. Have directions for use/administration readily available in all clinical areas where the antidotes, reversal agents, and rescue agents are used.
   - Identify which antidotes, reversal agents, and rescue agents can be administered immediately in emergency situations to prevent patient harm.

7. When compounding sterile preparations, perform an independent verification to ensure that the proper ingredients (medications and diluents) are added, including confirmation of the proper amount (volume) of each ingredient prior to its addition to the final container.
   - Except in an emergency, perform this verification in all locations where compounded sterile preparations are made, including patient care units.
   - Use technology to assist in the verification process, such as machine-readable coding (e.g., barcoding scanning, radio-frequency identification [RFID]) of ingredients, gravimetric verification, robotics, and IV workflow software, to augment the manual processes. When technology is in use, it is important that processes are in place to ensure it is maintained, the software is updated, and the technology is always used in a manner that maximizes the medication safety features of these systems.

8. Eliminate the prescribing of fentaNYL patches for opioid-naïve patients and/or patients with acute pain.

9. Eliminate injectable promethazine from the formulary.
   - Remove injectable promethazine from all areas of the organization including the pharmacy.
   - Classify injectable promethazine as a nonstocked, nonformulary medication.
   - Implement a medical staff-approved automatic therapeutic substitution policy to convert all injectable promethazine orders to another antiemetic.
   - Remove injectable promethazine from all medication order screens and from all order sets and protocols.

10. Seek out and use information about medication safety risks and errors that have occurred in other organizations outside of your facility and take action to prevent similar errors.
    - Identify reputable resources (e.g., ISMP, The Joint Commission, ECRI, patient safety organizations, state agencies) to learn about risks and errors that have occurred externally.
    - Determine appropriate actions to be taken to minimize the risk of these types of errors occurring in the hospital.
    - Document the decisions reached and gain approval for required resources as necessary.
    - Share the external stories of risk and errors with all staff, along with any changes that will be made in the hospital to minimize their occurrence, and then begin implementation.

11. Verify and document a patient's opioid status (naïve versus tolerant) and type of pain (acute versus chronic) before prescribing and dispensing extended-release and long-acting opioids.
    - Default order entry systems to the lowest initial starting dose and frequency when initiating orders for extended-release and long-acting opioids.
    - Alert practitioners when extended-release and long-acting opioid dose adjustments are required due to age or renal or liver impairment or when patients are prescribed other sedating medications.
    - Eliminate the prescribing of fentaNYL patches for opioid-naïve patients and/or patients with acute pain.
    - Eliminate the storage of fentaNYL patches in ADCs or as unit stock in clinical locations where acute pain is primarily treated.

12. Limit the variety of medications that can be removed from an ADC using the override function. Require a medication order (e.g., electronic, written, telephone, verbal) prior to removing any medication from an ADC, including those removed using the override function. Monitor ADC overrides to verify appropriateness, transcription orders, and documentation of administration. Periodically review for appropriateness of medications available using the override function.

13. Safeguard against errors with oxytocin use.
    - Require the use of standard order sets for prescribing oxytocin antepartum and/or postpartum.
    - Standardize to a single concentration/bag size for both antepartum and postpartum oxytocin infusions.
    - Standardize how oxytocin doses, concentration, and rates are expressed.
    - Provide oxytocin in a ready-to-use form.

14. Maximize the use of barcode verification prior to medication and vaccine administration by expanding use beyond inpatient care areas.
    - Target clinical areas with an increased likelihood of a short or limited patient stay, such as the emergency department and outpatient areas.
    - Regularly review compliance and other metric data to assess utilization and effectiveness of this safety technology.

15. Layer numerous strategies throughout the medication-use process to improve safety with high-alert medications.
    - Outline a robust set of processes for managing risk, impacting as many steps of the medication-use

process as feasible for each medication on the institution's high-alert medication.
- Ensure that the strategies address system vulnerabilities in each stage of the medication-use process (i.e., prescribing, dispensing, administering, and monitoring) and apply to prescribers, pharmacists, nurses, and other practitioners involved in the medication-use process.
- Ensure that the strategies address system vulnerabilities in each stage of the medication-use process (i.e., prescribing, dispensing, administering, and monitoring) and apply to prescribers, pharmacists, nurses, and other practitioners involved in the medication-use process.[7]

Safe preparation of compounded sterile preparations

Essential technology attributes

- ACDs are interfaced with the electronic health record to remove transcription errors.
- Clinical decision support
  - Is tailored to specific patient populations (e.g., adult, pediatric, neonatal)
  - Warns practitioners when solution contents are inappropriate or unstable
  - Warns practitioners when solution osmolarity comes close to maximum limits for peripheral administration
- Parenteral formulations are ordered in concentrations and dosing units that match those available in the ACD.
- Machine-readable coding (e.g., barcode scanning, RFID) is used to confirm additives on the ACD.
- ACDs should:
  - Maintain record of beyond-use dates of additives
  - Record lot numbers and expiration dates of additives
- Auxiliary product information (e.g., storage conditions, filter use during administration) should be incorporated in the ACD dispensing label.
- All practitioners granted access and to modify the ACD database have their own unique login and password.
- Staff are properly trained and demonstrate their ability to operate ACDs before using.
- The final preparation is visually inspected according to USP standards and applicable regulations/guidelines.
- Backup, emergency power is available to prevent an abrupt shutdown in the case of an unexpected power outage while the ACD is running.
- Defined downtime procedures exist and
  - Address standard workflow for both hardware and software failures.
  - Determine when a switch to manual processes is necessary.
  - Define documentation and labeling processes.

Safe pharmacy processes for ACDs

- ACDs are used for all compounded parenteral nutrition infusions.
- A workflow process is established to distinguish new products and input them into the ACD database before they are available for use.
- Staff with access to modify the ACD database is restricted.

- Staff permitted to change the ACD database are trained and their ability to perform database functions is evaluated.
- An independent double check anytime a change is made to the ACD database and is documented.
- All practitioners granted access to change the ACD database possess their own unique login and password.
- Staff are properly trained, and their competency for operating ACDs is evaluated before use.
- The final preparation is visually inspected according to USP standards, regulations, and guidelines.
- Backup, emergency power is available to prevent an abrupt shutdown in the case of an unexpected power outage while the ACD is running.
- Defined downtime procedures exist, and an annual tabletop stimulation is conducted to identify gaps and revise procedures as needed. Downtime procedures:
  - Address standard workflow for both hardware and software failures.
  - Determine when a switch to manual processes is necessary.
  - Define documentation and labeling processes.
- Tabletop simulations include assessment of users competency with manual SOPs.
- Vendor-suggested preventive maintenance is adhered to prevent unforeseen hardware and/or software downtime.

Safety gaps and associated best practices for automated compounding devices

Safety gap	Best practices
Connecting tubing to source products	A dedicated PEC is available for each ACD. If a dedicated PEC is not available when the ACD is in use, no other sterile compounding activities take place in the PEC.
	Policies and procedures define the steps required to set up the ACD before use and when tubing and source products need to be changed.
	Machine-readable code (e.g., barcode, RFID) verification and line tracing are used when setting up source products on the ACD.
	A second individual documents and verifies ACD setup steps, including machine-readable coding (e.g., barcode, RFID) verification for the connection of products to tubing and line tracing.
Using compounded stock solutions (e.g., diluted trace element solutions)	IV workflow management systems are used to prepare compounded solutions for use on the ACD.
Manually adding products (e.g., separately using a syringe) to a compounded sterile product prepared using an ACD	Use of the ACD is maximized to limit the number of products that must be added manually.

Safety gaps and associated best practices for automated compounding devices —cont'd	
Safety gap	Best practices
	If a product must be added manually to a sterile product prepared using an ACD, an IV workflow management system is used during the manual compounding step. If an IV workflow management system is not available, a second individual performs independent verification of manual additions to ensure that the proper medications (and diluents, if applicable) are added, including confirmation of the proper volume of each medication and diluent, if applicable) before addition to the final container.
	Machine-readable coding (e.g., barcode, RFID) is used to verify manually prepared additives.
	Policies define the order for adding manually prepared solutions to compounded sterile preparations to minimize the risk of precipitation.
Alert overrides	Organizations should define how overrides of system warnings or alerts are to be managed considering the overall goal is to limit overrides, building in a second verification before a warning is overridden, and being sensitive to operations that may unnecessarily lead to care delays.
	Limit warnings to those with the most value.
	Regularly review alert overrides to determine appropriateness and to facilitate process improvement.

ACD, automated compounding device; *PEC,* primary engineering control; *RFID,* radio-frequency identification.

Essential technology attributes in IV workflow management systems

- IV workflow management systems
  - Are interfaced with the electronic health record to eliminate order transcription from one system into another
  - Permit users to establish an MFR for non-patient-specific batch, stock solution, and patient-specific compounded sterile preparations
  - Maintain an electronic log of changes made to the database by users
  - Let users to customize the incoming order queue to prioritize work
  - Automatically perform calculations or conversions
  - Direct users through key steps in the compounding process
  - Record all steps and components of the compounding process
  - Provide beyond-use dating of opened or reconstituted products to warn practitioners and prevent use of an expired product
  - Permit customization of labels (e.g., tall man lettering [TML], color print, reverse print, electronic health record compatible barcode)
  - Regulate the printing of the dispensing label until the compounding process is finished
- MFR changes are time stamped, saved, and identify the user who made the modification.
- When a system update is available, IV workflow management system vendors ensure all customers receive and install the update in a reasonable time frame.

Safe pharmacy processes for IV workflow management systems

- Use of an IV workflow management system is the minimum safety standard for preparing compounded sterile preparations.
- A workflow process is in place to identify new products and enter them into the IV workflow management system database before they are available for use.
- When a new drug (or a new manufacturer of a drug that is already in the system) is entered into the IV workflow management system database, an assessment of information needed to ensure safe use of the drug is completed.
- The number of staff who have access to change the IV workflow management system database is limited.
- Staff who are granted access to change the IV workflow management system database are trained, and their competency to perform database functions is assessed.
- A second practitioner performs an independent double check anytime a change is made to the IV workflow management system database, and the check is documented in the system.
- When applicable, test changes made to the database (e.g., verifying that a newly entered barcode scans correctly).
- All practitioners approved to access and change the IV workflow management system database have their own unique login and password.
- MFRs are customized and include specific directions for each process step (e.g., volume of fluid to withdraw, volume of fluid to add, concentrations, formulations, special filters, tubing, diluents, supplies, storage instructions, protection from light guidance), and this information is presented to the user before initiation of the compounding process.
- Compounding staff prepare and label one patient-specific product at a time and avoid printing multiple patient-specific labels at once.
- The final label applied to the compounded sterile preparation is a dispensing label intended for the health care practitioner (or patient) who will be administering the medication.
- IV workflow management system hardware is set up in a manner that facilitates compounding without increasing the potential for frequent sterility breaches.
- Movement out of the PEC when using IV workflow management systems is minimized, decreasing the number of times gloves must be disinfected.

- At the completion of the compounding process, the final preparation is visually inspected according to USP standards and applicable regulations/guidelines. Documentation supports the visual inspection
- Routinely observe the compounding process to identify risks and ensure that IV workflow management systems are being used as designed and described in SOPs.
- Whenever a change to the workflow process is planned, the change is evaluated using simulation to identify gaps and revise procedures as necessary.
- Backup, emergency power is available to avoid an abrupt shutdown in case of an unexpected power outage while the IV workflow management system is running.
- Defined downtime procedures exist, and an annual table-top stimulation is conducted to identify gaps and revise procedures as needed. Downtime procedures:
  - Address standard workflow for both hardware and software failures
  - Determine when a switch to manual processes is necessary
  - Define documentation and labeling processes
- Tabletop simulations include assessment of users competency with manual SOPs.
- Vendor-suggested preventive maintenance is adhered to prevent unforeseen hardware and/or software downtime.

Safety gaps and associated best practices in IV workflow management systems

Safety gap	Best practices
Compounds that need multiple vials or infusion bags for preparation	Every vial or bag needed for compounding should have a machine-readable code (e.g., barcode, RFID) that is scanned during the compounding workflow process.
Tolerance limits when using gravimetric analysis	Users should follow guidance from product vendors when gravimetric analysis is used to determine the minimum volume that can be accurately measured by the integrated scale.
	Product vendors should communicate the minimum volume that can be accurately measured by the integrated scale to users and build this information into the IV workflow management system's master formulation records.
	Follow product vendors' recommendations for initial system settings and IV workflow management system setup.
	Drug manufacturers should publish and/or share densities of their drug products.
	Product vendors should supply densities if available and assist users in setting up tolerance limits.
	Users should partner with product vendors to support compounding process challenges (e.g., accuracy when measuring products in syringes, small dose accuracy, accounting for drug left in the hub of needles, quality of the integrated scale).

Safety gaps and associated best practices in IV workflow management systems—cont'd

Safety gap	Best practices
Alert overrides	Organizations should define how overrides of system warnings or alerts are to be managed considering the overall goal is to limit overrides, building in a second verification before a warning is overridden, and being sensitive to operations that may unnecessarily lead to care delays.
	Limit warnings to those with the most value.
	Regularly review alert overrides to determine appropriateness and to facilitate process improvement.
Label swapping	Prepare one product at a time, allowing dispensing labels to remain in the queue until the time of compounding to ensure the correct label is affixed to the product at the proper time.
	If separate production and dispensing labels are used, application of the dispensing label should be verified by machine-readable coding (e.g., barcode, RFID).
	Develop standard operating procedures to prevent unnecessary reprinting of production and/or dispensing labels.
Incomplete auxiliary product information	Auxiliary product information (e.g., storage conditions) should be incorporated in the IV workflow management system dispensing label

RFID, radio-frequency identification.

Essential technology attributes for IV robots

- IV robots are interfaced with the electronic health record to eliminate order transcription from one system not another.
  - IV robots are interfaced with IV workflow management systems if the IV workflow management system is used to compound solutions for use in the IV robot.
  - If a compounded sterile preparation has been discontinued before initiation of the compounding process, the system interface allows for the removal of these products from the queue.
- IV robots allow users to create an MFR for non-patient-specific batch, stock solution, and patient-specific compounded sterile preparations.
  - MFRs include additional steps required for IV robot setup and programming (e.g., needle angle, agitation time for reconstitution).
  - When MFRs are created, the IV robot prompts for an independent double check and the check is documented in the system.
  - IV robot MFRs are easily accessible, organized, and easy to maintain.
  - MFR changes are time-stamped and identify the user who made the modification.
- Machine readable coding (e.g., barcode scanning, RFID), and/or image capture for nonbarcoded items, is used to verify products, including diluents, during the compounding process.

- If a machine-readable code (e.g., barcode, RFID) is manually added to a product so that it can be used in the IV robot, a second individual verifies the code using an independent double check.
- At the completion of the compounding process, there is a gravimetric check of the preparation to ensure the correct volume of additives has been included.
- The IV robot applies a dispensing label to the completed compounded sterile preparation.
- IV robots allow for customization of labels (e.g., TML, color print, reverse printing, electronic health record-compatible barcode).
- IV robots prompt users when maintenance is needed.
- IV robot vendors supply a comprehensive user service agreement that specifically addresses, at a minimum, expectations related to service, hardware and software maintenance and update, training, and retraining of staff.
- When a system update is available, IV robot vendors ensure all customers receive and install the update in a reasonable time frame.

Safe pharmacy processes for IV robots

- IV robots are considered when preparing products with high volume of use and/or products that require large batch preparations.
- SOPs are defined for IV robot operations.
- Staff are adequately trained, and their competency for operating IV robots is assessed before use.
- Annual vendor-supported training is offered to all IV robot staff operators.
- Staff are assessed annually for their competence with IV robot operations.
- SOPs define the process required to program the IV robot.
- Staff who are granted access to program or change the IV robot database are trained, and their competency to perform database functions is assessed.
- All practitioners approved to access and change the IV robot database have their own unique login and password.
- The number of staff who have access to program or modify the IV robot database is limited. Modifications to the IV robot database are documented along with the reason the change was made.
- When modifications are made to the IV robot database, staff follow a defined change control process including an assessment of information required to ensure safe use of the new product. Drug-specific information in the IV robot database is reviewed and updated annually to ensure content is up-to-date.
- A second practitioner performs an independent double check anytime a change is made to the IV robot, and the check is documented in the system.
- When using the IV robot for large batches, staff attempt to secure a large volume of products from the same manufacturer production lot.
- Staff ensure that routine calibration and certification of IV robot equipment components are performed according to vendor requirements. Calibration and certification are documented.

- Maintenance, media fills, monthly surface sampling, and cleaning follow vendor recommendations, USP standards, and applicable regulations and guidelines.
- At the completion of the compounding process, the final preparation is visually inspected in compliance with USP standards and applicable regulations and guidelines.
- Backup, emergency power is available to avoid an abrupt shutdown in case of an unexpected power outage while the IV robot is running.
- Defined downtime procedures exist, and an annual table-top stimulation is conducted to identify gaps and revise procedures as needed. Downtime procedures:
  - Address standard workflow for both hardware and software failures
  - Determine when a switch to manual processes is necessary
  - Define documentation and labeling processes
- Tabletop simulations include assessment of users competency with manual SOPs.
- Vendor-suggested preventive maintenance is adhered to in order to prevent unforeseen hardware and/or software downtime.

Safety gap	Best practices
Machine-readable codes that are not readable	Users should avoid the use of products with difficult-to-read machine-readable codes (e.g., barcodes, RFID).
	Users should use IV workflow management systems to provide a product with reliable machine-readable codes (e.g., barcode, RFID).
Label swapping when the dispensing label is applied to the compounded sterile preparation manually	Label one product at a time immediately after generation of the dispensing label to ensure the correct label is affixed to the product.
	Application of the dispensing label is verified by machine-readable coding (e.g., barcode, RFID).
Incomplete auxiliary product information	Auxiliary product information (e.g., storage conditions) should be incorporated in the IV robot dispensing label.

RFID, radio-frequency identification.

Best practices for sterile compounding

- Sterile compounding outside the pharmacy should be minimized.
- To the extent possible, commercially manufactured parenteral products are used over manually compounded sterile preparations.
- Organizational practices employed for compounding sterile preparations follow USP standards and applicable regulations and guidelines.
- SOPs for compounding are defined and include QC, change control, and documentation.

- SOPs for labeling preparations are defined, sufficiently detailed, and used to prevent process variation among staff.
- SOPs for verification of compounded sterile preparations are defined, sufficiently detailed, and used to prevent process variation among staff.
- Staff who prepare and/or verify compounded sterile preparations are trained, and their competency to perform sterile compounding procedures is assessed annually.
  - Competency assessments for specific aspects of sterile compounding could include performing calculations, preparing dilutions, compounding base solutions, preparing medications for specific administration routes (e.g., intrathecal administration), demonstrating proper use of devices (e.g., filter needles/straws), and operating technology used in the compounding process.
  - Competency assessments must follow USP standards and applicable regulations and guidelines.
- Organizations include additional training and competency assessment for preparing chemotherapy, HDs, parenteral nutrition, neonatal and pediatric preparations, and high-risk compounding.
- All orders (or prescriptions) that are transcribed, including entry into a pharmacy information system, a chemotherapy dosing system, or an ACD, are verified by a pharmacist.
- MFRs are verified by a second individual using an independent double check before use.
- A process is in place (e.g., the use of bins) to allow for the separation of products and supplies used during the compounding process for each preparation or batch preparation.
- Compounding dose volume information is available on a production label, MFR, or other approved document to avoid the need for manual calculations.
- Production labels, if used, are not the final dispensing label.
- If multiple vials, bottles, bags, or syringes of a specific product are used during the preparation process, all vials, bottle, bags, and syringes, whether partially full or empty, are presented to the pharmacist as part of the final verification process.
- Clearly defined and segregated areas exist for products (and corresponding materials) awaiting verification by a pharmacist.
- In organizations that care for adult, pediatric, and neonatal patients, strategies are implemented to differentiate compounding productions (e.g., separate the timing for preparation of pediatric and neonatal patients from adult patients, prepare in different locations, adjust/customize labeling).
- Batch preparations are logged, and documentation includes the theoretical versus actual yield and all waste.
- Organizations consider outsourcing sterile compounding services as a strategic option to in-house compounding based on an in-depth assessment that considers organizational, operational, staffing, financial, quality, and regulatory issues.

- Organizations maintain a drug conservation policy to address and maintain the integrity and sterility of drugs in short supply during their handling and dispensing.
- Machine-readable coding (e.g., barcode, RFID) verification is used during replenishment and removal of medication stock used for sterile compounding.
- Pharmacists who practice primarily in sterile compounding should obtain advanced training (e.g., a certificate program).
- Pharmacists in charge of sterile compounding may consider Board of Pharmacy Specialties Board Certification in Compounded Sterile Preparations.
- Technicians expected to perform sterile compounding may consider PTCB Compounded Sterile Preparation Technician certification.
- Errors and close calls that occur during the preparation of compounded sterile preparations are documented through the organization's reporting system for analysis.
- Errors and close calls should be reported to the ISMP Medication Error Reporting Program or ISMP National Vaccine Errors Reporting Program for learning purposes and dissemination of prevention measures.

Recommendations

- Maximize the use of manufacturer-prepared products.
- Purchase products in patient-specific doses that are ready to administer.
- If a commercially manufactured product is not available, investigate the use of a commercially prepared product (e.g., from a compounding pharmacy or outsourcing facility). See reference section for American Society of Health System Pharmacists Guidelines on Outsourcing Sterile Compounding Services.
- When sterile compounding is performed in a pharmacy, multiple compounded sterile preparations of the same drug, dose, and administration route for one or multiple patients can be compounded at the same time.
- When sterile compounding is performed in a pharmacy (without use of compounding technology), the pharmacist independently verifies that the proper medications and diluents are added, including confirming the proper volume of each medication and/or diluent, before their addition to the final container.
- If compounding (e.g., dilution, reconstitution) must occur outside a pharmacy environment, aseptic techniques, processes and procedures, and USP standards for beyond-use dating, as well as other applicable regulations and guidelines, are followed.
- If compounding must occur outside a pharmacy environment, SOPs for compounding and labeling preparations are defined.
- If compounding must occur outside a pharmacy environment, have a second practitioner independently verify the proper medications (and diluents, where applicable) are added, including confirming each ingredient's proper volume before the addition to the final container.
- If compounding must occur outside a pharmacy environment, staff who prepare and/or verify compounded sterile preparations are trained, and their competency to perform sterile compounding and associated procedures is assessed annually.

- Errors and close calls that occur during the preparation of compounded sterile preparations are documented through the organization's reporting system for analysis.[8]

Look-alike/sound-alike medications with recommended tall man letters

The FDA issued a list of approved generic drug names using TML. TML is a method that utilizes lettering to distinguish look-alike drug names. Beginning on the left side of the drug name, TML emphasizes the differences between similar drug names by capitalizing unlike letters. In addition, TML can be utilized with color or boldfacing to draw awareness to the similarities between look-alike drug names.

FDA-approved list of generic drug names with tall man letters	
Drug name with tall man letters	Confused with
aceta**ZOLAMIDE**	aceto**HEXAMIDE**
aceto**HEXAMIDE**	aceta**ZOLAMIDE**
bu**PROP**ion	bus**PIR**one
bus**PIR**one	bu**PROP**ion
chlorpro**MAZINE**	chlorpro**PAMIDE**
chlorpro**PAMIDE**	chlorpro**MAZINE**
clomi**PHENE**	clomi**PRAMINE**
clomi**PRAMINE**	clomi**PHENE**
cyclo**SERINE**	cyclo**SPORINE**
cyclo**SPORINE**	cyclo**SERINE**
DAUNOrubicin	**DOXO**rubicin
dimenhy**DRINATE**	diphenhydr**AMINE**
diphenhydr**AMINE**	dimenhy**DRINATE**
DOBUTamine	**DOP**amine
DOPamine	**DOBUT**amine
DOXOrubicin	**DAUNO**rubicin
glipi**ZIDE**	gly**BURIDE**
gly**BURIDE**	glipi**ZIDE**
hydr**ALAZINE**	hydr**OXY**zine—**HYDRO**morphone
HYDROmorphone	hydr**OXY**zine—hydr**ALAZINE**
hydr**OXY**zine	hydr**ALAZINE**—**HYDRO**morphone
medroxy**PROGESTER**one	methyl**PREDNIS**olone—methyl**TESTOSTER**one
methyl**PREDNIS**olone	medroxy**PROGESTER**one—methyl**TESTOSTER**one
methyl**TESTOSTER**one	medroxy**PROGESTER**one—methyl**PREDNIS**olone
mito**XANTRONE**	Not specified
ni**CAR**dipine	**NIFE**dipine
NIFEdipine	ni**CAR**dipine
predniso**LONE**	predni**SONE**
predni**SONE**	predniso**LONE**
risperi**DONE**	r**OPINIR**ole

r**OPINIR**ole	risperi**DONE**
sulf**ADIAZINE**	sulfi**SOXAZOLE**
sulfi**SOXAZOLE**	sulf**ADIAZINE**
TOLAZamide	**TOLBUT**amide
TOLBUTamide	**TOLAZ**amide
vin**BLAS**tine	vin**CRIS**tine
vin**CRIS**tine	vin**BLAS**tine

Institute for Safe Medication Practices list of additional drug names with tall man letters

ISMP issues a list of look-alike drug names with recommended tall man letters containing drug name pairs and trios with recommended, bolded tall man (uppercase) letters to help draw attention to the dissimilarities in look-alike drug names. The list includes mostly generic-generic drug name pairs, although a few brand-brand or brand-generic name pairs are included.

ISMP provides a list of additional drug names with recommendations of the placement of tall man letters. The ISMP follows the CD3 rule. The methodology recommends working from the left of the drug name first by capitalizing all the characters to the right once two or more different letters are observed, and then, working from the right, returning two or more letters common to both words to lowercase letters. When the rule cannot be used because there are no common letters on the right side of the name, the procedure proposes capitalizing the central part of the word only. When use of this rule fails to lead to the best TML option (e.g., makes names appear too similar, makes names hard to read based on pronunciation), an alternative option is considered. It should be noted that this list is not approved by the FDA.

Drug name	Confused drug name
Aciphex	Accupril, Aricept
Actos	Actonel
Adderall	Adderall XR, Inderal
ALPRAZolam	clonazePAM, LORazepam
amiodarone	amantadine
amLODIPine	aMILopride
ARIPiprazole	proton pump inhibitors, RABEprazole
atorvastatin	atomoxetine
buPROPion	busPIRone
Cardizem	Cardene
CeleBREX	CeleXA, Cerebyx
cetirizine	sertraline, stavudine
clonazePAM	ALPRAZolam, clobazam, clonidine, clozapine, LORazepam
Cozaar	Colace, Zocor
Depakote	Depakote ER
DULoxetine	Dexilant, FLUoxetine, Paroxetine
gabapentin	gemfibrozil
glipiZIDE	glyBURIDE

(Continued)

Drug name	Confused drug name
HumaLOG	HumuLIN, NovoLOG
hydroCHLOROthiazide	hydrALAZINE, hydrOXYzine
HYDROcodone	oxyCODONE
Jantoven	Janumet, Januvia
Lantus	Latuda, Lente
levothyroxine	lamotrigine, Lanoxin, liothyronine
Lotronex	Protonix
medroxyPROGESTERone	HYDROXYprogesterone, methylPREDNISolone, methylTESTOSTERone
metFORMIN	metroNIDAZOLE
metoprolol succinate	metoprolol tartrate
NIFEdipine	niCARdipine, niMODipine
oxyCODONE	HYDROcodone, oxybutynin, OxyCONTIN, oxyMORphone
Paxil	Doxil, Plavix, Taxol
Plavix	Paxil, Pradaxa
Prandin	Avandia
prednisoLONE	predniSONE
propylthiouracil	Purinethol
PROzac	Prograf, PriLOSEC, Provera
SandIMMUNE	SandoSTATIN
SEROquel	Desyrel, SEROquel XR, Serzone, SINEquan
SINEquan	saquinavir, SEROquel, Singulair, Zonegran
SITagliptin	sAXagliptin, SUMAtriptan
SOLU-Medrol	DEPO-Medrol, Solu-CORTEF
Spiriva	Apidra, Inspra
sulfADIAZINE	sulfasalazine, sulfiSOXAZOLE
tacrolimus	tamsulosin
TEGretol	TEGretol XR, Tequin, TRENtal
Toujeo	Tradjenta, Tresiba, Trulicity
Tresiba	Tanzeum, Tarceva, Toujeo, Tradjenta
Trulicity	Tanzeum, Toujeo, Tradjenta, Tresiba
Zebeta	Diabeta, Zetia
Zestril	Zegerid, Zetia, ZyPREXA
Zetia	Bextra, Zebeta, Zestril
Zocor	Cozaar, ZyrTEC
Zyloprim	zolpidem
ZyPREXA	CeleXA, Reprexain, Zestril, ZyrTEC
ZyrTEC	Lipitor, Zerit, Zocor, ZyPREXA, ZyrTEC-D

Brand names start with an uppercase letter. Some brand names incorporate tall man letters in initial characters and may not be readily recognized as brand names. Brand names appear in black; generic names/other products appear in red.

A complete listing of FDA and ISMP Lists of Look-Alike Drug Names With Recommended Tall Man Letters can be accessed at https://www.ismp.org/sites/default/files/attachments/2017-11/tallmanletters.pdf.

A health care organization should implement processes to reduce the risk of potential errors involving look-alike and sound-alike medications. Examples of strategies used include using both the brand and generic names on prescriptions and labels; including the purpose of the medication on prescriptions; configuring computer selection screens to prevent look-alike names from appearing consecutively; and changing the appearance of look-alike product names to draw attention to their dissimilarities.

CHAPTER REVIEW QUESTIONS

1. Which organization is responsible for the safety, efficacy, and security of medications?
   a. Centers for Medicare and Medicaid Services
   b. DEA
   c. EPA
   d. FDA
2. Which USP standard addresses pharmaceutical compounding of nonsterile preparations?
   a. USP <795>
   b. USP <797>
   c. USP <800>
   d. USP <825>
3. Which legislation was enacted to improve the portability and continuity of health coverage in the group and individual markets?
   a. ACA
   b. Title II Drug Supply Chain Security Act
   c. FDCA
   d. HIPAA
4. Which organization is responsible for reducing the impact of substance abuse and mental illness in communities?
   a. DEA
   b. EPA
   c. NRC
   d. Substance Abuse and Mental Health Services Administration
5. Which of the following medications is an example of Schedule IV Controlled Substance?
   a. Acetaminophen with codeine
   b. Alprazolam
   c. Methylphenidate
   d. Pregabalin
6. How often must a pharmacy conduct a biennial inventory of all controlled substances?
   a. Every year
   b. Every 2 years
   c. Every 3 years
   d. Every 4 years
7. Which organization accredits specialty pharmacies?
   a. Accreditation Commission for Health Care
   b. Center for Pharmacy Practice Accreditation
   c. Joint Commission
   d. URAC
8. Which of the following is an example an organization that established pharmacy standards for compounding sterile products in the United States?
   a. Congress
   b. PTCB

c. State board of pharmacy

d. United States Pharmacopoeia (USP)

9. Which of the following is a legal document indicating an individual meets certain objective standards provided by a neutral organization?

    a. Certification

    b. Code

    c. Regulation

    d. Statute

10. Which legislation required every medications to be assigned an 11-digit number known as a NDC?

    a. Dietary Supplement Health and Education Act of 1994

    b. Drug Listing Act of 1972

    c. Kefauver-Harris Amendment to FDCA of 1962

    d. Prescription Drug Marketing Act of 1987

11. Which DEA document is used to order Schedule II Controlled Substances for a pharmacy?

    a. DEA Form 41

    b. DEA Form 106

    c. DEA Form 107

    d. DEA Form 222

12. Which of the following regulations should be checked prior to the disposal of HD waste?

    a. Federal regulations

    b. State regulations

    c. Local regulations

    d. All the above

13. When must a pharmacy provide a medication guide to a patient?

    a. When a medication is dispensed in a retail pharmacy

    b. When a drug is subject to a REMS as an element to assure safe use

    c. When the patient requests a medication guide

    d. All the above

14. Which of the following medications require a medication guide to be provided to a patient?

    a. Amoxicillin

    b. Celecoxib

    c. Cetirizine

    d. Famotidine

15. What is the maximum amount of pseudoephedrine that may be purchased in 1 day by a patient?

    a. 2.4 g

    b. 3.6 g

    c. 4.8 g

    d. 9 g

16. What is the minimum age for a patient to purchase pseudoephedrine?

    a. 14 years

    b. 16 years

    c. 18 years

    d. 21 years

17. Which of the following medications require a patient product insert be provided to a patient?

    a. Albuterol inhaler

    b. Diphenhydramine

    c. Hydrochlorothiazide

    d. Sulfamethoxazole/trimethoprim

18. The DEA is conducting an administrative inspection for a pharmacy. Which pharmacy records are subject for review?

    a. Biennial inventory

    b. Distribution records

    c. Dispensing records

    d. All the above

19. Which is an example of medication exempted from being dispensed in a child-resistant container?

    a. Furosemide

    b. Levothyroxine

    c. Nitroglycerin

    d. Warfarin

20. How often must a pharmacist or pharmacy technician demonstrate sterile compound competency and undergo written/electronic testing?

    a. At least every 3 months

    b. At least every 6 months

    c. At least every 12 months

    d. At least every 24 months

21. Which of the following is an area in nonsterile compounding that pharmacists or pharmacy technicians must demonstrate their competency?

    a. Achieving and or maintaining sterility

    b. Hand hygiene and garbing

    c. Proper use of PECs

    d. All the above

22. Which category CSP may be assigned a BUD of greater than 12 hours at controlled room temperature or more than 24 hours if refrigerated?

    a. Category 1

    b. Category 2

    c. Category 3

    d. Category 4

23. Prior to compounding a nonsterile compound, how long should people wash their hands and forearms?

    a. 15 seconds

    b. 30 seconds

    c. 45 seconds

    d. 60 seconds

24. A pharmacy technician has compounded a cream containing preservatives for a patient. Which BUD should be assigned to this compound?

    a. 14 days

    b. 35 days

    c. 90 days

    d. 180 days

25. Which of the following may be a root cause of a medication error?

    a. Human

    b. Organizational

    c. Technical

    d. All the above

26. A pharmacy technician forgets to provide a medication guide to a patient when they are picking up their prescription. What type of medication error is this?

    a. Adverse drug error

    b. Compliance error

    c. Documentation error

    d. Medication education error

27. Which temperature refers to a cold environment?
    a. −25°C and −10°C
    b. Not to exceed 8°C
    c. 8°C and 15°C
    d. 15°C and 30°C
28. When disposing of medication at home, which of the following may be mixed with the medication in a sealed plastic bag?
    a. Cat litter
    b. Coffee grounds
    c. Dirt
    d. All the above
29. Which of the following medications has the ISMP identified as a high-alert medication in a community pharmacy?
    a. CarBAMazepine
    b. Insulin U-100
    c. Insulin U-500
    d. Sacubitril/valsartan (ENTRESTO)
30. Which of the following has been identified by the ISMP as a best practice for a hospital?
    a. Dispense vinCRIStine and other vinca alkaloids in a syringe.
    b. Eliminate the prescribing of fentaNYL patches for opioid-tolerant patients and/or patients with acute pain.
    c. Limit the variety of medications that can be removed from an ADC using the override function.
    d. Weight the patient within 48 hours of being admitted.
31. Which organizations have issued lists of look-alike/sound-alike medications?
    a. DEA and FDA
    b. FDA and ISMP
    c. MedWatch and The Joint Commission
    d. All the above
32. Which strategy is used to reduce the risk of potential errors involving look-alike/sound alike medications?
    a. Configure the computer selection screens to prevent look-alike names from appearing consecutively.
    b. Identify the indication of the medication on the prescription.
    c. Use both brand and generic names on prescriptions and prescription labels.
    d. All the above.
33. Which is a behavior observed in a "Just Culture"?
    a. Human error
    b. At-risk behavior
    c. Reckless behavior
    d. All the above
34. Which type of Medicare requires participating pharmacies to implement a continuous quality improvement program?
    a. Part A
    b. Part B
    c. Part C
    d. Part D

REFERENCES

1. Code of ethics for pharmacists. Accessed June 16, 2022. https://www.ashp.org/-/media/assets/policy-guidelines/docs/endorsed-documents/code-of-ethics-for-pharmacists.ashx.
2. Pharmacy technician code of ethics. AAPT American Association of Pharmacy Technicians. Accessed June 16, 2022. https://www.pharmacytechnician.com/pharmacy-technician-code-of-ethics/
3. <795> Pharmaceutical compounding-non-sterile preparations. Accessed June 20, 2022. https://www.uspnf.com/sites/default/files/usp_pdf/EN/USPNF/usp-nf-commentary/795-commentary-20221101.pdf
4. High-alert medications in acute care settings. ISMP. Accessed June 14. 2022. https://www.ismp.org/recommendations/high-alert-medications-acute-list
5. High-alert medications in community/ambulatory care settings. ISMP. Accessed June 14, 2022. https://www.ismp.org/recommendations/high-alert-medications-community-ambulatory-list
6. High-alert medications in long-term care (LTC) settings. ISMP. Accessed June 14, 2022. https://www.ismp.org/recommendations/high-alert-medications-long-term-care-list
7. Targeted medication safety best practices for hospitals. ISMP. Accessed June 16, 2022. https://www.ismp.org/guidelines/best-practices-hospitals
8. ISMP guidelines for Sterile Compounding the safe use of sterile compounding. ISMP. Accessed June 17, 2022. https://www.ismp.org/resources/guidelines-sterile-compounding-and-safe-use-sterile-compounding-technology

Controlled Substances Diversion Prevention Certificate

Controlled substances diversion prevention domains

Controlled substance diversion (9%)
- Consequences of diversion (e.g., infection risks to patients, organizational liability, fines/indictments, fraud charges, loss of job and/or license)
- Signs of impaired health care workers (e.g., mood changes, agitation, dilated pupils, sudden declines in job performance)
- Motivations to divert controlled substances (CS) (e.g., addiction, financial gain, recreation)

Controlled substance diversion prevention program (30%)
- Areas of vulnerability in procurement, preparation and dispensing, prescribing, administration, and waste/removal processes
- Elements of a comprehensive and effective controlled substances diversion prevention program
- Types and functions of security control measures, devices, and software to detect and prevent diversion (e.g., locking storage, cameras, automatic dispensing cabinets, analytics software)
- High-risk areas of the pharmacy (e.g., anesthesia area, CS vault, IV room, will call, receiving)
- Chain of custody methods (e.g., regulation of access control, presence of witnesses for signing delivery sheets, use of tamper-evident containers)

Drug enforcement administration requirements (38%)
- Drug Enforcement Administration registration requirements (e.g., power of attorney, renewal)
- Procedures to validate Drug Enforcement Administration numbers (e.g., formula and component parts of the Drug Enforcement Administration number)
- Contents, appropriate usage, and record keeping for Drug Enforcement Administration Form 222
- Drug Enforcement Administration Controlled Substance Ordering System
- Contents, appropriate usage, and record keeping for Drug Enforcement Administration Form 41
- Contents, appropriate usage, and record keeping for Drug Enforcement Administration Form 106
- Knowledge of Drug Enforcement Administration scheduled medications and which are at high risk for diversion
- Drug Enforcement Administration requirements for conducting physical inventories and record keeping
- Contents, appropriate usage, and record keeping for Drug Enforcement Administration Form 107
- Actions to take during a robbery or theft event
- Procedures for sales of CS and restricted over-the-counter drugs (e.g., pseudoephedrine)

Surveillance and investigation (23%)
- Suspicious data patterns (e.g., waste buddy, night shift sedation, cancel removes, pocket inventory, anomalous usage)
- Surveillance practices and techniques (e.g., reconciliation of invoices to purchase history reports, checklist to verify all paperwork is complete, records audits)
- Signs of product tampering and/or alteration (e.g., vials tops that do not twist easily, chipped tablets, drug assay sampling)
- Signs of and methods to detect fraudulent prescriptions

Controlled substance diversion

Drug diversion can be defined as any criminal act or deviation that removes a prescription drug from its intended path from the manufacturer to the intended patient. Drug diversion can occur in all health care settings to include hospitals, clinics, physician offices, and pharmacies. Evidence indicates employees with the greatest access to controlled substances are at the highest risk for diversion.

Consequences of diversion

Controlled substance diversion may result in

- Putting the patient at risk of not receiving adequate pain relief
- Infection due to contaminated needles
- Inadequate care provided by an impaired health care provider
- Adverse publicity to the health care organization, resulting in damage to its reputation, that may result in both civil and criminal penalties
- Loss of job
- Felony prosecution, civil malpractice, professional licensing/certification being suspended/revoked of the health care worker
- Addiction and overdose
- Financial loss to a health care organization due to diversion
- Employee absenteeism
- Expensive drug diversion investigations
- Required reporting requirements that may become publicized and present negative publicity of the pharmacy

Signs of impaired health care workers

Behavioral signs of drug impairment

- Severe mood swings and personality changes
- Drowsiness, malaise, euphoria, anxiety, depression, insomnia, paranoia
- Frequent or unexplained tardiness, work absences, illness, or physical complaints
- Increasing isolation from coworkers
- Offering to check in narcotics or inventory them
- Excessive ordering of certain medications
- Increase in medication errors
- Employee underperformance
- Difficulty with authority and overreaction to criticism
- Wearing long sleeves when inappropriate
- Confusion and memory loss
- Difficulty concentrating or remembering details and instructions
- Inconsistent work performance and may suffer from mistakes made due to inattention, poor judgment, and bad decisions
- Heavy "wastage" of drugs
- Sloppy record keeping and drug shortages
- Normal tasks requiring greater effort and consuming more time
- Unable to keep appointments and missing deadlines
- Relationship problems with colleagues, family, and friends

Physical signs of drug impairment

- Bloodshot or glazed eyes
- Dilated or constricted pupils
- Deterioration in personal appearance
- Significant weight gain or loss
- Poor physical and dental hygiene
- Skin changes
- Track marks
- Visible intoxication
- Hand tremors
- Excessive perspiration
- Unusual body odor

Motivations for diversion

Most commonly abused drug classifications according to the Drug Enforcement Administration

- Opioids
- Depressants
- Hallucinogens
- Stimulants
- Anabolic steroids

Commonly diverted controlled substances

- Codeine
- Fentanyl
- Hydrocodone medication products
- Hydromorphone
- Meperidine
- Methadone
- Morphine
- Oxycodone
- Pentazocine
- Alprazolam
- Clonazepam
- Lorazepam

Opioid abuse is one of the major forces prompting drug diversion. The desire for prescription-controlled substances is increasing as a result of the growing population of drug abusers. Many of the opioids are available in injectable and oral dosage forms. Due to the purity and uniform strength of prescription-controlled substances, they are highly sought. The street value for prescription-controlled substances is higher than their retail value, and the financial gain from reselling these medications provides an incentive for drug diversion. High-cost antipsychotics such as aripiprazole, olanzapine, quetiapine, risperidone, and ziprasidone are highly desired even though they are not controlled substances

Controlled substance diversion prevention programs

Areas of vulnerability for controlled substances

Controlled substances can be diverted during the procurement, preparation and dispensing, prescribing, administration, and the handling of their disposal. Examples of drug diversion that occur during these processes include:

- Procurement
  - Purchase order and packing slip removed from records
  - Unauthorized individual orders for controlled substances on stolen Drug Enforcement Administration (DEA) Form 222
  - Product container compromised

- Preparation and dispensing
  - Controlled substances are replaced by product of similar appearance when prepackaging
  - Removing volume from premixed infusion
  - Multidose vial overfill diverted
  - Prepared syringe contents replaced with saline solution
- Prescribing
  - Prescription pads are diverted and forged to obtain controlled substances.
  - Prescriber self-prescribing controlled substances.
  - Verbal orders for control substances are created but not confirmed by the prescriber.
  - Patients alter written prescriptions.
- Administration
  - Controlled substances are withdrawn from automated distribution device on discharged or transferred patient.
  - Medication is documented as given but not being administered to the patient.
  - Waste is not witnessed and later diverted.
  - Substitute drug is removed and administered while control substance is diverted.
- Waste and removal
  - Controlled substances waste is removed from unsecure waste container.
  - Controlled substance waste in syringe is replaced with saline.
  - Expired controlled substances are removed from holding area.

Effective practices of a controlled substances diversion prevention program

A Controlled Substance Diversion Prevention Program should include administrative elements, core-level controls, and provider-level controls. Highlights of each of these controls are as follows.

Core administrative elements

Legal and regulatory requirements

- Institutional policy and procedures should indicate current legal and regulatory requirements to include:
  - Records retention, biennial inventory, DEA registration and power-of-attorney designations, procurement requirements and forms, prescription authentication, surveillance, investigation and reporting of controlled substance diversion or loss, authorization to access controlled substances, waste, and transfer
  - Self-monitoring practices to prevent, identify, and correct potential fraud, waste, or abuse of controlled substances within the organization
  - Policies and procedures in place for reporting controlled substance diversion
  - Maintaining controlled substance procurement and disposition records and inventories, surveillance findings, discrepancy investigations, and DEA; these documents must be accurate, complete and readily retrievable

- Practices in place for the disposition of patients' controlled substances, medical cannabis, marijuana, and illegal substances into a health care facility

Organization oversight and accountability

Organizational oversight involves the formation of a controlled substance management program that observes statutory and regulatory requirements and that prevents diversion and encourages accountability. An organization should:

- Create a Controlled Substance Diversion Prevention Program committee
  - To develop and implement polices/procedures addressing access to controlled substances
  - To review procedures regularly to ensure they are consistent with best industry practices
- Provide training on institutional policies, procedures, and regulatory requirements for controlled substances.
- Create a diversion response team to respond to suspected controlled substance diversion and provide findings to the respective individuals.

System-level controls

Human resource management should:

- Establish a written employee and provider substance abuse policy.
- Provide health care worker education on substance abuse.
- Establish supervisor training on substance abuse.
- Provide peer assistance to pharmacists and pharmacy technicians in recovery.
- Establish requirements for drug testing, for cause policy for drug testing and return-to work policies for health care workers.
- Implement sanctions for diversion violations.

Automation and technology controls

Automated technology controls should include automated dispensing and prepackaging devices and diversion monitoring software. Diversion monitoring software assists in managing the controlled substance inventory to include the documenting the removal, administration, and waste; billing; and auditing. Best practices involving automation and technology include that:

- The pharmacy is involved with choosing and implementing medication related automation systems.
- The pharmacy is responsible for approving access to controlled substances and for adding and removing users to automated dispensing devices.
- Automation and technology vendors should provide solutions that support control, surveillance, and auditing functions that address the entire chain of custody of control substances.
- Generated records are readily retrievable and contain the necessary information to perform investigations.
- Systems are utilized in high-risk areas, such as surgery or anesthesia and central pharmacy, which contain high-volume controlled substances.

- Integrated systems, to include auditing software and automated dispensing devices, are utilized in high-risk areas.
- Proper training is provided to health care workers in using automation and technology.
- Only authorized individuals have access to controlled substance in automated dispensing devices. A process is in place to suspend or withdraw access privileges to suspected individuals of diversion.
- Policies and procedures have been developed to address access, security, and documentation when automation and system failure occur.
- Policies and procedures specify when automated dispensing device overrides should be utilized.
- Downtime procedures are defined to maintain control, documentation, and accountability of controlled substances in an automated dispensing device or electronic vault.

Monitoring and surveillance

A health care organization should define, review, and audit appropriate data that could indicate possible controlled substance diversion and ensure these trends and variances are responded to in a timely manner and appropriate actions are taken.

Monitoring and surveillance cycle consists of

- Reviewing compliance appraisals
- Following trends of controlled substance usage
- Performing a complete investigation
- Taking appropriate action
- Implementing the necessary diversion prevention improvements

Appropriate processes and practices involved in monitoring and surveilling control substances should

- Address purchasing, inventory management, administration, waste and disposal, and documentation.
- Guarantee sufficient staff assist the pharmacist in surveillance monitoring.
- Ensure the verification of a perpetual inventory be conducted on a regular basis.
- Ensure prescribing practices are evaluated and when a substantial difference exists among health care providers it be reviewed.
- Review automated dispensing device reports at least monthly.
- Ensure processes exist to settle controlled substance discrepancies and that the pharmacy is involved in settling these differences.
- Ensure the pharmacy is responsible for reconciling controlled substances in high-risk areas of the facility.
- Mandate that high-risk medications are arbitrarily examined to include random testing of waste from high-risk or volume areas.

Investigation and reporting

A thorough investigation should occur when suspected diversion has occurred. Best practices involving the investigating and reporting of suspected diversions include:

- Investigating unresolved discrepancies or suspected diversions

- Considering any unresolved discrepancy be as a diversion
- Reporting and responding to a suspected diversion 24 hours a day/7 days a week
- A process for both reporting internal and external medication diversion incidents
- Parameters have been formulated and implemented to determine where a loss is "considered significant"; according to the DEA, factors to be considered for significant losses include:
  - Quantity of controlled substance lost in relation to the type of business
  - The specific controlled substances lost
  - Whether the loss of the controlled substances can be linked with access to those controlled substances by specific individuals, or whether the loss can be credited to unique activities that may take place involving the controlled substances
  - Whether the missing controlled substance are considered for diversion
  - Types of controlled substances losses
  - Patterns of losses over a period of time
  - Guidelines that exist as to when the DEA, state licensure boards, and local law enforcement should be notified

Provider-level controls
Chain of custody

Diversion control systems depend on utilizing retrievable evidence that the chain of custody is continued all times and at all points when the transfer of controlled substances occurs. Health care organizations must be able to audit the transfer of the controlled substances. Best practices employed to ensure proper chain of custody of controlled substances include:

- Only authorized health care workers are allowed to validate the dispensing and receipt of controlled substances.
- Tracking and reconciling electronically automated dispensing devices should be used for dispensing and storing of controlled substances.
- Pneumatic tube systems should never be used for delivering controlled substances unless the system possesses a secure transaction function. Generic passcodes should never be used in a health care facility.
- Transporting controlled substances should only be conducted by properly trained employees.
- Only secure, lockable, and tamper-evident delivery containers should be used when transporting controlled substances.

Storage and security

Practices utilized to ensure controlled substances are securely stored in a pharmacy should include:

- Controlled substances should be stored in a locked and secured location and only available to authorized individuals. When controlled substances are not under the direct physical control of an authorized individual, suitable practices are in place, which include:
  - Lockboxes are stored in a secure location when left unattended.

- Codes for electronic or keypad locks on cabinets or carts are not set at the manufacturer's default code and are protected using a strong code (*not* 6789).
- Procedures exist to track keys, secure keys after hours, replace lost keys, and change locks, and documentation exists indicating compliance.
- Guaranteeing lockout times for electronic locks on medication carts containing controlled substance are limited to a narrow window of time.

- Allow and reduce the number of authorized personnel to obtain controlled substances.
- Utilize key controls and passwords to access controlled substances.
- A chain of custody is maintained for keys, and a process exists to secure keys after hours.
- An employee's access to controlled substances is removed upon termination in real time and is documented.
- Only licensed pharmacy providers are permitted to verify monthly controlled substances counts. These counts include expired and unusable controlled substance awaiting disposal or transfer to a reverse distributor.
- Utilize automated dispensing technology in high volume-controlled substance areas.
- Identification and biometric authentication methods are utilized instead of passwords.
- Camera surveillance is used in high-risk areas, which include receiving areas, central pharmacy vault location, and approved waste receptacles.
- Procedures are followed to secure DEA storage of DEA forms and limiting their access. These include tracking the receipt and filling of DEA Form 222, along with blank DEA Form 222 listed consecutively on a log with the disposition and blank DEA Form 222 log stored separately from unused DEA forms.

Internal pharmacy procurement controls

Policies and procedures have been implemented involving the purchasing, preparing, and dispensing of controlled substances. Best pharmacy practices include:

- Obtaining all controlled substances from the pharmacy in a health care organization
- Limiting the number of authorized individuals to order controlled substances
- Electronic controlled substance ordering system (CSOS) files backed up, archived, and are readily retrievable
- DEA Form 222s secured and accounted through a control log containing the following:
  - DEA order form number
  - Date the form was received from the DEA
  - Date the form was issued
  - The vendor the DEA Form 222 issued
  - The initials or signature of the user
- Ordering and receiving duties of controlled substances conducted by different individuals
  - Two individuals should count and sign for receipt of controlled substances. The quantity on the packing slip should match what was ordered and invoiced.
  - A pharmacist should reconcile controlled substances received against what is indicated on the invoice and documents receipt; these documents should be signed and retained.

- Controlled substance purchase invoices are compared to orders and recorded into the pharmacy's perpetual inventory.
- Invoices should be reconciled to statements from the wholesaler to ensure all quantities have been received and accounted and not diverted.
- CSOS orders should be acknowledged as being received within 7 days of placing the order.
- Controlled substance inventory levels are reviewed regularly.

- Implementing processes to track and reconcile controlled substances when the product is obtained from a third-party vendor
- Establishing procedures for transferring controlled substances between pharmacies
- Using processes to address discrepancies in the procurement process

Internal pharmacy preparation and dispensing controls

Best practices employed in the preparation and dispensing of controlled substances in a pharmacy include:

- Maintaining a perpetual inventory of controlled substances by the pharmacy
- Limiting access to the controlled substance inventory to only authorized individuals
- Regularly checking controlled substances for alteration and tampering; researching any discrepancies
- Purchasing and dispensing controlled substances in unit dose packaging to reduce potential diversion during repackaging
- Using barcode scanning when refilling automated dispensing devices
- Verifying and auditing the delivery and receipt of controlled substances to patient care and procedural care locations
- Auditing and examining returns from the patient care for tampering

Prescribing and administration controls

Controlled substance prescription/medication orders can only be prescribed by a licensed practitioner with a valid DEA number. Controlled substance prescription/medication orders should be transmitted electronically with controlled access if permitted by state laws and regulations. Processes are in place to file written prescriptions. Best practices utilized during prescribing and administering control substances to reduce diversion include:

- A valid prescription/medication order exists from an authorized prescriber for all controlled substances prescribed.
- A process exists for identifying and confirming authorized prescribers using either an electronic or manual ordering system.
- Institutional policies exist to prevent a prescriber from prescribing controlled substances for themselves or their families.
- Require that pharmacists are responsible for verifying any prescription/medication orders for which they are unsure of the prescriber or any questions on the prescription/medication order.

- Obtain controlled substances from inventory as close to the schedule time of administration as possible.
- Secure controlled substances infusions in locked infusion pumps prior to being administered.
- Require controlled substance administration records contain the following information:
  - Date and time administered
  - Medication name
  - Medication strength
  - Dosage form
  - Dose administered
  - Signature of the health care worker who administered the dose
  - Amount wastes with cosignature
  - Proof of count verification per shift
  - Signature of health care worker who transferred the balance forward when transcribing to another controlled substance administration record

Returns, waste, and disposal controls

In an institutional setting, controlled substance should be stocked in ready-to-use forms and in the lowest commercially available doses to minimize waste. Waste includes products expiring, products prepared for administration but not administered to the patient, drug product remaining after a partial dose is removed from its packaged unit, overfill in vials, and drug product remaining in transdermal delivery systems. Chain of custody of controlled substances must be maintained to reduce the risk of diversion. Best practices include:

- Regularly monitoring inventory to identify chances to decrease the need to waste
- Requiring controlled substances be wasted immediately or as close to the time of administration as possible
- Involving a witness to observe the wasting and documentation of all controlled substances except when waste is being returned for analyzing and wasting
- Requiring a witness to observe the controlled substance being wasted and verifying the quantity noted on the document
- Ensuring a procedure exists for wasting fentanyl and that it adheres to DEA, FDA, Environmental Protection Agency, or state-specific guidelines
- Disposing of empty controlled substance containers in limited-access waste containers resulting in the waste being irretrievable
- Utilizing pharmaceutical waste containers to make controlled substances unrecoverable, irretrievable, and unusable
- Segregating expired and unusable controlled substance from other medications and monitoring until they are returned by a reverse distributor or disposed of properly
- Confirming the documentation provided by the reverse distributor corresponds with the pharmacy perpetual inventory record of expired and unusable controlled substances
- Reconciling medications returned through a reverse distributor with the reverse distribution log of controlled substances

Security control measures

Storage and security controls

There are many measures employed in health care organizations to prevent control substance diversion. These include adhering to an organization's policies and procedures, ensuring employees are properly trained, utilizing technology, and using surveillance and monitoring practices.

Hospital pharmacies

Controlled substances should be securely stored in a locked location such as safes, automated dispensing devices, locked cabinet/drawer, or refrigerator that can only be accessed by authorized individuals. Best security processes include:

- Ensuring codes for electronic or keypad locks on cabinets or carts are *not* set at the manufacturer's default code
- Requiring lockout times for electronic locks on controlled substance medication carts be limited to the narrowest window time frame
- Establishing a procedure to track keys, secure keys after hours, replace lost keys, and change locks with appropriate documentation
- Having windows present in storage medication rooms to permit visibility within the area
- Requiring employee belonging (e.g., backpacks, purses, and bags) *not* be permitted in the controlled substance storage area
- Permitting only authorized staff access to controlled substance storage areas
- Establishing policies/procedures for controlled substance access to include restrictions through assignment, key controls, and use of passwords
- Maintaining chain of custody for keys when key lock security is used and processes have been implemented to secure keys after hours
- Removing employee access to control substances of access in real time when employees have been terminated
- Verifying controlled substance inventory counts are conducted by two rotating, licensed, or otherwise authorized pharmacy personnel monthly
- Recommending user identification and biometric authentication be utilized rather than passwords
- Installing camera surveillance for high-risk areas, which includes receiving areas, central pharmacy vault location, approved waste receptacles, and remote areas
- Storing DEA forms securely, and limiting access to authorized individuals
- Implementing procedures for tracking the receipt and filling of DEA Form 222, logging the disposition of each DEA Form 222, and separating used/unused DEA Form 222
- Limiting access to prescription pads to authorized individuals in a health care facility
- Ensuring technology-generated prescription records are readily retrievable
- Training staff properly in the use of automation and technology
- Limiting access to controlled substances in automated dispensing devices to authorized individuals, and ensuring a process exists to withdraw their access privilege

- Ensuring the pharmacy department is responsible for approving access to controlled substances and for adding/removing users access to automated dispensing devices

Retail pharmacies

Retail pharmacies are faced with the risk of both internal and external diversion and the prospect of receiving fraudulent prescriptions from patents. Effective pharmacy security in retail pharmacy utilizes physical, policy, and technology to protect against diversions. Retail practices employed against controlled substance diversion include:

- Maintaining physical access controls, such as secured storage cabinets only accessible by badge or biometric access, by authorized employed personnel
- Utilizing security measures such as high-resolution cameras to monitor theft and provide a means for discrepancies to be resolved in a timely manner
- Installing chimes to ring every time the front door opens to draw attention to the customer
- Utilizing alarms systems with multiple panic buttons and remote triggers
- Dispersing Schedule III, IV, and V Controlled Substances throughout the pharmacy with noncontrolled medications
- Documenting and monitoring controlled substance inventory adjustments made by pharmacy employees, controlled substance prescriptions canceled and returned to stock, and controlled substance prescriptions left at will call past 10 days from processing
- Using e-prescribing to remove the opportunity of prescriptions pads being stolen, altered, or forged from a physician's office and presented at the pharmacy
- Investing in pharmacy automation systems that offer options for drug tracking and accounting
- Minimizing the use of temporary user and patient identifiers
- Guaranteeing the pharmacy's point-of-sale system is interfaced with prescription management software and has developed reports to identify discrepancies
- Auditing controlled substance purchases with drug utilization processes to identify discrepancies and trends
- Maintaining a system when accepting hard-copy controlled substance prescriptions that provides documentation of employee chain of custody and filing all prescriptions to include controlled substance prescriptions consecutively
- Maintaining a perpetual inventory of Schedule II Controlled Substances and auditing at least monthly
- Employing prescription management software to generate labels in developing a perpetual inventory log to identify the quantity of the Schedule II Controlled Substance dispensed
- Employing procedures for handling and documenting partial fills of controlled substances
- Greeting customers as they approach the pharmacy counter
- Screening potential employees by verifying reference checks and performing drug screening
- Maintaining a clutter-free workspace with minimal employee belongings such as purses, backpacks, and bags

Pharmacy high-risk areas

A "high-risk area" is defined as one where the same provider is prescribing, obtaining, preparing, and administering the medication. High-risk areas include surgery centers, operating rooms, procedural and anesthesia areas, and emergency departments. In addition, high-risk areas are locations where high volumes of controlled substances are ordered, prescribed, stored, and dispensed within the same location such as the pharmacy. Best pharmacy practices employed in high-risk pharmacy areas to minimize controlled substance diversion include:

- The pharmacist is responsible for all drugs and controlled substances dispensed and distributed in the health care setting.
- Documenting of doses administered to patients in the anesthesia and operating rooms should be found in the health record. Reconciling doses dispensed, waste, and return quantities as well as prescribed doses should also be documented.
- Reduce controlled drug inventory in surgical suites when a health care pharmacy has a satellite pharmacy.
- Staff the satellite pharmacy whenever surgery and procedural areas are staffed.
- Establish a process for providing an after-hours supply of medications if the satellite pharmacy is not open
- Implement systems to track drugs used, adjust par levels as needed, and monitor drug expiration dates should be used.
- Utilize controls to monitor pharmacy inventories for discrepancies.
- Manually inventory controlled substances located in the automated dispensing device vault monthly, to be performed by two licensed or authorized pharmacy employees.
- Conduct frequent verification audits of high risk or high volume to prevent or minimize inventory count discrepancies and the time to discover these discrepancies.
- Conduct a physical inventory of all controlled substances to include outdated and unusable at least monthly but preferably weekly in a pharmacy without an automated dispensing device vault.
- Inventory expired or recalled drugs pending return or transfer to a distributor for destruction, segregating them in a secure locker or safe until their transfer.
- Observe wasting and reconciling of specific high-risk controlled substances.
- Utilize automation and technology to facilitate security controls and surveillance.

Chain of custody methods

Federal and state laws and regulations oversee the procurement, prescribing, administration, and waste or removal of controlled substances. Organizational oversight addresses implementing best practices that guarantee the chain of custody and the health care worker being responsible for handling controlled substances at all times. The chain of custody takes into considerations all points where the transfer of controlled substance occurs between individuals, whether within or outside the pharmacy. Methods used to ensure chain of custody is maintained include:

- Identifying those health care workers who are authorized to access controlled substances
- Removing a health care worker's access to controlled substances immediately upon termination from the institution
- Requiring the presence of a witness for the delivery of controlled substances to a storage location and a signed confirmation of receipt of the delivery
- Using secure, lockable, and tamper-evident delivery containers, which should be traceable, when transferring controlled substances
- Utilizing tamper-evident packaging to stop an individual from accessing a medication, including taper enclosures, shrink-wrap, and tamper-evident caps for compounded medications
- Employing radiofrequency identification devices in high-risk settings, such as intensive care units and for IV medications

Drug Enforcement Administration requirements

Drug Enforcement Administration registration requirements

Every pharmacy dispensing a controlled substance must be registered with the DEA and must have a state license. The DEA Form 224 must be completed and should be completed online but may be submitted using a paper version of the DEA Form 224 (Application for New Registration Under Controlled Substance Act of 1970) by writing to the DEA. Upon receipt of the completed DEA Form 224, a DEA Form 223 (Certificate of Registration) is issued to the pharmacy and must be kept on site at the pharmacy and available for inspection. A renewal of the pharmacy's registration must be completed every 3 years using a DEA Form 224a (Application for Renewal of Registration Under the Controlled Substance Act of 1970).

A pharmacy may authorize one or more individuals to obtain and complete DEA Form 222 (US Official Order Form for Schedule I and II Controlled Substances) for the pharmacy by allowing them a power of attorney. The power of attorney must be signed by the registrant of the pharmacy and the individual to whom the power of attorney is being issued and by two witnesses. The power of attorney may be withdrawn at any time by the individual who signed the most current DEA registration or reregistration and two witnesses. The power of attorney must be kept with completed DEA Form 222.

Validating a Drug Enforcement Administration number

A practitioner's DEA may be verified by the pharmacy using the following link: https://apps.deadiversion.usdoj. gov/webforms2/spring/validationLogin?execution=e1s1.

A DEA number can be validated manually by remembering the following:

- New DEA registration numbers issued before 1985 to physicians, dentists, veterinarians, and other health care prescribers began with the letter A.
- New DEA registration numbers issued after 1985 began with either the letter B or F.
- A DEA number beginning with the letter M indicates the practitioner is a midlevel practitioner (physician assistant or nurse practitioner).
- Prescribers employed by a drug addiction treatment facility will have the letter X as the first letter of their DEA number.
- The letter G is assigned to prescribers under the Department of Defense.
- The second letter of the DEA registration number begins with the first letter of practitioner's last name.
- The first two letters are followed by a sequence of seven numbers. To determine if the DEA number is valid:
  - Add the first, third, and fifth numbers together.
  - Next add the second, fourth, and sixth numbers together. Multiply this sum by two.
  - Add the first and second set of numbers together. The number farthest from the left (one's column) should be same as seventh number in the DEA number.
    - Example: What should the seventh number in Dr. Andrew Shed's DEA number be if his DEA number begins with BS452589?
      Add 4 +2 + 8, which totals 14.
      Add 5 +5 + 9, which totals 19; multiply 19 by 2 and the product is 38.
      Add 14 + 38, which totals 52. The last number should be a 2.
      A valid DEA number for Dr. Andrew Shed would be BS4525892.

Using a hospital's Drug Enforcement Administration number

Practitioners, such as interns, residents, staff physicians, or midlevel practitioners, may prescribe controlled substances using the hospital's DEA registration number under the following conditions:

- Dispensing, administering, or prescribing is a part of their professional practice.
- The practitioner is licensed by the state.
- The hospital has confirmed the practitioner is licensed to administer, dispense, or prescribe controlled substances within the state.
- The hospital approves the practitioner to administer, dispense, or prescribe under its controlled substance registration and designates an internal code number to the practitioner.

Drug Enforcement Administration Form 222

Schedule I and II Controlled Substances may be ordered by using DEA Form 222 (Fig. 4.1). Effective October 31, 2021, the DEA Form 222 will be in a single-sheet format instead of a triplicate form. A DEA Form 222 is required for each distribution or transfer of a Schedule I or Schedule II Controlled

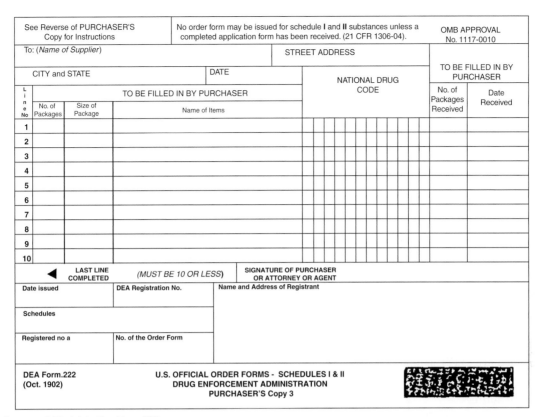

Fig. 4.1 Drug Enforcement Administration Form 222.

Substance. The pharmacy will request the DEA provide a limited number of DEA Form 222 to the pharmacy based upon the pharmacy's business activity. A DEA Form 222 contains an order form number; the name, address, and registration number of the pharmacy; and the schedules the pharmacy is authorized to dispense.

When completing a DEA Form 222, the purchaser must:

- Use a computer printer, pen, or indelible pencil.
- Only enter one item on each number line.
- Indicate the number of lines completed at the bottom of the form in its respective box.
- Enter the name and address for whom the controlled substances are being ordered must be on the DEA Form.
- Make a copy of the DEA Form and submit the original to the supplier.
- The form must be signed and dated by the individual who is authorized a registration application or have power of attorney.

In addition, the purchaser must:

- Upon receipt of the ordered medications, indicate the number of containers for each medication and the date they were received.
- Maintain a copy of the completed DEA form for a minimum of 2 years.
- Keep any defective DEA Forms for a minimum of 2 years.
- Retain all DEA Forms 222 separate from other pharmacy records.

Electronic copies of DEA Form 222 do not need to be stored on a different server.

A supplier of controlled substances may decline to honor a DEA Form 222 if the order is not complete or legible or is not properly prepared, executed, or endorsed. If the Form 222 shows any alteration, erasure, or change of any description, it should not be accepted. If for any reason the order cannot be filled, then the original DEA Form 222 must be returned to the purchaser with a reason for its return. A defective DEA Form 222 can be amended but a new DEA Form 222 must be issued in its place. In situations where a DEA Form 222 has been lost, the pharmacy must complete a new DEA Form 222 and provide a statement that the DEA Form 222 has been lost. If a pharmacy determines that a DEA Form 222 has been stolen, it must be promptly reported to the local DEA Diversion Field Office and provide the serial number(s) of the stolen form(s).

Drug Enforcement Administration Controlled Substance Ordering System

The CSOS is another method by which Schedule II Controlled Substances can be ordered. The CSOS allows secure electronic ordering of controlled substances without using a paper DEA Form 222. Using the CSOS, a pharmacy is able to order Schedule II Medications from controlled substance manufacturers, distributors, and pharmacies. Advantages of the CSOS include:

- Does not have a maximum number of line items per order
- CSOS certificates that include the same identification information as is found on a paper DEA Form 222, resulting in timely and accurate authentication by the supplier

- Allows just-in-time ordering resulting in smaller pharmacy inventories
- Reduces the number of ordering errors resulting in more accurate orders
- Lowers transaction costs for the pharmacy due to order accuracy and decreased paperwork

CSOS employs public key infrastructure technology, which offers secure online communication. Public key infrastructure technology offers a range of security ordering services, which include:

- Confidentiality, because only approved individuals have access to the data
- Authentication, which determines who is sending/receiving data
- Integrity, because the data have not been changed during transmission

All users of public key infrastructure technology are provided a digital certificate confirming their identity and right to place an electronic controlled substance order. CSOS digital certificates originate with the CSOS Certification Authority only after the pharmacy's information has been verified. All electronic controlled substance orders are signed using a digital certificate. Information contained in a CSOS Signing Certificate includes:

- Subscriber name
- Subscriber e-mail address
- Registrant location name as registered with the DEA
- Registrant location address as it is registered with DEA
- Registrant DEA number ("hashed" or encoded)
- Authorized ordering schedules
- Certificate validity period

A certificate will be canceled if the certificate holder is no longer permitted to sign Schedule II orders.

Electronic orders for controlled substances *will* not be filled if:
- The required data fields have not been filled in properly.
- The order is not signed using a digital certificate issued by DEA.
- The digital certificate used has ended or has been canceled prior to signature.
- The purchaser's public key will not authorize the digital certificate.
- The order is invalid for any reason.

A supplier must notify the purchaser and provide an explanation for not filling the order. Neither the purchaser nor the supplier can correct an electronic order for controlled substances, but instead a new order must be provided by the purchaser.

Drug Enforcement Administration Form 41

The DEA Form 41 (Registrant Record of Controlled Substances Destroyed) is used to request permission from the DEA to destroy controlled substances and is completed by DEA registrants. The DEA Form 41 is used to record nonrecoverable breakage or spillage. In situations in which a pharmacy uses a reverse distributor to destroy controlled substances, it is the reverse distributor's responsibility to submit the DEA 41. The DEA Form 41 requires the following information be included:

- Registrant information
  - Registered name
  - DEA registration number
    - Registered address (street, city, state, and zip code)
    - Telephone number
    - Contact information
- Item destroyed
  - Inventory
    - National Drug Code or DEA Controlled Substances Code Number
    - Batch number
    - Name of substance
    - Strength
    - Form
    - Package quantity
    - Number of full packages
    - Partial package count
    - Total destroyed
  - Collected substances
    - Returned mail-back package (yes or no)
    - Sealed inner liner (yes or no)
    - Unique identification number
    - Size of sealed inner liner
    - Quantity of package(s)/liner(s) destroyed
- Method of destruction such that the controlled substance is rendered to a condition that it is nonretrievable and meets all destruction requirements
  - Date of destruction
  - Method of destruction
  - Location or business name
  - Address (street, city, state, and zip code)
- Witnesses of the destruction
  - Printed name and signature of two witnesses
  - Date

The DEA Form 41 must be retained by the pharmacy for a minimum of 2 years.

Drug Enforcement Administration Form 106

The DEA Diversion Drug Theft Loss system has been replaced by the Theft Loss Reporting system (Fig. 4.2). The Theft Loss Reporting system provides the means for a registrant to submit a Form 106 and/or a Form 107. The Theft Loss Reporting system automatically determines which form(s) need to be produced and submitted depending on the type of registrant and the data entered. The DEA Diversion Drug Theft Loss system is used to electronically submit a DEA Form 106 (Report of Theft or Loss of Controlled Substances) and DEA Form 107 (Report of Theft or Loss of Listed Chemicals).

The DEA Form 106 (Report of Theft or Loss of Controlled Substances) is used in conveying the theft or loss of controlled substances, mail-back packages, and/or inner liners. A pharmacy must notify the area DEA in writing within 1 day of discovering the theft or significant loss of controlled substances by submitting a DEA Form 106 electronically. Information to be submitted on a DEA Form 106 includes:

- DEA registration number
- Name of business
- Address
- City, state, and zip code
- Point of contact
- Date of theft or loss
- Number of thefts and losses within the past 24 months
- Principal business of registrant

REPORT OF THEFT OR LOSS OF CONTROLLED SUBSTANCES

Federal Regulations require registrants to submit a detailed report of any theft or loss of Controlled Substances to the Drug Enforcement Administration.

Complete the front and back of this form in triplicate. Forward the original and duplicate copies to the nearest DEA Office. Retain the triplicate copy for your records. Some states may also require a copy of this report.

OMB APPROVAL
No. 1117-0001

1. Name and Address of Registrant (include ZIP Code) ZIP CODE	2. Phone No. (Include Area Code)

3. DEA Registration Number

2 ltr. prefix   7 digit suffix

4. Date of Theft or Loss

5. Principal Business of Registrant (Check one)

1 ☐ Pharmacy   5 ☐ Distributor
2 ☐ Practitioner   6 ☐ Methadone Program
3 ☐ Manufacturer   7 ☐ Other (Specify)
4 ☐ Hospital/Clinic

6. County in which Registrant is located

7. Was Theft reported to Police?
☐ Yes   ☐ No

8. Name and Telephone Number of Police Department (Include Area Code)

9. Number of Thefts or Losses Registrant has experienced in the past 24 months

10. Type of Theft or Loss (Check one and complete items below as appropriate)

1 ☐ Night break-in   3 ☐ Employee pilferage   5 ☐ Other (Explain)
2 ☐ Armed robbery   4 ☐ Customer theft   6 ☐ Lost in transit (Complete Item 14)

11. If Armed Robbery, was anyone:

Killed? ☐ No   ☐ Yes (How many) _____
Injured? ☐ No   ☐ Yes (How many) _____

12. Purchase value to registrant of Controlled Substances taken?
$

13. Were any pharmaceuticals or merchandise taken?
☐ No   ☐ Yes (Est. Value)
$

14. IF LOST IN TRANSIT, COMPLETE THE FOLLOWING:

A. Name of Common Carrier	B. Name of Consignee	C. Consignee's DEA Registration Number
D. Was the carton received by the customer? ☐ Yes ☐ No	E. If received, did it appear to be tampered with? ☐ Yes ☐ No	F. Have you experienced losses in transit from this same carrier in the past? ☐ No ☐ Yes (How Many) _____

15. What identifying marks, symbols, or price codes were on the labels of these containers that would assist in identifying the products?

16. If Official Controlled Substance Order Forms (DEA-222) were stolen, give numbers.

17. What security measures have been taken to prevent future thefts or losses?

FORM DEA - 106 (11-00) *Previous editions obsolete*

CONTINUE ON REVERSE

Fig. 4.2 Drug Enforcement Administration Form 106.

FORM DEA-106 (Nov. 2000) Pg. 2   **LIST OF CONTROLLED SUBSTANCES LOST**

Trade Name of Substance or Preparation	Name of Controlled Substance in Preparation	Dosage Strength and Form	Quantity
Examples: Desoxyn	Methamphetamine Hydrochloride	5 mg Tablets	3 x 100
Demerol	Meperidine Hydrochloride	50 mg/ml Vial	5 x 30 ml
Robitussin A-C	Codeine Phosphate	2 mg/cc Liquid	12 Pints
1.			
2.			
3.			
4.			
5.			
6.			
7.			
8.			
9.			
10.			
11.			
12.			
13.			
14.			
15.			
16.			
17.			
18.			
19.			
20.			
21.			
22.			
23.			
24.			
25.			
26.			
27.			
28.			
29.			
30.			
31.			
32.			
33.			
34.			
35.			
36.			
37.			
38.			
39.			
40.			
41.			
42.			
43.			
44.			
45.			
46.			
47.			
48.			
49.			
50.			

I certify that the foregoing information is correct to the best of my knowledge and belief.

_____   _____   _____

Signature   Title   Date

Fig. 4.2 cont'd

- Type of theft or loss (break-in/burglary, employee theft, hijacking of transport vehicle, packaging discrepancy, robbery, customer theft, loss in transit, or disaster)
- Theft reported to police to include responding officer's name and police report number
- Corrective measures taken to prevent future thefts or losses
- Listing and quantity of controlled substances lost or stolen

The DEA Form 106 must be maintained for 2 years.

Drug Enforcement Administration Form 107

The DEA Form 107 (Report of Theft or Loss of Listed Chemicals) is used to report any theft or loss of listed chemicals. The DEA has issued two lists of chemical, which are classified as List I and List II. List I and II chemicals are precursors in the manufacture of controlled substances. Examples of List I chemicals include ephedrine, ergocristine, ergotamine, and phenylpropanolamine. Acetone, benzyl chloride, ethyl ether, and potassium permanganate are examples of List II chemicals. DEA Form 107 should only be used for reporting any theft or loss of listed chemicals. When completing a DEA Form 107 the following information is required:

- The pharmacy's DEA number and your last name or the business name used to register for DEA number are required.
- CMEA registrants are compelled to provide the certificate ID number and the business name used to certify with the DEA.
- Background information regarding the loss or theft incident, to include the date and place, the type (night break-in, armed robbery, etc.), and the estimated value of the substances stolen must be provided.
- National Drug Code or chemical and quantity of the controlled substance being reported as a theft or loss. Quantity should be reported in milligrams, kilograms, milliliters, tablets, or capsules.
- DEA Form 107 is submitted electronically to the DEA. A copy of the DEA-107 must be maintained by the pharmacy for a minimum of 2 years.

Controlled substance schedules

Under the Controlled Substance Act of 1970, five drug schedules were created. A controlled substance is assigned a drug schedule based upon whether it has a currently accepted medical use in treatment in the United States and its relative potential and likelihood of causing dependence.

- Schedule I Controlled Substances
  - Have a high potential of abuse
  - No currently accepted medical use in the United States
  - Lack of accepted safety for use of the drug under medical supervision
  - Examples: heroin, lysergic acid diethylamide, marijuana (cannabis), 3,4-methylenedioxymethamphetamine ("ecstasy"), peyote, hashish, and "crack" cocaine

- Schedule II Controlled Substances
  - Have a high potential for abuse, which may lead to severe psychological or physical dependence
  - Have a currently accepted medical use in the United States with severe restrictions
  - Examples: morphine, codeine, opium, hydrocodone with acetaminophen, fentanyl, hydromorphone (Dilaudid), methadone, meperidine (Demerol), oxycodone (OxyContin), oxycodone with acetaminophen (Percocet), dextroamphetamine (Dexedrine), dextroamphetamine/amphetamine (Adderall), methylphenidate (Ritalin, Concerta), lisdexamfetamine (Vyvanse), and cocaine nasal (Goprelto)
- Schedule III Controlled Substances
  - Have a potential for abuse less than substance in Schedules I or II
  - Have a currently accepted medical use in the United States
  - Possibility of abuse leading to moderate or low physical dependence or high psychological dependence
  - Products containing not more than 90 milligrams og codeine per dosage unit
  - Examples: acetaminophen with codeine, buprenorphine, ketamine, and benzphetamine
- Schedule IV Controlled Substances
  - Have a low potential for abuse relative to substances in Schedule III
  - Have a currently accepted medical use with severe restrictions
  - Possibility of abuse leading to limited physical dependence or psychological dependence compared with substances in Schedule III
  - Examples: acetaminophen with alprazolam (Xanax), clonazepam (Klonopin), clorazepate (Tranxene T-Tab), diazepam (Valium), eszopiclone (Lunesta), lorazepam (Ativan), temazepam (Restoril)), tramadol, triazolam (Halcion), and zolpidem (Ambien)
- Schedule V Controlled Substances
  - Low potential for abuse relative to substances listed in Schedule IV
  - Have a currently accepted medical use in treatment in the United States
  - Possibility of abuse leading to limited physical dependence or psychological dependence compared with Schedule IV substances
  - Are often classified as antitussives and antidiarrheals
  - Cough preparations not containing more than 200 mg of codeine per 100 mL or per 100 g
  - Examples: codeine/guaifenesin (Cheratussin AC), diphenoxylate/atropine (Lomotil). pregabalin (Lyrica)

Drug Enforcement Administration physical inventories

An "inventory" is a complete and accurate list of all stocks and forms of controlled substances in the possession of the pharmacy as determined by an actual physical count for Schedule II Controlled Substances. The pharmacy may make an estimated count of all Schedule III, IV, or V substances for bottles containing less than 1000 tablets or capsules. An exact count must be made if the bottle contains more than 1000 tablets or capsules. All inventory counts of controlled substances must be retained at the pharmacy for a minimum of 2 years. Inventory records of Schedule II Controlled Substances must be kept separate from other pharmacy records while Schedule III, IV, and V records must be kept separate from other pharmacy records and are easily retrieved.

Initial inventory

- When issued a DEA registration the pharmacy must take an exact count of all controlled substances in the pharmacy during an initial inventory. Inventory information should include:
  - The date of the inventory
  - Whether the inventory was taken at the beginning or close of business
  - The name of each controlled substance inventoried
  - The finished form of each of the substances (e.g., 100-mg tablet)
  - The number of dosage units or volume in the manufacturer's container
  - The number of manufacturer's container of each finished form (e.g., five 100-tablet bottles)
  - Total count of the substance
- The initial inventory does not need to be submitted to the DEA but needs to be maintained by the pharmacy.
- Best practices indicate that an initial inventory record contains the name, address, pharmacy address, and signature of the individual taking the inventory.

Biennial inventory

- Is taken at least every 2 years
- Contains the same information taken during an initial inventory:
  - The date of the inventory
  - Whether the inventory was taken at the beginning or close of business
  - The name of each controlled substance inventoried
  - The finished form of each of the substances (e.g., 100-mg tablet)
  - The number of dosage units or volume in the manufacturer's container
  - The number of manufacturer's container of each finished form (e.g., five 100-tablet bottles)
  - Total count of the substance
- Biennial inventory does not need to be submitted to the DEA but does need to be maintained at the pharmacy.

Newly scheduled control substance inventory

- When a noncontrolled substance has been reclassified as a controlled substance, the medication must be inventoried if in stock on its effective date as a controlled substance.

Inventory for damaged substances

- If a controlled substance is damaged, defective, or adulterated and is being held for quality control purposes, an inventory must be conducted. Inventory information to be maintained includes:

- Name of substance
- Quantity of the substance to the nearest metric unit weight or total number units of the drug
- Reason for the medication to be maintained

Perpetual inventory

- A perpetual inventory indicates the actual quantity of a specific medication on hand at a specific time

Robbery or theft of controlled substances

During a robbery of controlled substances:

- Remain calm.
- Do as you are told.
- Do not resist.
- Do not attempt to apprehend the robber.
- Do not make sudden movements but move slowly and deliberate.
- Act as an eyewitness.
  - Observe the robber's physical characteristics.
    - Height
    - Build (skinny, heavy, muscular, etc.)
    - Approximate weight
    - Clothing (mask and type of mask)
    - Hair color and length
    - Tattoos
    - Scars
    - Facial features (beard, moustache, eye color, body piercings)
    - Any unique physical features such as walking with a limp
  - Pay attention to other aspects of the robbery.
    - Was a note used? If so, save for the police.
    - Was a weapon used? If so, what type was used?
    - Was there an accomplice? If so, note any unique physical characteristics.
    - Was a vehicle used to flee the scene? If so, note the vehicle's make, model, color, license number, and direction it was traveling.
    - Did the robber touch anything in the store? If so, inform the police.
- Activate alarm as soon as possible.
- Call police first and then your supervisor.
- Take charge.
  - Immediately obtain treatment for anyone who may be injured.
  - Lock the building down to prevent reentry and keep it closed until the police arrive.
  - Request customers to remain in the store to give a statement to the police.
  - Protect the crime scene. Stop others from touching anything touched by the suspect(s).
  - Promptly write down anything you observed.

After a burglary:

- Notify the local police department.
- Avoid touching or disturbing anything.
- After the police arrive, provide a detail list of what was stolen.
- Take the appropriate steps to improve security.

If controlled substances were taken:

- Report it to the local DEA office within 1 business day.
- Submit a completed DEA Form 106, Report of Theft or Loss of Controlled Substance, as soon as possible.
- File a report with the State Board of Pharmacy.

Sales of controlled substances and restricted over-the-counter medication

The Combat Methamphetamine Epidemic Act of 2005 (CMEA) established conditions to be followed in selling of Scheduled Listed Chemical Product (SLCP). A SLCP is any product that contains ephedrine, pseudoephedrine, or phenylpropanolamine and is marketed as a nonprescription (OTC) medication in the United States.

Requirements of the CMEA include:

- SLCPs are to be placed behind the counter or in locked cabinets.
- Purchaser's identity must be checked .
- Maintaining a log (paper or electronic) of all purchasers of SLCPs. Log requires
  - Purchaser's name and complete address
  - Purchaser's signature
  - Product sold
  - Quantity sold
  - Date and time
- Approved federal or state photoidentification of the purchaser. Approved federal government identification includes:
  - US passport
  - US Armed Forces military identification card
  - Foreign passport with a temporary I-551 stamp

Individuals 18 years of age or older may provide:

  - Driver's license or identification card with a photograph
  - School identification card with a photograph
  - Voter's registration card
  - US military card
  - Military dependent's identification card
  - Native American tribal documents
- The logbook must be maintained for 2 years.

Other SLCP requirements include:

- Pharmacy must train all employees selling SLCPs on CMEA requirements and indicate training has occurred.
- A maximum of 3.6 g of the chemical can be sold in 1 day.
- Product packaging is limited to blister packs with no more than two dosage units per blister.
- The maximum amount that can be purchased in 30 days is 9 g, of which no more than 7.5 g can be imported by private or commercial carrier or US Postal service.
- Annual self-certification of all sellers of SLCPs must take place, which indicates the seller is stating:
  - All employees have received SLCP training.
  - Training records are maintained.
  - Sales of SLCPs do not exceed 3.6 g per day to purchaser.
  - SLCPs are stored behind the counter or in a locked cabinet.
  - A written or electronic logbook is maintained.

Surveillance and investigation

Suspicious data patterns

According to the Joint Commission, the following trends in health care indicate drug diversion is accomplished by:

- Removing controlled substances
  - With no doctor's orders
  - For patients not assigned to the nurse
  - For recently discharged or transferred patients
- Compromising product containers
- Removing controlled substance and substituting with another product to the patient
- Creating a verbal order for controlled substances that is not verified by prescriber
- Diverting prescription pads forged to obtain controlled substances
- Self-prescribing controlled substances by prescriber
- Removing volume from premixed infusion
- Diverting multidose vial overfill
- Replacing prepared syringe contents with saline solution
- Altering written prescriptions
- Documenting medication is administered to the patient but is not
- Excessive pulling of as-needed medications for one provider compared with other providers
- Asking frequently for supplemental orders for controlled substances or pulling as-needed medications
- Noting drug dispensing machines show discrepancies or overrides
- Observing sloppy documentation, omissions, and care inconsistencies
- Wasting complete doses, wasting no doses, or heavy drug wasting
- Observing wasting is not adequately witnessed
- Failing to document waste
- Wasting medication that never reach the patient such as dropped medications, patient refusal, and discontinued orders
- Wasting medications with the same person as a witness (called a "waste buddy")
- Asking associates to sign off on "wasting" they did not witness
- Holding waste until the end of a shift or carrying medications in pockets
- Removing controlled substance waste from unsecure waste container
- Replacing controlled substance waste in syringe with saline
- Diverting expired controlled substances from holding area
- Observing patients continuing to complain about excessive pain, despite documented administration of pain medication
- Falsifying medical records by:
  - Late documentation of certain medications only
  - Coworkers assisting others in completing documentation
  - "Batching" assessments and treatments for pain
- Assisting other nurses administer pain medication
- Observing unauthorized individual orders for controlled substances on stolen DEA Form 222

- Paying extra attention to or entering patients' rooms who are receiving controlled substances
- Reviewing the medication orders of patients not assigned to them, helping colleagues medicate their patients, or volunteering to administer narcotics to patients
- Disappearing frequently during shift
- Volunteering for overtime or coming to work on days off

Surveillance practices and techniques

Surveillance processes are involved in all facets of the controlled substance management system, from purchasing to waste and disposal of these substances. Best surveillance practices include:

- Defining monitoring and surveillance measures, thresholds of variance that require action, reporting frequency, and surveillance procedures
- Conducting self-audits as well as regularly scheduled audits by individuals external to the area being audited
- Auditing human resources process to ensure:
  - Background checks are performed.
  - Training and competency requirements for authorized staff are documented.
  - Random drug testing requirements are complied with.
  - Licensure board reporting and rehabilitation program requirements are complied with.
- Monitoring drug purchase history through regularly scheduled audits to identify diversion through variations or changes in volume or pattern by:
  - Comparing controlled substance purchase invoices to controlled substance purchase orders and receipt into the pharmacy's perpetual inventory
  - Reconciling invoices to statements or wholesale purchase history reports to detect missing invoices
  - Identifying unusual peaks in quantity or frequency of controlled substance purchases
- Maintaining a perpetual inventory of all controlled substance on a regular basis consistent with the system being utilized by:
  - Verifying controlled substance counts from automated dispensing devices every time a controlled substance drawer is accessed, and a complete inventory for controlled substances in automated dispensing devices is conducted weekly by two authorized health care workers.
  - Delivering, replenishing, and stocking of controlled substances in patient care areas are performed by authorized pharmacy personnel and require an auditable verification of delivery and receipt
  - Counting controlled substance inventory in the pharmacy narcotic vault monthly.
  - Conducting a biennial physical inventory of all controlled substances and documenting it according to DEA requirements or per state requirements, depending on the most stringent requirement
- Monitoring automated dispensing device reports to guarantee overrides occur only as permitted by policies and procedures
- Reviewing automated dispensing device override reports daily to ensure an order exists during the time the medication was accessed from the automated dispensing device and corresponding documentation is in the medication administration record
- Implementing diversion monitoring software to support surveillance activities
- Reviewing reports that monitor controlled substance use in patient care areas at least monthly by pharmacy and patient care managers; process exists to generate control substance trend data and reports:
  - Tracking and trending of patient care usage
  - Comparing generated reports of automated dispensing device activity with the prescriber order and medication administration record
  - Comparing transaction activity to include inventory abnormalities, removal of quantities greater than prescribed dose, cancellations, returns, waste with that of peers
- Reviewing prescribing practices for unusual trends or patterns, such as variance compared with other prescribers
- Comparing controlled substance storage inventory transactions routinely with the medication administration record to ensure appropriate documentation of administration and waste
- Performing anesthesia-controlled substance audits on a regular basis
- Random testing of waste from all high-risk, high-volume areas, including areas for pharmacy sterile products preparation, anesthesia administration, and surgery
- Reconciling controlled substances dispensed in high-risk settings by the pharmacy against what controlled substances were documented as administered or wasted

Signs of product tampering and/or alteration

Signs of medication tampering

- The lot numbers on the vial and the box containing the product are different.
- The metal crimp on the vial is damaged.
- The flip top is missing.
- The product is discolored or cloudy or contains flakes or other foreign matter.
- Transaction patterns that have been associated with tampering include
  - Repeated canceled removals of a specific drug
  - Repeated returns of a specific drug
  - Frequent inventory counts, which permit access to the drug supply without registering a transaction
  - Excessively frequent access to patient-controlled analgesia (PCA) keys, or access to PCA keys for patients not under the care of the staff member

Methods to detect tampering

- Verifying the drug packaging is intact
- Ensuring that the medication does not appear to be adulterated
- Monitoring for canceled transactions and returns
- Monitoring for patterns for a specific drug

Methods to prevent medication tampering

- Ensuring medications are kept secure at all times
- Maintaining a regular schedule of controlled substance counts
- Requiring a witness be present for all inventory counts
- Limiting the number of PCA keys available to health care workers
- Storing PCA keys in a single access compartment in an automated drug cabinet
- Requiring a witness be present to prevent tampering from occurring
- Ensuring that all returns are placed in a specified return bin instead of returning directly to patient stock

Recommended actions to be taken in situations of tampering

- Documenting fully the tampering incident to include photographing the tampered medication
- Securing the medication and having it analyzed
- Determining if a patient has been harmed as a result of the tampering
- Reporting tampering to the FDA Office of Criminal Investigations, professional and pharmacy boards, law enforcement, and local public health officials upon confirmation of the tampering incident

Fraudulent prescriptions

A variety of methods are used to obtain fraudulent prescriptions, and they include:

- Altering a prescriber's original prescription
- Stealing legitimate prescription pads from a practitioner's office and/or hospitals
- Printing a legitimate prescriber's prescription pad using a different callback telephone number and manning the telephone number with an associate to verify the prescription
- "Doctor shopping"
- Calling in their own prescription and providing their own telephone number as a callback number
- Going to the emergency room and complaining of pain hoping for a prescription for a controlled substance
- Acquiring drugs that were legally prescribed to family members or friends
- Obtaining prescribed drugs illegally through the Internet
- Using a computer to create prescriptions for nonexistent prescribers

Prescriptions may be presented to the pharmacy such that they appear to be out of the scope practice for the practitioner. These include:

- The prescriber writing notably more prescriptions or in larger quantities compared with other practitioners in the same specialty
- The patient returning too frequently to have the controlled substance filled
- The prescriber writing prescriptions for antagonistic medications simultaneously

- The patient presenting prescriptions written for other individuals
- Multiple individuals appearing simultaneously with prescriptions from the same prescriber
- Noncommunity residents presenting prescriptions from the same prescriber

Characteristics of fraudulent prescriptions

- The prescription may be characterized by looking "too good" and the handwriting is too legible.
- The quantities, directions, or dosage differ from approved medical usage.
- The prescription does not conform with conventional abbreviations.
- It appears to be photocopied.
- Directions for use are written without abbreviations.
- The prescription is written in different-color inks or different handwriting.

Fraudulent prescriptions can be prevented by:

- Knowing the prescriber and recognizing their signature
- Knowing the prescriber's DEA registration number
- Knowing the patient
- Checking the date on the prescription to determine if it has been presented within a reasonable period time since being issued by the prescriber
- Contacting the prescriber for verification of the prescription if in doubt
- Requiring proper identification when a prescription is being picked up
- Being familiar with state and pharmacy regulations regarding new prescriptions for controlled substances
- Requiring pharmacy staff to undergo training to identify inappropriate prescriptions

CHAPTER REVIEW QUESTIONS

1. Which of the following may result as a consequence of drug diversion?
   a. Addiction
   b. Decreased risk of infection
   c. Loss of professional license or certification
   d. Both a and c
2. Which of the following is an example of a behavioral sign that may indicate the health care worker is impaired?
   a. Bloodshot eyes
   b. Hand tremors
   c. Significant weight loss
   d. Unreliable in meeting deadlines
3. Controlled substances can be diverted during the procurement, preparation and dispensing, prescribing, administration, and the handling their disposal. Which is an example of diversion occurring during dispensing?
   a. Altering a written prescription
   b. Replacing controlled substances by a product of similar appearance during prepackaging
   c. Removing expired controlled substances from holding area
   d. Ordering controlled substances on a stolen DEA Form 222

4. According to the DEA, which classification is frequently abused?
   a. Antibiotics
   b. Corticosteroids
   c. Diuretics
   d. Stimulants
5. Which of the following is an example of a system-level control for a Control Substance Diversion Prevention Program?
   a. Automation and technology
   b. Chain of custody control
   c. Legal and regulatory requirements
   d. Prescribing and administration
6. During which process is a drug product container compromised?
   a. Procurement
   b. Preparation and dispensing
   c. Prescribing
   d. Administration
7. Which system-level control would establish processes and practices addressing the purchasing, inventory management, administration, waste and disposal, and documentation of controlled substances?
   a. Automation and technology
   b. Human resource management
   c. Investigation and reporting
   d. Monitoring and surveillance
8. Which of the following is considered a "high-risk" area for controlled substance diversion?
   a. Anesthesia areas
   b. Emergency departments
   c. Operating rooms
   d. All the above
9. Which type of oversight refers to establishing best practices that ensure the chain of custody and the health care worker being responsible for handling-controlled substances at all times?
   a. Federal
   b. Organizational
   c. State
   d. All the above
10. A health care worker's access to controlled substances is removed immediately upon termination from the institution. What is this an example of?
    a. Completing a DEA Form 41
    b. Ensuring the chain of custody of controlled substances
    c. Preventing external diversion in a retail pharmacy
    d. All the above
11. Which DEA form is used to renew a pharmacy's registration with the DEA every 3 years?
    a. DEA Form 222
    b. DEA Form 223
    c. DEA Form 224
    d. DEA Form 224a
12. The first letter of DEA number is the letter M; what does it indicate?
    a. The prescriber received their DEA number before 1985.
    b. The prescriber is a midlevel practitioner.
    c. The prescriber is employed by the Department of Defense.
    d. The prescriber is employed by a drug addiction treatment facility.
13. Which health care practitioner may use a hospital's DEA number to prescribe controlled substances?
    a. Intern
    b. Resident
    c. Staff physician
    d. All the above
14. Which drug schedule can be ordered using a DEA Form 222?
    a. Schedule I
    b. Schedule II
    c. Schedule III
    d. Both a and b
15. Which is an advantage of using the CSOS?
    a. Eliminates the maximum number of line items per order
    b. Permits the electronic ordering of Schedule I, II, III, and IV Controlled Substances
    c. Results in lower transaction costs to the pharmacy
    d. All the above
16. How long must a pharmacy retain DEA Form 41?
    a. 1 year
    b. 2 years
    c. 5 years
    d. 7 years
17. Which DEA form is used to report the theft or loss of listed chemicals?
    a. DEA Form 41
    b. DEA Form 106
    c. DEA Form 107
    d. DEA Form 224
18. Which drug schedule has no currently accepted medical use in the United States?
    a. Schedule I
    b. Schedule II
    c. Schedule III
    d. Schedule IV
19. Which medication is classified as a Schedule III Controlled Substance?
    a. Acetaminophen with codeine
    b. Alprazolam
    c. Codeine/guaifenesin
    d. Hydrocodone with acetaminophen
20. Which type of inventory must be conducted every 2 years?
    a. Biennial inventory
    b. Initial inventory
    c. Inventory for damaged substances
    d. Newly scheduled control substance inventory
21. If the pharmacy is burglarized for controlled substances, what must be done?
    a. Report it to the local DEA office within 1 business day.
    b. Submit a completed DEA Form 41, Report of Theft or Loss of Controlled Substance, as soon as possible.
    c. File a report with the State Board of Pharmacy.
    d. All the above
22. What is the minimum age to purchase an SLCP?
    a. 14 years
    b. 16 years
    c. 18 years
    d. 21 years

23. According to the Joint Commission, which of the following may be a sign that drug diversion is occurring?
    a. A prescriber has received a written prescription for controlled substances from another physician.
    b. Controlled substance waste is being documented.
    c. Drug dispensing machines show discrepancies and overrides.
    d. All the above

24. What is the maximum amount of pseudoephedrine that can be purchased in 1 day by a qualified purchaser?
    a. 1.8 g
    b. 3.6 g
    c. 7.5 g
    d. 9 g

25. When monitoring the drug history purchase of a controlled substance, which of the following may identify drug diversion?
    a. Comparing controlled substance purchase invoices to controlled substance purchase orders and receipt into the pharmacy's perpetual inventory
    b. Identifying unusual peaks in quantity or frequency of controlled substance purchases
    c. Reconciling invoices to statements or wholesale purchase history reports to detect missing invoices
    d. All the above

5

Medication History Certificate

Eligibility requirements

- Must hold an active Pharmacy Technician Certification Board Certified Pharmacy Technician Certification
- Must fulfill one of the following:
  - Must complete a Pharmacy Technician Certification Board–Recognized Medication History Education/Training Program and have at least 6 months of experience conducting medication histories and/or similar experiences of patient-focused communication (such as intake of new patients/prescriptions and answering patient questions)
  - Must have at least 12 months of experience conducting medication histories and/or similar experiences of patient-focused communication (such as intake of new patients/prescriptions and answering patient questions)

Medication history domains

Concepts/terminology of medication history (45%)

- Definitions of key terms in the medication history process (e.g., medication allergy vs. medication intolerance, medication adherence)
- Translation between patient-friendly terms and medical terminology
- Adherence metrics and differences between primary and secondary nonadherence
- Common vaccinations and vaccination schedules Patient Safety and Quality Assurance Strategies (55%)
- Types of prescription/medication errors (e.g., abnormal doses, incorrect quantity, incorrect strength, incorrect drug, incorrect route of administration, incorrect directions, wrong timing, missing dose, misinterpretation of drug concentration)
- Potential impact of medication errors, including look-alike/sound-alike medications (e.g., ampicillin/amoxicillin)
- Patient factors that influence the ability to report medication information accurately and adhere to prescribed dosing schedules

- Health Insurance Portability and Accountability Act and best practices to maintain patient confidentiality during patient conversations
- Techniques or devices to assist with safe and consistent home medication use (e.g., pillboxes, medication calendars, medication alarms)
- Procedures to verify patient identity, including appropriate identifiers and knowledge of limitations for different identifiers

Concepts/terminology of medication history

Definitions of key terms in the medication history process

Adverse drug event (ADE): Harm experienced by a patient as a result of exposure to a medication or therapeutic agent

Adverse drug reaction: An unintended, harmful event attributed to the use of medicines—occurs as a cause of and during a significant proportion of unscheduled hospital admissions

Adverse event: Untoward incidents, therapeutic misadventures, or other adverse occurrences directly associated with care or services provided within the jurisdiction of a medical center, pharmacy, or other facility

Contraindication: A specific situation in which a medication, procedure, or surgery should not be used because it may have adverse effects on an individual

Dietary supplement: A product taken by mouth intended to supplement the diet, containing one or more dietary ingredients, including vitamins, minerals, herbs or other botanicals, amino acids, enzymes, tissues from organs or glands, or extracts of these (They are labeled as being a dietary supplement.)

Dosage form: The physical form in which a drug is produced and dispensed, such as a tablet, a capsule, or injectable

Dose: The amount of medicine taken at one time

Drug (medication): A substance intended for use in the diagnosis, cure, mitigation, treatment, or prevention of disease

Drug allergy (medication allergy): An abnormal reaction of the immune system to a drug (medication)

Drug (medication) intolerance (sensitivity): An inability to tolerate the adverse effects of a medication, generally at therapeutic or subtherapeutic doses

Family medical history (family history): A record of the relationships among family members along with their medical histories, including current and past illnesses (A family history may show a pattern of certain diseases in a family.)

Frequency: How often a medication is administered per unit of time

Herbal supplements (botanical): A type of dietary supplement containing one or more herbs

Idiopathic: A disease with no identifiable cause

Idiosyncratic reaction: Drug reactions that occur rarely and unpredictably among the population

Indication: The use of a medication for treating a particular disease or condition

Immunization (vaccination or inoculation): A process by which an individual becomes protected against a disease through vaccination

Medical condition: A disease, illness or injury; any physiologic, mental, or psychological condition or disorder

Medical history: Consists of past surgical history, family medical history, social history, allergies, and medications the patient is taking or may have recently stopped taking

Medication (drug): A substance intended for use in the diagnosis, cure, mitigation, treatment, or prevention of disease

Medication adherence: The extent to which patients take their medication as prescribed by their physicians (An individual is considered adherent if he or she takes 80% of the prescribed medications.)

Medication allergy (drug allergy): An abnormal reaction of the immune system to a medication (drug)

Medication history: A compilation of filled prescription information to include medication name, dosage, quantity, and date filled

Over-the-counter (OTC) medication: A medication that is safe and effective for use by the general public without a doctor's prescription

Prescription medication: A medication requiring a prescription from a licensed physician, physician assistant, or nurse prescription

Route of administration: The means by which a drug or agent enters the body to produce its effect

Schedule: When a drug is taken during its course of therapy

Social history: A summary of lifestyle practices and habits that may have a direct or indirect effect on their health (Lifestyle practices includes diet, exercise, sexual orientation, level of sexual activity and occupation. Habits take into consideration use of tobacco, alcohol, and other substances.)

Strength: Indicates how much of the active ingredient is present in each dosage

Vaccination (immunization or inoculation): A process by which an individual becomes protected against a disease through immunization

Vitamin: A group of substances that are needed for normal cell function, growth, and development

Translation between patient-friendly terms and medical terminology	
Medical terminology	Layman's term
Alopecia	Hair loss
Amblyopia	Reduction in vision
Amenorrhea	Absence of menstruation
Anemia	Decrease in red blood cells
Aneurism	Widening of the blood vessel
Angioplasty	Surgical repair of the vessel
Anorexia	Loss of appetite
Antacid	Relieves gastritis, ulcer pain, indigestion, and heartburn
Analgesic	Without pain, kills pain
Antianginal	Relieves heart pain
Antiarrhythmic	Prevents irregular heart rate
Antibiotic	Treats bacterial infection
Anticoagulant	Prevents blood clots
Anticonvulsant	Prevents seizure
Antidepressant	Prevents depression
Antidiabetic	Reduces blood glucose levels
Antidiarrheal	Stops diarrhea
Antiemetic	Prevents nausea and vomiting
Antifungal	Treats fungal infection
Antihistamine	Blocks effects of histamine
Antihyperlipidemic	Lowers high cholesterol levels
Antihypertensive	Reduces high blood pressure
Anti-inflammatory	Reduces inflammation
Antiparkinsonian	Treats Parkinson disease
Antipruritic	Prevents or relieves itching
Antiseptic	Topical antibacterial agent
Antispasmodic	Relieves intestinal cramping
Antitussive	Inhibits cough reflex
Antiviral	Treats viral infection
Anuresis	Inability to urinate
Anuria	Inability to produce urine
Aphagia	Inability to swallow
Aphasia	Inability to speak
Apnea	Temporary failure to breathe
Arthralgia	Joint pain
Arthritis	Joint inflammation
Astigmatism	Distorted vision
Atrophy	Process of shrinking muscle size
Bacteremia	Bacteria in the blood stream
Blepharitis	Inflammation of the eyelids
Bradycardia	Slow heart rate

(Continued)

Translation between patient-friendly terms and medical terminology —cont'd	
Medical terminology	**Layman's term**
Bradypnea	Slow breathing
Bronchitis	Inflammation of the bronchial membranes
Bronchodilator	Dilates bronchial tubes in the lung
Bursitis	Inflammation of the bursa
Cardiomyopathy	Decrease of the heart muscle
Cellulitis	Infection of the skin and subcutaneous tissue
Ceruminosis	Excessive earwax
Colitis	Inflamed or irritated colon
Colostomy	New opening in the colon
Condyloma	Genital wart
Conjunctivitis	Inflammation of the conjunctiva
Cyanosis	Abnormal blue skin color from lack of oxygen in the blood
Cystitis	Inflammation of the bladder
Dementia	Disorientation, confusion, loss of memory
Dermatitis	Skin inflammation
Diabetes	Pancreatic disorder of insufficient insulin production
Dialysis	Method of filtering impurities from blood
Diaphoresis	Excessive sweating
Diarrhea	Liquid or unformed bowel movement
Diplopia	Double vision
Dyslexia	Difficult reading
Dyspepsia	Condition of indigestion
Dyspnea	Labored breathing
Dystrophy	Progressive atrophy
Dysuria	Painful urination
Eczema	Chronic skin inflammation
Embolism	Obstruction of blood flow
Emphysema	Obstructive pulmonary disease
Encephalitis	Inflammation of the brain
Endocarditis	Inflammation of the heart muscle
Endocrine	Pertaining to glands that secrete hormones into the bloodstream
Endometriosis	Abnormal growth of uterine tissue
Enuresis	Involuntary urination
Epilepsy	Disorder characterized by recurrent seizures
Erythema	Skin redness
Fibromyalgia	Chronic pain in the muscles
Gastroenteritis	Inflammation of the stomach and intestinal tract
Glaucoma	Eye disease caused by increased intraocular pressure
Glycosuria	Glucose in the urine

Translation between patient-friendly terms and medical terminology —cont'd	
Medical terminology	**Layman's term**
Gynecology	Study of female reproductive organs
Hematoma	Liver tumor
Hernia	Protrusion of organ or tissue
Hyperglycemia	High blood sugar
Hyperlipidemia	High blood cholesterol
Hypertension	High blood pressure
Hyperthyroidism	Elevated thyroid levels
Hypertrophy	Process of increase in muscle size
Hypoglycemia	Low blood sugar
Hypothyroidism	Low thyroid levels
Hysterectomy	Removal of the uterus
Ichthyosis	Dry, scaly skin
Keratosis	Area of increased hardness of the skin
Leukemia	Increase in white blood cells
Mastectomy	Removal of the breast
Mastitis	Inflammation of the breast
Menorrhea	Prolonged bleeding in menopause
Myasthenia	Chronic muscular weakness
Myxedema	Swelling of the skin giving a waxy or slimy appearance
Nephralgia	Kidney pain
Neuralgia	Severe pain along a nerve
Onychomycosis	Fungal infection of the nail
Ostealgia	Bone pain
Osteoarthritis	Chronic bone and joint disease
Osteoporosis	Decreased bone density
Otalgia	Pain in the ear (earache)
Otorrhagia	Bleeding in the ear
Otitis	Inflammation of the ear
Paralysis	Breaking down of motor control
Phlebitis	Inflammation of the vein
Photophobia	Intolerance to light
Pneumonia	Bacterial infection of the lungs
Polyuria	Excessive urination
Prostatitis	Inflammation of the prostate
Pruritis	Intense itching
Psoriasis	Red, scaly patches that causes intense itching
Psychosis	Psychiatric disorder
Psychotropic	Changes mental states
Rhinitis	Inflammation of the nose; runny nose
Septicemia	Systemic blood infection
Splenectomy	Removal of the spleen
Tachycardia	Rapid heart rate

(Continued)

Translation between patient-friendly terms and medical terminology —cont'd	
Medical terminology	**Layman's term**
Tendonitis	Inflammation of a tendon
Tetany	Muscle twitches, cramps, convulsions
Thrombolytic	Dissolves blood clots
Thrombosis	Blood clots in the vascular system
Vasectomy	Removal of a segment of the vas deferens
Vasodilator	Dilates (opens) the blood vessels

Adherence metrics and differences between primary and secondary nonadherence

Adherence

- Adherence is defined as the extent to which patients take their medication as prescribed by their physicians.
- Individuals are considered adherent if they take 80% of their prescribed medication doses.
- Factors that affect adherence include patients getting their prescriptions filled, remembering to take their medication on time, and understanding the medication's instructions.

- Barriers to medication adherence consist of the patient's ability to pay for their medications, limited health literacy, a medication's adverse side effects, and polypharmacy.

Medication nonadherence

- Primary nonadherence: Occurs when a new medication is prescribed for a patient, but the patient fails to obtain the medication (or its appropriate alternative) within an acceptable period of time after it was initially prescribed
- Secondary nonadherence: Refers to a patient taking insufficient doses required to experience a therapeutic effect, missing doses or discontinuing their therapy early
- Intentional medication nonadherence: Active process whereby the patient chooses to deviate from the treatment regimen
- Unintentional medication nonadherence: Passive process in which the patient may be careless or forgetful about adhering to treatment regimen
- Nonadherence directly tied to increased morbidity, mortality, and avoidable health care costs
- Occurs when the patient takes less than 80% of their prescribed medications doses

Common vaccinations and vaccination schedules

Recommended Child and Adolescent Immunization Schedule (birth through 18 years), 2023					
Vaccine	**Abbreviation**	**Brand Name**	**Minimum Age**	**Series**	**Administered**
COVID-19	BNT162b2 mRNA-1273	Comirnaty (Pfizer-BioNTech) Spikevax (Moderna)	6 months	2 or 3 dose	**Primary series**: **Age 6 months–4 years**: 2-dose series at 0, 4-8 weeks (Moderna) or 3-dose series at 0, 3-8, 11-16 weeks (Pfizer-BioNTech) **Age 5–11 years**: 2-dose series at 0, 4-8 weeks (Moderna) or 2-dose series at 0, 3-8 weeks (Pfizer-BioNTech) **Age 12–18 years**: 2-dose series at 0, 4-8 weeks (Moderna) or 2-dose series at 0, 3-8 weeks (Pfizer-BioNTech)
Diphtheria, tetanus, and acellular pertussis	DTaP	Daptacel Infanrix	6 weeks	5-dose	2, 4, 6 and 15-18 months, 4-6 years
Diphtheria, tetanus	DT	No brand name	6 weeks-6 years old	5-dose	0.5 mL IM q4-8wk x3 doses, then 0.5 mL IM x1 at 15-18 month, then 0.5 mL IM x1 at 4-6 years old; Info: may give 4th dose as early as 12 months and 6 months after 3rd dose; 5th dose not needed if 4th dose given after 4th birthday and at least 6mo after 3rd dose
Haemophilus influenza type b vaccine	Hib (PRP-T), Hib (PRP-OMB)	ActHIB, Hiberix or Pentacel	6 weeks	4-dose	2, 4, 6, 12-15 months

(Continued)

Recommended Child and Adolescent Immunization Schedule (birth through 18 years), 2023—cont'd					
Vaccine	Abbreviation	Brand Name	Minimum Age	Series	Administered
		Pedvax	6 weeks	3-dose	2, 4, 12-15 months
Hepatitis A	HepA	Havrix, Vaqta	12 months	2-dose	Beginning at 12 months with 6- month interval at age 12-23 months
Hepatitis B	HepB	Engerix-B, Recombivax HB	Birth	3-dose	0, 1-2, 6-18 months
Human papillomavirus	HPV	Gardasil 9	9 years	2 or 3 dose	9-14 years at initial vaccination: 2-dose series at 0, 6-12 months (minimum interval: 5 months)
					15 years or older at initial vaccination: 3-dose series at 0, 1-2 months, 6 months (minimum intervals: dose 1 to dose 2: 4 weeks / dose 2 to dose 3: 12 weeks / dose 1 to dose 3: 5 months; repeat dose if administered too soon)
Influenza, (inactivated)	IIV	IIV-multiple manufacturers	6 months	1 or 2 doses based on patient age	2 doses, separated by at least 4 weeks, for children aged 6 months–8 years who have received fewer than 2 influenza vaccine doses before July 1, 2022 or whose influenza vaccination history is unknown (administer dose 2 even if the child turns 9 between receipt of dose 1 and dose 2).
					1 dose for children aged 6 months–8 years who have received at least 2 influenza vaccine doses before July 1, 2022.
					1 dose for all persons aged 9 years or older
Influenza (live, attenuated)	LAIV4	LAIV-FluMist Quadrivalent	2 years	1-dose	0.1 mL spray in each nostril one time annually
Measles, mumps, and rubella	MMR	M-M-R II	12 months	2-dose	12-15 months, 4-6 years.
Meningococcal serotype A-C-W-Y	MenACWY-CRM (Menveo) MenACWY-D (Menactra) MenACWY-TT (MenQuadfi)	Menveo Menactra MenQuadfi	Menveo-2 months Menactra-9 months MenQuadfi-2 years	2-dose	2-dose series at age 11–12 years and at 16 years
Meningococcal serotype B	MenB-4C (Bexsero) MenB-FHbp (Trumenba)	Bexsero Trumenba	10 years	2-dose	Bexsero: 2-dose series at least 1 month apart
					Trumenba: 2-dose series at least 6 months apart; if dose 2 is administered earlier than 6 months, administer a 3rd dose at least 4 months after dose 2.
Pneumococcal 13-valent conjugate	PCV13	Prevnar 13	6 weeks	4-dose	4- dose series at 2, 4, 6, 12–15 months
Pneumococcal 23 valent polysaccharide	PPSV23	Pneumovax	2 years	1-dose	0.5 mL SC/IM x1 dose; Info: give >8wk after PCV13

(Continued)

Recommended Child and Adolescent Immunization Schedule (birth through 18 years), 2023

Vaccine	Abbreviation	Brand Name	Minimum Age	Series	Administered
Poliovirus (inactivated)	IPV	IPOL	6 weeks	4-dose	4-dose series at ages 2, 4, 6–18 months, 4–6 years; administer the final dose on or after age 4 years and at least 6 months after the previous dose.
Rotavirus	RV1 RV5	RV1: Rotarix RV5: RotaTeq	6 weeks	Rotarix-2 dose. RotaTeq-3 dose.	Rotarix: 2-dose series at 2 and 4 months. RotaTeq: 3-dose series at 2, 4, and 6 months
Tetanus, diphtheria, and acellular pertussis	Tdap	Adacel, Boostrix	11 years	1-dose	Adolescents aged 11–12 years: 1 dose Tdap.
Tetanus and diphtheria vaccine	Td	Tenivac, TDvax	7 years	3-doses	0.5 mL IM x2 doses at least 4wk apart, then 0.5 mL IM x1 dose 6-12mo after prior dose
Varicella	VAR	Varivax	12 months	2-dose	2-dose series at 12–15 months, 4–6 years

Immunization schedule from: CDC. Child and adolescent immunization schedule. https://www.cdc.gov/vaccines/schedules/hcp/imz/child-adolescent.html. Accessed February 1, 2023

IM, intramuscular; *SC*, subcutaneous.

Recommended Adult Immunization Schedule for ages 19 years or older, 2023

Vaccine	Abbreviation	Brand Name	Routine Vaccine
COVID-19	BNT162b2	Comirnaty	Age 18 years and older: a 2-dose series where the second dose is administered every 21 days after the second shot. A booster, either Pfizer-BioNTech or Moderna may be administered 5 months after the second dose
	mRNA-1273	Spikevax	Age 18 years and older: a 2-dose series 28 days after the second shot. A booster, either Pfizer-BioNTech or Moderna may be administered 5 months after the second dose.
Haemophilus influenzae type B	Hib	ActHIB, Hiberix	For previously unvaccinated pts w/ asplenia, sickle cell disease; give at least 2wk prior to elective splenectomy; give 3-doses 4wk apart starting at 6-12mo after successful hematopoietic stem cell transplant.
Hepatitis A	HepA	Havrix, Vaqta	Not at risk but want protection from hepatitis A: 2-dose series HepA (Havrix 6–12 months apart or Vaqta 6–18 months apart [minimum interval: 6 months]) or 3-dose series HepA-HepB (Twinrix at 0, 1, 6 months [minimum intervals: dose 1 to dose 2: 4 weeks / dose 2 to dose 3: 5 months])
Hepatitis B	HepB	Engerix-B Recombivax HB Heplisav-B	Age 19 through 59 years: complete a 2- or 3-, or 4-dose series. 2-dose series only applies when 2 doses of Heplisav-B are used at least 4 weeks apart 3-dose series Engerix-B or Recombivax HB at 0, 1, 6 months [minimum intervals: dose 1 to dose 2: 4 weeks / dose 2 to dose 3: 8 weeks / dose 1 to dose 3: 16 weeks]) 3-dose series HepA-HepB (Twinrix at 0, 1, 6 months [minimum intervals: dose 1 to dose 2: 4 weeks / dose 2 to dose 3: 5 months]) 4-dose series HepA-HepB (Twinrix) accelerated schedule of 3 doses at 0, 7, and 21–30 days, followed by a booster dose at 12 months 4-dose series Engerix-B at 0, 1, 2, and 6 months for persons on adult hemodialysis (note: each dosage is double that of normal adult dose, i.e., 2 mL instead of 1 mL)
Human papillomavirus	HPV	Gardasil	HPV vaccination recommended for all persons through age 26 years: 2- or 3-dose series depending on age at initial vaccination or condition: Age 15 years or older at initial vaccination: 3-dose series at 0, 1–2 months, 6 months (minimum intervals: dose 1 to dose 2: 4 weeks / dose 2 to dose 3: 12 weeks / dose 1 to dose 3: 5 months; repeat dose if administered too soon)

(Continued)

Recommended Adult Immunization Schedule for ages 19 years or older, 2023—cont'd			
Vaccine	**Abbreviation**	**Brand Name**	**Routine Vaccine**
Influenza, inactivated	IIV	Multiple brands	Age 19 years or older: 1 dose any influenza vaccine appropriate for age and health status annually. Age 65 years or older: Any one of quadrivalent high-dose inactivated influenza vaccine (HD-IIV4), quadrivalent recombinant influenza vaccine (RIV4), or quadrivalent adjuvanted inactivated influenza vaccine (aIIV4) is preferred.
Measles, mumps, and rubella	MMR	M-M-R II	No evidence of immunity to measles, mumps, or rubella: 1 dose
Meningococcal	MenACWY	MenACWY-D MenACWY-CRM MenACWY-TT	First-year college students who live in residential housing (if not previously vaccinated at age 16 years or older) or military recruits: 1 dose MenACWY (Menactra, Menveo, or MenQuadfi)
Meningococcal serogroup B	MenB-C MenB-FHbp	Bexsero Trumenba	Adolescents and young adults age 16–23 years (age 16–18 years preferred) not at increased risk for meningococcal disease: Based on shared clinical decision-making, 2-dose series MenB-4C (Bexsero) at least 1 month apart or 2-dose series MenB-FHbp (Trumenba) at 0, 6 months (if dose 2 was administered less than 6 months after dose 1, administer dose 3 at least 4 months after dose 2); MenB-4C and MenB-FHbp are not interchangeable (use same product for all doses in series)
Pneumococcal 13-valent conjugate	PCV13	Prevnar 13	For high-risk pts 19 years old and older; may give to low-risk pts 65 years old and older based on shared clinical decision-making; follow w/ PPSV23 after >8wk in high-risk pts or after >1y in immunocompetent pts 65 years old and older; if prior PPSV23 but no PCV13 at 65 years old or older, give PCV13 >1y after last PPSV23 dose.
Pneumococcal 23-valent polysaccharide vaccine	PPSV23	Pneumovax 23	For high-risk pts <65 years old and all pts 65 years old and older per ACIP guidelines; give >8wk after PCV13 or PCV15 if high risk, otherwise give >1y after PCV13 or PCV15; repeat x1 after 5 years in high-risk pts or in pts 65 years old and older who received 1st dose when <65 years old and >5years ago.
Tetanus and diphtheria toxoids	Td	Tenivac, Tdvax	0.5 mL IM x2 doses at least 4wk apart, then 0.5 mL IM x1 dose 6-12mo after prior dose
Tetanus and diphtheria toxoids and acellular pertussis	Tdap	Adacel, Boostrix	Previously did not receive Tdap at or after age 11 years: 1 dose Tdap, then Td or Tdap every 10 years
Varicella	VAR	Varivax	No evidence of immunity to varicella: 2-dose series 4–8 weeks apart if previously did not receive varicella-containing vaccine (VAR or MMRV [measles-mumps-rubella-varicella vaccine] for children); if previously received 1 dose varicella-containing vaccine, 1 dose at least 4 weeks after first dose. Evidence of immunity: U.S.-born before 1980 (except for pregnant women and health care personnel [see below]), documentation of 2 doses varicella-containing vaccine at least 4 weeks apart, diagnosis or verification of history of varicella or herpes zoster by a health care provider, laboratory evidence of immunity or disease
Zoster, recombinant	RZV	Shingrix	Age 50 years or older: 2-dose series RZV (Shingrix) 2–6 months apart (minimum interval: 4 weeks; repeat dose if administered too soon), regardless of previous herpes zoster or history of zoster vaccine live (ZVL, Zostavax) vaccination (administer RZV at least 2 months after ZVL)

Immunization schedule from: CDC. Adult immunization schedule. https://www.cdc.gov/vaccines/schedules/hcp/imz/adult.html. Accessed February 1, 2023

ACIP, Advisory committee on immunization practices; *IM,* intramuscular; *MMRV,* measles-mumps-rubella-varicella vaccine, *SC,* subcutaneous.

Patient safety and quality assurance strategies

Types of prescription/medication errors

Five rights of patient safety

- The right drug
- The right dose
- The right dosage form
- The right route of administration
- The right time of administration

Medication Error

- According to the National Coordinating Council for Medication Error Reporting and Prevention, a "medication error is any preventable event that may cause or lead to inappropriate medication use or patient harm while the medication is in the control of the health care professional, patient, or consumer."

Root causes of medication errors

- Human: An error caused by an individual by not following procedures, missing or ignoring a step, or lack of training. For example, a pharmacy technician pulls a bottle of amoxicillin 250 mg from the shelf instead of amoxicillin 500 mg.
- Manufacturing: An error caused during manufacturing in which the medication is not manufactured according to specifications or the packaging or educational materials provided are incorrect.
- Organizational: The health care organization's policy and procedures lack appropriate directions for the staff to perform their jobs properly, to include training. An example would be the pharmacy is not following the current USP <795> standards for nonsterile compounding, USP <797> standards for sterile compounding, or USP <800> standards for handling hazardous drugs.
- Technical: The equipment used in processing or compounding a prescription is not working properly. For example, the pharmacy scale used to weigh ingredients is not calibrated properly or the automatic dispensing equipment is not working properly.

Types of prescription (medication) errors

- Medication errors maybe classified based upon the practitioner's role in the medication use process and they include prescribing, dispensing, and administering errors.
- Prescribing errors
  - Incorrect drug selection (based on indications, contraindications, known allergies, existing drug therapy, and other factors), dose, dosage form, quantity, route, concentration, rate of administration, or instructions for use of a drug product ordered or authorized by physician (or other legitimate prescriber)
  - Illegible prescriptions (medication orders) or misspellings on the e-script that lead to errors that reach the patient

  - Prescriber unaware of specific requirements of the drug such as risk evaluation and mitigation strategies being required prior to dispensing of medication
  - Use of abbreviations found on the Joint Commission Do Not Use list or Institute of Safe Medication Practices (ISMP) error-prone abbreviations, symbols, and dose designations
- Dispensing errors
  - Wrong formulation error occurs when a different dosage form or salt is dispensed without the prescriber's permission. An example would be dispensing metoprolol tartrate instead of metoprolol succinate.
  - Wrong drug error occurs when a drug was dispensed that is different than the drug prescribed.
  - Medication education error occurs when proper education material is not provided to the patient. An example is the failure of the pharmacist or pharmacy technician to provide a medication guide to the patient.
  - Adverse drug error occurs when a drug utilization review warning is missed or ignored. The pharmacy technician overrides a warning for warfarin in a 75-year-old patient and does not inform the pharmacist of the situation.
  - Wrong amount/dosage error occurs when the dose given is 5% greater or less than the dose prescribed. An example would be dispensing levothyroxine 0.025 mg instead of levothyroxine 0.125 mg.
  - Documentation error occurs when essential information is missing or incorrect. An example of this is when the medication list in the pharmacy information system is not updated with current information.
  - Compliance error occurs when a patient fails to adhere to the directions provided by their physician and pharmacist regarding taking their medication. An example would be a patient completing their 30-day therapy in 10 days, and the pharmacist failing to address the issue with the patient.
  - Monitoring error is a failure to review a prescribed regimen for appropriateness and detection of problems or failure to use appropriate clinical or laboratory data for adequate assessment of patient response to prescribed therapy. An example would be failing to monitor properly medications with narrow therapeutic indexes such as warfarin and levothyroxine.
  - Wrong drug preparation error occurs when the medication has been incorrectly formulated or manipulated before administration. An example would be using the incorrect diluent when preparing a sterile compound.
  - Deteriorated drug error occurs when a drug dispensed has expired or for which the physical or chemical dosage-form integrity has been compromised. An example would be dispensing a medication on September 30 when the label on the manufacturer's package indicates the expiration date is July 31 of that year. Another example would be dispensing a medication that has exceeded its beyond-use-date.
- Administering errors
  - Omission error is defined as the failure to administer an ordered dose to a patient before the next scheduled dose. An example is a nurse failing to administer a

patient's morning medication to them or patients at home forgetting to take their diuretic in the morning.

- Improper dose error is when the patient is administered a dose that is greater than or less than the amount ordered by the prescriber or administration of duplicate doses to the patient such as one or more dosage units in addition to those that were ordered. An example is when a nurse administers two tablets instead of one tablet as was prescribed or a patient at home taking an extra dose of amoxicillin in order shorten the time of the infection.
- Unauthorized drug error occurs when a medication is administered to a patient that has not been authorized by a legitimate prescriber for the patient.
- Wrong dosage form error occurs when a patient is administered a drug product in a different dosage form than ordered by the prescriber.
- Wrong time error occurs when the medication is administered outside a predefined time interval from its scheduled administration time. An example would be a nurse administering levothyroxine at noon instead of at 7 a.m. prior to breakfast.
- Wrong administration technique error occurs when an inappropriate procedure or improper technique is used in administering a medication. An example would be a nurse administering an injection subcutaneously instead of intramuscularly.
- A deteriorated drug error is when a drug being administered has expired or for which the physical or chemical dosage-form integrity has been compromised. An example would be dispensing a medication on September 30 when the label on the manufacturer's package indicates the expiration date is July 31 of that year. Another example would be administering a liquid antibiotic that has been left out at room temperature instead of being refrigerated.
- Wrong mixture with other drugs and supplements occurs when the nurse or patient do not follow the accompanying educational warnings regarding the medication. An example of this occur when a patient drinks grapefruit juice while taking a "statin."

Causes of dispensing errors

- Incomplete information causes a dispensing error as a result of a policy not being followed when completing a patient's medication profile such as allergies not being identified.
- Incorrect assumption not checked results in a dispensing error when wrong assumptions are made based upon missing or questionable information provided. An example is when the wrong drug is selected based upon the assumption you are able to interpret the prescriber's handwriting.
- Selection error occurs while reviewing a pull-down menu on the computer or on a pharmacy shelf when similar drug names are present, and you select the wrong drug. This is a common occurrence when dealing with look-alike/sound-alike (LASA) drug names. LASA drug names will be presented later in the chapter.
- Capture/habit error is the result of the pharmacist's or pharmacy technician's inattention due to distractions or the result of developing poor habits when filling a prescription. An example would be the pharmacy technician

is used to dispensing the usual adult dosage for a medication and fills the adults dose for the child and the pharmacist approves the prescription without noticing.

- Rushed error occurs when pressure is applied to satisfy patients or to meet quotas resulting in a medication error. Often, the error occurs as a result of not following institutional policies and procedures and taking shortcuts in filling a prescription. An example of a situation resulting in an error is not matching the National Drug Code number on the manufacturer's bottle with the National Drug Code on the prescription label.
- Distraction error is the result of an interruption during critical phases of the prescription filling process. A common distraction is the continuous telephone ringing in the pharmacy and no one answering it.
- Fear error occurs when an individual does not ask the pharmacist or another technician a question regarding a prescription or fails to provide input regarding a question affecting the pharmacy practice.

National Coordinating Council for Medication Error Reporting Index for Categorizing Medication Errors			
Category	Definition	Type of resulting error	Example
A	Circumstances occur that have potential for causing errors.	No error	N/A
B	Error occurred but did not reach patient.	Error, no harm	The pharmacy technician catches an error when the patient is picking up his or her prescription.
C	Error reached patient but did not cause harm.	Error, no harm	Multivitamin was not ordered on admission but the patient refused the medication.
D	Error reached patient, did not cause harm, but needed monitoring or intervention to prove no harm resulted.	Error, no harm	Regular-release metoprolol was ordered for patient instead of extended-release form.
E	Error occurred that may have contributed to or resulted in temporary harm to patient and patient required intervention.	Error, harm	Blood pressure medication was inadvertently omitted from order.
F	Error occurred that may have contributed to or resulted in temporary harm to patient and resulted in hospitalization.	Error, harm	Anticoagulant (warfarin) was ordered to be taken daily but the patient takes it every other day.

National Coordinating Council for Medication Error Reporting Index for Categorizing Medication Errors—cont'd			
Category	Definition	Type of resulting error	Example
G	Error occurred that may have contributed to or resulted in temporary or permanent harm to the patient.	Error, harm	Immunosuppressant medication was unintentionally ordered at one-fourth the recommended dose.
H	Error occurred that may have contributed to or resulted in harm to patient and required hospitalization to sustain life.	Error, harm	Anticonvulsant therapy was inadvertently omitted.
I	Error occurred that may have contributed or resulted in patient's death.	Error, death	Beta-blocker was not reordered postoperatively.
N/A, not applicable.			

Definitions

Harm: Impairment of the physical, emotional, or psychological function or structure of the body and/or pain resulting therefrom

Monitoring: To observe or record relevant or psychological signs

Intervention: May include change in therapy or active medical/surgical treatment

Intervention necessary to sustain life: Includes cardiovascular and respiratory support (e.g. CPR, defibrillation, intubation, etc.)

Potential impact of medication errors, including look-alike/sound-alike medications (e.g., ampicillin/amoxicillin)

The abbreviations, symbols, and doses designations listed on the following tables have been reported through the ISMP National Medication Errors Reporting Program. As a result of being misinterpreted, they have resulted in medication errors. According to the ISMP, "[T]hese abbreviations, symbols, and dose designations should NEVER be used when communicating medical information verbally, electronically, and/or in handwritten applications. This includes internal communications; verbal, handwritten, or electronic prescriptions; hand-written and computer-generated medication labels; drug storage bin labels; medication administration records; and screens associated with pharmacy and prescriber computer order entry systems, automated dispensing cabinets, smart infusion pumps, and other medication-related technologies."

Abbreviations for Doses/Measurement Units			
Error-prone abbreviations, symbols, and dose designation	Intended meaning	Misinterpretation	Best practice
cc	Cubic centimeters	Mistaken as u (units)	Use mL
IU[a]	International unit(s)	Mistaken as IV (intravenous) or the numeral 10	Use unit(s) (International units can be expressed as units alone)
l	Liter	Lowercase letter l mistaken as the numeral 1	Use L (uppercase) for liter
ml	Milliliter	Lowercase letter l mistaken as the numeral 1	Use mL (lowercase m, uppercase L) for milliliter
MM or M	Million	Mistaken as thousand	Use million
M or K	Thousand	Mistaken as million. M has been used to abbreviate both million and thousand (M is the Roman numeral for thousand)	Use thousand
Ng or ng	Nanogram	Mistaken as mg. Mistaken as nasogastric	Use nanogram or nanog
U or u[a]	Unit(s)	Mistaken as zero or the numeral 4, causing a 10-fold overdose or greater (e.g., 4 U seen as 40 or 4u seen as 44). Mistaken as cc, leading to administering volume instead of units (e.g., 4u seen as 4 cc)	Use unit(s)
μg	Microgram	Mistaken as mg	Use mcg

[a]On the Joint Commission's Do Not Use list.

Abbreviations for route of administration			
Error-prone abbreviations, symbols, and dose designation	Intended meaning	Misinterpretation	Best practice
AD, AS, AU	Right ear, left ear, each ear	Mistaken as OD, OS, OU (right eye, left eye, each eye)	Use right ear, left ear, or each ear
IN	Intranasal	Mistaken as IM or IV	Use NAS (all uppercase letters) or intranasal
IT	Intrathecal	Mistaken as intratracheal, intratumor, intratympanic, or inhalation therapy	Use intrathecal
OD, OS, OU	Right eye, left eye, each eye	Mistaken as AD, AS, AU (right ear, left ear, each ear)	Use right eye, left eye, or each eye
Per os	By mouth, orally	The os was mistaken as left eye (OS, oculus sinister)	Use PO, by mouth, or orally
SC, SQ, sq, or sub q	Subcutaneous(ly)	SC and sc mistaken as SL or sl (sublingual) SQ mistaken as "5 every" The q in sub q has been mistaken as "every"	Use SUBQ (all uppercase letters, without spaces or periods between letters) or subcutaneous(ly)

IM, intramuscular.

Abbreviation for frequency/instructions for use			
Error-prone abbreviations, symbols, and dose designation	Intended meaning	Misinterpretation	Best practice
HS hs	Half-strength At bedtime, hours of sleep	Mistaken as bedtime Mistaken as half-strength	Use half-strength Use HS (all uppercase letters) for bedtime
o.d. or OD	Once daily	Mistaken as right eye (OD, oculus dexter), leading to oral liquid medications administered in the eye	Use daily

Abbreviation for frequency/instructions for use —cont'd			
Error-prone abbreviations, symbols, and dose designation	Intended meaning	Misinterpretation	Best practice
Q.D., QD, q.d., or qd[a]	Every day	Mistaken as q.i.d., especially if the period after the q or the tail of a handwritten q is misunderstood as the letter i	Use daily
Qhs	Nightly at bedtime	Mistaken as qhr (every hour)	Use nightly or HS for bedtime
Qn	Nightly at bedtime	Mistaken as qh (every hour)	Use nightly or HS for bedtime
Q.O.D., QOD, q.o.d., or qod[a]	Every other day	Mistaken as qd (daily) or qid (four times daily), especially if the o is poorly written	Use every other day
qd	Daily	Mistaken as qid (four times daily)	Use daily
q6PM, etc.	Every evening at 6 p.m.	Mistaken as every 6 hours	Use daily at 6 p.m. or 6 p.m. daily
SSRI SSI	Sliding scale regular insulin Sliding scale insulin	Mistaken as selective-serotonin reuptake inhibitor Mistaken as strong solution of iodine (Lugol's)	Use sliding scale (insulin)
TIW or tiw BIW or biw	3 times a week 2 times a week	Mistaken as 3 times a day or twice in a week Mistaken as 2 times a day	Use 3 times weekly Use 2 times weekly
UD	As directed (ut dictum)	Mistaken as unit dose (e.g., an order for "dilTIAZem infusion UD" was mistakenly administered as a unit [bolus] dose	Use as directed

[a]On the Joint Commission's Do Not Use list.

Miscellaneous abbreviations associated with medication use			
Error-prone abbreviations, symbols, and dose designation	Intended meaning	Misinterpretation	Best practice
BBA BGB	Baby boy A (twin) Baby girl B (twin)	B in BBA mistaken as twin B rather than gender (boy) B at end of BGB mistaken as gender (boy) not twin B	When assigning identifiers to newborns, use the mother's last name, the baby's sex (boy or girl), and a distinguishing identifier for all multiples (e.g., Smith girl A, Smith girl B)
D/C	Discharge or discontinue	Premature discontinuation of medications when D/C (intended to mean discharge) on a medication list was misinterpreted as discontinued	Use discharge and discontinue or stop
IJ	Injection	Mistaken as IV or intrajugular	Use injection

Miscellaneous abbreviations associated with medication use —cont'd			
Error-prone abbreviations, symbols, and dose designation	Intended meaning	Misinterpretation	Best practice
OJ	Orange juice	Mistaken as OD or OS (right or left eye); drugs meant to be diluted in orange juice may be given in the eye	Use orange juice
Period following abbreviations (e.g., mg., mL.)[a]	Mg or mL	Unnecessary period mistaken as the numeral 1, especially if written poorly	Use mg, mL, etc., without a terminal period

[a]Relevant mostly in handwritten medication information.

Drug name abbreviations

Avoid abbreviating drug names completely to avoid confusion. Drug name abbreviations should never be used for any medications o the ISMP List of High-Alert Medications in Acute Care Settings, Community/Ambulatory Settings, and Long-Term Care Settings. The following drug name abbreviations have been involved in serious medication errors.

Error-prone abbreviations, symbols, and dose designation	Intended meaning	Misinterpretation	Best practice
Antiretroviral medications (e.g., DOR, TAF, TDF)	DOR: doravine TAF: tenofovir alafenamide TDF: tenofovir disoproxil fumarate	DOR: Dovato (dolutegravir and lamiVUDine) TAF: tenofovir disoproxil fumarate TDF: tenofovir alafenamide	Use complete drug names
APAP	Acetaminophen	Not recognized as acetaminophen	Use complete drug name
ARA A	Vidarabine	Mistaken as cytarabine ("ARA C")	Use complete drug name
AT II and AT III	AT II: angiotensin II (Giapreza) AT III: antithrombin III (Thrombate III)	AT II (angiotensin II) mistaken as AT III (antithrombin III) AT III (antithrombin III) mistaken as AT II (angiotensin II)	Use complete drug names
AZT	Zidovudine (Retrovir)	Mistaken as azithromycin, azaTHIOprine, or aztreonam	Use complete drug name
CPZ	Compazine (prochlorperazine)	Mistaken as chlorproMAZINE	Use complete drug name
DTO	Diluted tincture of opium or deodorized tincture of opium (Paregoric)	Mistaken as tincture of opium	Use complete drug name
HCT	Hydrocortisone	Mistaken as hydroCHLOROthiazide	Use complete drug name
HCTZ	hydroCHLOROthiazide	Mistaken as hydrocortisone (e.g., seen as HCT250 mg)	Use complete drug names
MgSO4[a]	Magnesium sulfate	Mistaken as morphine sulfate	Use complete drug name

(Continued)

Error-prone abbreviations, symbols, and dose designation	Intended meaning	Misinterpretation	Best practice
MS, MSO4[a]	Morphine sulfate	Mistaken as magnesium sulfate	Use complete drug name
MTX	Methotrexate	Mistaken as mitoXANTRONE	Use complete drug name
Na at the beginning of a drug name (e.g., Na bicarbonate	Sodium bicarbonate	Mistaken as no bicarbonate	Use complete drug name
NoAC	Novel/new oral anticoagulant	Mistaken as no anticoagulant	Use complete drug name
OXY	Oxytocin	Mistaken as oxyCODONE, OxyCONTIN	Use complete drug name
PCA	Procainamide	Mistaken as patient-controlled analgesia	Use complete drug name
PIT	Pitocin (oxytocin)	Mistaken as Pitressin, a discontinued brand of vasopressin still referred to as PIT	Use complete drug names
PNV	Prenatal vitamins	Mistaken as penicillin VK	Use complete drug name
PTU	Propylthiouracil	Mistaken as mercaptopurine (Purinethol)	Use complete drug name
T3	Tylenol with codeine No. 3	Mistaken as liothyronine, which is sometimes referred to as T3	Use complete drug name
TAC or tac	Triamcinolone or tacrolimus	Mistaken as tetracaine, Adrenalin, and cocaine; or as Taxotere, Adriamycin, and cyclophosphamide	Use complete drug names Avoid drug regimen or protocol acronyms that may have a dual meaning or may be confused with other common acronyms, even if defined in an order set
TNK	TNKase	Mistaken as TPA	Use complete drug name
TPA or tPA	Tissue plasminogen activator, alteplase (Activase)	Mistaken as TNK (TNKase, tenecteplase), TXA (tranexamic acid), or less often as another tissue plasminogen activator, Retavase (reteplase)	Use complete drug name
TXA	Tranexamic acid	Mistaken as TPA (tissue plasminogen activator)	Use complete drug name
ZnSO4	Zinc sulfate	Mistaken as morphine sulfate	Use complete drug name
[a]On the Joint Commission's Do Not Use list.			

Stemmed/coined drug names			
Error-prone abbreviations, symbols, and dose designation	Intended meaning	Misinterpretation	Beat practice
Nitro drip	Nitroglycerin infusion	Mistaken as nitroprusside infusion	Use complete drug name
IV vanc	Intravenous vancomycin	Mistaken as Invanz	Use complete drug name
Levo	Levofloxacin	Mistaken as norepinephrine (Levophed)	Use complete drug name
Neo	Neo-Synephrine, a well-known but discontinued brand of phenylephrine	Mistaken as neostigmine	Use complete drug name
Coined names for compounded products (e.g., magic mouthwash, banana bag, GI cocktail, half and half, pink lady)	Specific ingredients compounded together	Mistaken ingredients	Use complete drug/product names for all ingredients Coined names for compounded products should only be used if the contents are standardized and readily available for reference to prescribers, pharmacists, and nurses
Numeral embedded in drug name (not part of the official name) (e.g., 5-fluoro-uracil, 6-mercaptopurine)	Fluorouracil Mercaptopurine	Embedded numeral mistaken as the dose or number of tablets/capsules to be administered	Use complete drug names, without an embedded numeral if the numeral is not part of the official drug name
GI, gastrointestinal.			

Dose designations and other information			
Error-prone abbreviations, symbols, and dose designation	**Intended meaning**	**Misinterpretation**	**Best practice**
1/2 tablet	Half tablet	1 or 2 tablets	Use text (half tablet) or reduced font-size fractions (½ tablet)
Doses expressed as Roman numerals (e.g., V)	5	Mistaken as the designated letter (e.g., the letter V) or the wrong numeral (e.g., 10 instead of 5)	Use only Arabic numerals (e.g., 1, 2, 3) to express doses
Lack of a leading zero before a decimal point (e.g., .5 mg)[a]	0.5 mg	Mistaken as 5 mg if the decimal point is not seen	Use a leading zero before a decimal point when the dose is less than one measurement unit
Trailing zero after a decimal point (e.g., 1.0 mg)	1 mg	Mistaken as 10 mg if the decimal point is not seen	Do not use trailing zeros for doses expressed in whole numbers
Ratio expression of a strength of a single-entity injectable drug product (e.g., EPINEPHrine 1:1,000; 1:10,000; 1:100,000)	1:1,000: contains 1 mg/mL 1:10,000: contains 0.1 mg/mL 1:100,000: contains 0.01 mg/mL	Mistaken as the wrong strength	Express the strength in terms of quantity per total volume (e.g., EPINEPHrine 1 mg per 10 mL) Exception: combination local anesthetics (e.g., lidocaine 1% and EPINEPHrine 1:100,000)
Drug name and dose run together (problematic for drug names that end in the letter l [e.g., propranolol20 mg; TEGretol300 mg])	Propranolol 20 mg **TEG**retol 300 mg	Mistaken as propranolol 120 mg Mistaken as **TEG**retol 1300 mg	Place adequate space between the drug name, dose, and unit of measure
Numerical dose and unit of measure run together (e.g., 10 mg, 10Units)	10 mg 10 mL	The m in mg, or U in Units, has been mistaken as one or two zeros when flush against the dose (e.g., 10 mg, 10Units), risking a 10- to 100-fold overdose	Place adequate space between the dose and unit of measure
Large doses without properly placed commas (e.g., 100000 units; 1000000 units)	100,000 units 1,000,000 units	100000 has been mistaken as 10,000 or 1,000,000 1000000 has been mistaken as 100,000	Use commas for dosing units at or above 1,000 or use words such as 100 thousand or 1 million to improve readability Note: Use commas to separate digits only in the United States; commas are used in place of decimal points in some other countries

[a]On the Joint Commission's Do Not Use list.

Symbols			
Error-prone abbreviations, symbols, and dose designation	**Intended meaning**	**Misinterpretation**	**Best practice**
ℨ Symbol for Minim[a]	Dram Minim	Symbol for dram mistaken as the numeral 3 Symbol for minim mistaken as mL	Use the metric system
x1	Administer once	Administer for 1 day	Use explicit words (e.g., for 1 dose)
> and <	More than and less than	Mistaken as opposite of intended Mistakenly have used the incorrect symbol < mistaken as the numeral 4 when handwritten (e.g., <10 misread as 40)	Use more than or less than
↑ and ↓[a]	Increase and decrease	Mistaken as opposite of intended Mistakenly have used the incorrect symbol ↑ mistaken as the letter T, leading to misinterpretation as the start of a drug name, or mistaken as the numerals 4 or 7	Use increase and decrease
/ (slash mark)[a]	Separates two doses or indicates per	Mistaken as the numeral 1 (e.g., 25 units/10 units misread as 25 units and 110 units)	Use per rather than a slash mark to separate doses

(Continued)

Symbols —cont'd

Error-prone abbreviations, symbols, and dose designation	Intended meaning	Misinterpretation	Best practice
@[a]	At	Mistaken as the numeral 2	Use at
&[a]	And	Mistaken as the numeral 2	Use and
+[a]	Plus or and	Mistaken as the numeral 4	Use plus, and, or in addition to
°	Hour	Mistaken as a zero (e.g., q2° seen as q20)	Use hr, h, or hour
Φ or ∅[a]	Zero, null sign	Mistaken as the numerals 4, 6, 8, and 9	Use 0 or zero, or describe intent using whole words
#	Pound(s)	Mistaken as a number sign	Use the metric system (kg or g) rather than pounds. Use lb if referring to pounds

[a]Relevant mostly in handwritten medication information.

Apothecary or household abbreviations

Explicit apothecary or household measurements may *only* be safely used to express the directions for mixing dry ingredients to prepare topical products (e.g., dissolve 2 capfuls of granules per gallon of warm water to prepare a magnesium sulfate soaking aid). Otherwise, metric system measurements should be used.

Error-prone abbreviations, symbols, and dose designation	Intended meaning	Misinterpretation	Best practice
gr	Grain(s)	Mistaken as gram	Use the metric system (e.g., mcg, g)
dr	Dram(s)	Mistaken as doctor	Use the metric system (e.g., mL)
min	Minim(s)	Mistaken as minutes	Use the metric system (e.g., mL)
oz	Ounce(s)	Mistaken as zero or O_2	Use the metric system (e.g., mL)
tsp	Teaspoon(s)	Mistaken as tablespoon(s)	Use the metric system (e.g., mL)
Tbsp or Tbsp	Tablespoon(s)	Mistaken as teaspoon(s)	Use the metric system (e.g., mL)

Common abbreviations with contradictory meanings

Common abbreviations with contradictory meanings	Contradictory meaning	Correction
B	Breast, brain, or bladder	Use breast, brain, or bladder

Common abbreviations with contradictory meanings—cont'd

Common abbreviations with contradictory meanings	Contradictory meaning	Correction
C	Cerebral, coronary, or carotid	Use cerebral, coronary, or carotid
D or d	Day or dose (e.g., parameter-based dosing formulas using D or d [mg/kg/d] could be interpreted as either day or dose [mg/kg/day or mg/kg/dose]; or x3d could be interpreted as either 3 days or 3 doses)	Use day or dose
H	Hand or hip	Use hand or hip
I	Impaired or improvement	Use impaired or improvement
L	Liver or lung	Use liver or lung
N	No or normal	Use no or normal
P	Pancreas, prostate, pre-eclampsia, or psychosis	Use pancreas, prostate, pre-eclampsia, or psychosis
S	Special or standard	Use special or standard
SS or ss	Single strength, sliding scale (insulin), signs and symptoms, or ½ (apothecary) SS has also been mistaken as the numeral 55	Use single strength, sliding scale, signs and symptoms, or one-half or ½

Look-alike/sound-alike medications with recommended tall man letters

Both the FDA and ISMP have developed a list of confused drug names consisting of LASA medications as a result medication errors occurred involving these medications.

The FDA issued a list of approved generic drug names using tall man lettering (TML). TML is a method that utilizes lettering to distinguish look-alike drug names. Beginning on the left side of the drug name, TML emphasizes the differences between similar drug names by capitalizing unlike letters. In addition TML can be utilized with color or bold facing to draw awareness to the similarities between look-alike drug names.

FDA-Approved list of generic drug names with tall man letters	
Drug name with tall man letters	Confused with
aceta**ZOLAMIDE**	aceto**HEXAMIDE**
aceto**HEXAMIDE**	aceta**ZOLAMIDE**
bu**PROP**ion	bus**PIR**one
bus**PIR**one	bu**PROP**ion
chlorpro**MAZINE**	chlorpro**PAMIDE**
chlorpro**PAMIDE**	chlorpro**MAZINE**
clomi**PHENE**	clomi**PRAMINE**
clomi**PRAMINE**	clomi**PHENE**
cyclo**SERINE**	cyclo**SPORINE**
cyclo**SPORINE**	cyclo**SERINE**
DAUNOrubicin	**DOXO**rubicin
dimenhy**DRINATE**	diphenhydr**AMINE**
diphenhydr**AMINE**	dimenhy**DRINATE**
DOBUTamine	**DOP**amine
DOPamine	**DOBUT**amine
DOXOrubicin	**DAUNO**rubicin
glipi**ZIDE**	gly**BURIDE**
gly**BURIDE**	glipi**ZIDE**
hydr**ALAZINE**	hydr**OXY**zine—**HYDRO**morphone
HYDROmorphone	hydr**OXY**zine—hydr**ALAZINE**
hydr**OXY**zine	hydr**ALAZINE**—**HYDRO**morphone
medroxy**PROGESTER**one	methyl**PREDNIS**olone—methyl-**TESTOSTER**one
methyl**PREDNIS**olone	medroxy**PROGESTER**one—methyl**TESTOSTER**one
methyl**TESTOSTER**one	medroxy**PROGESTER**one—methyl**PREDNIS**olone
mito**XANTRONE**	Not specified
ni**CAR**dipine	**NIFE**dipine
NIFEdipine	ni**CAR**dipine
predniso**LONE**	predni**SONE**
predni**SONE**	predniso**LONE**
risperi**DONE**	r**OPINIR**ole
r**OPINIR**ole	risperi**DONE**
sulf**ADIAZINE**	sulfi**SOXAZOLE**
sulfi**SOXAZOLE**	sulf**ADIAZINE**
TOLAZamide	**TOLBUT**amide
TOLBUTamide	**TOLAZ**amide
vin**BLAS**tine	vin**CRIS**tine
vin**CRIS**tine	vin**BLAS**tine

Institute of Safe Medication Practices list of additional drug names with tall man letters

ISMP provides a list of additional drug names with recommendations of the placement of tall man letters. The ISMP follows the CD3 rule. The methodology recommends working from the left of the drug name first by capitalizing all the characters to the right once 2 or more different letters are observed, and then, working from the right, returning 2 or more letters common to both words to lowercase letters. When the rule cannot be used because there are no common letters on the right side of the name, the procedure proposes capitalizing the central part of the word only. When use of this rule fails to lead to the best TML option (e.g., makes names appear too similar, makes names hard to read based on pronunciation), an alternative option is considered. It should be noted that this list is not approved by the FDA.

Drug name	Confused drug name
Aciphex	Accupril, Aricept
Actos	Actonel
Adderall	Adderall XR, Inderal
ALPRAZolam	clonazePAM, LORazepam
amiodarone	amantadine
amLODIPine	aMILopride
ARIPiprazole	proton pump inhibitors, RABEprazole
atorvastatin	atomoxetine
buPROPion	busPIRone
Cardizem	Cardene
CeleBREX	CeleXA, Cerebyx
cetirizine	sertraline, stavudine
clonazePAM	ALPRAZolam, clobazam, clonidine, clozapine, LORazepam
Cozaar	Colace, Zocor
Depakote	Depakote ER
DULoxetine	Dexilant, FLUoxetine, Paroxetine
gabapentin	gemfibrozil
glipiZIDE	glyBURIDE
HumaLOG	HumuLIN, NovoLOG
hydroCHLOROthiazide	hydrALAZINE, hydrOXYzine
HYDROcodone	oxyCODONE
Jantoven	Janumet, Januvia
Lantus	Latuda, Lente
levothyroxine	lamotrigine, Lanoxin, liothyronine
Lotronex	Protonix
medroxyPROGES-TERone	HYDROXYprogesterone, methylPRED-NISolone, methylTESTOSTERone
metFORMIN	metroNIDAZOLE
metoprolol succinate	metoprolol tartrate
NIFEdipine	niCARdipine, niMODipine
oxyCODONE	HYDROcodone, oxybutynin, OxyCONTIN, oxyMORphone

(Continued)

Drug name	Confused drug name
Paxil	Doxil, Plavix, Taxol
Plavix	Paxil, Pradaxa
Prandin	Avandia
prednisoLONE	predniSONE
propylthiouracil	Purinethol
PROzac	Prograf, PriLOSEC, Provera
SandIMMUNE	SandoSTATIN
SEROquel	Desyrel, SEROquel XR, Serzone, SINEquan
SINEquan	saquinavir, SEROquel, Singulair, Zonegran
SITagliptin	sAXagliptin, SUMAtriptan
SOLU-Medrol	DEPO-Medrol, Solu-CORTEF
Spiriva	Apidra, Inspra
sulfADIAZINE	sulfasalazine, sulfiSOXAZOLE
tacrolimus	tamsulosin
TEGretol	TEGretol XR, Tequin, TRENtal
Toujeo	Tradjenta, Tresiba, Trulicity
Tresiba	Tanzeum, Tarceva, Toujeo, Tradjenta
Trulicity	Tanzeum, Toujeo, Tradjenta, Tresiba
Zebeta	Diabeta, Zetia
Zestril	Zegerid, Zetia, ZyPREXA
Zetia	Bextra, Zebeta, Zestril
Zocor	Cozaar, ZyrTEC
Zyloprim	zolpidem
ZyPREXA	CeleXA, Reprexain, Zestril, ZyrTEC
ZyrTEC	Lipitor, Zerit, Zocor, ZyPREXA, ZyrTEC-D

Brand names start with an uppercase letter. Some brand names incorporate tall man letters in initial characters and may not be readily recognized as brand names. Brand names appear in black; generic names/other products appear in red.

A complete listing of the ISMP List of Look-Alike Drug Names with Recommended Tall Man Letters can be accessed at https://www.ismp.org/sites/default/files/attachments/2017-11/tallmanletters.pdf

A health care organization should implement processes to reduce the risk of potential errors involving LASA medications. Examples of strategies include using both the brand and generic names on prescriptions and labels; including the purpose of the medication on prescriptions; configuring computer selection screens to prevent look-alike names from appearing consecutively; and changing the appearance of look-alike product names to draw attention to their dissimilarities.

Patient factors that influence the ability to report medication information accurately and adhere to prescribed dosing schedules

Medication adherence

An individual is considered adherent if they take 80% of their prescribed medication doses. Terminology associated with adherence includes

- Primary nonadherence: Occurs when a new medication is prescribed for a patient, but the patient fails to obtain the medication (or its appropriate alternative) within an acceptable period of time after it was initially prescribed.
- Secondary nonadherence: Occurs when a patient fills a prescription but does not take the medication as it was intended and/or prescribed.
- Intentional medication nonadherence: Active process whereby the patient chooses to deviate from his or her treatment regimen.
- Unintentional medication nonadherence: Passive process in which the patient may be careless or forgetful about adhering to treatment regimen.
- Nonadherence can be directly tied to increased morbidity, mortality, and avoidable health care costs.

Factors affecting medication adherence
Health literacy

- Health literacy requires a patient to be able to read, listen, communicate, and comprehend, and follow a medication regimen.
- Low health literacy skills hinder patients' ability to build knowledge about their illness and therapy, resulting in nonadherence.
- Differences in education, English proficiency, socioeconomic status, and situational circumstances can affect an individual's health literacy.
- Identifying low health literacy in patients can be demonstrated by observing:
  - The patient provides incomplete filled-out forms.
  - The patient misses medication refills for chronic conditions.
  - The patient refers to the medications by their shapes or colors.
  - The patient avoids reading printed medication materials when in front of a pharmacist.
  - The patient mispronounces words.
  - The patient uses a child to interpret what the pharmacist is when counseling the patient.

Medication cost

- High out-of-pocket medication costs have a negative impact on medication adherence since
  - Patients may not fill even the initial prescription, let alone refills.
  - Patients may skip doses or cut pills in half to stretch their dwindling supply if they do not have the money for a refill due to high copays.
  - Patients may seek lower-cost therapies, use alternative ones, or buy medication from unreliable online sources or from sources outside of the country where quality can be a concern.
    - A lack of availability and immediacy of health benefits or other assistance programs is related to a greater decrease in medication adherence in any population group.
    - Cost-related nonadherence increases when a patient is taking multiple medications for one or more conditions.

Polypharmacy

- Refers to when a patient is being prescribed at least five medications
- Types of polypharmacy
  - Excessive polypharmacy: Concurrent use of 10 or more different drugs
  - Polypharmacy: The use of five to nine drugs
  - No polypharmacy: Taking four or less drugs (included those taking no medicines)
- Risk factors contributing to polypharmacy
  - Multiple medical conditions being managed by multiple physicians
  - Patient's age (extremely common in patients 6 years of age and older)
  - Patients having chronic mental health conditions
  - Filling prescriptions in multiple pharmacies
  - Patients residing in long-term care facilities
- Polypharmacy concerns
  - ADEs: Refers to an injury resulting from the use of a drug and refers to harm caused by a drug at usual dosages. Preventable ADEs occur as a result of inappropriate medication use in older patient. Drug classification associated with preventable ADE include cardiovascular, anticoagulants, hypoglycemics, diuretics and nonsteroidal antiinflammatory drugs.
  - Drug interactions: Use of multiple medications increases the potential for drug-drug interactions. Common ADEs includes hypertension, hypotension, and renal failure.
  - Prescribing cascades: Using additional drugs to treat the ADEs is associated with other drugs by misinterpreting the ADE as a new medical condition
  - Inappropriate therapy or nonadherence is common in patients with visual or cognitive decline.
  - Use of over-the-counter and complementary medications can result in herb-drug interactions.
  - Changes in pharmacokinetics (absorption, distribution, metabolism, and elimination) are associated with aging increase the risk of adverse drug reactions.
  - Unintentional overdose can occur.
  - Polypharmacy may result in a patient's death.

Health Insurance Portability and Accountability Act and best practices to maintain patient confidentiality during patient conversations

- Designate a counseling area away from the dispensing area and other patients. If possible, the counseling area should be in a private room away from pharmacy activities, other patients, and other distractions such as noise.
- Monitor your voice level so that other individuals cannot hear what you are saying to the patient.
- When speaking to a patient over the phone regarding medication, make sure that you confirm the identity of the patient's name, birth date, and address.
- Require all staff to undergo Health Insurance Portability and Accountability Act training when hired and on an annual basis.

Techniques or devices to assist with safe and consistent home medication use (e.g., pillboxes, medication calendars, medication alarms)

- Educate the patient regarding potential outcomes. The failure of the pharmacist to inform the patient of potential outcomes may cause the patient to stop taking the medication. If the patient begins to feel better, he or she may stop taking the medication and conversely if the patient does not see the intended effects, he or she may stop taking the medication without consulting a physician.
- E-prescribing has been demonstrated to increase first-fill medication adherence by 10% compared with using paper prescriptions.
- Synchronize patients' medication to allow them to refill all of their medications at the same time.
- Some e-prescribing software has the ability to monitor prescriptions dispensed or unfilled in real time and can send prompts when a new or refill prescription is available.
- Utilize comprehensive medication review summaries to discuss medication adherence or nonadherence with patients.
- Assist patients to customize their support tools. Examples of support tools include
  - Pillboxes (pill container or pill case): A pillbox is a container used to organize a patient's medication doses for a certain length of time. Using a pillbox is very helpful for patients if they need to take a few different medications. It will help them avoid missing doses of their medications. Pillboxes come in many different sizes. They can hold medication doses for up to 14 days and have up to four spaces per day.
  - Medication calendar: A reminder of the regular intake of medicines at prescribed times. A medication calendar will improve medication adherence by helping patients take their medication at the right time. A medication calendar can provide patients with documentation to provide to their physician.
  - Medication alarms: A medication reminder alarm is a tool that uses an alarm cue to prompt users to take medication. Some case studies have revealed that such devices may be effective in enhancing medication adherence in the elderly patients with mild dementia.
  - PillPack: PillPack is a service provided by online pharmacies whereby all the medications are packaged indicating the date and time on the package.
  - MedMinder: MedMinder provides alerts that are both visual and auditory. The beeps can be easily heard and the lights flash on and off to get a patient's attention. The system also provides automatic phone calls as reminders in situations that the lights and beeps do not prompt taking the scheduled medication.

Procedures to verify patient identity, including appropriate identifiers and knowledge of limitations for different identifiers

It is the responsibility of health care workers to check the identity of patients and match the correct patients with the correct care (e.g., laboratory results, specimens, procedures) before that care is administered. The Joint Commission requires at least two identifiers be provided by the patient prior to administering the point-of-care testing. Acceptable identifiers include

- The individual's name
- An assigned identification (such as a medical record number)
- Telephone number or another person-specific identifier
- Electronic identification technology coding, such as bar coding or radio-frequency identification, that includes two or more person-specific identifiers

Clear protocols exist for identifying patients who lack identification and for distinguishing the identity of patients with the same name. The labeling of containers used for blood and other specimens should be done in the presence of the patient and requires two identifiers. The practice of prelabeling blood tubes prior to seeing the patient and matching them at the time of collection is not acceptable. In situations when a labeled container is not used due to failure of the patient to provide a urine specimen, it must be discarded immediately.

CHAPTER REVIEW QUESTIONS

1. Which term refers to when a medication should not be used because it may cause adverse effects on the patient?
   a. Contraindication
   b. Drug allergy
   c. Drug intolerance
   d. Idiosyncratic reaction
2. Which of the following is a summary of lifestyle practices?
   a. Family medical history
   b. Medical history
   c. Medication history
   d. Social history
3. A patient is reading a prescription and asks, "What is hypertension?" How would you respond?
   a. Hypertension is high blood sugar levels.
   b. Hypertension is high blood cholesterol levels.
   c. Hypertension is high blood pressure.
   d. Hypertension is high thyroid levels.
4. After reading the patient product insert accompanying the filled prescription, a patient asks, "What is dermatitis?" How would you respond?
   a. Dermatitis is inflammation of the heart muscle.
   b. Dermatitis is inflammation of the colon.
   c. Dermatitis is inflammation of the skin.
   d. Dermatitis is inflammation of the vein.

5. A patient is reviewing the medical history on his electronic health records and observes the term "fibromyalgia." What does fibromyalgia mean?
   a. Bone pain
   b. Chronic muscle pain
   c. Kidney pain
   d. Nerve pain
6. A patient is prescribed furosemide for edema in her ankles. The patient does not have the prescription filled. Which type of medication nonadherence is the patient exhibiting?
   a. Intentional medication nonadherence
   b. Primary nonadherence
   c. Secondary nonadherence
   d. Unintentional medication nonadherence
7. For a patient to be compliant with his medication therapy, what percentage of his prescribed doses must the patient take?
   a. 75%
   b. 80%
   c. 85%
   d. 90%
8. What is the minimum age for measles, mumps, and rubella vaccination for a pediatric patient?
   a. Birth
   b. 6 weeks of age
   c. 6 months of age
   d. 12 months of age
9. A pediatric patient is prescribed Prevnar 13. How many doses will they receive?
   a. 1
   b. 2
   c. 3
   d. 4
10. A 21-year-old patient wishes to receive the Comirnaty vaccine indicated for COVID-19. It is a 2-dose series. What is the earliest the patient may receive the second dose?
    a. 14 days after the first dose
    b. 21 days after the first dose
    c. 28 days after the first dose
    d. 35 days after the first dose
11. What is the maximum age for an adult to receive the Gardasil vaccine for human papillomavirus?
    a. 18 years of age
    b. 22 years of age
    c. 24 years of age
    d. 26 years of age
12. Which is the brand name for Zoster (recombinant) vaccine?
    a. Gardasil
    b. Shingrix
    c. Trumenba
    d. Varivax
13. Which vaccine is recommended for first-year college students residing in residential housing for the first time who have not been previously vaccinated?
    a. Hepatitis A
    b. Human papillomavirus
    c. Meningococcal serotype A-C-W-Y
    d. COVID-19 mRNA-1273

14. What type of error occurs if abbreviations found on the do not use list or error-prone abbreviations are used?
    a. Administration
    b. Dispensing
    c. Prescribing
    d. All the above

15. A pharmacy's automatic dispensing machine malfunctions and may result in a medication error. Which root cause classification would this be considered?
    a. Human
    b. Manufacturing
    c. Organizational
    d. Technical

16. The pharmacy technician fails to provide a medication guide to a patient receiving warfarin. What type of medication error has occurred?
    a. Compliance error
    b. Documentation error
    c. Medication education error
    d. Wrong drug error

17. A pharmacy technician is processing a prescription of warfarin for a 75-year-old patient and fails to inform the pharmacist of the drug utilization review message appearing on the computer screen. What type of dispensing would this be considered?
    a. Adverse drug error
    b. Deteriorated drug error
    c. Mislabeling error
    d. Wrong formulation error

18. Prior to handing a patient a filled prescription, the pharmacy technician observes the wrong medication has been dispensed. According to National Coordinating Council for Medication Error Reporting Index for Categorizing Medication Errors, which category of medication error would this be classified?
    a. Category A
    b. Category B
    c. Category C
    d. Category D

19. Instead of using the abbreviation "OD" on a prescription, how should the physician write the expression?
    a. Left ear
    b. Left eye
    c. Right ear
    d. Right eye

20. A physician is writing a prescription for an oral liquid for a patient. Which system should be used in expressing the volume?
    a. Apothecary
    b. Avoirdupois
    c. Household
    d. Metric

21. How are the drugs buPROPion and busPIRone classified?
    a. Controlled substances
    b. Medications with confused drug names
    c. Medications that should not be crushed
    d. Proprietary drug names

22. A physician prescribes a new prescription for levothyroxine for a patient; however, the patient fails to have the prescription filled. Which form of nonadherence is the patient displaying?
    a. Intentional medication nonadherence
    b. Primary nonadherence
    c. Secondary nonadherence
    d. Unintentional medication nonadherence

23. Which is the minimum number of medications prescribed for a patient whereby excessive polypharmacy exists?
    a. 4
    b. 5
    c. 10
    d. 15

24. Which of the following is *not* a component of health literacy?
    a. Patients' ability to comprehend the directions on their prescription label
    b. Patients' ability to communicate with their health care provider
    c. Patients' ability to read the directions on their prescription label
    d. Patients' ability to pay for their medication

25. According to the Joint Commission, how many identifier(s) should a patient provide to confirm their identity prior to point of care testing?
    a. 1
    b. 2
    c. 3
    d. 4

6

Medication Therapy Management Certificate

Medication therapy management domains

Medications and medical concepts (40%)
- Medication strengths/dose, drug class, dosage forms, routes of administration, special handling/storage and administration instructions, and duration of drug therapy
- Interchangeable drug classes and dosage forms (i.e., to identify cost-saving opportunities)
- Patient-friendly terms for medical terminology
- Definitions of key terms in a medication history process (e.g., medication allergy vs. medication intolerance, medication adherence)
- Definitions of key terms for medical history (e.g., medical conditions, social history, immunizations)
- Common medication-related problems (e.g., side effects, nonadherence, affordability, gap in therapy)
- Laboratory measures (e.g., A1C, potassium, blood pressure) and related medical terms

Patient safety and quality assurance strategies (36%)
- Calculate adherence (e.g., days' supply, quantity, dose, proportion of days covered)
- Systematical review of information for accuracy and completeness (e.g., components of medication-related action plan, comprehensive medication review documentation, personal medication record, required medication therapy management billing fields)
- Types of prescribing errors and inappropriate prescribing (e.g., abnormal doses, incorrect strength, incorrect drug, incorrect route of administration, incorrect directions, wrong timing, missing dose)
- Potential impact of prescribing errors and medication problems (e.g., inappropriate dosing schedule, inappropriate therapy, duplicate therapy, interactions or conflicting therapies)

Medication therapy management administration and management (24%)
- Definition and purpose of medication therapy management programs and core service elements (medication therapy review, personal medication record, medication-related action plan, intervention and/or referral, documentation, and follow-up)
- Centers for Medicare and Medicaid Services requirements for offering medication therapy management services
- Decision making and prioritization (e.g., recently discharged patients, follow-up versus new outreach, serious errors identified) when tracking stages of service (pending, in progress, complete) and maintainwing schedules and timelines for documentation, follow-up, and billing for medication therapy management services

Medications and medical concepts

Medications

Drug class
- May be broken down based upon the body system they affect, pharmacology, intent of use, route of administration, and mechanism of action

Body system	Drug classification
Cardiovascular	Angiotensin-converting enzyme inhibitor, angiotensin II receptor antagonists, antihyperlipidemics, antihypertensives, beta blockers, calcium channel blockers, diuretics, and vasodilators

(Continued)

Body system	Drug classification
Circulatory	Anticoagulants, antihemorrhagics, antiplatelets, and thrombolytics
Endocrine	Antithyroid agents, corticosteroids, hypoglycemic agents, hypothalamic-pituitary hormones, sex hormones, and thyroid hormones
Gastrointestinal	Antacids, antidiarrheals, antiemetics, H_2 antagonists, laxatives, and proton pump inhibitors
Immune	Antibiotics, anticancer agents, antifungals, antiparasitics, antivirals, immunomodulators, and vaccines
Integumentary	Antipruritics, emollients, and medicated dressings
Musculoskeletal	Anabolic steroids, antirheumatics, bisphosphonates, corticosteroids, muscle relaxants, and nonsteroidal antiinflammatory drugs
Nervous	Analgesics, anesthetics, anticonvulsants, antidepressants, antiparkinsonian drugs, antipsychotics, and stimulants
Reproductive	Fertility agents, progestins, estrogens, and sex hormones
Respiratory	Bronchodilators, cough suppressants, decongestants, and H_1 antagonists
Other	Antidotes, contrast media, and radiopharmaceuticals

Strengths/dose

- Amount of medication taken at a specific time to produce a therapeutic effect
- Solid doses commonly expressed as milligrams (mg) or in some cases micrograms (mcg)
- Liquid doses normally expressed as milligrams/milliliter (mg/mL) or micrograms/milliliter (mcg/mL)
- International units used to measure the activity of specific vitamins (vitamin D_3) and specific medications (insulin and heparin)

Dosage forms

- "Dosage forms" refers to the means by which a drug is available for use or the vehicle by which the drug is delivered.
- Dosage forms are administered either enterally or parenterally. An enteral medication involves a medication that travels from the mouth through the alimentary canal to the rectum. A parenteral medication is administered in a manner other than through the mouth.
- Enteral dosage forms:
  - Tablet: A hard formulation in which the drugs and other ingredients are machine compressed into a shape. They vary in size, weight, hardness, thickness, and disintegration and dissolution rates. Tablets may be film coated, sugar coated, compressed, and effervescent. Other forms of tablets include:
    - Chewable tablet: An oral dosage form intended to be chewed and then swallowed by the patient rather than swallowed whole (e.g., carbamazepine)
    - Delayed-release tablet: The dosage form formulated so that the drug is released slowly over time (e.g., pantoprazole)
    - Enteric-coated tablets: A tablet coated with a material that permits transit through the stomach to the small intestine before the medication is released (e.g., enteric-coated aspirin)
    - Sublingual tablet: A tablet that dissolves when placed beneath the tongue and absorbs into the blood through tissue there (Sublingual dosage form are used when results must occur quickly, e.g., nitroglycerin.)
    - Troche: A tablet is administered buccally between the gums and the inner lining of the mouth cheek (e.g., clotrimazole oropharyngeal).
  - Capsule: A solid dosage form in which the drug is enclosed in a hard or soft soluble container, usually of a form of gelatin. They range in sizes from a 000 (largest) to 5 (smallest). The gelatin shell dissolves in the stomach and releases the medication from the capsule. Many capsules are intended to be swallowed; however, sprinkles are capsules where the contents are sprinkled over food. Fluoxetine is an example of a capsule and Depakote is available as a sprinkle dosage form.
  - Caplet: A smooth, coated, oval-shaped medicinal tablet in the general shape of a capsule (e.g., acetaminophen)
  - Lozenge: Various-shaped solid dosage forms, usually containing a medicinal agent and a flavoring substance, that are intended to be dissolved slowly in the oral cavity for localized or systemic effects
  - Bulk powders: Contain the active ingredient in a small powder paper or foil envelope. The patient empties the envelope into a glass of water or juice and drinks it. Examples include cholestyramine and psyllium.
  - Solution: A clear liquid made up of one or more ingredients dissolved in a solvent.
    - Aqueous solution: Water is used as the solvent.
    - Nonaqueous solution: A solution that predominantly contains solvents other water
  - Syrup: A concentrated solutions of sugar in water or other aqueous liquid. They are more viscous than water and contain less than 10% alcohol.
  - Elixir: A sweetened hydroalcoholic (water and alcohol) liquids for oral use. They are less viscous than a syrup and have an alcohol content of 5%–40%.
  - Emulsion: An emulsion is a two-phase system in which one liquid is dispersed in the form of small globules throughout another liquid. The dispersed liquid is known as the internal phase, whereas the dispersion medium as the external or continuous phase. Emulsions contain a stabilizing agent known as an emulsifier.
    - Oil-in-water: Oil is the dispersed phase and an aqueous solution is the continuous phase.
    - Water-in-oil: Water is the dispersed phase and oil is the continuous phase.
  - Suspension: A coarse dispersion containing finely divided insoluble material suspended in a liquid medium. Oral suspensions are flavored and sweetened. Some oral suspensions are packaged as a lyophilized powder and are reconstituted with water.

- Parenteral dosage forms:
  - Sprays: A collection of drops dispersed in a gas
  - Inhalant solution: A solution of a drug or combination of drugs for administration as a nebulized mist intended to reach the respiratory tree
  - Enemas: A liquid injected into the rectum for therapeutic or diagnostic purposes
  - Aerosol: Suspension of tiny particles or droplets in the air, such as dusts, mists, or fumes, which may be inhaled or absorbed by the skin
  - Spray: A jet of liquid in fine drops, coarser than a vapor, produced by forcing the liquid from the minute opening of an atomizer, mixing it with air
  - Nebulizer: A medical device that converts a liquid medication to a mist, which allows it to be inhaled
  - Creams: An emulsion of oil and water in approximately equal proportions; lotions: a liquid for topical application that contains insoluble solids or liquids
  - Ointments: A homogenous, viscous, semisolid preparation, which is most commonly a greasy, thick oil (oil 80% and water 20%) with a high viscosity that is intended for external application to the skin or mucus membranes
  - Gel: A two-phase system containing an extremely fine solid particle that, when mixed, is difficult to distinguish between the two phases and is considered a semisolid form, containing a gelling agent to increase the viscosity of the compound
  - Pastes: A semisolid dosage form that contain a large proportion of solid component, which differ from ointments in their consistency, as they contain larger amounts of solids and consequently are thicker and stiffer
  - Transdermal patch: A medicated patch applied to the skin
  - Lotion: A low- to medium-viscosity medicated or non-medicated topical preparation, intended for application to unbroken skin
  - Tincture: A dilute solution consisting of a medicinal substance in alcohol or in alcohol and water, usually 10% to 20% by volume
  - Liniment: A solutions or mixture of various substances in oil, alcoholic solution of soap, or emulsions, intended for external application
  - Implant: A drug delivery system that provides controlled delivery of a drug over a period of time at the site of implantation
  - Suppository: A form of medicine contained in a small piece of solid material, such as cocoa butter or glycerin, that melts at body temperature (A suppository is inserted into the rectum, vagina, or urethra and the medicine is absorbed into the bloodstream.)
  - Solutions, suspensions, emulsions that are available as parenteral dosage forms but have been specifically formulated based upon their route of administration

Routes of administration

- Enteral route of administration:
  - Oral dosage forms are swallowed from the mouth and absorbed in the stomach and intestine. Examples of oral dosage forms include tablets, capsules, bulk powders, solutions, suspensions, elixirs, syrups and emulsions.
  - Sublingual medications are placed and absorbed under the tongue. Sublingual dosage forms include tablets and lozenges. An example of a sublingual dosage form is nitroglycerin.
  - Buccal dosage forms are placed and absorbed against the cheek. Examples of buccal dosage forms include tablets, troches.
  - Rectal dosage forms are inserted and absorbed in the rectum. Examples of rectal dosage forms include suppositories, ointments, and solutions.
- Parenteral routes of administration:
  - IV medications are injected into a vein using a syringe and needle and is absorbed into the veinous circulatory system. An IV injection may be either large volume or small volume. It may have a rapid onset of action. IV dosage forms include solutions and suspensions. Examples of intravenous solutions include normal saline and dextrose 5% in water.
  - Intramuscular medications are injected and absorbed into the muscle tissue. They have a slower onset but longer duration of action compared with an IV injections. Intramuscular dosage forms include solutions and suspensions. Olanzapine and ziprasidone are examples of medications that may be injected intramuscularly.
  - Intradermal medications are injected and absorbed into the dermal area of the skin. Intradermal dosage forms include solutions and suspensions.
  - Subcutaneous medications are injected and absorbed into the subcutaneous tissue of the skin and have slower absorption rates than intramuscular administration but faster than oral administration. Subcutaneous dosage forms include solutions, suspensions, emulsion, and implants. Examples of medications administered subcutaneously include insulin, heparin, and enoxaparin.
  - Dermal medications are applied and absorbed through the skin. Dermal dosage forms include solutions, suspensions, tinctures, collodions, liniments, creams, gels, lotions, pastes, aerosols, and transdermal patches.
  - Intranasal medications are inhaled and absorbed through the nose. Intranasal dosage forms include solutions, suspensions, ointment, and gels.
  - Inhalation medications are inhaled and absorbed through the lungs and include solutions and aerosols.
  - Intraocular drugs are instilled and absorbed through the eyes and include solutions, suspensions, and ointments.
  - Otic medications are instilled and absorbed through the ear and include solutions and suspensions.
  - Vaginal drugs are inserted and absorbed through the vagina. Vaginal dosage forms include solutions, creams, suppositories, and tablets.

Storage

- Medications should be stored in their original packaging, at the recommended temperature, proper humidity, and away from sunlight.
- Effects of improper storage can:
  - Result in both physical and chemical changes of the medication
  - Alter the medication's taste

- Change the medication's appearance
- Alter the medications smell
- Change the viscosity of liquid formulations
- Result in drug precipitation of liquid formulations
- Cause a loss of drug potency

USP <1079> in the practice of pharmacy

- Room temperature: 20°C–25°C
- Controlled room temperature: 20°C–25°C
- Cool storage: 8°C–15°C
- Refrigerator storage: 2°C–8°C
- Freezer storage: −25°C–10°C

Commonly refrigerated medicines	
Brand name	**Generic name**
Augmentin	Amoxicillin/clavulanic acid
Avonex	Interferon beta-1a
Enbrel	Etanercept
Foradil	Formoterol
Humalog	Insulin lispro
Humira	Adalimumab
Lantus	Insulin glargine
Levemir	Insulin detemir
Xalatan	Latanoprost

Vaccine storage		
Vaccine	**Indication**	**Storage requirements**
DTaP	Diphtheria, tetanus, and pertussis	Refrigeration
Engerix-B	Hepatitis B	Refrigeration
Havrix	Hepatitis A	Refrigeration
MMR	Measles, mumps, and rubella	Refrigeration
MMRV: ProQuad	Measles, mumps, rubella, and varicella	Freezer
Varivax	Varicella (chickenpox)	Freezer
Zostavax	Herpes zoster, shingles	Freezer

Medication sensitivities	
Medication	**Sensitivity**
Cyclosporine capsules	Light sensitive
Dipyridamole	Moisture sensitive
Dabigatran	Moisture sensitive
Etanercept	Light sensitive
Golimumab	Light sensitive
Nitroglycerin sublingual tablets	Light and moisture sensitive
Oxcarbazepine oral solution	Light sensitive
Ritonavir capsules	Light and moisture sensitive

Beyond-use dates for nonsterile compounded preparations

- Nonaqueous formulations: The beyond-use date (BUD) is not later than the time remaining until the earliest expiration date of any active pharmaceutical ingredient or 6 months, whichever is earliest.
- For water-containing formulations: The BUD is not later than 14 days when stored at controlled cold temperature.
- For water-containing topical/dermal and mucosal liquid and semisolid formulations: The BUD is not later than 30 days.

Special considerations for insulin

- Insulin should not be stored near extreme heat or cold.
- Insulin should not be stored in the freezer, direct sunlight, or the glove compartment of a car.
- Insulin products contained in vials or cartridges supplied by the manufacturers (opened or unopened) may be left unrefrigerated at a temperature between 59 °F and 86 °F for up to 28 days.
- An insulin product that has been altered for the purpose of dilution or by removal from the manufacturer's original vial should be discarded within 2 weeks.

Administration instructions
Oral medications

- Take the medication by mouth and swallow.
- Should not be chewed unless the patient has been instructed to chew it.

Sublingual medications

- Place the sublingual dosage form under the tongue and allow it to dissolve.

Buccal medications

- Place the buccal medication between the gum and cheeks and allow it to dissolve.

Parenteral medications
Injectable medications

- Use a syringe and needle to inject the medication into the body.

Routes of Administration for Injectable Medications			
Route of administration	**Needle gauge**	**Needle length (inches)**	**Angle of injection (degrees)**
Intravenous	16–20	1–1.5	15–35
Intramuscular	19–22	1–1.5	90
Subcutaneous	24–27	⅜–1	45–90
Intradermal	25–26	⅜	5–15

Metered dose inhaler

- Prime the inhaler by removing the cap of the metered dose inhaler, shaking the inhaler, and spraying it in the air away from you.
- Take off the cap and shake the inhaler.
- Breathe out all the way.
- Hold the inhaler in one of these two ways:

- If using a spacer/valved-holding chamber, place the inhaler into the end with the hole and the mouthpiece end in your mouth.

Or

- If not using a spacer, hold inhaler 1 to 2 inches (or two finger widths) in front of your open mouth.

■ As you start breathing in slowly through your mouth, press down on the inhaler one time. If you are using a spacer or valved-holding chamber, press down on the inhaler before starting to breathe in. Breathe in slowly.
■ Keep on breathing in slowly, as deeply as you can.
■ Hold your breath as you count to 10 slowly.
■ For inhaled quick-relief medications, wait about 1 minute between puffs. There is no need to wait between puffs for other mediations.

Dry powder inhaler

■ Follow your device instructions to load the medication dose.
■ Stand or sit up straight and breathe out completely.
■ Put the mouthpiece into your mouth, close your lips tightly around it, and breathe in quickly and forcefully.
■ Take the dry powder inhaler out of your mouth, hold your breath for 5–10 seconds, then exhale slowly.
■ If the treatment plan calls for a second dose, reload and repeat the steps.
■ When using a capsule device, open the chamber and check to see if the powder has been fully inhaled. If you see remaining powder, close the device, exhale fully, close your mouth around the mouthpiece, and inhale again. When the capsule is empty, remove and discard it.
■ Close the device and store in a dry place. Do not wash with water; use only a dry cloth to wipe the mouthpiece.

Topical medications

■ Wash hands.
■ Wear nonsterile gloves unless skin is broken; if skin is broken, wear sterile gloves.
■ Wash, rinse, and dry the affected area with a water and a clean cloth.
■ Place required amount of medication in palm of hands apply evenly over the affected area.

Ophthalmic drops

■ Wash hands before instilling eye drops.
■ Tilt your head back and look up.
■ With one hand, pull your lower eyelid down and away from your eyeball pocket.
■ Squeeze the prescribed number of eye drops into the pocket.
■ For at least 1 minute, close your eye and press your finger lightly on your tear duct.

Ophthalmic ointment

■ Sit down comfortably and put your head back.
■ Pull your lower lid down.
■ Apply ointment into the pocket formed by your lid pulled away from your eye. You can put in about half-inch strip of ointment. If you are having trouble releasing the ointment from the tube, you can apply the ointment to the tip of a cotton swab, and then insert it into the eyelid pocket. Try not to touch the tip of the tube to the lids.

■ Blinking the eyes will spread the ointment to the upper lids as well.
■ Wipe off the excess with a clean tissue.

Otic

■ Hold the bottle in your hands for 1 or 2 minutes to warm up the solution before putting it in your ear. Otherwise, putting cold solution in your ear could cause you to become dizzy.
■ Wash your hands with soap and water.
■ Gently clean any discharge that can be removed easily from the outer ear, but do not insert any object or swab into the ear canal.
■ If you are using the eardrops for a middle ear infection: Drop the medicine into the ear canal. Then, gently press the tragus of the ear (see the diagram in the medication guide) four times in a pumping motion. This will allow the drops to pass through the hole or tube in the eardrum and into the middle ear.
■ If you are using the eardrops for an ear canal infection: Gently pull the outer ear up and back for adults (down and back for children) to straighten the ear canal. This will allow the eardrops to flow down into the ear canal.
■ Keep the ear facing up for about 5 minutes to allow the medicine to come into contact with the infection.
■ If both ears are being treated, turn over after 5 minutes, and repeat the application for the other ear.
■ To keep the medicine as germ free as possible, do not touch the applicator tip to any surface (including the ear). Also, keep the container tightly closed.

Duration of drug therapy

■ Patients should take their medication as instructed by their physician and should not discontinue it unless told to do so by their physician.
■ If patients experience adverse effects, they should notify their physician, who will determine whether the medication should be discontinued.
■ Most antibiotics should be taken for 7–14 days.
■ Topical medications should be applied to the affected area as outlined on the prescription label.

Interchangeable drug classes and dosage forms

■ Pharmaceutical equivalents:
  • Contain the same active ingredient (to include the same salt form)
  • Contain the same quantity of active ingredient
  • Same dosage form
  • May have different inactive ingredients
  • May have different shapes, release mechanisms, packaging, or expiration dates
■ Pharmaceutical alternatives:
  • Contain the same active ingredient but different salt form
  • May have different amounts of active ingredient
  • May have different dosage forms
  • May have different inactive ingredients
  • May have different shapes, release mechanisms, packaging, or expiration dates

- Therapeutic equivalents:
  - Produce the same therapeutic effect and have the same safety profile
  - Must meet the following FDA criteria:
    - Are safe and effective
    - Are pharmaceutical equivalents
    - Are bioequivalent and do not pose a known or potential problem and have demonstrated an suitable bioequivalence standard
    - Are labeled properly
    - Comply with Current Good Manufacturing Practices regulations

- Bioequivalence:
  - Compares the bioavailability between two dosage forms

FDA *Approved Drug Products with Therapeutic Equivalence Evaluations* (commonly known as the Orange Book) provides information on the therapeutic equivalence of brand and generic drugs.

- 'A' drug products that are considered by the FDA therapeutically equivalent to other pharmaceutically equivalent products, i.e., drug products for which there are no known or suspected bioequivalence problems. These are designated AA, AN, AO, AP, or AT, depending on the dosage form; or actual or potential bioequivalence problems have been resolved with adequate in vivo and/or in vitro evidence supporting bioequivalence. These are designated AB. AA: Products not presenting bioequivalence problems in conventional dosage forms, AB: Products meeting necessary bioequivalence requirements, AN: Solutions and powders for aerosolization, AO: Injectable oil solutions, AP: Injectable aqueous solutions and, in certain instances, intravenous non-aqueous solutions, AT: Topical products.
- 'B' drug products are considered[1] not to be therapeutically equivalent to other pharmaceutically equivalent products, i.e., drug products for which actual or potential bioequivalence problems have not been resolved by adequate evidence of bioequivalence. Often the problem is with specific dosage forms rather than with the active ingredients. These are designated BC, BD, BE, BN, BP, BR, BS, BT, BX, or B*. B: Drug products requiring further FDA investigation and review to determine therapeutic equivalence, BC: Extended-release dosage forms (capsules, injectables and tablets), BD: Active ingredients and dosage forms with documented bioequivalence problems, BE: Delayed-release oral dosage forms, BN: Products in aerosol-nebulizer drug delivery systems, BP: Active ingredients and dosage forms with potential bioequivalence problems, BR: Suppositories or enemas that deliver drugs for systemic absorption, BS: Products having drug standard deficiencies, BT: Topical products with bioequivalence issues, BX: Drug products for which the data are insufficient to determine therapeutic equivalence.

Medical terminology

Medical terminology	Layman's term
Alopecia	Hair loss
Amblyopia	Reduction in vision

Medical terminology	Layman's term
Amenorrhea	Absence of menstruation
Anemia	Decrease in red blood cells
Aneurism	Widening of the blood vessel
Anorexia	Loss of appetite
Antacid	Relieves gastritis, ulcer pain, indigestion, and heartburn
Analgesic	Kills pain
Antianginal	Relieves heart pain
Antiarrhythmic	Prevents irregular rhythm
Antibiotic	Treats bacterial infection
Anticoagulant	Prevents blood clots
Anticonvulsant	Prevents seizure
Antidepressant	Prevents depression
Antidiabetic	Reduces blood glucose levels
Antidiarrheal	Stops diarrhea
Antiemetic	Prevents nausea and vomiting
Antifungal	Treats fungal infection
Antihistamine	Blocks effects of histamine
Antihyperlipidemic	Lowers high cholesterol levels
Antihypertensive	Reduces high blood pressure
Antiinflammatory	Reduces inflammation
Antiparkinsonian	Treats Parkinson's disease
Antipruritic	Prevents or relieves itching
Antiseptic	Topical antibacterial agent
Antispasmodic	Relieves intestinal cramping
Antitussive	Inhibits cough reflex
Antiviral	Treats viral infection
Anuresis	Inability to urinate
Anuria	Inability to produce urine
Aphagia	Inability to swallow
Aphasia	Inability to speak
Apnea	Temporary failure to breathe
Arthralgia	Joint pain
Arthritis	Joint inflammation
Atrophy	Process of shrinking muscle size
Bacteremia	Bacteria in the blood stream
Blepharitis	Inflammation of the eyelids
Bradycardia	Slow heart rate
Bradypnea	Slow breathing
Bronchitis	Inflammation of the bronchial membranes
Bronchodilator	Dilates bronchial tubes in the lung
Bursitis	Inflammation of the bursa
Cardiomyopathy	Decrease of the heart muscle
Cellulitis	Infection of the skin and subcutaneous tissue

(Continued)

Medical terminology	Layman's term
Colitis	Inflamed or irritated colon
Colostomy	New opening in the colon
Conjunctivitis	Inflammation of the conjunctiva
Cyanosis	Abnormal blue skin color from lack of oxygen in the blood
Cystitis	Inflammation of the bladder
Dementia	Disorientation, confusion, loss of memory
Dermatitis	Skin inflammation
Dialysis	Method of filtering impurities from blood
Diaphoresis	Excessive sweating
Diplopia	Double vision
Dyslexia	Difficult reading
Dyspepsia	Condition of indigestion
Dyspnea	Labored breathing
Dystrophy	Progressive atrophy
Dysuria	Painful urination
Eczema	Chronic skin inflammation
Embolism	Obstruction of blood flow
Emphysema	Obstructive pulmonary disease
Encephalitis	Inflammation of the brain
Endocarditis	Inflammation of the heart muscle
Endometriosis	Abnormal growth of uterine tissue
Enuresis	Involuntary urination
Epilepsy	Disorder characterized by recurrent seizures
Erythema	Skin redness
Fibromyalgia	Chronic pain in the muscles
Gastroenteritis	Inflammation of the stomach and intestinal tract
Glycosuria	Glucose in the urine
Gynecology	Study of female reproductive organs
Hematoma	Liver tumor
Hyperglycemia	High blood sugar
Hyperlipidemia	High blood cholesterol
Hypertension	High blood pressure
Hyperthyroidism	Elevated thyroid levels
Hypertrophy	Process of increase in muscle size
Hypoglycemia	Low blood sugar
Hypothyroidism	Low thyroid levels
Hysterectomy	Removal of the uterus
Keratosis	Area of increased hardness of the skin
Leukemia	Increase in white blood cells
Mastectomy	Removal of the breast
Mastitis	Inflammation of the breast
Menorrhea	Prolonged bleeding in menopause
Myasthenia	Chronic muscular weakness

Medical terminology	Layman's term
Myxedema	Swelling of the skin giving a waxy or slimy appearance
Nephralgia	Kidney pain
Neuralgia	Severe pain along a nerve
Onychomycosis	Fungal infection of the nail
Ostealgia	Bone pain
Otalgia	Pain in the ear (earache)
Otorrhagia	Bleeding in the ear
Otitis	Inflammation of the ear
Paralysis	Breaking down of motor control
Phlebitis	Inflammation of the vein
Photophobia	Intolerance to light
Polyuria	Excessive urination
Prostatitis	Inflammation of the prostate
Pruritis	Intense itching
Psychotropic	Changes mental states
Rhinitis	Inflammation of the nose; runny nose
Septicemia	Systemic blood infection
Splenectomy	Removal of the spleen
Tachycardia	Rapid heart rate
Tendonitis	Inflammation of a tendon
Thrombosis	Blood clots in the vascular system
Vasectomy	Removal of a segment of the vas deferens

Medication history process terminology

Adverse drug event (ADE): Harm experienced by a patient as a result of exposure to a medication or therapeutic agent

Adverse drug reaction: An unintended, harmful event attributed to the use of medicines that occurs as a cause of and during a significant proportion of unscheduled hospital admissions

Adverse event: Untoward incidents, therapeutic misadventures, or other adverse occurrences directly associated with care or services provided within the jurisdiction of a medical center, pharmacy, or other facility

Dietary supplement: A product taken by mouth intended to supplement the diet, containing one or more dietary ingredients, including vitamins, minerals, herbs or other botanicals, amino acids, enzymes, tissues from organs or glands, or extracts of these (They are labeled as being a dietary supplement.)

Dosage form: The physical form in which a drug is produced and dispensed, such as a tablet, a capsule, or injectable

Dose: The amount of medicine taken at one time

Drug (medication): A substance intended for use in the diagnosis, cure, mitigation, treatment, or prevention of disease

Drug allergy (medication allergy): An abnormal reaction of the immune system to a drug (medication)

Drug (medication) intolerance (sensitivity): Refers to an inability to tolerate the adverse effects of a medication, generally at therapeutic or subtherapeutic doses

Family medical history (family history): A record of the relationships among family members along with their medical histories, including current and past illnesses, which may show a pattern of certain diseases in a family

Frequency: How often a medication is administered per unit of time

Herbal supplements (botanical): A type of dietary supplement containing one or more herbs

Idiosyncratic drug reaction: An adverse effect that cannot be explained by the known mechanisms of action by a medication

Indication: The use of a medication for treating a particular disease or condition

Immunization (vaccination or inoculation): A process by which an individual becomes protected against a disease through vaccination

Medication (drug): A substance intended for use in the diagnosis, cure, mitigation, treatment, or prevention of disease

Medication allergy (drug allergy): An abnormal reaction of the immune system to a medication (drug)

Medication adherence: The extent to which patients take their medication as prescribed by their physicians (Patients are considered adherent if they take 80% of their prescribed medications.)

Medical condition: A disease, illness or injury; any physiologic, mental, or psychological condition or disorder

Over-the-counter medication: A medication that is safe and effective for use by the general public without a doctor's prescription

Prescription medication: A medication requiring a prescription from a licensed physician, physician assistant, or nurse prescription

Route of administration: The means by which a drug or agent enters the body to produce its effect

Schedule: When a drug is taken during its course of therapy

Social history: A summary of lifestyle practices and habits that may have a direct or indirect effect on their health, including diet, exercise, sexual orientation, level of sexual activity, and occupation (Social habits take into consideration use of tobacco, alcohol, and other substances.)

Strength: Indicates how much of the active ingredient is present in each dosage

Vaccination (immunization or inoculation): A process by which an individual becomes protected against a disease through immunization

Medical history terminology

Medical history

- Goals of a medical history:
  - To understand the state of health of the patient further and to determine within the history is related to any acute complaints to direct you toward a diagnosis
  - To gain information to prevent potential harm to the patient during treatment such as avoiding medications

to which the patient has an allergy or avoiding administering or prescribing a medication the patient has previously taken and had an adverse reaction
  - To identify the relevant chronic illnesses and other prior disease states for which the patient may not be under treatment but may have had lasting effects on the patient's health
- Components of a medical history include:
  - Chief complaint is a statement from the patient indicating the reason why the patient is seeking medical attention. Examples include shortness of breath, runny nose, rapid heart rate, and difficulty sleeping.
  - Symptoms are a physical or mental problem that a person experiences that may indicate a disease or condition; often they may not be detected by a medical test or laboratory work. Examples include rash, headache, frequent urination, and muscle pain.
  - Medication history is obtained to become familiar with the medications a patient is taking and to avoid potential drug-drug interactions.
  - Medication allergy is the abnormal reaction of the immune system to as a result of a medication such as penicillin or a sulfonamide.
  - Family history may reveal potential indicators of genetic predisposition to disease such as cardiac diseases or depression.
  - Surgical history provides a list of all invasive procedures an individual has undergone such as a mastectomy or a tonsillectomy.
  - Social history is a summary of lifestyle practices that may have a direct or indirect effect on an individual's heath. A social history includes an individual's occupation, exercise habits, diet, hobbies, substance use, sexual orientation, sexual behavior, and firearms in household.
  - Immunization history provides information on the vaccines an individual has received such as measles, mumps, and rubella.

Medical conditions terminology

- Addison disease: A condition that occurs when adrenal glands do not produce enough of the hormones cortisol and aldosterone
- Alzheimer disease: A progressive mental deterioration that can occur in middle or old age, due to generalized degeneration of the brain
- Anaphylaxis: An acute allergic reaction to an antigen (e.g., a bee sting) to which the body has become hypersensitive
- Angina: A condition marked by severe pain in the chest, often also spreading to the shoulders, arms, and neck, caused by an inadequate blood supply to the heart
- Asthma: A chronic (long-term) condition that affects the airways in the lungs
- Atherosclerosis: A disease of the arteries characterized by the deposition of plaques of fatty material on their inner walls
- Attention-deficit hyperactivity disorder: Any of a range of behavioral disorders occurring primarily in children, including such symptoms as poor concentration, hyperactivity, and impulsivity
- Benign prostatic hyperplasia: Enlargement of the prostate

- Bipolar disorder: A mental condition marked by alternating periods of elation and depression
- Chronic obstructive pulmonary disease: A chronic inflammatory lung disease that causes obstructed airflow from the lung
- Constipation: A condition in which there is difficulty in emptying the bowels, usually associated with hardened feces
- Depression: A mood disorder that causes a persistent feeling of sadness and loss of interest
- Diarrhea: The passage of three or more loose or liquid stools per day
- Dysrhythmia: An abnormal rhythm of the heart
- Eczema: A group of conditions in which the skin becomes inflamed, forms blisters, and becomes crusty, thick, and scaly
- Edema: Buildup of flood in the body tissues
- Epilepsy: A central nervous system (neurological) disorder in which brain activity becomes abnormal, causing seizures or periods of unusual behavior and sensations and sometimes loss of awareness
- Erectile dysfunction: Inability of a male to maintain an erection
- Gastroesophageal reflux disease: A condition which occurs when stomach acid repeatedly flows back into the tube connecting the mouth and the stomach (esophagus). This backwash (acid reflux) can irritate the lining of your esophagus
- Glaucoma: A condition in which there is a buildup of fluid in the eye, which presses on the retina and the optic nerve
- Graves' disease: An immune system disorder that results in the overproduction of thyroid hormones (hyperthyroidism)
- Hyperlipidemia: A condition in which there are high levels of fat particles (lipids) in the blood
- Hypertension: A disease that develops when blood flows through your arteries at higher-than-normal pressures
- Hypotension: Low blood pressure
- Hypothyroidism: A condition in which the thyroid gland does not produce enough of certain crucial hormones
- Myocardial infarction: A blockage of blood flow to the heart muscle
- Osteoarthritis: A form of arthritis that only affects the joints, usually in the hands, knees, hips, neck, and lower back
- Osteoporosis: A decrease in the amount and thickness of bone tissue
- Parkinson disease: A brain disorder that causes unintended or uncontrollable movements, such as shaking, stiffness, and difficulty with balance and coordination
- Pelvic inflammatory disease: Inflammation of the female genital tract accompanied by fever and lower abdominal pain
- Peptic ulcer: A sore in the lining of the stomach or duodenum, the first part of the small intestine
- Pneumonia: A severe inflammation of the lungs in which the alveoli (tiny air sacs) are filled with fluid
- Psoriasis: A chronic disease of the skin marked by red patches covered with white scales
- Psychosis: A severe mental disorder in which a person loses the ability to recognize reality or relate to others
- Rheumatoid arthritis: An autoimmune disease that causes pain, swelling, and stiffness in the joints and may cause severe joint damage, loss of function, and disability

- Rhinitis: Irritation and swelling of the mucous membrane in the nose
- Schizophrenia: A group of severe mental disorders in which a person has trouble telling the difference between real and unreal experiences, thinking logically, having normal emotional responses to others, and behaving normally in social situations
- Stroke: A loss of blood flow to part of the brain, which damages brain tissue
- Systemic lupus erythematosus: A chronic, inflammatory, connective tissue disease that can affect the joints and many organs, including the skin, heart, lungs, kidneys, and nervous system
- Tuberculosis: A disease caused by a specific type of bacteria that spreads from one person to another through the air
- Type 1 diabetes mellitus: A situation where the pancreas does not make insulin resulting in blood glucose levels that are too high
- Type 2 diabetes mellitus: A chronic condition that affects the way the body processes blood sugar (glucose)
- Urinary incontinence: Inability to hold urine in the bladder
- Urinary tract infection: Bacterial or fungal infection of the urinary tract

Common medication-related problems
Side effects
- Secondary undesirable effects can occur during medication therapy that may lead to nonadherence.
- Side effects can appear as a result on an inappropriate dose, incorrect administration, bodily reaction, and drug interactions.
- Patients who experience side effects may stop taking their medications, self-adjust their regimen to counter the side effects, or not start their regimen at all.
- Examples of common side effects include headache, nausea, vomiting, constipation, diarrhea, upset stomach, rhinitis, itchy skin, and rash.

Nonadherence
- Primary nonadherence: Occurs when a new medication is prescribed for a patient but the patient fails to obtain the medication (or its appropriate alternative) within an acceptable period of time after it was initially prescribed
- Secondary nonadherence: Happens when a patient fills a prescription but does not take the medication as it was intended and/or prescribed
- Intentional medication nonadherence: Active process whereby the patient chooses to deviate from the treatment regimen
- Unintentional medication nonadherence: Passive process in which the patient may be careless or forgetful about adhering to treatment regimen
- Can be directly tied to increased morbidity, mortality, and avoidable health care costs

Affordability
- High out-of-pocket medication costs have a negative impact on medication adherence since:
  • Patients may not fill even the initial prescription, let alone refills.

- Patients may skip doses or cut pills in half to stretch their dwindling supply if they do not have the money for a refill due to high copays.
- Patients may seek lower-cost therapies, use alternative ones, or buy medication from unreliable online sources or from sources outside of the country where quality can be a concern.
- A lack of availability, immediacy of health benefits, or other assistance programs are related to a greater decrease in medication adherence in any population group.
- Cost-related nonadherence increases when a patient is taking multiple medications for one or more conditions

Low health literacy

- Health literacy refers to the degree to which individuals have the ability to find, understand, and use information and services to inform health-related decisions and actions for themselves and others.
- Health literacy requires a patient to be able to read, listen, communicate, and comprehend to follow a medication regimen.
- Low health literacy skills hinder patients' ability to build knowledge about their illness and therapy resulting in nonadherence.
- Differences in education, English proficiency, socioeconomic status, and situational circumstances can affect an individual's health literacy.
- Identifying low health literacy in patients can be demonstrated by observing:
  - Incompletely filled-out forms
  - Missing medication refills for chronic conditions
  - Medications referred to by their shapes or colors
  - Avoidance of reading printed material when in front of a pharmacist
  - Mispronouncing words

Patient skills

- Skill levels that impact adherence include the ability to use drug-delivery devices, communication issues, forgetfulness/memory retention, lack of confidence and physical capabilities.
  - Understanding how to use drug delivery devices properly.
  - Communication skills can also negatively affect medication adherence, especially when a patient is unable to recall a prescriber's directions. A patient's inability to accurately communicate directions affects how the patient relays his or her care instructions to other health care providers. In addition, it inhibits asking appropriate question that could affect the accuracy of therapy.
  - Forgetfulness and memory-retention skills are common sources of medication nonadherence. Memory retention of learned knowledge decreases over time unless it is continuously reviewed.
  - Confidence-building skills that increase a patient's perception are correlated with better medication adherence among various disease states. A patient's failure to correctly follow a prescribed medication regimen is worsened when a patient does not ask their providers questions due to a feeling of apprehension or intimidation.
  - Patient physical skills

Polypharmacy

- Refers to multiple medications being prescribed to treat the same condition
- Types of polypharmacy:
  - Excessive polypharmacy: Concurrent use of 10 or more different drugs
  - Polypharmacy: The use of five to nine drugs
  - No polypharmacy: Taking four or fewer drugs (included those taking no medicines)
- Risk factors contributing to polypharmacy:
  - Multiple medical conditions being managed my multiple physicians
  - Patient's age (extremely common in patients 60 years of age and older)
  - Patients having chronic mental health conditions
  - Filling prescriptions in multiple pharmacies
  - Patients residing in long-term care facilities
- Polypharmacy concerns:
  - Adverse drug events (ADEs): Refers to an injury resulting from the use of a drug and refers to harm caused by a drug at usual dosages. Preventable ADEs occurs as a result of inappropriate medication use in older patient. Drug classification associated with preventable ADE include cardiovascular, anticoagulants, hypoglycemics, diuretics, and nonsteroidal antiinflammatory drugs.
  - Drug interactions: Use of multiple medications increases the potential for drug-drug interactions. Common ADEs includes hypertension, hypotension, and renal failure.
  - Prescribing cascades: Using additional drugs to treat the ADEs is associated with other drugs by misinterpreting the ADE as a new medical condition.
  - Inappropriate therapy or nonadherence is common in patients with visual or cognitive decline.
  - Use of over-the-counter and complementary medications can result in herb-drug interactions.
  - Changes in pharmacokinetics (absorption, distribution, metabolism, and elimination) that are associated with aging increase the risk of adverse drug reactions.
  - Unintentional overdose may result.
  - Patient death may result.

Laboratory measures

Diabetes

- This chronic endocrine disease is associated with hyperglycemia.
- Symptoms of diabetes include polyuria (frequent urination), polydipsia (abnormal thirst), polyphagia (excessive hunger), weight loss, blurred vision, numbness or tingling in feet and fingers, tiredness, and dry skin.
- Types of diabetes:
  - Type 1 diabetes mellitus:
    - Caused by a destruction or a defect in the beta cells of the pancreas
    - Results in the pancreas being unable to synthesizes and secrete insulin and therefore the patient must use exogenous insulin
    - Common symptoms include polyuria (frequent urination), polydipsia (excessive thirst), and polyphagia (increased appetite)

- Type 2 diabetes mellitus:
  - Occurs as a result of insulin resistance or a decrease ability of tissues to respond to insulin
  - Insulin resistance increases in overweight or obese individuals
  - Occurs in patients older than 45 years of age
  - Is considered a metabolic disorder
  - Conditions associated with type 2 diabetes mellitus include obesity, hypertension, and hyperlipidemia
- Gestational diabetes mellitus:
  - Occurs in patients during pregnancy; blood glucose levels return to normal after pregnancy
  - Occurs as a result of weight gain during pregnancy and an increase in estrogen concentrations
  - Failure to monitor gestational diabetes mellitus properly during pregnancy may result in pregnancy complications and health problems for the child after birth
- A1C (hemoglobin A1C or HbA1c test) is a blood test for type 2 diabetes and prediabetes. It measures average blood glucose, or blood sugar, level over the past 3 months.

Interpreting diabetes laboratory tests		
Test	**Reading**	**Category**
A1C	<5.7%	Normal
	5.7%–6.4%	Prediabetes
	≥6.5%	Diabetes
Fasting plasma glucose (fasting for at least 8 h)	<100 mg/dL (5.5 mmol/L	Normal
	100–125 mg/dL (5.5–6.9 mmol/L)	Prediabetes
	≥126 mg/dL (7 mmol/L)	Diabetes
2 h after meals	<140 mg/dL (7.8 mmol/L)	Normal
	140–199 mg/dL (7.8–11.1 mmol/L)	Prediabetes
	≥200 mg/dL (11.1 mmol/L)	Diabetes

Hypertension

- Hypertension is also known as high blood pressure.
- Individuals with hypertension are asymptomatic and are unaware that they have the condition.
- Types of hypertension:
  - Essential hypertension occurs when the cause for hypertension cannot be determined.
  - Secondary hypertension occurs when the cause for hypertension can be determined.
- Blood pressure readings:
  - Systolic blood pressure (the first number) indicates how much pressure an individual's blood is exerting against the artery walls when the heart beats.
  - Diastolic blood pressure (the second number) indicates how much pressure an individual's blood is exerting

against the artery walls while the heart is resting between beats.

Hypertension classifications	
Blood pressure (mm Hg)	**Category**
<120/≤80	Normal
120–129/<80	Elevated
130–139/80–89	High blood pressure stage 1 hypertension
≥140/≥90	High blood pressure stage 2 hypertension
>180/>120	Hypertensive crisis

Hyperlipidemia (hypercholesterolemia)

- Hyperlipidemia is an abnormal high level or concentration of fats or lipids in the blood.
- Patients with hyperlipidemia are unaware that they have the condition.
- Terminology:
  - Cholesterol: Non-water-soluble lipid, which is transported in lipoprotein particles, which are water soluble
  - Low-density lipoprotein cholesterol: Known as the "bad" cholesterol, which is the main source of blockages in the arteries
  - High-density lipoprotein cholesterol: Considered the "good" cholesterol and helps remove "bad" low-density lipoprotein cholesterol
  - Very low-density lipoprotein cholesterol: Particles in the blood that carry triglycerides
  - Apolipoprotein B: The primary protein contained within low-density lipoprotein and very low-density lipoprotein
  - Total cholesterol: A measure of the total amount of cholesterol in the blood that includes both low-density lipoprotein cholesterol and high-density lipoprotein cholesterol
  - Triglycerides: The dominant form of body-stored fat consisting of three fatty molecules and a molecule of the alcohol glycerol

Types of hyperlipidemia			
Type	**Lipoprotein(s) elevated**	**Serum cholesterol level**	**Serum triglyceride level**
I	Chylomicrons	Normal to mildly increased	Very severely increased
IIa	LDL	Moderately increased	Normal
IIb	LDL and VLDL	Moderately increased	Moderately increased
III	IDL	Moderately increased	Severely increased
IV	VLDL	Normal to mildly increased	Moderately increased
V	VLDL and chylomicrons	Normal to mildly increased	Very severely increased

IDL, Intermediate density lipoprotein; *LDL*, low-density lipoprotein; *VLDL*, very low-density lipoprotein.

Desired lipid levels

Lipid	Measurement in mg/dL (mmol/L)
Total cholesterol	<200 (5.2)
	200–239 (5.2–6.2)
	≥240 (6.2)
LDL	<100 (3.4)
	100–189 (3.4–4.9)
	≥190 (4.9)
HDL	≥60 (1.6)
	40–59 (1–1.5) (men)
	50–59 (1.3–1.5) (women)
	<40 (1) (men)
	<50 (1.3) (women)
Triglycerides	<150 (1.7)
	150–499 (1.7–5.6)
	≥500 (5.6)

LDL, low-density lipoprotein; *HDL*, high-density lipoprotein.

Normal laboratory values

Complete blood count

Test acronym	Meaning	Normal range values (male)	Normal range values (female)
WBC	Number of white blood cells	0–5 cells/μL	0–5 cells/μL
RBC	Number of red blood cells	25–35 mL/kg body weight	20–30 mL/kg body weight
HGB	Hemoglobin level	14–18 g/dL	12–16 g/dL
HCT	Hematocrit	42%–50%	37%–47%
	Plasma	44 mL/kg body weight	43 mL/kg body weight
PLT	Number of platelets	25–44 mL/kg body weight	28–43 mL/kg body weight

Normal range values from: American Board of Internal Medicine. Published January 2023. https://www.abim.org/Media/bfijryql/laboratory-reference-ranges.pdf

White blood cell differential

Test	Normal range values
Leukocyte count	4000–11,000/μL
Neutrophils (Neut)%	40-60%
Lymphocytes (Lymph)%	30%–45%
Monocytes (Mono)%	0%–6%
Eosinophils (Eos)%	0%–3%
Basophils (Baso)%	0%–1%
Absolute neutrophil count (ANC)	2000–825 μL

Normal range values from: American Board of Internal Medicine. Published January 2023. https://www.abim.org/Media/bfijryql/laboratory-reference-ranges.pdf.

Chemistry and serum —cont'd

Test	Normal range values
Sodium (Na)	136–145 mEq/L
Potassium (K)	3.5–5.0 mEq/L
Chloride (Cl)	98–106 mEq/L
Magnesium (Mg), serum	1.6–2.6 mEq/L
Bicarbonate (CO_2)	23–28 mEq/L
Calcium	9–10.5 mg/dL
Serum glutamic pyruvic transaminase or Alanine transaminase	10–40 U/L
Phosphorous, serum	3.0–4.5 mg/dL
Alkaline phosphatase	30–120 U/L
Bilirubin (direct)	0–0.3 mg/dL
Bilirubin (total)	0.3–1.2 mg/dL
Creatine	Men: 0.7–1.2 mg/dL Women: 0.5–1.0 mg/dL
Blood urea nitrogen	8–20 mg/dL
Albumin	3.5–5.5 g/dL
Globulin	2.0–3.5 g/dL
Total protein	15–45 mg/dL
Thyroxine (T_4), total	5–12 μg/dL
Thyroxine (T_4), free	0.8–1.8 ng/dL
Triiodothyronine (T3), total	80–180 ng/dL
Triiodothyronine (T3), reverse	20–40 ng/dL
Triiodothyronine (T3), free	2.3–4.2 pg/mL
Immunoglobulin A	90–325 mg/dL
Immunoglobulin E	<380 IU/mL
Immunoglobulin G	800–1500 mg/dL
Immunoglobulin M	45–150 mg/dL

Normal range values from: American board of internal medicine. Published January 2022. Accessed February 3, 2022. https://www.abim.org/Media/bfijryql/laboratory-reference-ranges.pdf.

Patient safety and quality assurance strategies

Adherence

- According to the American Medical Association, "A patient is considered adherent if they take 80% of their prescribed medicine(s). If patients take less than 80% of their prescribed medication(s), they are considered nonadherent."
- Methods to calculate adherence:
  - Proportion of days covered: Ratio of the number of days the patient is covered by the medication to the number of days the patient is eligible to have the medication on hand
  - Medication possession ratio: Ratio of the amount of days a patient has medication on hand to the amount of days a patient is eligible to have the medicine on hand

- Days' supply:
  - Days' supply for tablets (capsules, caplets, etc.): Total quantity dispensed/total quantity taken per day
  - Days' supply for oral liquids: Total quantity dispensed (mL)/total quantity (mL) taken per day
  - Days' supply for inhalers: Total number of inhalations per container/total number of inhalations taken each day
  - Days' supply for ophthalmic solution: To calculate use the conversion that 1 mL is equal to 20 drops: Total volume of container × 20 drops per mL ÷ number of drops instilled each day.

Information review

Medication-related action plan (MAP), also known as the therapeutic action plan, is a patient-centric document containing a list of actions for the patient to use in tracking progress for self-management. Information contained in the MAP may include:

- Patient name
- Primary care physician (name and telephone number)
- Pharmacy name and telephone number
- Date the MAP was created
- Action steps for the patient
- Notes for the patient
- Appointment information

Medication therapy review (MTR) is a systematic process of collecting patient-specific information, assessing medication therapies to identify medication-related problems, developing a prioritized list of medication-related problems, and creating a plan to resolve them. An MTR may be either a comprehensive or a targeted medication review. A comprehensive medication review consists of:

- Collecting patient-specific information
- Assessing medication therapies to identify medication therapy problems
- Developing a prioritized list of medication therapy problems
- Creating a plan to resolve the identified medication therapy problems with the patient, caregiver, and/or prescriber
- Providing a live, interactive medication review and consultation with the patient or caregiver in person, virtually, or over the phone

A targeted medication review addresses an actual or potential medication-related problem associated with a specific medication and can take place any time outside of a comprehensive medication review.

Personal medication record (PMR), also known as the personal medication list, is a comprehensive record of the patient's medications (prescription and nonprescription medications, herbal products, and other dietary supplements). The PMR is intended for patients to use in medication self-management. Patients should be educated to carry the PMR with them at all times and share it at all health care visits and at all admissions to or discharges from institutional settings to help ensure that all health care professionals are aware of their current medication regimen. Information contained in the PMR may include:

- Patient name
- Patient birthdate

- Patient phone number
- Emergency contact information (name, relationship, and phone number)
- Primary care physician (name and phone number)
- Pharmacy (name and phone number)
- Patient allergies
- Other patient medication-related problems
- Date PMR last updated
- Date last reviewed by pharmacist, physician, or other health care professional
- Patient signature
- Health care provider's signature
- For each medication:
  - Medication name and strength
  - Indication
  - Instructions for use
  - Start date
  - Stop date
  - Ordering prescriber
  - Special instructions

The pharmacy technician plays an important role with the PMR by:

- Participating in the initial patient interviews
- Gathering information regarding the medications the patient is taking
- Collecting information how the medications are being used
- Updating the patient's PMR
- Verifying the patients medications through a second reliable source such as a caregiver
- Providing updated PMR to prescribers and other members of the health care team
- Explaining to patients how to use the PMR

Prescribing error

A prescribing error occurs when there is "an unintentional significant reduction in the probability of treatment being timely and effective or increase in the risk of harm when compared with generally accepted practice."[2] An prescribing error can result from an incorrect drug selection (based on indications, contraindications, known allergies, existing drug therapy, and other factors), dose, dosage form, quantity, route, concentration, rate of administration, instructions for use of a drug product ordered or authorized by physician (or other legitimate prescriber), or illegible prescriptions or medication orders that lead to errors that reach the patient.

Types of medication errors[a]	
Type	**Definition**
Prescribing error	Incorrect drug selection (based on indications, contraindications, known allergies, existing drug therapy, and other factors), dose, dosage form, quantity, route, concentration, rate of administration, or instructions for use of a drug product ordered or authorized by physician (or other legitimate prescriber); illegible prescriptions or medication orders that lead to errors that reach the patient
Omission error[b]	The failure to administer an ordered dose to a patient before the next scheduled dose, if any

Types of medication errors[a] —cont'd

Type	Definition
Wrong time error	Administration of medication outside a pre-defined time interval from its scheduled administration time (This interval should be established by each individual health care facility.)
Unauthorized drug error[c]	Administration to the patient of medication not authorized by a legitimate prescriber for the patient
Improper dose error[d]	Administration to the patient of a dose that is greater than or less than the amount ordered by the prescriber or administration of duplicate doses to the patient (i.e., one or more dosage units in addition to those that were ordered)
Wrong dosage form error[e]	Administration to the patient of a drug product in a different dosage form than ordered by the prescriber
Wrong drug preparation error[f]	Drug product incorrectly formulated or manipulated before administration
Wrong administration technique error[g]	Inappropriate procedure or improper technique in the administration of a drug
Deteriorated drug error[h]	Administration of a drug that has expired or for which the physical or chemical dosage form integrity has been compromised
Monitoring error	Failure to review a prescribed regimen for appropriateness and detection of problems, or failure to use appropriate clinical or laboratory data for adequate assessment of patient response to prescribed therapy
Compliance error	Inappropriate patient behavior regarding adherence to a prescribed medication regimen
Other medication error	Any medication error that does not fall into one of above predefined categories

[a]The categories may not be mutually exclusive because of the multidisciplinary and multifactorial nature of medication errors.

[b]Assumes no prescribing error. Excluded would be (1) a patient's refusal to take the medication or (2) a decision not to administer the dose because of recognized contraindications. If an explanation for the omission is apparent (e.g., patient was away from nursing unit for tests or medication was not available), that reason should be documented in the appropriate records.

[c]This would include, for example, a wrong drug, a dose given to the wrong patient, unordered drugs, and doses given outside a stated set of clinical guidelines or protocols.

[d]Excluded would be (1) allowable deviations based on preset ranges established by individual health care organizations in consideration of measuring devices routinely provided to those who administer drugs to patients (e.g., not administering a dose based on a patient's measured temperature or blood glucose level) or other factors such as conversion of doses expressed in the apothecary system to the metric system and (2) topical dosage forms for which medication orders are not expressed quantitatively.

[e]Excluded would be accepted protocols (established by the pharmacy and therapeutics committee or its equivalent) that authorize pharmacists to dispense alternate dosage forms for patients with special needs (e.g., liquid formulations for patients with nasogastric tubes or those who have difficulty swallowing), as allowed by state regulations.

[f]This would include, for example, incorrect dilution or reconstitution, mixing drugs that are physically or chemically incompatible, and inadequate product packaging.

[g]This would include doses administered (1) via the wrong route (different from the route prescribed), (2) via the correct route but at the wrong site (e.g., left eye instead of right), and (3) at the wrong rate of administration.

[h]This would include, for example, administration of expired drugs and improperly stored drugs.

From American Society of Hospital Pharmacists: ASHP guidelines on preventing medication errors in hospitals. *Am J Hosp Pharm*. 1993;50:305–314. © 1993, American Society of Health-System Pharmacists, Inc. All rights reserved. Reprinted with permission.

Prescribing errors effect

Inappropriate prescribing may result in:

- The patient condition not being treated properly
- Patient injury or death
- Adverse drug reactions
- ADEs
- Patient nonadherence
- Polypharmacy

Category	Definition	Type of resulting error
A	Circumstances that have potential for causing errors	No error
B	Error occurred but did not reach patient	Error, no harm
C	Error reached patient but did not cause harm	Error, no harm
D	Error reached patient, did not cause harm but needed monitoring or intervention to prove no harm resulted	Error, no harm
E	Error occurred that may have contributed to or resulted in temporary harm to patient and patient required intervention	Error, harm
F	Error occurred that may have contributed to or resulted in temporary harm to patient and resulted in hospitalization	Error, harm
G	Error occurred that may have contributed to or resulted in temporary or permanent harm to the patient	Error, harm
H	Error occurred that may have contributed to or resulted in harm to patient and required hospitalization to sustain life	Error, harm
I	Error occurred that may have contributed or resulted in patient's death	Error, death

Medication therapy management administration and management

Medication therapy management

The American Pharmacist Association defined medication therapy management (MTM) "as a distinct service or group of services that optimize therapeutic outcomes for individual patients." MTM services are independent of but can provide medications to a patient. Some of the MTM services provided to patients include:

- Conducting or obtaining necessary appropriate assessments of the patient's health status
- Developing a medication treatment plan

- Selecting, starting, altering, or administering medication therapy
- Observing and assessing the patient's response to therapy, including safety and effectiveness
- Executing a comprehensive medication review to identify, resolve, and prevent medication-related problems, including ADEs
- Recording the care delivered and communicating fundamental information to the patient's other primary care providers
- Delivering verbal education and training intended to improve patient understanding and proper use of their medications
- Offering information, support services, and resources intended to improve patient adherence with their medication regimens
- Organizing and incorporating MTM services with other health care management services being offered to the patient

MTM:

- Is patient centered rather than product centered
- Focuses on overall regimen rather than individual medication
- Involves collaboration between pharmacists and other health care providers

The goals of MTM involve:
- Reducing preventable adverse events and associated costs
- Decreasing medication-related morbidity and mortality
- Cutting health care costs due to duplicate or unnecessary prescriptions

As a result the outcomes associated with MTM must demonstrate an:

- Increase in the patient's understanding and self-management skills of their medications
- Improvement in patient adherence, thereby increasing an efficacy of their medications
- Increase in adherence to Centers for Medicare and Medicaid Services (CMS) quality performance standards

MTM covers a broad range of professional activities and responsibilities within the licensed pharmacist's, or other qualified health care provider's, scope of practice. Based upon the individual needs of the patient, these services may include[3] MTR, PMR (also known as a personal medication list), MAP, intervention or referral, and documentation.

Medication therapy review

MTR is a systematic process of collecting patient-specific information, assessing medication therapies to identify medication-related problems, developing a prioritized list of medication-related problems, and creating a plan to resolve them. The MTR's goal is to improve patients' knowledge of their medications, address problems or concerns they may have, and encourage patients to self-manage their medications and their health condition(s). MTR may either a comprehensive medication review or targeted medication review. The following activities may take place during an MTR:

- Interviewing the patient to gather data including demographic information, general health and activity status, medical history, medication history, immunization history, and patients' thoughts or feelings about their conditions and medication use
- Evaluating all clinical information available to the pharmacist, including the patient's physical and overall health status, including current and previous conditions
- Assessing the patient's values, preferences, quality of life, and goals of therapy
- Evaluating the patient's cultural issues, education level, language barriers, health literacy level, and communication abilities that could affect outcomes
- Assessing the patient to identify symptoms that could be associated with adverse events caused by any of their current medications
- Interpreting, monitoring, and assessing patient's laboratory results
- Assessing, identifying, and prioritizing medication related problems related to:
  - The appropriateness of each medication prescribed for the patient, including benefit versus risk
  - The appropriateness of the dose and dosing regimen of each medication, including consideration of indications, contraindications, potential adverse effects, and potential problems with concomitant medications
  - Therapeutic duplication or other unnecessary medications
  - Adherence to the therapy
  - Untreated diseases or conditions
  - Medication cost considerations
  - Health care/medication access considerations
- Designing a plan to address each identified medication related problem
- Furnishing education and training on the appropriate use of medications and monitoring devices and their relationship to medication adherence
- Mentoring patients to be able to manage their medications
- Monitoring and evaluating the patient's response to therapy, including safety and effectiveness
- Communicating appropriate information to the physician or other health care professionals, including consultation on the selection of medications, suggestions to address identified medication problems, updates on the patient's progress, and recommended follow-up care

Pharmacist and pharmacy technician's role in participating in a medication therapy review		
Medication therapy review	Pharmacist	Pharmacy technician
Scheduling eligible patients for MTM consultations with the pharmacist		X
Collecting data from patient profiles		X
Requesting patients to bring all over-the-counter medications, including supplements, to the consultation		X
Encouraging patients to bring copies of recent laboratory work		X

Pharmacist and pharmacy technician's role in participating in a medication therapy review—cont'd		
Medication therapy review	Pharmacist	Pharmacy technician
Requesting patients bring immunization records to the consultation		X
Interviewing the patient to gather data	X	X
Evaluating patient clinical information	X	
Assessing patient symptoms	X	
Interpreting and monitoring patient's laboratory results	X	X
Interpreting, monitoring, and assessing patient's laboratory results	X	
Assessing, identifying, and prioritizing medication-related problems	X	
Designing a plan to address each identified medication-related problem	X	
Providing training on the proper use of medications and monitoring devices	X	X
Mentoring patients to be able to manage their medications	X	X
Monitoring and evaluating the patient's response to therapy, including safety and effectiveness	X	
Communicating appropriate information to the physician or other health care professionals, including consultation on the selection of medications, suggestions to address identified medication problems, updates on the patient's progress, and recommended follow-up care	X	

MTM, medication therapy management.

Personal medication record

PMR, also known as the personal medication list, is a comprehensive record of the patient's medications (prescription and nonprescription medications, herbal products, and other dietary supplements). In MTM, medication reconciliation is one of steps involved in developing the PMR. Medication reconciliation is the process of identifying the medications a patient has been prescribed and comparing it to what the patient taking. It is quite common that differences will be found between these two lists. During medication reconciliation incorrect or missing doses are uncovered. In addition, it may be noted that frequency of the dose is incorrect or the presence of duplicate therapies. The PMR is intended for patient to use in medication self-management. Patients should be educated to carry the PMR with them at all times and share it at all health care visits and at all admissions to

or discharges from institutional settings to help ensure that all health care professionals are aware of their current medication regimen. Information contained in the PMR includes:

- Patient name
- Patient birth date
- Patient phone number
- Emergency contact information (name, relationship, telephone number)
- Primary care physician (name and telephone number)
- Pharmacy/pharmacist (name and telephone number)
- Allergies
- Other medication-related problems (e.g., What medication caused the problem? What was the problem the patient had?)
- Potential questions for patients to ask about their medications (e.g., When you are prescribed a new drug, ask your doctor or pharmacist...)
- Date last updated
- Date last reviewed by the pharmacist, physician, or other health care professional
- Patient's signature
- Health care provider's signature
- For each medication, include the following:
  - Medication (e.g., drug name and dose)
  - Indication (e.g., what the medication is being taken to treat)
  - Instructions for use (e.g., When does the patient take the medication? How much medication does the patient take?)
  - Start date
  - Stop date
  - Ordering prescriber/contact information (e.g., prescriber's name and telephone number)
  - Special instructions (e.g., take with food or take on an empty stomach)

Whenever a patient is prescribed a new medication; has a current medication discontinued by their prescriber; has received changes in the directions taking their medication; starts using a new prescription or nonprescription medication, herbal product, or other dietary supplement; or has any other changes to the medication regimen, the patient should update the PMR to help ensure a current and accurate record. The pharmacist, physician, and other health care professionals can actively assist the patient with the PMR revision process. Pharmacists may use the PMR to communicate and collaborate with physicians and other health care professionals to achieve optimal patient outcomes. Widespread use of the PMR will support uniformity of information provided to all health care professionals and enhance the continuity of care provided to patients while facilitating flexibility to account for pharmacy- or institution-specific variations.

Pharmacist and pharmacy technician's role in developing a patient's personal medication record		
Developing a patient's personal medical record	Pharmacist	Pharmacy technician
Contacting the patient to remind him or her of the MTM meeting		X

(Continued)

Pharmacist and pharmacy technician's role in developing a patient's personal medication record—cont'd		
Developing a patient's personal medical record	Pharmacist	Pharmacy technician
Gather information during the patient interview	X	X
Medication reconciliation	X	X
Gather information about how the medications are being used	X	X
Begin filling in the PMR	X	X
Updating the PMR	X	X
Providing copies of the PMR to the health care team	X	X
Explaining to patient how to use the PMR	X	X
Communicate and collaborate with physicians and other health care professionals to achieve optimal patient outcomes by using the PMR	X	
MTM, medication therapy management; *PMR*, personal medication record.		

Medication-related action plan

MAP, also known as the therapeutic action plan, is a patient-centric document containing a list of actions for the patient to use in tracking progress for self-management. Goals of MAP include:

- Help encourage the patient to assist in managing their own health.
- Establish practical steps for both the patient and health care team to follow.
- Recognize and remedy problems or errors related to medication safety.
- Investigate ways to lower costs: reduce waste, improve adherence, provide less-expensive drug alternatives when possible.

The care plan is developed by the pharmacist and is utilized by the patient in managing their medication therapy. The MAP is a valuable component of the documentation outlined in the MTM service model. The patient's MAP includes only items that the patient can act on that are within the pharmacist's scope of practice or that have been agreed to by relevant members of the health care team. The MAP should not include outstanding action items that still require physician or other health care professional review or approval. The patient can use the MAP as a simple guide to gauge their progress. The MAP may contain the following:

- Patient name
- Primary care physician (doctor's name and telephone number)
- Pharmacy/pharmacist (pharmacy name/pharmacist name and telephone number)
- Date of MAP creation (date prepared)
- Action steps for the patient ("What I need to do...")
- Notes for the patient ("What I did and when I did it...")

- Appointment information for follow-up with pharmacist, if applicable

The pharmacy technician plays a vital role in following up with patients regarding their MAP. The pharmacy technician:

- May schedule follow-up MTM appointments or calls.
- May keep track of essential actions for patients. For example, telephone, email, or text messaging reminders to the patient to schedule necessary laboratory tests or follow-up physician visits.
- Follows pharmacy protocols associated with MTM. For example, the pharmacy technician may review patient records to see if refills are being made on a timely basis. The pharmacy technician may offer to synchronize the patient's medication refills to ensure they are being refilled at the same time and saving the patient trips to the pharmacy.
- Communicates effectively with the patient by being clear what might be expected before their next follow-up call pr visit.
- Maintains clear, organized, and updated patient records. Communicates and collaborates with members of the health care team to include pharmacists, physician's practices, and other health care providers.

Pharmacist and pharmacy technician's role in developing a medication-related action plan		
Developing a MAP	Pharmacist	Pharmacy technician
Assisting with patient interviews	X	X
Assessing patient	X	
Developing MAP	X	
Updating MAP	X	X
Scheduling MTM meetings		X
Tracking patient actions		X
Reviewing patient refills	X	X
MAP, medication-related action plan; *MTM*, medication therapy management.		

Intervention and/or referral

As problems are identified by the pharmacist, some can be intervened on and handled directly by the pharmacist. The level of pharmacist intervention depends on the pharmacist's clinical practice setting. Pharmacists working in an ambulatory care clinic under a collaborative practice agreement (CPA) or collaborative drug therapy management) with a physician may be able to provide a different level of problem intervention than a pharmacist working in a community setting without such an agreement. In addition, a pharmacist in a community setting would have the ability to intervene when vaccinations are warranted for the patient, while a pharmacist providing telephonic services would not have such abilities. Some patients' medical conditions or medication therapy may be highly specialized or complex, and the patient's needs may extend beyond the core elements of

MTM service delivery. In such cases, pharmacists may provide additional services according to their expertise or refer the patient to a physician, another pharmacist, or other health care professional. The communication of appropriate information to the physician or other health care professional, including consultation on the selection of medications, suggestions to address medication problems, and recommended follow-up care, is integral to the intervention component of the MTM service model.

A CPA or collaborative drug therapy management is a formal agreement between a pharmacist or pharmacy group and a licensed prescriber. It provides the advantage of permitting the pharmacist to operate under protocol to make immediate changes in drug therapy and to provide immediate, on-site delivery of care to patients (such as ordering of pertinent laboratory tests). The progression from typical pharmacist–provider interaction and a CPA is as follows:

1. Pharmacist dispenses prescriber's prescriptions.
2. Pharmacist and prescriber ask questions and exchange information.
3. Pharmacist suggests recommendations; prescriber considers and often accepts recommendations.
4. Prescriber delegates responsibilities under a CPA.[4]

According to CMS guidelines, a "collaborative practice protocol" consists of a written document that identifies drug therapy management actions that a pharmacist is authorized to perform for a patient.[5] CMS maintains that this document should be created jointly by the pharmacist and the physician and should include a description of the terms of agreement, including[5]:

- Identify each physician and pharmacist permitted to participate in a patient's collaborative drug therapy management, including all covering physicians and/or pharmacists.
- Establish the method by which the physician and/or pharmacist will be informed about covering practitioners for collaborative practice purposes.
- Identify responsibilities, including the scope of practice and authority, to be performed by the pharmacist.
- Indicate any restrictions placed on the use of certain types or classes of drugs or drug therapies.
- Identify any diagnosis or types of conditions that are specifically included or excluded.
- Incorporate copies of all protocols to be used in the collaborative practice.
- Indicate effective date for the agreement.
- signed and dated by physician(s) and pharmacist(s).

Each state determines what is permitted under a CPA. The magnitude of services that can be performed by pharmacists within the CPA also differs from state to state. Some states have strict limitations, and others permit more of the decision making up to the discretion of the provider. Once a state has allowed CPA and has defined the specific terms, individual organizations can decide what they will permit pharmacists to do. Services performed by pharmacists under CPAs are not limited to modification of drug therapy and monitoring of laboratory tests. States may require credentialing for pharmacists to participate in CPAs, while other states may stipulate specific continuing education or completion of a certificate training program.

Situations that may require referral include:

- A patient may demonstrate future problems discovered during the MTR that may necessitate referral for evaluation and diagnosis.
- A patient may require disease management education to help him or her manage chronic diseases such as diabetes or coagulation.
- A patient may require monitoring for high-risk medications (e.g., warfarin, phenytoin, lithium, or methotrexate).

The intent of intervention and/or referral is to optimize medication use, enhance continuity of care, and encourage patients to avail themselves of health care services to prevent future adverse outcomes.

Pharmacist and pharmacy technician's role in intervening or referring patients for medication therapy review services		
Intervening or referring patient's for MTM services	Pharmacist	Pharmacy technician
Developing a collaborative agreement	X	
Responsible for communicating appropriate information to the physician or other health care professional	X	
Assisting in developing written communication to physician or other health care professional		X
Consulting on the selection of medications	X	
Suggestions to address medication problems	X	
Recommending follow-up care	X	
MTM, medication therapy review.		

Documentation

Follow-up MTM services are documented in a consistent manner and must be maintained for 10 years according to CMS regulations. Follow-up MTM visits are planned based upon the patient's medication-related needs or in situations where the patient is transitioned from one health care setting to another. Following-up with the patient or on issues identified in the interview is an important part of the final core element. The time involved in follow-up is patient specific and depends on what problems were identified during the review. Follow-up within a few days of the review may be necessary for urgent issues, whereas follow-up may not be necessary for a month or longer for other issues. At minimum, follow-ups should occur at least every 3 months to review the patient's medication record and to determine if any previously identified problems were resolved and if any problems have arisen since the previous review. The pharmacy technician's role in MTM follow-up includes:

- Scheduling follow-up patient appointment calls for MTM visits

- Keeping track of necessary actions for patients such as scheduling required laboratory tests or physician appointments
- Reviewing patient records to determine if refills are being done are on a timely basis

Technology has made documentation of provided MTM services much easier and more efficient for health care providers. The ultimate goal for MTM documentation software is to offer pharmacists their choice of an integrated documentation and billing system for their practice. A documentation system would allow integration with dispensing systems for pharmacists providing MTM services in a community setting, permit for interoperability between various systems, and improve efficiency and effectiveness, especially regarding standardization, billing, tracking outcome information, and meeting necessary reporting requirements. Documentation systems currently being used in MTM services include Cerner, Epic, MTMPath, MirixaPro, OutcomesMTM, Nexus AG, PharmMD, QAS/1 and RxCompanion.

Proper documentation of MTM services may be used to:

- Facilitate communication between the pharmacist and the patient's other health care professionals regarding recommendations intended to resolve or monitor actual or potential medication-related problems.
- Improve patient care and outcomes.
- Augment the continuity of patient care among health care providers and settings.
- Guarantee adherence with federal, state, and local laws and regulations for the maintenance of patient records.
- Protect against professional liability.
- Identify services provided to the patient for billing or reimbursement purposes (e.g., payer audits).
- Demonstrate the value of pharmacist provided MTM services.
- Display clinical, economic, and humanistic outcomes.

MTM documentation includes creating and maintaining an ongoing patient-specific record that contains, in chronological order, a record of all provided care in an established standard health care professional format (e.g., the SOAP [subjective observations, objective observations, assessment, and plan] note.)

Documentation should be completed electronically; however, it may be done manually. Incorporating the PMR, MAP, and other practice-specific forms will assist the pharmacist in maintaining appropriate professional documentation. The use of consistent documentation will help facilitate collaboration among members of the health care team while accommodating practitioner, facility, organizational, or regional variations.

Documentation elements for the patient record	
Documentation category	**Examples**
Patient demographics	Basic information: address, phone, email, gender, age, ethnicity, education status, patient's special needs, health plan benefit/insurance coverage

Documentation elements for the patient record —cont'd	
Documentation category	**Examples**
Subjective observations	Pertinent patient-reported information: previous medical history, family history, social history, chief complaints, allergies, previous adverse drug reactions
Objective observations	Known allergies, diseases, conditions, laboratory results, vital signs, diagnostic signs, physical examination results, review of systems
Assessment	Problem list, assessment of medication-related problems
Plan	A care plan is the health care professional's course of action for helping a patient achieve specific health goals
Education	Instruction provided to the patient with verification of understanding
Collaboration	Communication with other health care professionals: recommendations, referrals, and correspondence with other professionals (cover letter, SOAP note)
PMR	Documentation of all medications, including prescription and nonprescription medications, dietary supplements and herbal product
MAP	Documentation containing a list of patient actions used in tracking progress for self-management
Follow-up	Transition plan or scheduling of next follow-up visit
Billing	Time spent on patient care, complexity of the care, and the amount charged

MAP, medication-related action plan; *PMR*, personal medication record; *SOAP*, subjective observations, objective observations, assessment, and plan.

Pharmacist and pharmacy technician's role in documenting MTM services		
Documenting MTM services	**Pharmacist**	**Pharmacy technician**
Patient demographics	X	X
Subjective observations	X	X
Objective observations	X	
Assessment	X	
Plan	X	
Education	X	X
Collaboration	X	
PMR	X	X
MAP	X	X
Follow-up	X	
Billing		X

MAP, medication-related action plan; *MTM*, medication therapy review; *PMR*, personal medication record.

Centers for Medicare and Medicaid Services requirements for offering medication therapy management services

MTM programs:

- Must ensure optimum therapeutic outcomes for targeted beneficiaries through improved medication use
- Must reduce the risk of adverse events
- Must be developed in cooperation with licensed and practicing pharmacists and physicians
- Must describe the resources and time required to implement the program if using outside personnel and establishes the fees for pharmacists or others
- May be furnished by pharmacists or other qualified providers
- May distinguish between services in ambulatory and institutional settings
- Must be coordinated with any care management plan established for a targeted individual under a chronic care improvement program

Medication therapy management criteria (effective 2021)

- Multiple chronic conditions (the minimum threshold can be set at two or three conditions; however, plans cannot require *more* than three chronic conditions as the minimum number)
- Multiple Part D drugs (plans can set the minimum threshold anywhere between two and eight, but plans cannot require *more* than eight drugs as the minimum number)
- Likely to incur annual costs for medications of at least $4376

Core chronic conditions covered under medication therapy management

- Alzheimer's disease
- Bone disease/arthritis (e.g., osteoporosis, osteoarthritis, rheumatoid arthritis)
- Chronic heart failure
- Diabetes
- Dyslipidemia (abnormal amount of lipids, such as cholesterol or fat, in the blood)
- End-stage renal disease
- Hypertension
- Mental health disorder (e.g., depression, schizophrenia, bipolar disorder, chronic or disabling disorder)
- Respiratory disease (e.g., asthma, chronic obstructive pulmonary disease, or chronic obstructive pulmonary disease or chronic lung disorder)

Decision making and prioritization

Opportunities for the identification of patients targeted for MTM services may result from many sources including, but not limited to, pharmacist identification, physician referral, patient self-referral, and health plan or other payer referral.

Pharmacists may wish to notify physicians or other health care professionals in their community or physicians within their facility, if applicable, of their MTM services, so that physicians may refer patients for MTM services.

To aid in prioritizing who may benefit most from MTM services, pharmacists, health plans, physicians, other health care professionals, and health systems may consider using one or more of the following factors to target patients who are likely to benefit most from MTM services:

- Patient has experienced a transition of care, and their regimen has changed.
- Patient is receiving care from more than one prescriber.
- Patient is taking five or more chronic medications (including prescription and nonprescription medications, herbal products, and other dietary supplements).
- Patient has at least one chronic disease or chronic health condition (e.g., heart failure, diabetes, hypertension, hyperlipidemia, asthma, osteoporosis, depression, osteoarthritis, chronic obstructive pulmonary disease).
- Patient has laboratory values outside the normal range that could be caused by or may be improved with medication therapy.
- Patient has demonstrated nonadherence (including underuse and overuse) to a medication regimen.
- Patient has limited health literacy or cultural differences, requiring special communication strategies to optimize care.
- Patient has experienced a loss or significant change in health plan benefit or insurance coverage.
- Patient has recently experienced an adverse event (medication-related or non-medication-related) while receiving care.
- Patient is taking high-risk medication(s), including narrow therapeutic index drugs (e.g., warfarin, phenytoin, lithium, levothyroxine, methotrexate).
- Patient wants or needs to reduce out-of-pocket medication costs.
- Patient self-identifies and demonstrates an observed need for MTM services.

Required medication therapy management billing fields

- The CMS requires that pharmacists who wish to bill for MTM obtain a National Provider Identifier.
- Pharmacies and organizations must maintain a separate National Provider Identifier from that of individual pharmacists.
- Current Procedural Technology (CPT) codes are used for billing MTM.

CPT 99605	Medication therapy management service(s) provided by pharmacist, individual, face-to-face with patient, with assessment and intervention if provided; new patient visit, initial 15 min
CPT 99606	Medication therapy management service(s) provided by pharmacist, individual, face-to-face with patient, with assessment and intervention if provided; established patient visit, initial 15 min
CPT 99607	Additional 15-min increments (use with either CPT 99605 or CPT 99606)

CHAPTER REVIEW QUESTIONS

1. A patient receives a prescription for an angiotensin-converting enzyme inhibitor. A condition in which body system is being treated?
   a. Cardiovascular system
   b. Circulatory system
   c. Endocrine system
   d. Respiratory system

2. Which dosage form consists of a concentrated solution of sugar in water or other aqueous liquid?
   a. Emulsion
   b. Suspension
   c. Syrup
   d. Tincture

3. Which of the following is an example of a parenteral dosage form?
   a. Bulk powder
   b. Ophthalmic solution
   c. Rectal suppository
   d. Sublingual tablet

4. What temperature classification is 20°C to 25°C?
   a. Cool
   b. Cold
   c. Room temperature
   d. Excessive heat

5. Which medication must be refrigerated?
   a. Enbrel
   b. Spikevax
   c. Synthroid
   d. Zostavax

6. What is the maximum number of days an opened vial of insulin be stored at room temperature?
   a. 14 days
   b. 21 days
   c. 28 days
   d. 42 days

7. At what angle should a patient administer their dose of insulin?
   a. 5–15 degrees
   b. 15–35 degrees
   c. 45–90 degrees
   d. 90 degrees

8. How would you respond to a patient who asks you, "What is pruritis?"
   a. An ear ache
   b. Intense itching
   c. Runny nose
   d. Skin redness

9. A patient has read the patient product insert and observes the term "tachycardia." How would you explain the meaning of tachycardia?
   a. Bone pain
   b. Glucose in the urine
   c. Painful urination
   d. Rapid heart rate

10. Which term refers to an abnormal reaction of the immune system to a medication?
   a. ADE
   b. Drug intolerance
   c. Idiosyncratic drug reaction
   d. Medication (drug) allergy

11. Which of the following is a component of an individual's medical history?
   a. Exercise
   b. Family history
   c. Religion
   d. Substance use

12. Which form of nonadherence occurs when a new medication is prescribed for a patient but the patient fails to obtain the medication?
   a. Intentional nonadherence
   b. Primary nonadherence
   c. Secondary nonadherence
   d. Unintentional nonadherence

13. The pharmacy technician measures a patient's blood pressure and observes it is 115/70. How would the patient's blood pressure be classified?
   a. Hypertensive crisis
   b. Elevated
   c. Normal
   d. Stage 1 hypertension

14. Which substance is a non-water-soluble lipid, which is transported in lipoprotein particles, which are water-soluble?
   a. Apolipoprotein B
   b. Cholesterol
   c. Triglycerides
   d. Very low-density lipoprotein cholesterol

15. Which of the following is a demonstrated outcome associated with MTM?
   a. Cutting health care costs due to duplicate or unnecessary prescriptions
   b. Decreasing medication-related morbidity and mortality
   c. Increasing patients' understanding and self-management skills of their medication
   d. Reducing preventable adverse events

16. Which of the following activities can a pharmacy technician perform with an MTR?
   a. Assess, identify, and prioritize medication-related problems
   b. Design a plan to address each identified medication related problem
   c. Provide suggestions to address a patient's identified medication problems to the physician
   d. Schedule eligible patients for MTM consultations

17. Which medications are listed in a patient's PMR?
   a. Herbal products
   b. Nonprescription medications
   c. Prescription medications
   d. All of the above

18. Which of the following tasks may a pharmacy technician perform in developing a patient's MAP?
   a. Remind patients of follow-up physician appointments
   b. Remind patients of scheduled laboratory tests
   c. Review patient refill history
   d. All of the above

19. What task may a pharmacy technician perform during the intervening/referring a patient phase for MTM services?
   a. Assisting in developing written communication to physician or other health care professional

b. Consulting the physician on the selection of medications

c. Developing a collaborative agreement with a physician

d. Providing suggestions to the physicians to address medication problems

20. Who determines what is covered under a CPA between a physician and a pharmacist?
    a. CMS
    b. FDA
    c. National Association of Boards of Pharmacy
    d. State

21. Which of the following is a chronic condition covered under MTM according to CMS enrolled in Medicare Part D?
    a. Herpes zoster (shingles)
    b. Hypertension
    c. Hypothyroidism
    d. Pneumonia

22. Which CPT code is used in in billing for MTM for a pharmacist's services for a new patient?
    a. CPT 99064
    b. CPT 99065
    c. CPT 99606
    d. CPT 99607

23. A patient presents a prescription for a proton pump inhibitor. Which body system is being treated?
    a. Cardiovascular
    b. Circulatory
    c. Endocrine
    d. Gastrointestinal

24. Which type of oral dosage form is formulated so that it travels through the stomach to the small intestine before the medication is released?
    a. Capsule
    b. Enteric coated tablet
    c. Sublingual table
    d. Troche

25. Which condition affects the patient's airways in the lungs?
    a. Asthma
    b. Dysrhythmia
    c. Edema
    d. Pneumonia

REFERENCES

US Food and Drug Administration. Orange book preface. Accessed August 1, 2022. https://www.fda.gov/drugs/development-approval-process-drugs/orange-book-preface

Velo, G. P., & Minuz, P. (2009). Medication errors: prescribing faults and prescription errors. *Br J Clin Pharmacol*, *67*(6), 624–628. https://doi.org/10.1111/j.1365-2125.2009.03425.x.

Council on Credentialing in Pharmacy, Albanese, N. P., & Rouse, M. J. (2003). Scope of contemporary pharmacy practice: roles, responsibilities, and functions of pharmacists and pharmacy technicians. *J Am Pharm Assoc*, *2010*(50), e35–e69.

Centers for Disease Control and Prevention (CDC), Published 2017. Accessed June 2, 2022. https://www.cdc.gov/dhdsp/pubs/docs/CPA-Team-Based-Care.pdf

Centers for Medicare and Medicaid Services. CMS physician/non-physician collaborative practice plan guidelines. Accessed June 2, 2022. http://www.cms.org/uploads/CollabPracticePlan.pdf

RESOURCES

Medication Adherence: Improve Patient Outcomes and Reduce Costs, Accessed March 24, 2023. https://edhub.ama-assn.org/steps-forward/module/2702595

The American Pharmacists Association. Accessed March 24, 2023. https://www.aphafoundation.org/medication-therapy-management

7

Immunization Administration Certificate

Immunization administration domains

Concepts/terminology of vaccine administration (30%)

- Roles of pharmacy technicians in supporting immunizations
- Definition of key terms in the immunization process (e.g., active vs. passive immunity, inactivated vs. live attenuated vaccine)
- Common vaccinations and vaccination schedules (e.g., influenza; zoster; pneumococcal; tetanus, diphtheria, and acellular pertussis)

Vaccine safety and administration (50%)

- Preparation for vaccine administration, including supply selection (e.g., reconstitution, needle length)
- Procedures for vaccine administration: subcutaneous, intramuscular, inhalation
- Safety considerations during vaccine administration (e.g., handling and disposal of sharps)

Documentation, product handling, and adverse reaction management for vaccines (20%)

- Procedures for immunization-related documentation (e.g., Vaccine Information Statement forms)
- Procedures for receiving, storing, and handling of vaccines (e.g., cold chain, disposal)
- Managing vaccine-related adverse reactions and emergency situations (e.g., localized reactions, syncope, anaphylaxis, Vaccine Adverse Event Reporting System vs. Vaccine Error Reporting Program)

Concepts/terminology of vaccine administration

Pharmacy technician role

The pharmacist is responsible for verifying the vaccine order, reviewing the immunization screening questions, ensuring the vaccine is appropriate for the patient, counseling the patient, and answering medical questions. Prior to 2017, pharmacy technicians were responsible for providing administrative tasks, screening such as preparing supplies, selecting the correct needle and syringe, drawing up vaccine doses into a syringe, documenting, monitoring vaccine inventory, billing of immunizations, addressing emergency situations, reporting of adverse events, calling and scheduling patients, and screening patients.[1] Since 2017, several states (Idaho, Michigan, Rhode Island, and Utah) amended their scope of practice rules and regulations, which now permit pharmacy technicians to immunize patients. In those states that permit pharmacy technicians to immunize patients, it is the pharmacist responsibility to delegate this task to the qualified pharmacy technician.

In August 2020, the Department of Health and Human Services amended the Public Readiness and Emergency Preparedness Act, which permits pharmacy technicians to administer immunizations if they have met specific requirements in all states.

Requirements to permit pharmacy technicians to perform immunizations	
Category	Public Readiness and Emergency Preparedness Act requirement[2]
Pharmacist requirements	■ Vaccination must be ordered by supervising qualified pharmacist. ■ The pharmacist must be available for the immunizing qualified pharmacy technician.

(Continued)

Requirements to permit pharmacy technicians to perform immunizations —cont'd	
Category	Public Readiness and Emergency Preparedness Act requirement[2]
Vaccine requirements	■ Vaccine must be FDA authorized or FDA licensed. ■ For COVID-19 vaccines, vaccination must be ordered and administered according to ACIP's COVID-19 vaccine recommendations. ■ Vaccinations must be ordered and administered according to ACIP's standard immunization schedule.
Technician requirements	■ Qualified pharmacy technician/state-authorized pharmacy intern must satisfactorily complete a practical training program approved by ACPE. The program must include a hands-on injection technique and recognition and treatment of emergency reactions to vaccines. ■ The qualified pharmacy technician/pharmacy intern must have a current certificate in basic cardiopulmonary resuscitation. ■ The qualified pharmacy technician must complete a minimum of 2 hours of ACPE-approved, immunization-related continuing pharmacy education during the state licensing period(s).
Requirements for reporting, record keeping, and referral	■ Supervising qualified pharmacist must comply with record-keeping and reporting requirements of the state in which they administer vaccines. This includes notifying the patient's primary care provider when available and submitting required immunization information to state/local information system (vaccine registry). ■ Suervising pharmacist is responsible for adhering to requirements for reporting adverse events. They must review vaccine registry or other vaccination records prior to ordering vaccination to be administered by qualified pharmacy technician/state-authorized pharmacy intern. ■ Qualified pharmacy technician/state-authorized pharmacy intern must, if patient is <18 years of age, inform patient and adult caregiver accompanying patient of importance of a well-child visit with a pediatrician or other licensed primary care provider and refer patients as appropriate. ■ Supervising qualified pharmacist must comply with any applicable requirements according to CDC's COVID-19 vaccination provider agreement an any other federal requirements that apply to administration of COVID-19 vaccines.

CDC, Centers for Disease Control and Prevention.

Immunization terminology

■ Adjuvants: A substance found in a vaccine used to help boost the body's response to the vaccine (e.g., aluminum salts).

■ Active immunity: Immunity as a result of exposure to a disease organism that triggers the immune system to produce antibodies to that disease.

■ Anaphylaxis: An acute, potentially life-threatening, immunoglobulin E-mediated allergic reaction that occurs in previously sensitized people when they are reexposed to the sensitizing antigen. Symptoms can include stridor, dyspnea, wheezing, and hypotension.

■ Antibodies: Complex molecules (immunoglobulins) made in response to an antigen's presence (e.g., a protein of bacteria or other infecting organism) that neutralizes a foreign substance's effect.

■ Antigen: A substance that causes antibody production, resulting in an immune response.

■ Antigen-presenting cell: An immune system cell that presents antigens to lymphocytes to activate an immune response.

■ Attenuated: An altered or weakened live vaccine made from the disease organism against which the vaccine protects.

■ Cold chain: A temperature-controlled supply chain that includes all vaccine-related equipment and procedures. The cold chain begins with the cold storage unit at the manufacturing plant and includes the transportation, delivery of the vaccine, and proper storage at the provider facility and ends when the vaccine is administered to the patient.

■ Cytokine: A protein that signals cells of the immune system.

■ Humoral immunity: The immune response mediated by antibodies.

■ Immunity: An infection resistance type caused by the body's immune response after exposure to antigens or vaccine administration.

■ Immunization: A process by which a person becomes protected against a disease through vaccination.

■ Inactivated vaccine: A vaccine composed of dead or inactivated viruses and bacteria.

■ Innate immunity: Natural immunity.

■ Lyophilization: A process in which water is removed from a product after it is frozen and placed under a vacuum, allowing the ice to change directly from solid to vapor without passing through a liquid phase.

■ Live attenuated vaccine: A disease-causing virus or bacterium that is weakened in a laboratory so it cannot cause disease.

■ Natural immunity: Immunity acquired from exposure to the disease organism through infection with actual disease.

■ Passive immunity: Immunity as a result of a patient being administered antibodies to a disease rather than producing them through their own immune system.

■ Preservative: A substance found in a vaccine to prevent contamination. An example is thimerosal.

■ Stabilizers: A substance found in a vaccine to keep vaccine effective after it is manufactured. Sugars and gelatin are examples of stabilizers.

■ Toxoid: A chemically modified toxin from a pathogenic microorganism, which is no longer toxic but is still antigenic and can be used as a vaccine.

■ Vaccination: The act of introducing a vaccine into the body to produce protection from a specific disease.

- Vaccine: A preparation that is used to stimulate the body's immune response against diseases.
- Vaccine-induced immunity: Immunity acquired through the introduction of a killed or weakened form of the disease organism through vaccination.
- Virion: A virus particle.

- Virus: A microscopic, nonliving organism that replicates exclusivity inside the host's cell using parts of the host cell, including DNA, ribosomes, and proteins.

Common vaccinations and vaccination schedules

Recommended child and adolescent immunization schedule (birth through 18 years)					
Vaccine	**Abbreviation**	**Brand**	**Minimum age**	**Series**	**Administered[3]**
COVID-19 (Pfizer-BioNTech)	COVID 19 mRNA-1273	Comimaty (Pfizer-BioNTech) Spikevax (Moderna)	6 months	2 or 3 dose series (individuals 12 years of age and older should receive a booster)	Primary series: • Age 6 months–4 years: 2-dose series at 0, 4-8 weeks (Moderna) or 3-dose series at 0, 3-8, 11-16 weeks (Pfizer-BioNTech) • Age 5–11 years: 2-dose series at 0, 4-8 weeks (Moderna) or 2-dose series at 0, 3-8 weeks (Pfizer-BioNTech) • Age 12–18 years: 2-dose series at 0, 4-8 weeks (Moderna) or 2-dose series at 0, 3-8 weeks (Pfizer-BioNTech)hange
Diphtheria, tetanus, and acellular pertussis	DTaP	Daptacel Infanrix	6 weeks	5 doses	2, 4, 6, and 15–18 months, 4–6 years
Diphtheria, tetanus	DT	No brand name	6 weeks to 6 years	5 doses	0.5 mL IM q 4–8 weeks ×3 doses, then 0.5 mL IM ×1 at 15–18 month, then 0.5 mL IM ×1 at 4–6 years old; info: may give 4th dose as early as 12 months and 6 months after 3rd dose; 5th dose not needed if 4th dose given after 4th birthday and at least 6 months after 3rd dose
Haemophilus influenzae type b	Hib (PRP-T) Hib (PRP-OMB)	ActHIB, Hiberix, or Pentacel	6 weeks	4 doses	2, 4, 6, 12–15 months
		Pedvax	6 weeks	3 doses	2, 4, 12–15 months
Hepatitis A	HepA	Havrix, Vaqta	12 months	2 doses	Beginning at 12 months with 6-month interval
Hepatitis B	HepB	Engerix-B, Recombivax HB	Birth	3 doses	0, 1–2, 6–18 months
Human papillomavirus	HPV	Gardasil 9	11–12 years (can start at 9 years)	2- or 3-dose series	9–14 years at initial vaccination: 2-dose series at 0, 6–12 months (minimum interval: months) 15 years or older at initial vaccination: 3-dose series at 0, 1–2 months, 6 months (minimum intervals: dose 1 to dose 2: 4 weeks; dose 2 to dose 3: 12 weeks; dose 1 to dose 3: 5 months; repeat dose if administered too soon
Influenza (inactivated)	IIV	IIV-multiple manufacturers	6 months	1 or 2 doses based on patient age	2 doses, separated by at least 4 weeks, for children aged 6 months to 8 years who have received fewer than 2 influenza vaccine doses before July 1, 2020, or whose influenza vaccination history is unknown (administer dose 2 even if the child turns 9 between receipt of dose 1 and dose 2) 1 dose for children aged 6 months to 8 years who have received at least 2 influenza vaccine doses before July 1, 2020 1 dose for all persons aged 9 years or older
Influenza (live, attenuated)	LAIV4	LAIV-FluMist Quadrivalent	2 years	1 dose	0.1 mL spray in each nostril one time annually

(Continued)

Recommended child and adolescent immunization schedule (birth through 18 years)—cont'd

Vaccine	Abbreviation	Brand	Minimum age	Series	Administered[3]
Measles, mumps, and rubella	MMR	M-M-R II	12 months	2 doses	12–15 months, 4–6 years; 2nd dose may be administered as early as weeks after dose 1
Meningococcal serotype A-C-W-Y	MenACWY-CRM (Menveo) MenACWY-D (Menactra) MenACWY-TT (MenQuadfi)	Menveo, Menactra, MenQuadfi	Menveo, 2 months; Menactra, 9 months' MenQuadfi, 2 years	2 doses	2-dose series at age 11–12 years and at 16 years
Meningococcal serotype B	MenB-4C (Bexsero); MenB-FHbp (Trumenba)	Bexsero, Trumenba	10 years	2 doses	Bexsero: 2-dose series at least 1 month apart Trumenba: 2-dose series at least 6 months apart; if dose 2 is administered earlier than 6 months, administer a 3rd dose at least 4 months after dose 2
Pneumococcal 13-valent conjugate	PCV13	Prevnar 13	6 weeks	4 doses	4-dose series at 2, 4, 6, 12–15 months
Pneumococcal 23-valent polysaccharide	PPSV23	Pneumovax	2 years	1 dose	0.5 mL SC/IM ×1 dose; info: give >8 weeks after PCV13; repeat ×1 in 5 years if sickle cell disease, hemoglobinopathy, asplenia, immunocompromised
Poliovirus (inactivated)	IPV	IPOL	6 weeks	4 doses	4-dose series at ages 2, 4, 6–18 months, 4–6 years; administer the final dose on or after age 4 years and at least 6 months after the previous dose
Rotavirus	RV1 RV5	RV1: Rotarix RV5: RotaTeq	6 weeks	Rotarix, 2 doses; RotaTeq, 3 doses	Rotarix: 2-dose series at 2 and 4 months RotaTeq: 3-dose series at 2, 4, and 6 months
Tetanus, diphtheria, and acellular pertussis	Tdap	Adacel Boostrix	11 years	1 dose	Adolescents aged 11–12 years: 1 dose Tdap Pregnancy: 1 dose Tdap during each pregnancy, preferably during the early part of gestational weeks 27–36
Tetanus and diphtheria vaccine	Td	Tenivac TDvax	7 years	3 doses	0.5 mL IM ×2 doses at least 4 weeks apart, then 0.5 mL IM × 1 dose 6–12 months after prior dose
Varicella	VAR	Varivax	12 months	2 doses	2-dose series at 12–15 months, 4–6 years

IM, intramuscular; *q*, every; *SQ*, subcutaneous.

Combination vaccinations

Vaccine	Abbreviation	Trade names
DTaP, hepatitis B, and inactivated poliovirus vaccine	DTaP-HepB-IPV	Pediarix
DTaP, inactivated poliovirus, and Haemophilus influenzae type B vaccine	DTaP-IPV/Hib	Pentacel
DTaP and inactivated poliovirus vaccine	DTaP-IPV	Kinrix, Quadracel
DTaP, inactivated poliovirus, Haemophilus influenzae type b, and hepatitis B vaccine	DTaP-IPV-Hib-HepB	Vaxelis
Measles, mumps, rubella, and varicella vaccines	MMRV	ProQuad

Recommended adult immunization schedule for ages 19 years or older

Vaccine	Abbreviation	Brand name	Routine vaccine[4]
COVID-19	BNT162b2	Comirnaty	Age 16 years and older: a 2-dose series where the second dose is administered every 21 days after the second shot; a booster, either Pfizer-BioNTech or Moderna, may be administered 5 months after the second dose
	mRNA-1273	Spikevax	Age 18 years and older: a 2-dose series 28 days after the second shot; a booster, either Pfizer-BioNTech or Moderna, may be administered 5 months after the second dose

(Continued)

Recommended adult immunization schedule for ages 19 years or older—cont'd			
Vaccine	Abbreviation	Brand name	Routine vaccine[4]
	JNJ-78436735		One dose; booster should be either Pfizer-BioNTech or Moderna and be received at least 2 months after receiving dose
Haemophilus influenzae type B	Hib	ActHIB Hiberix	For previously unvaccinated patients with asplenia, sickle cell disease; give at least 2 weeks prior to elective splenectomy; give 3 doses 4 weeks apart starting at 6–12 months after successful hematopoietic stem cell transplant
Hepatitis A	HepA	Havrix Vaqta	Not at risk but want protection from hepatitis A: 2-dose series HepA (Havrix 6–12 months apart or Vaqta 6–18 months apart [minimum interval: 6 months]) or 3-dose series HepA-HepB (Twinrix at 0, 1, 6 months [minimum intervals: dose 1 to dose 2: 4 weeks; dose 2 to dose 3: 5 months])
Hepatitis B	HepB	Engerix-B Recombivax HB Heplisav-B	Age 19 through 59 years: complete a 2- or 3-, or 4-dose series 2-dose series only applies when 2 doses of Heplisav-B* are used at least 4 weeks apart 3-dose series Engerix-B or Recombivax HB at 0, 1, 6 months (minimum intervals: dose 1 to dose 2: 4 weeks; dose 2 to dose 3: 8 weeks; dose 1 to dose 3: 16 weeks) 3-dose series HepA-HepB (Twinrix at 0, 1, 6 months [minimum intervals: dose 1 to dose 2: 4 weeks; dose 2 to dose 3: 5 months]) 4-dose series HepA-HepB (Twinrix) accelerated schedule of 3 doses at 0, 7, and 21–30 days, followed by a booster dose at 12 months 4-dose series Engerix-B at 0, 1, 2, and 6 months for persons on adult hemodialysis (Note: each dosage is double that of normal adult dose, i.e., 2 mL instead of 1 mL.)
Human papillomavirus	HPV	Gardasil	HPV vaccination recommended for all persons through age 26 years: 2- or 3-dose series depending on age at initial vaccination or condition: Age 15 years or older at initial vaccination: 3-dose series at 0, 1–2 months, 6 months (minimum intervals: dose 1 to dose 2: 4 weeks; dose 2 to dose 3: 12 weeks; dose 1 to dose 3: 5 months; repeat dose if administered too soon) Age 9–14 years at initial vaccination and received 1 dose or 2 doses less than 5 months apart: 1 additional dose Age 9–14 years at initial vaccination and received 2 doses at least 5 months apart: HPV vaccination series complete, no additional dose needed
Influenza, inactivated	IIV	Multiple brands	Age 19 years or older: 1 dose any influenza vaccine appropriate for age and health status annually
Measles, mumps, and rubella	MMR	M-M-R II	No evidence of immunity to measles, mumps, or rubella: 1 dose
Meningococcal serogroups A, C, W, Y	MenACWY	MenACWY-D MenACWY-CRM MenACWY-TT	First-year college students who live in residential housing (if not previously vaccinated at age 16 years or older) or military recruits: 1 dose MenACWY (Menactra, Menveo, or MenQuadfi)
Meningococcal serogroup B	MenB-C MenB-FHbp	Bexsero Trumenba	Adolescents and young adults age 16–23 years (age 16–18 years preferred) not at increased risk for meningococcal disease: based on shared clinical decision-making, 2-dose series MenB-4C (Bexsero) at least 1 month apart or 2-dose series MenB-FHbp (Trumenba) at 0, 6 months (if dose 2 was administered less than 6 months after dose 1, administer dose 3 at least 4 months after dose 2); MenB-4C and MenB-FHbp are not interchangeable (use same product for all doses in series)
Pneumococcal 13-valent conjugate	PCV13	Prevnar 13	For high-risk patients 19 years old and older; may be given to low-risk patients 65 years old and older based on shared clinical decision-making; follow with PPSV23 after >8 weeks in high-risk patients or after >1 year in immunocompetent pts 65 years old and older; if prior PPSV23 but no PCV13 at 65 years old or older, give PCV13 >1 year after last PPSV23 dose
Pneumococcal 23-valent polysaccharide vaccine	PPSV23	Pneumovax 23	For high-risk patients <65 years old and all patients 65 years old and older per ACIP guidelines; give >8 weeks after PCV13 or PCV15 if high risk, otherwise give >1 year after PCV13 or PCV15; repeat ×1 after 5 years in high-risk patients or in patients 65 years old and older who received 1st dose when <65 years old and >5 years ago
Tetanus and diphtheria toxoids	Td	Tenivac Tdvax	0.5 mL IM ×2 doses at least 4 weeks apart, then 0.5 mL IM ×1 dose 6–12 months after prior dose

(Continued)

Recommended adult immunization schedule for ages 19 years or older—cont'd			
Vaccine	**Abbreviation**	**Brand name**	**Routine vaccine[4]**
Tetanus and diph-theria toxoids and acellular pertussis	Tdap	Adacel Boostrix	Previously did not receive Tdap at or after age 11 years: 1 dose Tdap, then Td or Tdap every 10 years
Varicella	VAR	Varivax	No evidence of immunity to varicella: 2-dose series 4–8 weeks apart if previously did not receive varicella-containing vaccine (VAR or MMRV [measles-mumps-rubella-varicella vaccine] for children); if previously received 1 dose varicella-containing vaccine, 1 dose at least 4 weeks after first dose Evidence of immunity: US-born before 1980 (except for pregnant women and health care personnel [see below]), documentation of 2 doses varicel-la-containing vaccine at least 4 weeks apart, diagnosis or verification of history of varicella or herpes zoster by a health care provider, laboratory evidence of immunity or disease
Zoster, recombinant	RZV	Shingrix	Age 50 years or older: 2-dose series RZV (Shingrix) 2–6 months apart (min-imum interval: 4 weeks; repeat dose if administered too soon), regardless of previous herpes zoster or history of zoster vaccine live (ZVL, Zostavax) vaccination (administer RZV at least 2 months after ZVL)

ACIP, Advisory Committee of Immunization Practices; *IM*, intramuscular.

Vaccine safety and administration

Vaccine administration preparation

Infection control

- Hand hygiene should be conducted prior to vaccine preparation, between patients, and any time hands become soiled (e.g., when diapering).
- Hands should be washed with a waterless, alcohol-based hand rub or soap and water. When hands are visibly dirty or contaminated with blood or other body fluids, they should be washed thoroughly with soap and water.

Reconstituting vaccines

Refer to package inserts for complete instructions on reconsti-tuting specific vaccines.

1. For single-dose vaccine products (except Rotarix), select a syringe and needle of proper length to be used for both reconstitution and administration of the vaccine. For Rotarix, refer to the package insert.
2. Before reconstituting, check labels on both the lyophilized vaccine vial and the diluent to verify that
   - They are the appropriate products to mix together.

- The diluent is the correct volume.
- Neither the vaccine nor the diluent has expired.
3. Reconstitute vaccine just prior to use by:
   - Removing the protective caps and cleaning each stopper with an alcohol swab
   - Inserting the needle of the syringe into diluent vial and withdrawing the entire contents
   - Injecting diluent into lyophilized vaccine vial and rotating or inverting to carefully mix the lyophilized powder
4. Check the appearance of the reconstituted vaccine.
   - Reconstituted vaccine may be used if the color and appearance correspond to the description on the package insert.
   - If there is discoloration, extraneous particulate matter, obvious lack of resuspension, or the vaccine cannot be thoroughly mixed, mark the vial as "Do Not Use," return it to proper storage conditions, and contact the local health department immunization program or the vaccine manufacturer.
5. If reconstituted vaccine is not used immediately or comes in a multidose vial, be sure to:
   - clearly mark the vial with the date and time then vaccine was reconstituted,
   - maintain the product at 2°C–8°C (36°F–46°F); do not freeze, and
   - use only within the time indicated on chart above.

Vaccines with diluents[5]				
Vaccine product name	**Lyophilizedvaccine (powder)**	**Liquid diluent (may contain vaccine)**	**Time allowed between reconstitution and use, as stated in package insert**	**Diluent Storage environment**
ActHIB (Hib)	Hib	0.4% sodium chloride	24h	Refrigerator
Hiberix (Hib)	Hib	0.9% sodium chloride	24h	Refrigerator or room temp
Imovax (RABHDCV)	Rabies virus	Sterile water	Immediately	Refrigerator
M-M-R II (MMR)	MMR	Sterile water	8h	Refrigerator or room temp

(Continued)

Vaccines with diluents[5]—cont'd				
Vaccine product name	Lyophilizedvaccine (powder)	Liquid diluent (may contain vaccine)	Time allowed between reconstitution and use, as stated in package insert	Diluent Storage environment
Menveo (MenACWY)	MenA	MenCWY	8 h	Refrigerator
Pentacel (DTaP-IPV/Hib)	Hib	DTaP-IPV	Immediately	Refrigerator
ProQuad (MMRV)	MMRV	Sterile water	30 min	Refrigerator or room temp
RabAvert (RABPCECV)	Rabies virus	Sterile water	Immediately	Refrigerator
Rotarix (RV1)	RV1	Sterile water, calcium carbonate, and xanthan	24 h	Refrigerator or room temp
Shingrix (RZV)	RZV	AS01B§ adjuvant suspension	6 h	Refrigerator
Varivax (VAR)	VAR	Sterile water	30 min	Refrigerator or room temp
YF-VAX (YF)	YF	0.9% sodium chloride	60 min	Refrigerator or room temp

Remember when preparing a vaccine to:

- Adhere to strict aseptic medication preparation practices.
- Perform hand hygiene prior to preparing vaccines.
- Use a specific, clean medication area that is not close to areas where contaminated items are placed.
- Avoid distractions.
- Prepare medications for one patient at a time.
- Always adhere to the manufacturer's directions found on the package inserts.

Remember when filling a syringe, *never*:

- Enter a vial with a previously used syringe or needle.
- Mix different vaccine products in the same syringe.
- Transfer vaccine from one syringe to another syringe.
- Mix partial doses from separate vials to get a full dose.

Subcutaneous injection

The following vaccines are administered subcutaneously:

- Measles, mumps and rubella (MMR)
- Varicella (VAR)
- Zoster, live (ZVL)

Administration by subcutaneous route		
Age	Needle length	Injection site
Infants (1–12 months)	5/8″	Fatty tissue over antero-lateral thigh muscle
Children 12 months or older, adolescents, and adults	5/8″	Fatty tissue over antero-lateral thigh muscle or fatty tissue over triceps

Intramuscular injections

The following vaccines are administered intramuscularly (IM):

- Diphtheria-tetanus-pertussis (DTaP, Tdap)
- Diphtheria-tetanus (DT, Td)

- *Haemophilus influenzae* type b (Hib)
- Hepatitis A (HepA)
- Hepatitis B (HepB)
- Human papillomavirus (HPV)
- Inactivated influenza (IIV)
- Meningococcal serogroups A, C, W, Y (MenACWY)
- Meningococcal serogroup B (MenB)
- Pneumococcal conjugate (PCV13)
- Zoster, recombinant (RZV)

Intramuscular administration for children and adolescents		
Age	Needle size and gauge	Injection site
Newborn (0–28 days)	5/8″; 22–25 gauge	Anterolateral thigh muscle
Infant (1–12 months)	1″; 22–25 gauge	Anterolateral thigh muscle
Toddler (1–2 years)	1–1¼″; 22–25 gauge	Anterolateral thigh muscle
	5/8–1″; 22–25 gauge	Alternate site: deltoid muscle of arm if muscle mass is adequate
Children (3–10 years)	5/8–1″; 22–25 gauge	Deltoid muscle
	1–1¼″; 22–25 gauge	Alternate site: anterolateral thigh muscle
Children and adults (11 years and older)	5/8–1″; 22–25 gauge	Deltoid muscle
	1–1½″; 22–25 gauge	Alternate site: anterolateral thigh muscle

Intramuscular administration for adults (19 years or older)		
Age and gender	Needle length and gauge	Injection site
Less than 130 pounds (60 kg)	1″; 22–25 gauge	Deltoid muscle
130–152 pounds (60–70 kg)	1″; 22–25 gauge	Deltoid muscle
Men: 153–260 pounds (70–118 kg)	1–1.5″; 22–25 gauge	Deltoid muscle
Women: 153–200 pounds (70–90 kg)	1–1.5″; 22–25 gauge	Deltoid muscle
Men: greater than 260 pounds (118 kg)	1.5″; 22–25 gauge	Deltoid muscle
Women: greater than 200 pounds (90 kg)	1.5″; 22–25 gauge	Deltoid muscle

Remember needle selection is based upon the:

- Route of administration
- Patient's age
- Patient's gender and weight
- Injection site
- Injection technique

Vaccine administration procedures

Subcutaneous

The following vaccines are administered subcutaneously:

- Measles, mumps, and rubella (MMR)
- Varicella (VAR)
- Zoster, live (ZVL)

To administer a subcutaneous injection to an infant (Fig. 7.1):

1. Perform proper hand hygiene.
2. Clean the skin with a sterile alcohol swab.
3. Squeeze the subcutaneous tissue to prevent injecting into the muscle.
4. Before administering the vaccine, it is not necessary to aspirate (pull back on the syringe plunger) after needle insertion.
5. Insert needle at 45-degree angle into the fatty tissue of the anterolateral thigh.
6. Withdraw the needle.
7. Apply an adhesive bandage to the injection site of there if there is any sign of bleeding.

To administer a subcutaneous injection to a child (after their first birthday) and adults (Fig. 7.2):

1. Perform proper hand hygiene.
2. Clean the skin with a sterile alcohol swab.
3. Squeeze the subcutaneous tissue to prevent injecting into the muscle.
4. Before administering vaccine, it is not necessary to aspirate after needle insertion.

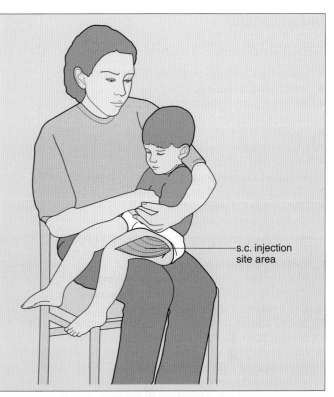

Fig. 7.1 Subcutaneous injection site for toddlers into the fatty area of anterolateral thigh. (From Keystone JS, Kozarsky PE, Freedman DO et al: *Travel Medicine*, 3rd ed. Elsevier; 2019.)

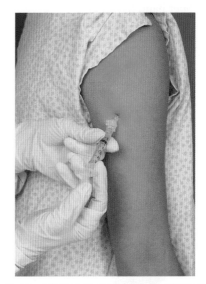

Fig. 7.2 Subcutaneous injection site for adult in the triceps muscle. (From Skidmore-Roth *Mosby's® Drug Guide for Nursing Students*, 15th ed. Elsevier; 2023.) (From Perry AG, Potter PA, and Elkin MK. *Nursing Interventions & Clinical Skills*, 5th ed. Mosby; 2012.) *Mosby's® Drug Guide for Nursing Students*, 15th ed. Elsevier; 2023.)

5. Insert needle at 45-degree angle into the fatty tissue covering the triceps muscle.
6. Withdraw the needle.
7. Apply an adhesive bandage to the injection site of there if there is any sign of bleeding.

Intramuscular

The following vaccines are administered IM:

- Diphtheria-tetanus-pertussis (DTaP, Tdap)
- Diphtheria-tetanus (DT, Td)
- *Haemophilus influenzae* type b (Hib)
- Hepatitis A (HepA)
- Hepatitis B (HepB)
- Human papillomavirus (HPV)
- Inactivated influenza (IIV)
- Meningococcal serogroups A, C, W, Y (MenACWY)
- Meningococcal serogroup B (MenB)
- Pneumococcal conjugate (PCV13)
- Zoster, recombinant (RZV)

To administer a vaccine IM for an infant or toddler (Fig. 7.3):

1. Perform proper hand hygiene.
2. Identify the appropriate administration site.
3. Clean the skin with a sterile alcohol swab.
4. Use a needle long enough to reach deep into the muscle.
5. Before administering an injection of vaccine, it is not necessary to aspirate after needle insertion.
6. Insert needle at a 90-degree angle into the anterolateral thigh muscle with a quick thrust.
7. Withdraw the needle.
8. Apply an adhesive bandage to the injection site of there if there is any sign of bleeding.

To administer a vaccine IM to a child or adult (Fig. 7.4):

1. Perform proper hand hygiene.
2. Identify the appropriate administration site.
3. Clean the skin with a sterile alcohol swab.
4. Use a needle long enough to reach deep into the muscle.

5. Before administering an injection of vaccine, it is not necessary to aspirate after needle insertion.
6. Insert needle at a 90-degree angle into the central and thickest portion of the deltoid muscle—above the level

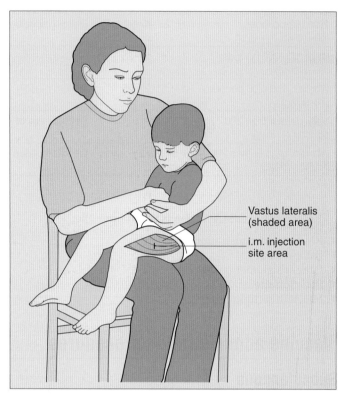

Fig. 7.3 **Intramuscular injection for toddler in the anterolateral thigh muscle.** (From Keystone JS, Kozarsky PE, Freedman DO et al. *Travel Medicine*, 3rd ed. Elsevier; 2019.)

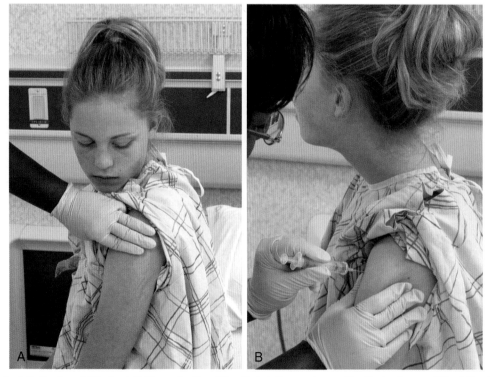

Figure 7.4 **Intramuscular injection for adult in the deltoid muscle.** (From Lilley LL et al. *Pharmacology and the Nursing Process*, 10th ed. Elsevier; 2023.)

of the armpit and two to three fingerbreadths (2 inches) below the acromion process—with a quick thrust. To avoid causing an injury, do not inject too high (near the acromion process) or too low.

7. Withdraw the needle.
8. Apply an adhesive bandage to the injection site of there if there is any sign of bleeding.

Inhalation for live attenuated influenza vaccine

FluMist is a live attenuated influenza vaccine administered intranasally. To administer an intranasal vaccine:

1. Perform proper hygiene.
2. Remove the rubber tip protector. Do not remove the dose-divider clip at the other end of the sprayer.
3. With the patient in a vertical position, place the tip just inside the nostril to ensure influenza (live, attenuated) vaccine is released into the nose. The patient should breathe normally.
4. With a single motion, push the plunger as quickly as possible until the dose-divider clip prevents you from going further.
5. Pinch and remove the dose-divider clip from the plunger.
6. Place the tip just inside the other nostril, and with a single motion, depress plunger as quickly as possible to release the remaining vaccine.
7. Dispose of the applicator in a sharps container.

Oral drops

Rotarix is an oral drop vaccine indicated for rotavirus. To administer an oral vaccine available in drops:

1. Perform proper hand hygiene.
2. Remove the cap of the vial and push the transfer adapter onto the vial (lyophilized vaccine).
3. Shake the diluent in the oral applicator. Connect the oral applicator to the transfer adapter.
4. Push the plunger of the oral applicator to transfer the diluent into the vial. The suspension will appear white and cloudy.
5. Withdraw the vaccine into the oral applicator.
6. Twist and remove the oral applicator from the vial.
7. Administer the dose by gently placing the applicator plunger into the infant's mouth toward the inner cheek and gently expelling the contents until the applicator is empty. The vaccine should not be administered directly into the throat since it may cause the patient to cough or gag, resulting in the vaccine being expelled.
8. Allow the patient to swallow.
9. Dispose the empty vial, cap, and oral applicator in an approved biological waste container according to local regulations.

Rotavirus vaccine

Rotateq

1. Tear open the pouch and remove the dosing tube. Clear the fluid from the dispensing tip by holding the tube vertically and tapping the cap.

2. Open the dosing tube in two easy motions:
   * Puncture the dispensing tip by turning the cap clockwise until it becomes tight.
   * Remove the cap by turning it counterclockwise.
3. Administer the dose by gently squeezing liquid into infant's mouth toward the inner cheek until dosing tube is empty.
4. Dispose of the empty tube and cap in an approved biological waste container according to local regulations.

Multiple vaccinations

When multiple parenteral vaccinations are administered at the same time, keep the following in mind:

- Administer combination vaccines if available.
- Administer each vaccine in a different injection site. The injection site should be 1 inch or more away from the other site.
- Vaccines that are highly reactive and have demonstrated the ability to cause an injection site reaction, such as DTaP, PCV13, should be administered in different limbs.
- For infants and younger children, if more than two vaccines are being injected into the same limb, the thigh is the preferred site due to its greater muscle mass. In older children and adults, the deltoid muscle can be used for multiple IM injections.
- Vaccines that have been identified to be painful when injected, such as HPV and MMR, should be administered after other vaccines.
- If both a vaccine and an immune globulin medication are prescribed such as Td/Tdap and tetanus immune globulin or hepatitis B vaccine and hepatitis B immune globulin, the vaccine should be administered in a separate limb from the immune globulin.

Vaccine administration safety

While administering a vaccination to a patient, if you experience a needlestick or sharps injury or an exposure to patient blood or other body fluids, the following should be done:

- Wash needlesticks and cuts with soap and water.
- Flush splashes to the nose, mouth, or skin with water.
- Irrigate eyes with clean water, saline, or sterile irrigants.
- Report the incident to your supervisor.
- Immediately seek medical treatment.

Sharps are defined as objects capable of piercing the skin and consist of contaminated needles, lancets, infusion needle sets, connection needles, and autoinjectors. To protect yourself from needlestick injuries when administering vaccines:

- Place sharps disposal containers as close as possible to you or within arm's reach (Fig. 7.5). If a wall mount is not possible, place the container on a table or a cart in an upright position. Sharps disposal containers should *not* be placed on the floor or the ground.
- Immediately after using a sharp, engage any safety feature, and place it in a sharps disposal container that is closable, puncture-resistant, leakproof on the sides and bottom, and biohazard labeled or color-coded.

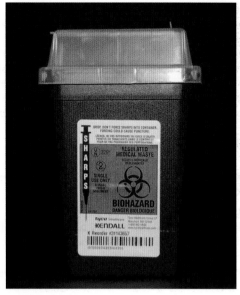

Fig. 7.5 Sharps container. (From VanMeter KC, Hubert RJ. *Microbiology for the Healthcare Professional*, 3rd ed. Elsevier; 2022.)

- Do *not* remove, recap, break, or bend contaminated needles or separate contaminated needles from syringes before disposing of them into a sharps disposal container. It is safest to immediately place the connected needle and syringe into the sharps disposal container.
- Sharps containers should be used to discard needles and other sharps contaminated with blood or other potentially infectious material.
- Close the container when it is filled to the clearly marked fill line or when it is ¾ full if it does not have a marked fill line.
- Do not overfill sharps disposal containers.

  It is important to remember that:

- Only needles and sharps are placed in sharps disposal containers.
- Anything that can be placed in regular waste containers such as uncontaminated trash, gauze, alcohol pads, needle caps, and gloves should *not* be placed in a sharps disposal container.
- Place nonsharp contaminated material, such as gauze contaminated with blood or other potentially infectious material, in a red biohazard waste disposal bag.

Sharps container disposal

Sharp containers may be disposed of by:

- Dropping them off at a drop box, a supervised collections sites or public household hazardous waste collection sites.
- Mailing back FDA-cleared sharps disposal containers to a collection site by following the manufacturer's instructions included with the disposal container.
- Arranging for special waste pickup services.

Documentation, product handing, and adverse reaction management for vaccines

Immunization-related documentation

Vaccine Information Statements (VISs) are information sheets produced by the Centers for Disease Control and Prevention (CDC). VISs describe both the benefits and risks of a vaccine to adult vaccine recipients and the parents or legal representatives of vaccinees. Federal law requires that VISs be dispensed before each dose whenever certain vaccinations are administered.

VISs must be provided when administering the following vaccines:

- DTaP
- Td and Tdap
- Hepatitis A
- Hepatitis B
- Hib
- HPV
- Influenza (inactivated and live, intranasal)
- MMR and MMRV
- Meningococcal (MenACWY, MenB)
- Pneumococcal conjugate
- Polio
- Rotavirus
- Varicella (chickenpox)

Under the National Childhood Vaccine Injury Act (i.e., adenovirus, anthrax, dengue, Japanese encephalitis, pneumococcal polysaccharide, rabies, typhoid, yellow fever, and zoster), health care providers are not compelled by federal law to use VISs unless they have been purchased under CDC contract. However, CDC recommends that VISs be used whenever these vaccines are given.

Dates of current Vaccine Information Statements (December 17, 2021)			
Vaccine	Date	Vaccine	Date
Adenovirus	January 8, 2020	MMR	August 6, 2021
Anthrax.	January 8, 2020	MMRV	August 6, 2021
Cholera	October 30, 2019	Multivaccine	October 15, 2021
Dengue	December 17, 2021	PCV13	August 6, 2021
DTaP	August 6, 2021	PPSV23	October 30, 2019
Hepatitis A	October 15, 2021	Polio	August 6, 2021
Hepatitis B	October 15, 2021	Rabies	January 8, 2020

(Continued)

Dates of current Vaccine Information Statements (December 17, 2021)—cont'd			
Vaccine	Date	Vaccine	Date
Hib	August 6, 2021	Rotavirus	October 15, 2021
HPV	August 6, 2021	Td	August 6, 2021
Influenza	August 6, 2021	Tdap	August 6, 2021
Japanese enceph	August 15, 2019	Typhoid	
MenACWY	August 6, 2021	Varicella	August 6, 2021
MenB	August 6, 2021	Yellow fever	April 1, 2020
		Zoster	October 30, 2019

DTaP, diphtheria-tetanus-pertussis; *Hib, Haemophilus influenzae* type b; *HPV*, Human papillomavirus; *MenACWY*, Meningococcal serogroups A, C, W, Y; *MENB*, Meningococcal serogroup B.

Things to remember about Vaccine Information Statements

- VIS must be given:
  - Prior to the vaccination (and prior to each dose of a multidose series)
  - Regardless of the age of the vaccinee
  - Regardless of whether the vaccine is administered
- Prior to vaccination, VIS may be:
  - Provided as a paper copy
  - Offered on a permanent, laminated office copy
  - Downloaded by the vaccinee (parent/legal representative) to a smartphone or other electronic device
  - Made available to be read before the office visit (These patients must still be provided during the immunization visit, as a reminder.)
- Federal law mandates the use of VISs in both public and private sector settings, regardless of the source of payment for the vaccine.
- A VIS is required in both public and private sector health care settings.
- A current VIS must be provided before a vaccine is administered to the patient.
- If a combination vaccine (e.g., Kinrix, Quadracel, Pediarix, Pentacel, Twinrix) is administered and does not have a stand-alone VIS, the patient should be provided with an individual VIS for the component vaccines, or use the multivaccine VIS. The multivaccine VIS may be used in place of the individual VISs for DTaP, Hib, hepatitis B, polio, and pneumococcal when two or more of these vaccines are administered during the same visit. They may be used for infants as well as children through 6 years of age. The multivaccine VIS should *not* be used for adolescents or adults.
- When possible, VISs should be provided in a language/format that the recipient can understand.
- Federal law does *not* require signed consent for a person to be vaccinated; however, some states may require it.

- To verify that a VIS was given, providers must record in the patient's medical record (or permanent office log or file) the following information:
  - The edition date of the VIS
  - The office address and name and title of the person who administers the vaccine
  - The date the VIS is provided
  - The date the vaccine is administered
  - The vaccine manufacturer and lot number
- VISs should not be altered before giving them to patients, but you can add some information.

Receiving, storing, and handling of vaccines[6]

A cold chain is a temperature-controlled supply chain that includes vaccine-related equipment and procedures. The cold chain starts with the cold storage unit at the manufacturing facility, includes the transportation and delivery of the vaccine and proper storage at the provider facility, and ends with administration of the vaccine to the patient.

A health care facility that administers vaccines must develop and maintain clearly written, detailed, and current storage and handling standard operating procedures (SOPs). The SOPs should address the following:

- General information—include contact information for vaccine manufacturers and equipment service providers. Other information to be considered includes important facility staff, job descriptions, training requirements, and frequently used forms.
- Routine storage and handling—include information for all aspects of vaccine inventory management, from ordering to monitoring storage conditions.
- Emergency vaccine storage, handling, and transport—outline steps to be taken in the event of equipment malfunctions, power failures, natural disasters, or other emergencies that might affect vaccine storage conditions.
- Employee training in the proper storage and handling of vaccines. Training should occur when an individual is hired, when new vaccines are added to the institution's formulary, and when Advisory Committee of Immunization Practices (ACIP) vaccine recommendations are updated.

Vaccine coordinator/alternate vaccine coordinator responsibilities

- Ordering vaccines
- Supervising proper receipt and storage of vaccine deliveries
- Documenting vaccine inventory information
- Coordinating and checking vaccines inventory management to include proper vaccine rotation and removing expired vaccines
- Placing temperature monitoring devices (TMDs) and ensuring daily temperatures are recorded
- Addressing temperature excursions (out-of-range temperatures) and equipment failures
- Supervising vaccine transport
- Directing emergency preparations

Receiving vaccines

Best practices for unpacking deliveries include:

- Examining the shipping container and contents for signs of damage
- Comparing the contents against the packing list
- Confirming that lyophilized vaccines arrive with the correct type and quantity of diluents
- Examining vaccine and diluent expiration dates to guarantee there are no expired or soon-to-expire products
- Inspecting the cold chain monitor for any temperature excursion
- Recording any differences between the contents and the packing list or other concerns about the contents to the vaccine manufacturer immediately
- Labeling any vaccine as "Do Not Use" if a temperature excursion is suspected

Storing vaccines

The CDC recommends the following types of refrigerators and freezers:

- Purpose-built or pharmaceutical-grade units that either refrigerate or freeze vaccines. These may be compact or under-the-counter style of large units.
- A stand-alone, household-grade unit may be an acceptable option in some practice settings; however, only the refrigerated compartment of this type of refrigerator be used since temperature variances may occur.

Storage units should:

- Be positioned in a well-ventilated room, leaving space between the unit, ceiling, and any wall
- Be level and its door should open and close smoothly
- Be placed in a room with a temperature between 20°C and 25°C (68°F and 77°F)
- Have capacity to store the largest inventory during the busiest time of the year

Temperatures

- May take 2 to 7 days to stabilize temperatures in a new or repaired refrigerator.
- Freezers may require 2–3 days to stabilize temperature.
- Prior to using a storage unit the minimum and maximum temperature must be checked and recorded daily for 2 to 7 days. If the temperatures are unable to be recorded digitally, they must be recorded a minimum of two times each day. The storage unit may be used after having two consecutive days of recorded temperatures within the recommended range.

The storage unit's power supply must be protected, and this can be accomplished by:

- Plugging in only one storage unit per electrical outlet
- Using a safety-lock plug or an outlet cover to prevent the unit from being unplugged
- Posting "Do Not Unplug" warning signs at outlets and on storage units

- Labeling fuses and circuit breakers to alert people not to turn off power to storage units
- Using caution when using power outlets that can be tripped or switched off
- Avoiding using built-in circuit switches, outlets activated by a wall switch, and multioutlet power strips

Temperature monitoring devices

- TMDs are required for all vaccine storage units, emergency transport, and backup storage units.
- The CDC suggests and the vaccines for children require the use of a continuous monitoring and recording device known as a "digital data logger" (DDL) set at recording the temperature at least every 30 minutes.

Characteristics of DDLs include:

- Detachable probe that reflects vaccine temperatures
- Alarm for out-of-range temperatures
- Low-battery indicator
- Current, minimum, and maximum temperature display
- Recommended uncertainty of ±0.5°C (±1 °F)
- Logging interval (or reading rate) that can be programmed by the user to measure and record temperatures at least every 30 minutes

DDLs must have a current and valid Certificate of Calibrations; calibration testing must be performed every 1 to 2 years depending on the manufacturer's recommendation. Information contained on the Certificate of Calibration Testing includes:

- Model/device name or number
- Serial number
- Date of calibration
- Confirmation that the instrument passed testing
- Recommended uncertainty of ±0.5°C (±1 °F) or less

Temperatures

- Refrigerators should maintain temperatures between 2°C and 8°C (36 °F and 46 °F).
- Freezers should keep temperatures between −50°C and 15°C (58 °F and +5 °F).
- The storage unit's minimum and maximum temperatures should be checked and recorded at the start of each workday.
- If a TMD is being utilized and does not display minimum and maximum temperatures, then the current temperature should be checked and recorded a minimum of two times (at the start and end of the workday).
- A temperature monitoring log sheet should be positioned near each storage unit door.

The following information should be recorded on a temperature monitoring log:

- Minimum/maximum temperature
- Date
- Time
- Name of the individual who checked and recorded the temperature

- Any actions taken for a temperature excursion (outside the temperature range established by the manufacturer)

In situations where a temperature excursion occurs:

- Notify the vaccine coordinator immediately.
- Label exposed vaccines "Do Not Use," and place them in a separate container away from other vaccines in the storage unit.
- Document the details of the incident.
- Follow the institution's SOP for temperature excursions to include checking the temperature monitoring device.
- Contact the vaccine manufacturer.
- Document actions taken and results of the actions.

Storage units and TMDs require maintenance, which can be accomplished by:

- Inspecting the storage unit door seals frequently for signs of wear and tear.
- Examining the door hinges and correct so that the door opens and closes easily and fits appropriately against the body of the unit.
- Cleaning unit coils and motor according to manufacturer instructions.
- Cleaning inside of units to prevent bacterial and fungal growth.
- Defrost manual-defrost freezers when the frost is greater than 1 cm or the manufacturer's recommended limit.
- Temperature monitoring devices undergoing "drift" over time that affects accuracy. If calibration testing reveals the device is no longer accurate within ±0.5°C (±1 °F), it should be replaced.

Vaccine inventory management

- Should be inventoried at least once a month and prior to ordering additional vaccines and diluents.
- Should be rotated and checked for expired doses consistently.
- Expired vaccines and diluents should be removed immediately to avoid accidentally administering them.
- Vaccines with an expiration date listed as a month and year may be used until the last day of the month of that year.
- When a drug manufacturer designates a beyond-use date (BUD), the vaccines must be used prior to the expiration date on the label. The BUD is determined based on the date the vial is first punctured and the storage information in the package insert. When a vaccine does not have a BUD, the vaccine should be used by the expiration date indicated by the manufacturer.
- The BUD replaces the expiration date and should be recorded on the label, along with the initials of the person performing the calculation.

Important things to remember regarding beyond-use dates

- Once a reconstituted vaccine is mixed with a diluent, you should refer to the medication's package insert.
- Once a multidose vial vaccine has been entered, refer to the medication's package insert to determine the BUD.

- Manufacturer-shortened expiration dates may apply when vaccine is exposed to inappropriate storage conditions.
- Some multidose vials have a specific number of doses that can be withdrawn. Once the maximum number of doses has been removed, discard the vial and any residual vaccine.

Best practices in storing vaccines

- Store vaccines in their original packaging with lids closed in separate containers until ready for administration to protect them from light and provide additional thermal stability/protection.
- Place vaccines and diluents with the earliest expiration dates in front of those with later expiration dates.
- Store vaccines and diluents with similar packaging or names or with pediatric and adult formulations on different shelves.
- Store diluent with the corresponding refrigerated vaccine whenever possible; never store diluents in a freezer.
- Place vaccines and diluents 2 to 3 inches from the unit walls, ceiling, floor, and door.
- Position vaccines and diluents in rows and allow space between them to promote air circulation.
- Avoid storing vaccines and diluents in any part of a household-grade storage unit that may not provide stable temperatures or sufficient air flow.
- Position water bottles on the top shelf, the floor, and in the door racks of a household-grade storage unit to help provide a stable temperatures.
- Avoid storing any items other than vaccines, diluents, and water bottles inside storage units.
- IF other medications must be stored in the refrigerator, they must be clearly marked and stored separately from vaccines.
- The TMD should be placed in the center of the unit and surrounded by the vaccines. The DDL should be set to measure temperature at least every 30 minutes.

Handling of vaccines

- Vaccines should be drawn up only at the time of administration.
- If a vaccine must be predrawn:
  - Establish a separate administration station for each vaccine type to prevent medication errors.
  - Draw up vaccines only after arriving at the site.
  - An individual administering vaccines should not draw up more than one multidose vial or 10 doses at one time.
  - Observe patient traffic to avoid drawing up unnecessary doses.
  - Predraw reconstituted vaccine into a syringe *only* when it is ready for administration.
  - If a predrawn vaccine is *not* used within 30 minutes of being reconstituted, adhere to manufacturer guidelines for storage and time limits.
- Any remaining vaccine in predrawn syringes should be disposed at the end of the day.
- Never transfer a predrawn, reconstituted vaccine back into a vial.

Disposal

- In some situations, unused vaccine and diluent doses, unopened vials, expired vials, and potentially compromised vaccine may be returned for credit.
- Open and broken vials and syringes, manufacturer-filled syringes that have been initiated and vaccines predrawn by providers cannot be returned; they should be discarded according to state requirements.
- After use, all syringe/needle devices should be discarded in biohazard containers that are closable, puncture-resistant, leakproof on sides and bottom, and labeled or color-coded.

- Never recap, cut, or detach used needles from syringes before disposal.
- Empty, expired, or compromised vaccine vials do not require disposal in a biomedical waste container since they are not considered hazardous or pharmaceutical waste.
- Follow all state regulations regarding proper disposal.

Managing vaccine-related adverse reactions

After the administration of a vaccine, the patient may experience adverse reaction to it. Common adverse reactions include localized reactions, syncope and anaphylaxis.

Reaction	Signs and symptoms	Management
Localized	Soreness, redness, itching, or swelling at the injection site	Apply a cold compress to the injection site. Analgesic and antipruritic medications may be taken to address the symptoms.
	Slight bleeding	Apply pressure and an adhesive compress over the injection site.
	Continuous bleeding	Place thick layer of gauze pads over site and maintain direct and firm pressure: raise the bleeding injection site (e.g., arm) above the level of the patient's heart.
Psychological fright, presyncope, and syncope	Fright before injection is given	Have patient sit or lay down for the vaccination.
	Patient feels "faint" (e.g., light-headed, dizzy, weak, nauseated, or has visual disturbance)	Have patient lie flat. Loosen any tight clothing and maintain open airway. Apply cool, damp cloth to patient's face and neck. Keep patient under close observation until full recovery.
	Fall, without loss of consciousness	Examine the patient to determine if injury is present before attempting to move the patient. Place patient flat on back with feet elevated.
	Loss of consciousness	Check to determine if injury is present before attempting to move the patient. Place patient flat on back with feet elevated. Call 911 if patient does not recover immediately.
Anaphylaxis	Skin and mucosal symptoms such as generalized hives, itching, or flushing, swelling of lips, face, throat, or eyes	Using an Epi-Pen: 1. Remove the auto-injector from the clear carrier tube. 2. Flip open the of the carrier rube. 3. Tip and slide the auto-injector out of carrier tube. 4. Hold the auto-injector in your fist with the orange tip pointing downward. 5. With your other hand, remove the safety release by pulling straight up without bending or twisting it. 6. Place the orange tip against the middle of the outer thigh at a right angle to the thigh. 7. Swing and push the auto injector firmly until iot clicks. 8. Hold firmly in place for 3 seconds. 9. Remove the auto-injector from the thigh. 10. Massage the auto injection area for 10 seconds.
	Respiratory symptoms such as nasal congestion, change in voice, sensation of throat closing, shortness of breath, wheeze or cough	
	Gastrointestinal symptoms such as nausea, vomiting, diarrhea, and cramping abdominal pain	
	Cardiovascular symptoms such as collapse, dizziness, tachycardia and hypotension	

Emergency medical protocol for managing anaphylactic reactions in adults

- If itching and swelling are limited to the vaccine injection, observe patient carefully for the development of generalized symptoms.
- For generalized symptoms, call 911 and have the secondary health care professional alert the patient's physician. The primary health care professional should evaluate the patient's airway, breathing, circulation, and their level of consciousness. Vital signs should be observed continuously.
- Use epinephrine in a 1.0 mg/mL aqueous solution (1:1000 dilution) to treat anaphylaxis. A 0.3 mg dose should be administered IM using a prefilled syringe or an autoinjector in the mid-outer thigh. The recommended dose of epinephrine is 0.01 mg/kg, ranging for adults from 0.3 mg to maximum dose of 0.5 mg. A dose of epinephrine may be repeated 2 additional times every 5–15 minutes (or sooner as needed) while waiting for emergency medical services to arrive.

Age group	Range of weight (pounds)	Range of weight (kg)	1.0 mg/mL aqueous solution (1:1000 dilution); intramuscular. minimum dose: 0.05 mL	Epinephrine autoinjector or prefilled syringe (0.1 mg, 0.15 mg, 0.3 mg)
1–6 months	9–19	4–8.5	0.05 mL (or mg)	Off-label
7–36 months	20–32	9–14.5	0.1 mL (or mg)	0.1 mg
37–59 months	33–39	15–17.5	0.15 mL (or mg)	0.15 mg/dose
5–7 years	40–56	18–25.5	0.2–0.25 mL (or mg)	0.15 mg/dose
8–10 years	57–76	26–34.5	0.25–0.3 mL (or mg)	0.15 mg or 0.3 mg/dose
11–12 years	77–99	35–45	0.35–0.4 mL (or mg)	0.3 mg/dose
13 years & older	100+	46+	0.5 mL (or mg) – max. dose	0.3 mg/dose

- A 1–2 mg/kg dose of diphenhydramine may be administered every 4–6 hours up to a maximum single dose of 100 mg to treat itching and hives.

Age group	Range of weight (pounds)	Range of weight (kg)	Liquid: 12.5 mg/5 mLTablets: 25 mg or 50 mg
7–36 months	20–32	9–14.5	10–15 mg/dose
37–59 months	33–39	15–17.5	15–20 mg/dose
5–7 years	40–56	18–25.5	20–25 mg/dose
8–12 years	57–99	26–45	25–50 mg/dose
13 years and older	100+	46+	50 mg/dose (up to 50 mg or 100 mg single dose)

- Observe the patient closely until emergency medical services arrives. If necessary, perform cardiopulmonary resuscitation, and maintain an open airway. Keep patient lying flat on their back unless they are experiencing breathing difficulty. If breathing is difficult, patient's head may be elevated, provided blood pressure is sufficient to prevent loss of consciousness. If the patient's blood pressure is low, elevate their legs. Monitor blood pressure and pulse every 5 minutes.
- Record the patient's reaction (e.g., hives, anaphylaxis) to the vaccine, all vital signs, medications administered to the patient, including the time, dosage, response, and the name of the medical personnel who administered the medication, and other relevant clinical information.
- Notify the patient's primary care physician.
- Report the incident to the Vaccine Adverse Event Reporting System (VAERS) at https://vaers.hhs.gov/esub/index.jsp.

Vaccine Adverse Event Reporting System

VAERS is a national system to detect safety problems in US-licensed vaccines. VAERS is a postlicensure vaccine safety monitoring program. The goals of VAERS are to:

- Evaluate the safety of newly licensed vaccines.
- Detect new, unusual, or rare vaccine adverse events.
- Monitor increases in known adverse events.
- Identify potential patient risk factors for particular types of adverse events.
- Identify whether specific vaccine lots have demonstrated a higher incidence of adverse reactions.
- Assess the safety of newly licensed vaccines.
- Determine and address reporting clusters.
- Recognize persistent safe-use problems and administration errors.
- Provide a national safety monitoring system that extends to the entire general population for response to public health emergencies.

Anyone can report an adverse event associated with a vaccine through VAERS. Health care professionals are required to report any adverse event listed in the VAERS Table of Reportable Events and any adverse event listed by the vaccine manufacturer as a contraindication. Health care providers are strongly urged report any adverse event after the administration of a vaccine, whether it is or is not clear that the vaccine caused the adverse event, and any vaccine administration errors.

An individual may submit a report to VAERS by:

- Using the online reporting tool at https://vaers.hhs.gov/esub/index.jsp or
- Downloading the writable PDF form (located at https://vaers.hhs.gov/uploadFile/index.jsp) to your computer, completing it, and then returning to the VAERS website to upload the completed form

Information collected through the VAERS includes:

- The type of vaccine received
- The date of the vaccination
- When the adverse event(s) began
- The patient's current illness(es) and medications
- The patient's medical history
- The patient's past history of adverse events associated with vaccinations
- Demographic information

VAERS **Vaccine Adverse Event Reporting System**
www.vaers.hhs.gov

Adverse events are possible reactions or problems that occur during or after vaccination. Items **2, 3, 4, 5, 6, 17, 18** and **21** are **ESSENTIAL** and should be completed. Patient identity is kept confidential. Instructions are provided on the last two pages.

INFORMATION ABOUT THE PATIENT WHO RECEIVED THE VACCINE (Use **Continuation Page** if needed)

1. Patient name: (first) ____ (last) ____
Street address: ____
City: ____ State: ____ County: ____
ZIP code: ____ Phone: ( ) ____ Email: ____
2. Date of birth: (mm/dd/yyyy) ____
3. Sex: ☐ Male ☐ Female ☐ Unknown
4. Date and time of vaccination: (mm/dd/yyyy) ____ Time: hh:mm ☐AM ☐PM
5. Date and time adverse event started: (mm/dd/yyyy) ____ Time: hh:mm ☐AM ☐PM
6. Age at vaccination: ___ Years ___ Months
7. Today's date: (mm/dd/yyyy) ____
8. Pregnant at time of vaccination?: ☐ Yes ☐ No ☐ Unknown
(If yes, describe the event, any pregnancy complications, and estimated due date if known in item 18)
9. Prescriptions, over-the-counter medications, dietary supplements, or herbal remedies being taken at the time of vaccination:
10. Allergies to medications, food, or other products:
11. Other illnesses at the time of vaccination and up to one month prior:
12. Chronic or long-standing health conditions:

INFORMATION ABOUT THE PERSON COMPLETING THIS FORM

13. Form completed by: (name) ____
Relation to patient: ☐ Healthcare professional/staff ☐ Patient (yourself) ☐ Parent/guardian/caregiver ☐ Other: ____
Street address: ____ ☐ Check if same as item 1
City: ____ State: ____ ZIP code: ____
Phone: ( ) ____ Email: ____
14. Best doctor/healthcare professional to contact about the adverse event: Name: ____ Phone: ( ) ____ Ext: ____

INFORMATION ABOUT THE FACILITY WHERE VACCINE WAS GIVEN

15. Facility/clinic name: ____
Fax: ( ) ____
Street address: ____ ☐ Check if same as item 13
City: ____
State: ____ ZIP code: ____
Phone: ( ) ____
16. Type of facility: (Check one)
☐ Doctor's office, urgent care, or hospital
☐ Pharmacy or store
☐ Workplace clinic
☐ Public health clinic
☐ Nursing home or senior living facility
☐ School or student health clinic
☐ Other: ____
☐ Unknown

WHICH VACCINES WERE GIVEN? WHAT HAPPENED TO THE PATIENT?

17. Enter all vaccines given on the date listed in item 4: (Route is HOW vaccine was given, Body site is WHERE vaccine was given) Use **Continuation Page** if needed

Vaccine (type and brand name)	Manufacturer	Lot number	Route	Body site	Dose number in series
select			select	select	select
select			select	select	select
select			select	select	select
select			select	select	select

18. Describe the adverse event(s), treatment, and outcome(s), if any: (symptoms, signs, time course, etc.)
Use **Continuation Page** if needed
19. Medical tests and laboratory results related to the adverse event(s): (include dates)
Use **Continuation Page** if needed
20. Has the patient recovered from the adverse event(s)?: ☐ Yes ☐ No ☐ Unknown
21. Result or outcome of adverse event(s): (Check all that apply)
☐ Doctor or other healthcare professional office/clinic visit
☐ Emergency room/department or urgent care
☐ Hospitalization: Number of days (if known) ____
Hospital name: ____
City: ____ State: ____
☐ Prolongation of existing hospitalization (vaccine received during existing hospitalization)
☐ Life threatening illness (immediate risk of death from the event)
☐ Disability or permanent damage
☐ Patient died – Date of death: (mm/dd/yyyy) ____
☐ Congenital anomaly or birth defect
☐ None of the above

ADDITIONAL INFORMATION

22. Any other vaccines received within one month prior to the date listed in item 4: Use **Continuation Page** if needed

Vaccine (type and brand name)	Manufacturer	Lot number	Route	Body site	Dose number in series	Date Given
select			select	select	select	
select			select	select	select	

23. Has the patient ever had an adverse event following any previous vaccine?: (If yes, describe adverse event, patient age at vaccination, vaccination dates, vaccine type, and brand name)
☐ Yes ____ ☐ No ☐ Unknown
24. Patient's race: (Check all that apply) ☐ American Indian or Alaska Native ☐ Asian ☐ Black or African American ☐ Native Hawaiian or Other Pacific Islander ☐ White ☐ Unknown ☐ Other: ____
25. Patient's ethnicity: ☐ Hispanic or Latino ☐ Not Hispanic or Latino ☐ Unknown
26. Immuniz. proj. report number: (Health Dept use only) ____

COMPLETE ONLY FOR U.S. MILITARY/DEPARTMENT OF DEFENSE (DoD) RELATED REPORTS

27. Status at vaccination: ☐ Active duty ☐ Reserve ☐ National Guard ☐ Beneficiary ☐ Other: ____
28. Vaccinated at Military/DoD site: ☐ Yes ☐ No

FORM FDA VAERS 2.0 (02/23)

Fig. 7.6 Vaccine Adverse Event Reporting System (VAERS) form. (From Vaccine Adverse Event Reporting System, https://vaers.hhs.gov/, 2023. VAERS is cosponsored by the Centers for Disease Control and Prevention and the FDA, agencies of the US Department of Health and Human Services.)

Advantages of Vaccine Adverse Event Reporting System

- Anyone may submit a report to VAERS.
- VAERS collects information about the individual receiving the vaccine, the vaccine, and the adverse events.
- All data *except* patient information are made public.

Disadvantages of Vaccine Adverse Event Reporting System

- VAERS is a passive reporting system requiring an individual who experienced or is aware of adverse event must report it.
- VAERS reports may lack specific details or be erroneous.

- VAERS data alone cannot determine if the vaccine caused the reported adverse event.

Under VAERS, a determination is not made whether a vaccine caused an adverse event. If VAERS identifies a pattern of adverse events, follow-up studies are conducted by the medical community to decide of the vaccine (Fig. 7.6).

Vaccine Error Reporting Program

The National Coordinating Council for Medication Error Reporting and Prevention defines a vaccine medication error as "any preventable event that may cause or lead to inappropriate medication use or patient harm." A preventable event is one that is due to an error that could be avoided. Vaccine administration errors may result in insufficient immunological protection, patient injury, cost, convenience, and diminished faith in the health care system. According to the CDC common vaccine administration errors include:

- Doses administered too early (e.g., before the minimum age or interval)
- Wrong vaccine (e.g., Tdap instead of DTaP)
- Wrong dosage (e.g., pediatric formulation of hepatitis B vaccine administered to an adult)
- Wrong route (e.g., MMR given by IM injection)
- Vaccine administered outside the approved age range
- Expired vaccine or diluent administered
- Improperly stored vaccine administered
- Vaccine administered to a patient with a contraindication
- Wrong diluent used to reconstitute the vaccine or only the diluent was administered.[7]

Prevention of vaccine errors	
Error type	**Preventative action[8]**
Wrong vaccine, route, site, or dosage	Circle important information on the packaging to emphasize the difference between the vaccines.
	Include the brand name with the vaccine abbreviation whenever possible (e.g., PCV13 [Prevnar13]) in orders, medical screens).
	Separate vaccines into bins or other containers according to type and formulation. Use color-coded identification labels on vaccine storage containers.
	Store look-alike vaccines in different areas of the storage unit (e.g., pediatric and adult formulations of the same vaccine on different shelves in the unit).
	Do not list vaccines with look-alike names sequentially on computer screens, order forms, or medical records, if possible.
	Consider using "name alert" or "look-alike" stickers on packaging and areas where these vaccines are stored.
	Establish "Do Not Disturb" or no-interruption areas or times when vaccines are being prepared or administered.
	Prepare vaccine for one patient at a time. Once prepared, label the syringe with vaccine name.
	Do not administer vaccines prepared by someone else.
	Triple-check work before administering a vaccine and ask another staff member to check.
	Keep reference materials on recommended sites, routes, and needle lengths for each vaccine used in your facility in the medication preparation area.
	Clearly identify diluents if the manufacturer's label could mislead staff into believing the diluent is the vaccine itself.
	Integrate vaccine administration training into orientation and other appropriate education requirements.
	Provide education when new products are added to inventory or recommendations are updated.
	Use standing orders, if appropriate.
Wrong patient	Verify the patient's identity before administering vaccines.
	Educate staff on the importance of avoiding unnecessary distractions or interruptions when staff is administering vaccine.
	Prepare and administer vaccines to one patient at a time. If more than one patient needs vaccines during the same clinical encounter (e.g., parent with two children), assign different providers to each patient, if possible. Alternatively, bring only one patient's vaccines into the treatment area at a time, labeled with vaccine and patient name.
Documentation orders	Do not use error-prone abbreviations to document vaccine administration (e.g., use intranasal route [NAS] to document the intranasal route—not IN, which is easily confused with IM [intramuscular]).
	Use ACIP vaccine abbreviations.
	Change the appearance of look-alike names or generic abbreviations on computer screens, if possible.
Improperly stored and/or handled vaccine administrated (e.g., vaccine doses in a series)	Integrate vaccine storage and handling training based on manufacturer guidance and/or requirements.

(Continued)

Prevention of vaccine errors—cont'd	
Error type	**Preventative action[8]**
	Rotate vaccines so those with the earliest expiration dates are in the front of the storage unit. Use these first.
	Remove expired vaccines/diluents from storage units and areas where viable vaccines are stored
	Isolate vaccines exposed to improper temperatures and contact the state or local immunization program and/or the vaccine manufacturer.
Scheduling errors (e.g., vaccine doses in a series administered too soon)	Use standing orders, if appropriate.
	Create procedures to obtain a complete vaccination history using the immunization information system, previous medical records, and personal vaccination records.
	Integrate vaccine administration training, including timing and spacing of vaccines, into orientation and other appropriate education requirements.
	For children, especially infants, schedule immunization visits after the birthday.
	Post current immunization schedules for children and adults that staff can quickly reference in clinical areas where vaccinations may be prescribed and administered.
	Post reference sheets for timing and spacing in your medication preparation area. CDC has vaccine catch-up guidance for DTaP, Tdap, Hib, PCV13, and polio vaccines to assist health care personnel in interpreting the catch-up schedule for children.
	Counsel parents and patients on how important it is for them to maintain immunization records

ACIP, Advisory Committee of Immunization Practices; *CDC*, Centers for Disease Control and Prevention; *DTaP*, diphtheria, tetanus, and acellular pertussis; *Hib*, *Haemophilus influenzae* type b; *PCV13*, pneumococcal 13-valent conjugate; *Tdap*, tetanus, diphtheria, and acellular pertussis.

Some vaccine administration errors require revaccination and others do not. Those that require revaccination include:

- Hepatitis B vaccine is administered by any route other than IM injection, or in adults at any site other than the deltoid or anterolateral thigh.
- HPV vaccine is administered by any route other than IM injection.
- Influenza vaccine is administered subcutaneously.
- Any vaccination using less than the appropriate dose does not count and the dose should be repeated according to age unless serological testing reveals a satisfactory response has developed. It should be noted that if two half-volume formulations of vaccine are administered on the same clinic day, these two doses can count as one valid dose.
- A partial dose of an injectable vaccine is administered because the syringe or needle leaks or the patient jerks away.

Revaccination is not required when a vaccine administration error involves:

- Any vaccination using more than the appropriate dose should be counted if the minimum age and minimum time interval have been met.
- Hepatitis A vaccine and meningococcal conjugate vaccine being administered by the subcutaneous route if the minimum patient age and minimal time interval have been met.
- Administering a dose 4 or fewer days earlier than the minimum time interval or age is unlikely to have a negative effect on the immune response to that dose. Vaccine doses administered during this 4-day grace period, or before the minimum interval or age, are considered valid. When in doubt, refer to state or local regulations for guidance.

The Vaccine Error Reporting Program (VERP) collects information about preventable vaccine administration errors.

VERP is administered by the Institute of Safe Medication Practices and is a national surveillance program that allows health care providers and consumers to report vaccine errors, investigates the causes and severity of the error, informs the health care community of error, and helps prevent future errors by working with the FDA, drug manufacturers, standards organizations, and the health care community to provide proactive risk assessments and educational material to health care facilities. Health care practitioners may submit a vaccine error using https://www.ismp.org/form/verp-form. Patients and consumers may report a vaccine error using https://www.ismp.org/form/cmerp-form.

CHAPTER REVIEW QUESTIONS

1. Which of the following immunization tasks may a pharmacy technician perform?
   a. Counsel the patient.
   b. Determine the appropriateness of the vaccine.
   c. Document the immunization.
   d. Verify the vaccine order.
2. Which term refers to a preparation that is used to stimulate the body's immune response against diseases?
   a. Antibody
   b. Antigen
   c. Cytokine
   d. Vaccine
3. Which vaccine is administered may be administered at birth to the patient?
   a. Hepatitis A
   b. Hepatitis B
   c. Measles, mumps, and rubella
   d. Varicella

4. How many doses are in a series for DTaP?
   a. 2
   b. 3
   c. 4
   d. 5
5. What is the brand name for the human papillomavirus vaccine?
   a. Bexsero
   b. Engerix-B
   c. Gardasil 9
   d. Prevnar 13
6. What is the maximum age for a patient to receive the human papillomavirus vaccine?
   a. 19 years
   b. 23 years
   c. 26 years
   d. 50 years
7. At what frequency after a patient receives their first dose of Tdap vaccine should they receive subsequent vaccinations of this vaccine?
   a. Yearly
   b. Every 2 years
   c. Every years
   d. Every 10 years
8. What temperatures should a reconstituted multidose be stored?
   a. 0°C–2°C
   b. 2°C–8°C
   c. 10°C–16°C
   d. 16°C–20°C
9. Which vaccine, after being reconstituted, must be used immediately?
   a. Hib
   b. MMR
   c. RZV
   d. VAR
10. What size needle should be used to administer a varicella vaccine subcutaneously to an adolescent?
    a. 5/8″
    b. 1″
    c. 1¼″
    d. 1½″
11. Which diluent is used to reconstitute the Shingrix (RZV) vaccine?
    a. AS01B§ adjuvant suspension
    b. 0.4% sodium chloride
    c. 0.9% sodium chloride
    d. Sterile water
12. Which vaccine is administered IM?
    a. HPV
    b. MMR
    c. VAR
    d. ZVL
13. To administer a vaccine IM into an adult, what angle should the needle be inserted?
    a. 45 degrees
    b. 60 degrees
    c. 75 degrees
    d. 90 degrees
14. Which vaccine is administered intranasally to a patient?
    a. FluMist Quadrivalent
    b. Prevnar 13

   c. Rotarix
   d. Trumenba
15. When should a sharps container be replaced in a healthcare facility?
    a. When it is a quarter filled
    b. When it is half-filled
    c. When it is three-quarters filled
    d. When it is completely filled
16. What is the first thing that should be done if you experience a needlestick injury?
    a. Wash the needlestick injury with clean water.
    b. Wash the needlestick injury with saline.
    c. Wash the needlestick injury with sterile irrigants.
    d. Wash the needlestick injury with soap and water.
17. What should be used to clean the skin prior to administering a vaccine subcutaneously or IM?
    a. Alcohol swab
    b. Hydrogen peroxide
    c. Merthiolate
    d. Sterile water
18. The diluent for which vaccine may be stored either at room temperature or in the refrigerator?
    a. Menveo
    b. RabAvert
    c. Shingrix
    d. Varivax
19. Which vaccine is administered as an oral drop?
    a. Gardasil
    b. Measles, mumps, and rubella
    c. Prevnar 13
    d. Rotarix
20. An adult is receiving an IM injection. What is the primary site of injection?
    a. Anterolateral thigh muscle
    b. Biceps muscle
    c. Deltoid muscle
    d. Triceps muscle
21. Which of the following must appear on a patient's medical record when a vaccine is administered?
    a. The date of when the next dose of the vaccine is to be administered
    b. The name and title of the individua administering the vaccine
    c. The original date of the VIS
    d. The vaccine manufacturer, the lot number, and expiration date of the vaccine
22. Prior to storing vaccines in the storage unit, how many consecutive days of temperature being recorded within the recommended range?
    a. 2
    b. 4
    c. 5
    d. 7
23. What temperature should freezers be maintained?
    a. −50°C and −30°C
    b. −50°C and −15° C
    c. −40°C and −10°C
    d. −40° and 0°C
24. What is the first thing that should be done if a temperature excursion occurs?
    a. Contact the vaccine manufacturer.
    b. Document the details of the incident.

    c. Label exposed vaccines "Do Not Use" and segregate.

    d. Notify the vaccine coordinator.

25. Which document should be used when reporting an adverse event as a result of a vaccine?

    a. MERP

    b. VAERS

    c. VERP

    d. VIS

REFERENCES

Demarco M, Carter C, Houle SKD, Waite NM, JAPHA. The role of pharmacy technicians in vaccination services: a scoping review. Published October 2, 2021. Accessed February 1, 2022. https://www.japha.org/article/S1544-3191(21)00386-1/fulltext.

Hohmeier KC, McKeiman K. Pharmacy technicians are valued more than ever: insights into a team-centered immunization approach. Pharmacy Times. Published July 2021. Accessed February 1, 2021. https://www.pharmacytimes.com/view/pharmacy-technicians-are-valued-more-than-ever-insights-into-a-team-centered-immunization-approach.

Centers for Disease Control and Prevention (CDC). Child and adolescent immunization schedule by age. Accessed February 1, 2023. https://www.cdc.gov/vaccines/schedules/hcp/imz/child-adolescent.html.

Centers for Disease Control and Prevention. Adult Immunization schedule by age. Accessed February 1, 2023. https://www.cdc.gov/vaccines/schedules/hcp/imz/adult.html.

Vaccines with diluents: how to use them. Accessed February 1, 2022. https://www.immunize.org/catg.d/p3040.pdf.

Centers for Disease Control and Prevention. Vaccine handling and storage. Accessed February 1, 2022. https://www.cdc.gov/vaccines/pubs/pinkbook/vac-storage.html.

Centers for Disease Control and Prevention. Vaccine administration, Wolicki J and Miller E. Accessed February 1, 2022. https://www.cdc.gov/vaccines/pubs/pinkbook/vac-admin.html.

Centers for Disease Control and Prevention. Vaccine administration: preventing vaccine administrative errors. Accessed February 1, 2022. https://www.cdc.gov/vaccines/hcp/admin/downloads/vaccine-administration-preventing-errors.pdf.

8

Point-of-Care Testing Certificate

Eligibility requirements

- Must hold an active Pharmacy Technician Certification Board Certified Pharmacy Technician Certification
- Must complete a Pharmacy Technician Certification Board–Recognized Point-of-Care Testing Education/Training Program

Point-of-care domains

Safety and precautions (16%)

- Roles of pharmacists and pharmacy technicians in point-of-care (POC) testing
- Occupational Safety and Health Administration Bloodborne Pathogen Standard and related safety considerations
- Biohazard waste handling and disposal
- Personal protective equipment necessary to protect patients and those administering tests
- Need for and methods to confirm patient identity

Diseases and specimens (34%)

- Basic anatomical and physiological terms related to tests
- Common specimen types (e.g., whole blood, saliva) and their location on/in the body
- Signs, symptoms, and characteristics of common chronic disease states (e.g., hypertension, diabetes, hypercholesterolemia) where POC testing may be relevant
- Signs, symptoms, and characteristics of common acute infections where POC testing may be relevant
- Collecting a focused health history (e.g., acute symptoms [e.g., Centor Score], medication allergies, signs of disease [e.g., swelling, bruising])

Clinical Laboratory Improvement Amendments–waived tests (30%)

- Clinical Laboratory Improvement Amendments (CLIA) of 1988 as it pertains to POC tests
- CLIA waiver process, CLIA Certificate of Compliance, and CLIA Certificate of Accreditation

- Devices and technology used in common POC tests
- Conditions and uses for common tests (e.g., prothrombin time, influenza, streptococcus, A1C, HIV, hepatitis C, COVID-19, glucose, cholesterol)
- Understanding and following manufacturer instructions for tests

Test results, quality control, and recording (20%)

- Qualitative and quantitative test results and their characteristics and related concepts (e.g., time since exposure, terms "false positive" and "false negative")
- Requirements and best practices in recording results
- Identifying invalid or anomalous results
- Labeling and documentation requirements for patient samples
- Quality control testing methods (i.e., external, internal) and when they should be used

Safety and precautions

Roles of pharmacists and pharmacy technicians in point-of-care testing

Role	Task	Pharmacist	Pharmacy technician
Laboratory manager			
	Maintaining logs as required by federal and state laws	X	X
	Ensuring appropriate storage of tests and reagents	X	X
	Running external controls as required	X	X

(Continued)

Role	Task	Pharmacist	Pharmacy technician
	Maintaining current copies of manufacturers' instructions	X	X
Patient intake			
	Welcoming patients and explain the point-of-care service	X	X
	Identifying qualified patients for point-of-care test	X	X
	Collecting demographic, consent forms and payments for the service	X	X
Physical assessment			
	Obtaining vital sign(s) from patient, if required	X	X
	Performing patient physical assessment, if required	X	X
	Screening patient for inclusion/exclusion criteria	X	X
Specimen collection			
	Collecting patient specimen(s) according to manufacturer's instructions, including storage and handling of specimen	X	X
Run test			
	Running test(s) according to manufacturer's instructions	X	X
	Performing quality control according to manufacturer's instructions	X	X
Interpret results			
	Interpreting test results according to the manufacturer's instructions	X	
Record results			
	Recording test results legibly in a log and adhering to facility's policies. Retain results as a permanent record	X	X
Patient assistance			

Role	Task	Pharmacist	Pharmacy technician
	Referring patient for confirmatory testing if required by state/local requirements	X	X
Disease reporting			
	Reporting results of positive testing of specific infectious disease to public health agencies, if required	X	X

Occupational Safety and Health Administration Bloodborne Pathogens Standard and related safety considerations

The Occupational Safety and Health Administration (OSHA) Bloodborne Pathogens Standard affects sites where workers have potential occupational exposure to blood and infectious materials. OSHA's Bloodborne Pathogens Standard must address:

- Exposure control plan:
  - An Exposure Control Plan is a document, used as a source of information for answering blood-borne pathogen (BBP)-related questions and to help ensure exposure control activities are in place for an organization.
  - It must recognize job classifications, tasks, and procedures where occupational exposure exists.
  - A written Exposure Control Plan must be provided to employees.
  - It must be reviewed and updated annually.
- Safety devices:
  - Evaluate medical devices with engineered sharps injury protections (safety devices).
  - Use appropriate, effective, and commercially available safety devices.
  - Utilize frontline employees in the evaluation and selection process.
  - Document the evaluation and selection of safety devices annually.
- Hepatitis B vaccination:
  - Offer free hepatitis B vaccinations to all employees with occupational exposure to blood or other potentially infectious materials.
- Controls:
  - Ensure employees comply with universal precautions.
  - Utilize engineering and work practice controls to remove or reduce employee exposure.
  - Provide and guarantee the use of appropriate personal protective equipment, to include gloves, gowns, laboratory coats, face shields or masks, and eye protection.
  - Ensure that contaminated sharps are disposed of properly in the appropriate sharps containers.
- Postexposure incident procedures:
  - Establish a procedure for postexposure evaluation and follow-up.

- Record the route of exposure and other circumstances. Identify the source individual where feasible.
- Offer postexposure medical evaluation by a health care professional at no cost to employees.
- Test the source individual's blood for BBPs where possible and test the exposed employee's blood after consent is obtained.
- Ensuring the provision of postexposure medication when medically required according to the Department of Health and Human Services.
- Training:
  - Employees must be trained annually by a knowledgeable individual.
  - Training must include:
    - An accessible copy of the Bloodborne Pathogen Standard (29 CFR 1910.1030)
    - Information on the epidemiology and symptoms of blood-borne diseases
    - Information on modes of transmission of BBPs
    - Description of the employer's Exposure Control Plan
    - Distinguishing tasks that may involve exposure to blood or other potentially infectious materials
    - Use and limitations of methods to reduce exposure, including engineering controls, work practices, and personal protective equipment
    - Information on the hepatitis B vaccine
    - What to do and whom to contact after an exposure occurs
    - Information on postexposure evaluation and follow-up
    - An opportunity for interactive questions and answers

Best practices to reduce the risk of blood-borne exposure during point-of-care testing

- Provide safety training for handling blood, exposure to blood-borne pathogens, and other infectious materials.
- Handle all blood and body fluids as if they are infectious.
- Use required personal protective equipment (PPE) and safety devices.
- Do not eat, drink, or apply cosmetics in the testing area.
- Prohibit storage of food in refrigerators where testing supplies or specimens are stored.
- Be cautious of exposure to mucous membranes such as eyes, nostrils, and mouth.
- Wear goggles or face shields.
- Avoid the use of needles and lancets if safe and effective alternatives are available.
- Never reuse single-use devices such as needles and lancets.
- Avoid recapping needles, transferring a body fluid between containers, and opening blood tubes.
- Dispose of used sharps properly in puncture-proof sharps containers.
- Ensure proper equipment is available for the safe handling and disposal of hazardous waste to include properly labeled or color-coded sharps containers and biohazard trash bags and bins.

- Report all occupational exposures promptly to ensure that you receive appropriate follow-up care.
- Report any real or potential hazards you observe to the person who directs or oversees testing.
- Participate in training related to infection prevention.
- Obtain a hepatitis B vaccination.
- Post safety information for employees and patients.

Biohazard waste handling and disposal

Biohazardous waste, also known as infectious or biomedical waste, is any waste containing infectious materials or potentially infectious substances such as blood. Examples of biohazardous waste:

- Human blood and blood products
  - Plasma
  - Serum
  - Blood components
- Human body fluids
  - Amniotic fluid
  - Cerebral spinal fluid
  - Pericardial fluid
  - Peritoneal fluid
  - Saliva
  - Semen
  - Synovial fluid
  - Vaginal secretions

During point-of-care (POC) testing:

- Biohazard bags and sharps containers are used for disposal of contaminated materials. These containers should be placed as close to the testing area as possible and standing upright. The containers should be replaced routinely and not overfilled.
- Biohazardous containers:
  - Should be constructed to contain all contents and prevent leakage of fluids during handling, storage, transport, and/or shipping.
  - Are color-coded to indicate the hazardous material:
    - Red—biohazardous waste
    - White with blue lid—pharmaceutical waste
    - Yellow—chemotherapy waste
    - Black—Resource Conservation and Recovery Act hazardous waste
  - Should be closed prior to removal to prevent spillage.
- Hazardous waste cannot be disposed of with regular trash.
- Refer to and follow the manufacturer's directions for handling and disposing of reagents, specimen, cartridges, and other test materials

Personal protective equipment (PPE)

Standard precautions are to be adhered to during point-of-care testing and include:

- Hand hygiene: Cleaning your hands by using either handwashing (washing hands with soap and water), antiseptic hand wash, antiseptic hand rub (i.e., alcohol-based hand sanitizer including foam or gel), or surgical hand antisepsis.

- Use PPE whenever there is an expectation of possible exposure to infectious material. Appropriate PPE includes laboratory coats or gowns, gloves, and eye protection.
- Respiratory hygiene/cough etiquette:
  - Cover your mouth and nose with a tissues when coughing or sneezing.
  - Use the nearest waste receptacle to dispose of the tissue after use.
  - Perform hand hygiene.
  - Provide tissues and no-touch receptacles for used tissue disposal.
  - Provide conveniently located dispensers of alcohol-based hand rub; where sinks are available, ensure that supplies for handwashing (i.e., soap, disposable towels) are consistently available.
- Properly handle, clean, and disinfect patient care equipment and instruments/devices and the surrounding environment.
- Use sharps safety (engineering and work practice controls).
- Use sterile instruments and devices.
- Clean and disinfect environmental surfaces.

Patient confirmation

It is the responsibility of health care workers to check the identity of patients and match the correct patients with the correct care (e.g., laboratory results, specimens, procedures) before that care is administered. The Joint Commission requires at least two identifiers be provided by the patient prior to administering the point-of-care testing. Acceptable identifiers include:

- Individual's name
- Assigned identification (such as a medical record number)
- Telephone number or another person-specific identifier
- Electronic identification technology coding, such as bar coding or radio-frequency identification, that includes two or more person-specific identifiers

Clear protocols for identifying patients who lack identification and for distinguishing the identity of patients with the same name are outlined. The labeling of containers used for blood and other specimens should be done in the presence of the patient and requires two identifiers. The practice of prelabeling blood tubes prior to seeing the patient and matching them at the time of collection is not acceptable. In situations where a labeled container is not used due to failure of the patient to provide a urine specimen, it must be discarded immediately.

Diseases and specimens

Basic anatomical and physiological terminology terms related to tests

Common terminology

- Chief complaint: A description of the symptoms that caused a patient to seek medical care.
- History of present illness: A description of the onset and symptoms associated with the chief complaint
- Past medical history: A summary of patient's diagnoses, medications, surgeries, immunizations and allergies

Physical assessment

- Inspection: process of collecting information about the patient's well-being using your senses
- Vital signs: parameters intended to provide insight into the body's most basic functions (e.g., body temperature, heart rate, respiration rate, blood pressure, oxygen saturation)
- Systolic blood pressure: the maximum blood pressure during one heartbeat and the top number in a blood pressure reading
- Diastolic blood pressure: the minimum pressure between heartbeats and the bottom number in a blood pressure reading

Patient assessment (inspection)

- Visual inspection
- Auditory inspection
- Tactile inspection
- Olfactory inspection

Physical assessment

- Vital signs
  - Body temperature
    - Interpretation
      - Normal: 97°F (36.1°C) to 99°F (37.2°C)
      - Fever: 100.4°F (38°C)
      - Concerning: 103.0°F (39.4°C)
        - Factors affecting body temperature
          - Medications such as acetaminophen, nonsteroidal antiinflammatory drugs or corticosteroids may lower an individual's temperature.
          - The temperature of recently ingested food or beverage can affect an individual's body temperature.
          - Exposure to extreme external temperatures or precipitation can affect assessment of temperature.
  - Heart rate: also known as the pulse, the number of times the heart beats in 1 minute
    - Pulse may be measured manually placing your fingers over an artery and counting the beats over 15 or 30 seconds and multiplying by 4 or 2 to get beats per minute.
    - Pulse may be measured by automatic blood pressure cuffs or pulse oximeters.
    - Interpretation
      - Normal: 60 to 100 beats per minute (BPM)
      - Concerning: <50 BPM or >110 BPM
    - Factors affecting the heart rate
      - Weather
        - The pulse may go up a bit in higher temperatures and humidity levels.
      - Standing up
        - Heart rate might spike for about 20 seconds after standing up from sitting.
      - Emotions
        - Stress and anxiety can raise the heart rate.
      - Body size
        - Individuals who are severely obesity can have a slightly faster pulse.

- Medications
  - Beta blockers slow the heart rate and too much thyroid medicine can speed the heart up.
- Caffeine and nicotine
  - Coffee, tea, tobacco, and soda can accelerate the heart rate.
- Infection may increase or decrease heart rate.
- Exercise
  - Regular exercise can lower the resting heart rate.
  - Recent exercise may increase the heart rate.
- Dehydration
  - Low body water can increase the heart rate.
- Respiration rate: number of breaths an individual takes in 1 minute
  - Can be determined by counting the number of inhalations an individual takes in 30 seconds and multiplying by 2 to get breaths per minute.
  - Interpretation
    - Normal: 12 to 20 breaths per minutes
    - Concerning: <10 breaths per minutes or >24 breaths per minutes
      - Factors affecting the respiration rate
        - Weather
          - Respiratory rate may go up in high and low temperatures.
        - Emotions
          - Stress and anxiety can raise the respiratory rate.
        - Body size
          - Obese individuals can have a faster respiratory rate.
        - Caffeine and nicotine
          - Coffee, tea, tobacco, and soda can raise your respiratory rate.
        - Infection
          - It may increase respiratory rate.
        - Exercise
          - Recent exercise can increase respiratory rate.
- Blood pressure: the measure of the pressure that results from the heart pumping blood through the circulatory system
  - Reported as systolic pressure/diastolic pressure
    - Systolic measurement—maximum pressure during one heartbeat
    - Diastolic measurement—minimum pressure between heartbeats
      - Can be determined using a manual or automatic blood pressure cuff
      - Interpretation
  - Normal: less than 120/80 mm Hg
  - Concerning: systolic: <100 mm Hg or >160 mm Hg; diastolic: <50 mm Hg or >100 mm Hg
    - Factors affecting blood pressure
      - Medications
        - They may increase or decrease blood pressure.
      - Pain
        - It may increase blood pressure.
      - Emotions
        - Stress and anxiety can increase blood pressure.

- Caffeine and nicotine
  - Coffee, tea, tobacco, and soda can increase blood pressure.
- Infection
  - Infection may increase or decrease blood pressure.
- Exercise
  - Recent exercise can increase blood pressure.
- Oxygen saturation: a measure of how much oxygen is being carried by the blood, and indicates how well the lungs are working; measured using an oximeter
  - Interpretation
    - Normal: >94%
    - Concerning: <90%
  - Factors affecting oxygen saturation
    - Existing lung disease
      - Individuals with chronic obstructive lung disease may have a lower pulse oximetry.
    - Smoking
      - Smokers may have falsely high levels because of carbon monoxide in the blood.
    - Weather
      - Cold temperatures can construct blood vessels resulting in low readings.
    - Dark nail polish
      - It may result in low readings.
    - Infection
      - It may result in low readings.
- Vital statistics: used to assess the patient's general state of health and consist of the patient's age, height, and weight.

Common specimen types

When a test is approved for both waived and nonwaived testing, the manufacturer's instructions may include instructions that could be performed using more than one type of sample. Unprocessed samples can only be used in processing waived tests. Examples of unprocessed samples include:

- Whole blood
- Urine
- Throat swab, nasopharyngeal swab, nasal wash
- Saliva and oral fluids
- Stool

Signs, symptoms, and characteristics of common chronic disease states

Hypertension

- Hypertension is sustained elevation of resting systolic blood pressure (≥130 mm Hg), diastolic blood pressure (≥80 mm Hg), or both.
- Types:
  - Primary: no known cause
  - Secondary: has a known cause
- Causes include sleep apnea, chronic kidney disease, primary aldosteronism, diabetes, or obesity.
- Patients with hypertension are normally asymptomatic. Patients with hypertension have been known to complain of experiencing fizziness, facial flushing, headache, fatigue, epistaxis, and nervousness.

- Diagnosis:
  - Multiple measurements of blood pressure to confirm presence of hypertension at two or three different times. Hypertension is diagnosed and classified by sphygmomanometry. Other diagnostic tests may be performed to determine etiology of hypertension ands potential damage to organs.
- Patient monitoring to include blood pressure, pulse, and weight

Blood pressure (mm Hg)	Category of hypertension
<120/≤80	Normal
120–129/<80	Elevated
130–139/80–89	High blood pressure stage 1 hypertension
≥140/≥90	High blood pressure stage 2 hypertension
>180/>120	Hypertensive crisis

- Hypertension treatments:
  - Pharmacological classifications prescribed include:
    - Diuretics:
      - Thiazide: hydrochlorothiazide
      - Loop: furosemide
    - Angiotensin-converting enzyme inhibitors (e.g., lisinopril and enalapril)
    - Angiotensin II receptor blockers (e.g., losartan and valsartan)
    - Beta-adrenergic antagonist (beta blockers) (e.g., metoprolol and atenolol)
    - Calcium channel blockers (e.g., amlodipine and diltiazem)
  - Behavioral modification:
    - Increased physical activity with a structured exercise program
    - Weight loss if overweight or obese
    - Healthy diet rich in fruits, vegetables, whole grains, and low-fat dairy products, with reduced saturated and total fat content
    - Reduced dietary sodium to < 500 mg/day
    - Enhanced dietary potassium intake, unless contraindicated due to chronic kidney disease or use of drugs that reduce potassium excretion
    - Moderation in alcohol intake
    - Smoking cessation if applicable)

Diabetes

- Diabetes occurs as a result of impaired insulin secretion and peripheral insulin resistance leading to hyperglycemia
- Types:
  - Diabetes mellitus type I
  - Diabetes mellitus type II
- Symptoms include polydipsia (excess thirst), polyphagia (excess hunger), polyuria (frequent urination), and blurred vision.
- Causes:
  - Diabetes mellitus type I occurs as a result of absent insulin production due to autoimmune pancreatic beta-cell destruction.
- Diabetes mellitus type II is due to inadequate insulin secretion because patients have developed resistance to insulin.
- Diagnosis:
  - Fasting plasma glucose levels
  - Glycosylated hemoglobin (HbA1C)
  - Oral glucose tolerance testing
- Patient monitoring to include blood pressure, pulse, and weight

Diabetes testing		
Test	**Reading**	**Category of diabetes**
A1C	<5.7%	Normal
	5.7% to 6.4%	Prediabetes
	≥6.5%	Diabetes
Fasting plasma glucose(fasting for at least 8 hours)	<100 mg/dL (5.5 mmol/L)	Normal
	100–125 mg/dL (5.5–6.9 mmol/L)	Prediabetes
	≥126 mg/dL (7 mmol/L)	Diabetes
2 hours after meals	<140 mg/dL (7.8 mmol/L)	Normal
	140–199 mg/dL (7.8–11.1 mmol/L)	Prediabetes
	≥200 mg/dL (11.1 mmol/L)	Diabetes

- Diabetes treatments:
  - Pharmacological classifications prescribed:
    - Insulin (e.g., Lantus)
    - Alpha-glucosidase inhibitors (e.g., acarbose)
    - Biguanide (e.g., metformin)
    - Dipeptidyl peptidase-4 inhibitors (e.g., sitagliptin)
    - Glucagon-like peptide-1 receptor agonists (e.g., exenatide and liraglutide)
    - Sodium-glucose transporter 2 inhibitors (e.g., canagliflozin and empagliflozin)
    - Sulfonylureas (e.g., glyburide and glipizide)
    - Thiazolidinediones (e.g., rosiglitazone and pioglitazone)
  - Behavioral modifications:
    - Exercise
    - Diet modification
    - Weight loss
    - Smoking cessation
    - Reduce alcohol consumption

Dyslipidemia

- Dyslipidemia is the elevation of plasma cholesterol, triglycerides, or both, or a low high-density lipoprotein cholesterol level that contributes to the development of atherosclerosis.
- Types of dyslipidemia:
  - Primary: Caused by genetic factors
  - Secondary: Caused by lifestyle behaviors
- Symptoms: None.

- Causes of dyslipidemia include a sedentary lifestyle with excessive dietary intake of total calories, saturated fat, cholesterol, and trans fats. Secondary causes include diabetes mellitus, chronic kidney disease, and hypothyroidism.
- Diagnosis is made by measuring total cholesterol, triglycerides (TG), and high-density lipoprotein (HDL) cholesterol and calculated low-density lipoprotein (LDL) cholesterol and very low density lipoproteins (VLDL) cholesterol.

Lipid	Measurement in mg/dL (mmol/L)
Total cholesterol	<200 (5.2)
	200–239 (5.2–6.2)
	≥240 (6.2)
LDL	<100 (3.4)
	100–189 (3.4–4.9)
	≥190 (4.9)
HDL	≥60 (1.6)
	40–59 (1–1.5) (men) 50–59 (1.3 to 1.5) (women)
	<40 (1) (men)<50 (1.3) (women)
Triglycerides	<150 (1.7)
	150–499 (1.7–5.6)
	≥500 (5.6)

HDL, high-density lipoprotein; *LDL*, low-density lipoprotein.

- Dyslipidemia treatments:
  - Pharmacological classification prescribed
    - 3-hydroxy-3-methylglutaryl coenzyme A reductase inhibitors (e.g., atorvastatin and simvastatin)
    - Niacin
    - Bile acid sequestering resins (e.g., colestipol and cholestyramine)
    - Fibrates (e.g., fenofibrate and gemfibrozil)
    - Omega-3 acid ethyl esters
  - Behavioral modifications:
    - Exercise
    - Diet modification
    - Weight loss
    - Smoking cessation
    - Reduce alcohol consumption

Signs, symptoms, and characteristics of common acute infections

COVID-19

- Disease is caused by the SARS-CoV-2 virus.
- Virus is spread from an infected person's mouth or nose in small liquid particles when they cough, sneeze, speak, sing, or breathe.
- Symptoms include fever or chills, cough, shortness of breath or difficulty breathing, fatigue, muscle or body aches, headache, new loss of taste or smell, sore throat, congestion or runny nose, nausea or vomiting and diarrhea.
- Rapid tests used in POC settings can be nucleic acid amplification test (NAAT), antigen, or antibody tests.
- Rapid tests are used to rule in or rule out COVID-19.

Influenza

- A respiratory tract infection caused by the influenza virus
- Transmitted through inhalation of respiratory droplets by coughing and sneezing
- Symptoms: fever, myalgia (muscle aches, headache), tiredness and fatigue, nonproductive cough and rhinitis (runny nose)
- Can be detected using rapid influenza diagnostic tests, which detect viral antigens
- Fingerstick blood specimens used to identify individuals with prior infection or immunization

Influenza-like illness

- Transmitted by person-to-person contact, particularly with respiratory secretions
- Symptoms: fever >101 °F (38.7°C) and cough and/or sore throat without known cause other than influenza

Acute pharyngitis

- It is commonly caused by *Streptococcus pyogenes*, also known as Group A Streptococcus (GAS)
- It is spread through direct person-to-person transmission by saliva or nasal secretions from an infected person.
- Symptoms include sudden onset of sore throat, fever, headache, swelling of the tonsils, creamy white patches on the tonsils, redness at the back of the throat, tender lymph nodes, nausea, vomiting, and abdominal pain.
- Centor Score is used as a screening tool to identify individuals with GAS pharyngitis.
- POC testing involves either a rapid antigen detection test or throat culture to confirm GAS pharyngitis.

Chlamydia

- It is caused *Chlamydia trachomatis*.
- It is transmitted through sexual contact with the penis, vagina, mouth, or anus of an infected partner.
- Symptoms include discharge, burning sensation during urination, unusual sores, and rash.
- POC testing involves vaginal swab for women and urine sample for men.

Gonorrhea

- It is caused by *Neisseria gonorrhoeae*.
- It is transmitted through sexual contact with the penis, vagina, mouth, or anus of an infected partner.
- Symptoms:
  - Men: dysuria or a white, yellow, or green urethral discharge
  - Women: dysuria, increased vaginal discharge, or vaginal bleeding between periods
- POC testing involves vaginal swab for women and urine sample for men.

Syphilis

- It is caused by *Treponema pallidum*.
- It is transmitted by direct contact with a syphilitic sore (chancre), commonly found on or around the external genitals, in the vagina, around the anus, in the rectum, or in or around the mouth.
- Chancres appear during the first stage of syphilis. Skin rashes and/or mucous membrane lesions (sores in the mouth, vagina, or anus) may be present during the second stage of condition.
- POC testing is performed on fingerstick blood.

Bacterial vaginosis

- It is caused by a change in in the normal balance of bacteria in the vagina.
- Patient maybe asymptomatic; however, symptoms may be present, which include:
  - A thin white or gray vaginal discharge
  - Pain, itching, or burning in the vagina
  - Presence of a strong fishlike odor, especially after sex
  - Burning sensation during urination
  - Itching around the outside of the vagina
- POC testing is performed using a vaginal swab.

Collecting a health history

Collecting an individual health history consists of obtaining a complete medical history. Components of a medical history include the following:

- Chief complaint is a statement from the patient indicating the reason why they are seeking medical attention. Examples include shortness of breath, runny nose, rapid heart rate, and difficulty sleeping.
- Symptoms are a physical or mental problem that a person experiences that may indicate a disease or condition; often they may not be detected by a medical test or laboratory work. Examples include rash, headache, frequent urination, and muscle pain.
- History of present illness involves collecting information related to the current condition for which the patient is seeking help.
- Medication history is obtained to become familiar with the medications a patient is taking and to avoid potential drug-drug interactions.
- Medications allergy is the abnormal reaction of the immune system to as a result of a medication, such as penicillin or a sulfonamide.
- Family history is a record of the relationships among family members along with their medical histories. It may reveal potential indicators of genetic predisposition to disease such as cardiac diseases or depression.
- Surgical history provides a list of all invasive procedures an individual has undergone such as a mastectomy or a tonsillectomy.
- Social history is a summary of lifestyle practices that may have a direct or indirect effect on an individual's heath. A social history includes an individual's occupation, exercise habits, diet, hobbies, substance use, sexual orientation, sexual behavior, and firearms in household.

- Immunization history provides information on the vaccines an individual has received such as measles, mumps, and rubella.

Centor score

- The score is a symptom-based screening tool that is used to help identify individuals with GAS pharyngitis.
- The Centor criteria include:
  - Fever
  - Tonsillar exudate
  - Tender anterior cervical adenopathy
  - Fever
- One point is awarded for each of the criteria met. In addition, age is taken into consideration:
  - 3–14 years of age: add 1 point.
  - 15–44 years of age: add 0 points.
  - 45 years of age and older: subtract 1 point.
  - Scores may range from −1 though 5:
    - −1, 0, or 1 point—no antibiotic or throat culture necessary (risk of streptococcal infection <10%)
    - 2 or 3 points—should receive a throat culture and treat with an antibiotic if culture is positive (risk of streptococcal infection 32% if 3 points, 15% if 2 points)
    - 4 or 5 points—consider rapid strep testing and or culture

Clinical Laboratory Improvement Amendments—waived tests

Clinical Laboratory Improvement Amendments of 1988 as it pertains to point-of-care tests

The Clinical Laboratory Improvement Amendments (CLIA) Program regulates laboratories testing human specimens and confirms they deliver accurate, reliable, and timely patient test results regardless of where the test is performed. CLIA applies to all laboratories testing "materials derived from the human body with the intent of providing information for the diagnosis, prevention, or treatment of any disease or impairment of, or the assessment of the health of, human beings." CLIA applies to all institutions providing clinical laboratory services and mandates these laboratories meet applicable federal requirements and have a current CLIA certificate. CLIA requirements also apply to laboratories in physician offices.

Clinical Laboratory Improvement Amendments administration responsibilities

Centers for Medicare and Medicaid Services (CMS)

- Approves and reapproves private accreditation organizations doing inspections
- Approves state exemptions
- Collects user fees
- Conducts laboratory inspections

- Enforces regulatory compliance
- Issues laboratory certificates
- Oversees laboratory proficiency testing performance and approves proficiency testing programs
- Develops, implements, and publishes CLIA rules and regulations

Food and Drug Administration (FDA)

- Develops CLIA complexity categorization rules and guidance
- Categorizes tests based on complexity
- Reviews requests for waiver
- Reviews in Vitro Diagnostic applications for marketing devices

Centers for Disease Control and Prevention (CDC)

- Performs laboratory quality improvement studies
- Develops and distributes professional information and educational resources
- Creates technical standards and laboratory practice guidelines, including cytology guidelines and standards
- Conducts laboratory quality improvement studies
- Manages CLIA Committee
- Monitors proficiency testing practices
- Provides analysis, research, and technical help

Clinical Laboratory Improvement Amendments waiver process and certifications

The CLIA defines a laboratory "as a facility that performs applicable testing on materials derived from the human body for the purpose of providing information for the diagnosis, prevention, or treatment of any disease or impairment of, or assessment of the health of, human beings." According to the CLIA, a waived test is classified as "simple laboratory examinations and procedures that have an insignificant risk of an erroneous result."

The CLIA waiver process involves the following steps

- Enroll the laboratory in the CLIA program by completing an application (Form CMS-116)
- Submit the application process to your local state agency. An application must be submitted for each laboratory location and each laboratory must have their own certificate.
- Pay the certificate fee every 2 years.
- Follow the manufacturer's instructions for the waived tests the pharmacy is performing. This involves following all of the instructions in the package insert from "intended use" to "limitations of the procedure." Following the manufacturer's instructions includes:
  - Observing storage and handling requirements for the test system components
  - Adhering to the expiration date of the test system and reagents, as applicable
  - Performing quality control (QC), as required by the manufacturer

- Performing function checks and maintenance of equipment
- Training testing personnel in the performance of the test, if required by the manufacturer
- Reporting patients' test results in the units described in the package insert
- Sending specimens for confirmatory tests, when required by the manufacturer
- Ensuring that any test system limitations are observed.
- Notify your state agency of any changes in ownership, name, address or laboratory director within 30 days, or if you wish to add tests that are more complex.
- Check with the state agency for any other state-specific requirements.

Certificate of Waiver (CoW)

- A CoW permits a laboratory to administer tests the FDA categorizes as waived tests. A waived tests is one that is classified as a simple, low-risk test for an incorrect result or with no reasonable risk of harm. Examples of waived tests include
  - Certain glucose and cholesterol testing methods
  - Fecal occult blood tests
  - Pregnancy tests
  - Select urine tests
- Laboratories that conduct only waived tests must:
  - Enroll in the CLIA program.
  - Pay applicable certificate fees every 2 years.
  - Adhere to manufacturer's test instructions.
- Laboratories with CoW are not surveyed every 2 years.
- Laboratories with CoW are only surveyed:
  - If a complaint has been made
  - If the testing is beyond the scope of the certificate
  - If there is a risk of harm due to incorrect testing
  - To collect waived test information

CLIA Certificate of Registration (COR)

- Prior to applying for Certificate of Compliance (CoC) or Certificate of Accreditation (CoA), a laboratory must obtained a Certificate of Registration (CoR).
- A CoR is temporary and permits a laboratory to conduct moderated and high-complexity tests until the laboratories is surveyed to verify it meets CLIA regulations.
- For laboratories applying for a CoA or CoC, a CoR shows registration with the CLIA program and permits to operate until compliance is evaluated
- A CoR is valid for 2 years.

CLIA Certificate of Compliance (CoC)

- A laboratory gets a CoC after an on-site survey finds it complies with all applicable CLIA regulations.
- Surveys occur every 2 years at CoC laboratories performing moderate and high-complexity testing.
- Surveys assist laboratories to improve patient care through education and stress requirements directly affecting the laboratory's quality test performance.
- A CoC determines the laboratory's compliance to CIA regulations.

CLIA Certificate of Accreditation (CoA)

- CoAs are awarded to laboratories that perform moderate and high complexity tests and comply with the standards of a private nonprofit Accreditation Organization (AO) approved by CMS
- To obtain approval, a nonprofit AO's standards must meet or exceed CLIA regulatory requirements
- An AO inspection takes place once every 2 years.
- Every 6 years or sooner, an institution reapplies for continued permission to confirm its standards meet or exceed CLIA's requirements.

Provider-Performed Microscopy (PPM) Procedures Certificate

- Consists of moderate complex tests that are performed by physicians, midlevel practitioners, or dentists during a patient's visits.
- Uses a bright-field or phase-contrast microscope in conducting the test
- Laboratories with a Provider-Performed Microscopy Procedures Certificate are not surveyed every 2 years. They are only surveyed:
  - If a complaint has been made
  - If the testing is beyond the scope of the certificate
  - If there's a risk of harm due to incorrect testing
  - To collect Provider-Performed Microscopy Procedures Certificate test information

Point-of-care technology

Lateral flow

- Lateral flow assays are used to detect antigens, antibodies, and chemicals in a sample.
- Lateral flow assays function by binding an analyte to a colorimetric probe.
- When the probe is bound to the analyte, it is captured by markers adhered to a nitrocellulose membrane. This results in a visible line being formed in the test region and is read as a positive test.
- If an analyte is not present in a sample, the probes do not attach in this region and the test is read as negative.
- Examples of POC tests using lateral flow include SARS-CoV-2 antigen test, influenza test, GAS test, and home pregnancy tests.

Advantages	Disadvantages
One-step assay; no washing steps required	One-step assay
Fast, low cost, and low sample volume	Qualitative results (positive/negative)
Qualitative (on/off) and semi-quantitative result	Inaccurate sample volume reduces precision
Relatively short development time brings applications faster to market	Restriction on test volume in test gives a limit of sensitivity
Simple test procedure	No possibility to enhance the response by enzyme reaction
Applications at point of care	Good antibody preparation is required

Advantages	Disadvantages
Proteins, haptens, nucleic acids, and amplicons can be detected	Analysis time is dependent on nature of the sample, e.g., viscosity
Individual tests can be used or an array format for the mid throughput screening	Obstruction of pores due to matrix components
Long shelf life, no need to refrigerate, and batches can be prepared in advance	Sample pretreatment is not needed for nonfluid samples
For fluid samples, pretreatment is often not necessary	

Molecular Nucleic Acid Amplification Tests (NAAT)

- Includes polymerase chain reaction
- Magnifies pathogen-specific genetic targets from a sample
- Can be highly sensitive and specific, but may not be able to differentiate between live and dead organisms or those that are colonizing a patient versus those that might be causing infection
- Examples of NAAT include SARS-CoV-2 antigen test, influenza test, and sexually transmitted infections

Advantages	Disadvantages
High sensitivity and specificity	Expensive reagents
Capable of detecting low levels of pathogens	Require specialized equipment
Can even be self-administered at home	Prone to contamination
Some are considered rapid tests	May require longer to get results
If POC NAATs do not deliver presumptive results, they can be used for confirmatory testing	Do not differentiate between viable organisms and genetic fragments from nonviable remnants

NAAT, nucleic acid amplification test; *POC*, point of care.

Serum chemistry analyzers

- Analyzers are used to perform tests on whole blood, serum, plasma, or urine samples to determine concentrations of analytes (e.g., cholesterol, electrolytes, glucose, calcium, metabolites, and drugs).
- A photometer is often used to measure analyte concentrations of a sample. A photometer measures masses of organic or inorganic materials in a solution or liquid.

Blood glucose monitor (glucometer)

- Measures the amount of glucose in the blood normally from a finger stick
- Professional use—blood glucose monitoring systems:
  - Possesses more stringent performance characteristics, especially at high and low value
  - Planned to be used on multiple patients
  - Can be used in individuals without a diagnosis of diabetes

- Home use—self-monitoring blood glucose test systems:
  - Available as over-the-counter blood glucose meters
  - Not intended to be used on multiple patients due to possibility of transmission of blood-borne pathogens
  - Not used in pharmacies for POC testing

HgbA1c analyzers

- They provide quantitative determination of glycated hemoglobin (% hemoglobin A1c, HgbA1c).
- The measurement of % HgbA1c is recommended as a marker of long-term metabolic control in persons with diabetes mellitus.
- They can report the concentration of hemoglobin in a blood or urine sample in g/L, g/dL, or mol/L.
- Capillary or venous whole blood is used as a sample.

International normalized ratio analyzers

- Measures blood-clotting time (prothrombin time [PT]) for people who are taking anticoagulation medications such as warfarin
- International normalized ratio (INR) analyzers display both the PProthT and calculated INR.
- Analyzer uses fingerstick blood as sample.
- Accuracy of results may decrease with higher INRs.

Common point-of-care tests conditions and uses for common tests (e.g., prothrombin time, influenza, Streptococcus, A1C, HIV, hepatitis

A1C (also known as the hemoglobin A1C or HbA1c test)

- Measures a patient's average blood sugar levels over the past 3 months
- Used to diagnose prediabetes and diabetes
- Normal A1C level: below 5.7%; level of 5.7% to 6.4% indicates prediabetes; and level of 6.5% or more indicates diabetes (Within the 5.7% to 6.4% prediabetes range, the higher a patient's A1C, the greater their risk is for developing diabetes mellitus type II.)
- Sample drawn from a vein in the arm
- Quantitative test

Prothrombin Time/international Normalized Ratio (PT)

- Measures how long it takes for a clot to form in a blood sample drawn from either the vein or finger tip
- Indicated to assess warfarin therapy
- Desired therapeutic goal:
  - 2–3 for most indications
  - 2.5–3.5 for individuals with prosthetic heart valves
- Quantitative test

Cholesterol

- Uses whole blood as a sample
- Quantitative test

Lipid panel

- Requires fingerstick blood sample
- Quantitative test

Screening tests

COVID-19

- Detects the presence of SARS-CoV-2 virus
- Types of POC testing:
  - NAATs
  - Antigen tests
- Specimens may be collected using a nasal swab or fingertip stick
- Positive test results must be reported to the state government
- Qualitative test

HIV

- Detects the presence of HIV antibodies
- Transmitted through blood and fluids
- Is a screening test where results are referred to as reactive and nonreactive; patients with reactive test results should be referred to appropriate programs
- Samples obtained through a fingerstick blood or oral fluid specimen

Hepatitis C

- Detects the presence of hepatitis C antibodies
- Transmitted from person-to-person through contact with blood and less commonly by sexual contact
  - Requires a fingerstick blood specimen
  - Is a screening test where results are referred to as reactive and nonreactive

Home pregnancy

- Measures urine sample for presence of human chorionic gonadotropin
- Qualitative test

Manufacturer instructions

The manufacturer's instructions for performing the test means to follow all of the instructions in the package insert from "intended use" to "limitations of the procedure." The manufacturer's instructions can be found in the package insert for each and should be read before testing begins. It is important the package insert is current for the test system in use, the correct specimen type is used, the proper reagents (testing solutions) are added in the correct order, and the test is performed according to the step-by-step procedure outlined in the package insert. Failing to use the current instructions might cause inaccurate results that may result in a misdiagnosis or delay in proper treatment of a patient. If in doubt whether you have current instructions, contact the manufacturer at the telephone number listed in the package insert.

Components of manufacturer instructions	
Component	**Information provided**
Intended use	Describes the test purpose, substance detected or measured, test methodology, appropriate specimen type, and FDA-cleared conditions for use. Additionally, might include if the test is diagnostic or for screening a target population and if it is intended for professional use or self-testing.
Summary	Explains what the test detects; a short history of the methodology, the disease process or health condition detected or monitored; the response to disease, symptoms and severity, and disease prevalence and appropriate references.
Test principle	A description of the test methodology and technical reactions of the test and the interactions with the sample to detect or measure a specific substance.
Precautions	Alerts the user of practices or conditions affecting the test, potential hazards and safety precautions (toxic reagents, handling infectious samples or biohazardous waste). Warnings to not mix components from different lot numbers or use products beyond the expiration date are often included.
Storage and stability	The recommended conditions for storing reagents or kits; temperature ranges and other physical requirements (humidity, exposure to light) affecting the stability of reagents or test components.
Reagents and materials supplied	A list of reagents and materials included in the test kit, the concentration, and major ingredients in reagents.
Materials required but not provided	A description of any additional materials necessary to perform the test that are not provided with the test kit.
Sample collection and preparation	A detailed procedure for collecting the appropriate sample including storage and handling instructions. Conditions affecting the acceptability of the sample may be described.
Test procedure	Step-by-step instructions and information critical to correctly performing the test are provided in this section.
Interpretation of results	An explanation of how to read or interpret the test results, often includes visual aids. Instructions for dealing with invalid results, precautions against reporting results when supplementary or confirmatory testing is required
QC	Instructions for performing QC, what aspects of the test are monitored by internal and/or external QC, and when to perform QC testing.
Limitations	Describes the conditions that can affect test results, or circumstances for which the test was not intended, such as interference from medical conditions, drugs or other substances; limitations for testing with certain samples or populations; more specific testing may be required; warnings that the test does not differentiate between active infection and carrier states, or warnings that test results should be considered with clinical signs, history, and other information.
Expected values	Describes the test results normally expected, how results can vary with disease prevalence or seasonality. Studies leading to the expected results might be included.
Performance characteristics	Details of the studies done to evaluate the overall performance of the test, including the data for determining accuracy, precision, sensitivity, specificity and reproducibility are present. Additional information from studies of cross-reactivity with interfering substances is included.
QC, quality control.	

Test results, quality control, and recording

Qualitative and quantitative test results

Qualitative

- Results are interpreted as positive, negative; reactive, nonreactive; or invalid.
- These results identify the presence or absence of a particular substance, condition, or microbial organism.
- For visual read tests, the result may be indicated by the presence of a colored line or dot.
- Examples of qualitative tests include COVID-19 and pregnancy tests.

Quantitative

- Number results produced by the test device or instrument.

- These results identify the quantity of substance being measured and are reported in specific measurement units.
- Interpreting the rest requires comparison to clinically relevant values.
- Examples of quantitative include PT/INR and A1c.

Test performance

The perfect diagnostic test would identify the disease in all patients that do have it, and does not detect the disease in patients that do not have it

	Disease present	Disease absent
Positive test result	True positive (TP)	False positive (FP)
Negative test result	False negative (FN)	True negative (TN)

Sensitivity

- The proportion of patients who *do* have the disease that test positive

- Sensitivity can be calculated using the following equation:

$$\text{Sensitivity} = [\text{True Positives} \div (\text{True Positives} + \text{True Negatives})] \times 100$$

- Increases as the number of false-negative results decreases; decreases as the number of false-negative results increases

False negative

- A false-negative result is when a patient with the underlying disease tests negative.
- Example: If 100 patients with influenza with a test with a sensitivity of 90%, we would expect 10 patients to test negative. If the test had a sensitivity of 75%, we would expect 25 patients to test negative.

Specificity

- The proportion of patients that *do not* have the disease that test negative.
- Specificity can be calculated using the following equation:

$$\text{Specificity} = [\text{True Negatives} \div (\text{True Positives} + \text{True Negatives})] \times 100$$

- Specificity increases as the number of false-positive results decreases; specificity decreases as number of false-positive results increase.

False positive

- A false-positive result is when a patient without the underlying disease tests positive.
- Example: If a pharmacy tested 100 patients without COVID-19 with a test with a specificity of 80%, we would expect 20 patients to test positive. If the test had a specificity of 65%, we would expect 35 patients to test positive.

Positive predictive value

- Positive predictive value (PPV) is the probability that a patient who tested positive actually has the disease.

$$\text{PPV} = [\text{True Positives} \div (\text{True Positives} + \text{False Positives})] \times 100$$

- PPV increases as the incidence of the disease increases.

Negative predictive value

- Negative predictive value (NPV) is the probability that a patient who tested negative truly does *not* have the disease.

$$\text{NPV} = [\text{True Negatives} \div (\text{True Negatives} + \text{False Negatives})] \times 100$$

- NPV increases as the disease incidence decreases.

Time since exposure

- Time since exposure (incubation periods) refers to the time from exposure to development of symptoms. Depending on the condition being tested, it may take several days or even week for symptoms to appear in an individual.

- In some situations, a patient may continue to test positive for months after they have been exposed/infected even when they are no longer contagious.

Recording results

Requirements

- Record test results legibly in a log or following the testing site's policy and keep as a permanent record. These records should have enough detail for easy retrieval of information. Guidelines for recording results include:
  - Quantitative (numerical) results should be recorded in the appropriate units of measurement.
  - Qualitative results should be recorded using words or abbreviations rather than symbols. For example use: "Positive" or "Pos," "Reactive" or "R" instead of "+" and "Negative" or "Neg," "Nonreactive" or "NR" instead of "−".

Results of log-qualitative test

- Record the facility information and test name on the top of the form.
- Enter the date of the test, sample number, patient name or identification, test results, lot number, and expiration date of test.
- The person performing the test should initial the results after verifying all of the information has been entered correctly.

Results of log-quantitative test

- Record the facility information, test name, and reportable range for the test on the top of the form.
- Enter the date of the test, sample number, patient name or identification, test results, lot number, and expiration date of test.
- The person performing the test should initial the results after verifying all of the information has been entered correctly.

Results log with quality control-qualitative test

- Record the facility information and test name on the top of the form.
- Record the QC material lot number, expiration date, positive and negative control result.
- If the results are acceptable, QC passes and patient results can be reported.
- If the results are not acceptable, QC fails. Troubleshoot (check expiration dates, storage condition etc.), retest the QC, and document the corrective action taken.

Results log with quality control-quantitative test

- Record the facility information and test name on the top of the form.
- Record the QC material lot number, expiration date, positive and negative control result.
- If the results are acceptable, QC passes and patient results can be reported.

- If the results are not acceptable, QC fails. Troubleshoot (check expiration dates, storage condition etc.), retest the QC and document the corrective action taken.

Results log with multiple test

- Record the facility information on the top of the form.
- Record the date, sample number, patient identification, test name, reportable range (if applicable), test result, lot number, expiration date, and the initials of the individual performing the test.

Best practices

- Make sure patient reports are legible and reported in a timely manner.
- Make sure reports are standardized and easily distinguishable from referral laboratory test reports.
- Report patient test results only to authorized persons.
- Document verbal reports, followed by a written test report.

Invalid test results

If test results are invalid, compromised, or disagree with the patient's clinical information, then the test should be repeated. Additionally, testing should be repeated when:

- Quantitative (numerical) results have values beyond the measuring range of the instrument.
- The test system gives an "invalid" result or prevents the display of the result.

The manufacturer's instructions for test performance should include steps for handling high or low results that cannot be accurately measured. Test results should not be reported until the problem(s) are identified and corrected.

Labeling and documentation

- Be sure to label the sample as soon as it is collected with a unique identifier such as name and date of birth to prevent sample mix-up.
- Sample labels may also include the date and time of collection and who collected the sample.
- For tests in which the sample is applied directly to the test device (for example: test strip or cassette), label the test device with the patient identifier before collecting the sample.

Quality control testing methods

QC involves procedures used to identify unfavorable environmental conditions and discrepancies in operator performance that occur due to test system failures. QC involves monitoring the accuracy and precision of the test performed. The benefits associated with of quality assessment includes reduced errors, better patient outcomes, improved patient and employee safety, and reduced costs.

Analytic system quality assessment

- Internal controls are processes for staff performing and overseeing testing to evaluate their current practices, including:
  - Performing and documenting QC procedures and results
  - Reviewing QC records and test results
  - Reviewing room and refrigerator log sheets for complete documentation
  - Documenting and reviewing problems and establishing a plan to improve processes
  - Documenting and reviewing injury/incident reports
- External controls are performed by outside organizations to evaluate current practices to include:
  - Undergoing voluntary inspections by individuals who would evaluate testing practices and documentation systems and offering suggestions for improvement
  - Subscribing voluntarily to proficiency testing programs (The use of a CLIA proficiency testing program is not a CIA requirement.)
  - Exchanging samples with other testing sites using the same test method(s) to compare results

Proficiency testing

- Proficiency testing is not normally required for waived testing; however, there are many benefits of participating in a proficiency testing program. They include:
  - A regular, external check on the quality of testing
  - An incentive to improve performance
  - A comparison of performance with that of other participating sites (peers)
  - A chance to receive feedback and technical advice from programs that offer proficiency testing
  - Help in evaluating methods and instrumentation
  - Support with staff education, training, and competence monitoring
  - An opportunity for in recognizing areas needing improvement
- Personnel competency assessments
- Calibration verification
- Temperature log:
  - The CLIA requires a waived testing site follow the current manufacturer's instructions provided with the test. The manufacturer's instructions will give storage conditions for the product and a temperature range for storing reagents, controls, and patient specimens.
  - A refrigerator used to store patient samples is kept between +2°C and +8°C. A freezer used for sample storage is often kept between −25°C and −15°C. The acceptable temperature range for a freezer or refrigerator is determined by the temperature range indicated for the reagents, controls, and patient specimens that are stored in it.
  - Recording temperatures requires:
    - Posting a temperature log on the refrigerator and/or freezer door
    - Reading the thermometer(s) in the refrigerator and/or freezer daily

- Checking for separated columns, gas bubbles, and cracks each time the thermometer is read, as applicable
- Recording the temperature(s) of the refrigerator and/or freezer
- Dating and initialing/signing the temperature log

- Noting on the temperature log when the pharmacy is closed
- Blank log entry remaining blank if a temperature reading is missed (Do not make up or guess what the temperature was for that reading.)

Sample temperature log					
Date	Temperature	Checked by	Date	Temperature	Checked by
1			17		
2			18		
3			19		
4			20		
5			21		
6			22		
7			23		
8			24		
9			25		
10			26		
11			27		
12			28		
13			29		
14			30		
15			31		
16					

Signature   Date

- Documenting action taken when the temperature in the refrigerator and/or freezer falls outside the recommended range for storage

Corrective action for out-of-range temperature		
Date	Action taken	Initials

Signature   date

- The person who directs or supervises the testing reviewing and signing when the temperature log is completed for the month
  - Records
  - Log books or electronic files can be used to maintain records. Examples of records include:
    - Test orders, test results, results from confirmatory or additional testing
    - QC results
    - Lot numbers, dates used and received, and expiration dates of reagents, kits, and QC material
    - Daily temperature checks, test system or equipment function checks, and maintenance
    - Test system failures, troubleshooting, and corrective action taken when problems have been identified
    - Test or product recall notices
    - Personnel training and competency assessments
    - Results of proficiency testing or other external quality assessment activities

CHAPTER REVIEW QUESTIONS

1. Which of the following tasks may only the pharmacist perform?
   a. Collecting demographic, social, and clinical data and consent forms, insurance, and payments from the patient
   b. Ensuring appropriate storage of tests and reagents
   c. Interpreting test results according to manufacturer's instructions
   d. Recording test results in a log
2. How often must an institution's exposure control plan be reviewed and updated?
   a. Every year
   b. Every 2 years
   c. Every 3 years
   d. Every 4 years
3. Which vaccination must an institution provide free to all employees with occupational exposure to blood or other potentially infectious materials?
   a. Hepatitis A
   b. Hepatitis B
   c. Hepatitis C
   d. All the above
4. How often must employees receive blood-borne pathogen training?
   a. Every 6 months
   b. Every year
   c. Every 2 years
   d. Every 3 years

5. Which of the following substances may contain biohazardous waste?
   a. Amniotic fluids
   b. Saliva
   c. Serum
   d. All the above

6. Which color container indicates it contains biohazardous waste?
   a. Black
   b. Red
   c. White with a blue lid
   d. Yellow

7. Which is the minimum number of identifier(s) the Joint Commission requires a patient provide to the POC testing site prior to administering the POC test?
   a. 1
   b. 2
   c. 3
   d. 4

8. The pharmacy technician is taking a patient's blood pressure and the reading is 133/81. What category of hypertension does the patient have?
   a. Normal
   b. Elevated
   c. Stage 1 hypertension
   d. Hypertensive crisis

9. A patient is diagnosed with stage 2 hypertension. Which of the following drug classifications are *not* indicated for this condition?
   a. Angiotensin-converting enzyme inhibitors
   b. Beta-adrenergic antagonists
   c. Diuretics
   d. 3-Hydroxy-3-methylglutaryl coenzyme A reductase inhibitors

10. Which condition is an A1C test used to diagnose?
    a. Diabetes
    b. Dyslipidemia
    c. Hypertension
    d. Hypothyroidism

11. Which condition is caused by the SARS-CoV-2 virus?
    a. Acute pharyngitis
    b. COVID-19
    c. Influenza
    d. Syphilis

12. Which term refers to the physical or mental a problems an individual is experiencing?
    a. Chief complaint
    b. Family history
    c. Medication allergy
    d. Symptom

13. Which condition may a Centor Score be used as a screening tool to identify?
    a. Chlamydia
    b. Gonorrhea
    c. GAS pharyngitis
    d. Influenza-like illness

14. Which organization conducts laboratory inspections for facilities providing POC testing?
    a. Centers for Disease Control and Prevention (CDC)
    b. CMS

c. Drug Enforcement Administration
d. FDA

15. If a facility wishes to participate in a the CLIA Waiver Process, which of the following must be done?
    a. Enroll the laboratory in the CLIA program by completing an application (Form FDA-116).
    b. Follow the manufacturer's instructions for the waived tests the pharmacy is performing.
    c. Pay the certificate fee every year.
    d. Submit the application process to Health and Human Services at the federal government.

16. Which of the following is a true statement regarding a facility which has been issued a CoW?
    a. Are not required to enroll in the CLIA program
    b. Are not surveyed
    c. Permits a facility to administer waived tests
    d. All of the above

17. What would a facility be measuring if they were using an INR analyzer?
    a. Blood glucose
    b. Cholesterol
    c. Glycated hemoglobin
    d. Prothrombin time

18. Which of the following tests is a qualitative test?
    a. A1C
    b. Cholesterol
    c. COVID-19
    d. Lipid panel

19. You have been asked to review the manufacturer's instructions prior to administering a POC test. Under which section would you find what the test detects?
    a. Intended use
    b. Precautions
    c. Summary
    d. Test principle

20. Which term refers to the proportion of patients who do have the disease that test positive?
    a. False-negative result
    b. False-positive result
    c. Sensitivity
    d. Specificity

21. How should you record the results of a quantitative test?
    a. Use +
    b. Use Neg
    c. Use Positive
    d. Use a number with the correct units

22. Who should initial the results of a quantitative test after verifying the information is correct?
    a. Manager of the laboratory
    b. Person performing the test
    c. Pharmacist
    d. Pharmacy technician

23. Which is the appropriate temperature range for storing a patient's sample in the refrigerator?
    a. 0 and + 4°C
    b. +2°C and +8°C
    c. +4°C and +10°C
    d. +6°C and +12°C

24. Which of the following is (are) required when recording temperatures?
    a. Dating and initialing/signing the temperature log
    b. Posting a temperature log on the refrigerator and/or freezer door
    c. Reading and recording the thermometer(s) in the refrigerator and/or freezer daily
    d. All the above

25. Which is (are) an example(s) of records that must be maintained by a POC?
    a. Daily temperature checks, test system or equipment function checks, and maintenance
    b. QC results
    c. Test or product recall notices
    d. All the above

9

Billing and Reimbursement Certificate

Billing and reimbursement domains

Programs and eligibility (20%)
- Programs and eligibility terminology
- Third-party reimbursement types (e.g., pharmacy benefit mangers, medication assistance programs, self-pay)
- Health care reimbursement systems in different settings (e.g., home health, long-term care, home infusion, health systems, community pharmacy, and ambulatory clinics)
- Eligibility requirements for private and/or federally funded insurance programs (e.g., Medicare, TRICARE, Medicaid)
- Eligibility for patient assistance through available programs (e.g., a 340B-eligible program)

Claims processing and adjudication (48%)
- Pharmacy/medical claim processing terminology
- Information needed to submit pharmacy/medical claims
- General pharmacy claim submission process (e.g., data entry, verification, adjudication)
- Third-party claim rejection troubleshooting and resolution
- Methods for determining drug cost and sale prices (e.g., average wholesale price, dispensing fees, gross and net profit, acquisition cost
- Coordination of benefits or plan limitations to determine each party's responsibility

- Reimbursement policies for all plans being billed, regardless of contracted payers, HMOs, PPO, CMS, or commercial plans
- Identification of formulary coverage or alternatives
- 340B terminology

Prior authorization (20%)
- Prior authorization terminology
- Information needed to submit medical/pharmacy prior authorization (e.g., patient and prescriber information, drug, dose)
- General process of prior authorization (e.g., from formulary alternatives to contacting the provider, then through payer to patient)
- Third-party prior authorization rejection troubleshooting and resolution

Audits and compliance (12%)
- Audit and compliance terminology
- Contract documentation for claims billed to specific insurance plans (e.g., International Classification of Diseases-10 codes, provider feedback, and authorizations to change medications)
- Federal laws/regulations regarding audits (e.g., mandated audits by Centers for Medicare and Medicaid Services for all government funded programs)
- Accrediting bodies and surveys (e.g., Utilization Review Accreditation Commission, The Joint Commission, Centers for Medicare and Medicaid Services, Det Norske Veritas)

Programs and eligibility

Programs and eligibility terminology

Pharmacy benefit managers
- Third-party administrators of prescription drug programs that process and pay prescription drug claims
- Responsible for developing and maintaining the prescription plan's formulary
- Contact with pharmacies to provide pharmacy services for subscribers

- Negotiate discounts and rebates from drug manufacturers
- May establish exclusive contracts with large organizations, managed care organizations, or independent entities
- Often own their own mail order service

  Examples: CVS, Cigna, United Healthcare, Humana

Types of eligibility commercial insurance

- Group health plans cover employees or group members and their dependents.
- Individual plans covers individual and family or dependents.

Eligibility commercial insurance considerations

- Lifetime maximum or limits: The maximum dollar amount that a health insurance company agrees to pay on behalf of a member for services
- Qualifying event: An event such a divorce or death of the employee or termination of employment that will trigger changes in a member's health coverage
- Dependent coverage: Spouse and children up to the age of 26
- Domestic partners: Varies with state

Commercial health insurance

- Conventional indemnity plan: Permits the participant the choice of any provider without effect on reimbursement. Reimburse as expenses are incurred.
- PPO: Coverage is provided through a network of selected health care providers. Enrollees may go outside network the beneficiary incurs larger costs.
- Exclusive provider organization: A more restrictive type of preferred provider organization plan. Beneficiaries must use providers from the specified network. There is no coverage for care received from a non-network provider except in an emergency.
- HMO: Beneficiaries must use providers from the specified network. There is no coverage for care received from a nonnetwork provider except in an emergency. In an HMO the primary care physician acts a gatekeeper to any other services in the network.
- Self-funded health insurance plan: A plan that is funded by an employer rather than through a health insurance company. A health insurance company, however, will typically handle plan administration.
- High-deductible health plan: A plan with requires greater out-of-pocket spending, often with lower premiums. For 2022, the Internal Revenue Service defines a high-deductible health plan as any plan with a deductible of at least $1400 for an individual or $2800 for a family. A high-deductible health plan's total yearly out-of-pocket expenses (including deductibles, copayments, and coinsurance) cannot be more than $7050 for an individual or $14,100 for a family.
- Point-of-service: An "HMO/PPO" hybrid. Requires an in network primary care physician to make referrals for all services. It allows referrals outside of network; however, the beneficiary incurs larger costs like a PPO.
- Medigap Supplemental Plans: Pays the Medicare deductibles, copayments, and other expenses for Medicare Part A and B.

Comparison of major health plan types			
Plan type	Provider options	Cost containment	Functions
PPO	Network or out of network providers	Referral not required for specialists	Higher cost for out-of-network providers
		Fees are discounted	Preventative care coverage varies
		Preauthorization for some procedures	
HMO	Network only	Primary care physician paid by contract or capitation	Only network provider visits covered
		Specialists paid according to a contractual agreement	Covers preventative care
		No payment for out-of-network nonemergency services	
Point-of-service	Network providers or out-of-network providers	Within network, primary care physician manages care	Lower copayments for network providers
			Higher costs for out-of-network providers
			Covers preventative care
Indemnity	Any provider	Little or none	Higher costs
		Preauthorization required for some procedures	Deductibles
			Coinsurance
			Preventative care not usually covered
Consumer-driven health plan	Similar to PPO	Increases patient awareness of health care costs	High deductible
		Patient pays directly until high deductible is met	Low premium

Third party reimbursement types

Patient assistance programs

- Created by pharmaceutical and medical supply manufacturers to help financially needy patients purchase necessary medications and supplies

- Prescription medications may be made available at no cost or at a minimal fee for individuals who do not have insurance or are underinsured

Manufacturer-sponsored prescription coupons (manufacture discount programs)

- Are provided by pharmaceutical companies to encourage use of specific medications
- Are commonly combined with commercial insurance to lower copayments for a certain period of time
- Disadvantage: the patient may not be able to continue using the brand medication after the manufacturer coupon expires and the prescription savings are no longer available

Drug discount cards

- They do not provide an insurance benefit but they provide the patient the ability to purchase medications at a contracted provider rate.
- They are normally free of charge to the patient; however, they may charge a fee to use the card.
- Patients can compare medication prices offered by the various free prescription discount cards either online or via mobile apps to determine the most cost-effective option.
- Examples include GoodRx, SingleCare, Blink Health, ScriptSave, WellRx, and RxSaver

Health savings account

- A type of savings account that permits the patient to set aside money on a pretax basis to pay for qualified medical expenses.
- To qualify for health savings account, one must:
  - Not be claimed as a dependent on anyone else's tax return
  - Not be enrolled in Medicare
  - Be covered under a high-deductible health plan
- Can be used to pay for deductibles, copayments, and coinsurance
- Unspent funds may be transferred to the next year
- The account is owned by the individual.

Flexible spending account

- A flexible spending account (FSA) is also known as a flexible spending arrangement.
- It is a special account that the patient puts money into to pay for certain out-of-pocket health care costs.
- Taxes are not paid on this money.
- FSA funds can be used to pay deductibles and copayments, but not for insurance premiums.
- FSA funds may be used on prescription medications, as well as over-the-counter medicines with a doctor's prescription.
- Reimbursements for insulin are allowed without a prescription.

- Funds may be used to cover costs durable medical expenses (DME), supplies like bandages, and diagnostic devices like blood sugar test kits.
- Funds must be used within the plan year; however, employers may provide a "grace period" of up to 2½ extra months to use the money in the FSA or permit the individual to carry over up to $570 per year to use in the following year.

Self-pay

- Patient does not have insurance coverage and is responsible for paying for the prescription.
- Patient pays with either cash, check, credit card, or debit card.

Health care reimbursement systems

Community pharmacy

- Reasonable and customary consists of the acquisition cost and the markup to cover the operating costs needed to dispense a medication.
- Usual and customary, also known as usual, customary, and reasonable, is the maximum amount of payment for a given prescription determined by the insurer.
- Capitation is a fixed amount of money per patient per unit of time paid in advance to the physician (or health care provider) for the delivery of health care services. The capitation rate is established either as per member, per month or per member, per year.

Ambulatory payment classification

- Ambulatory payment classifications (APCs) are the government's method of paying facilities for outpatient services for the Medicare program.
- APCs are an outpatient prospective payment system for hospital patients applicable only to hospitals and have no impact on physician payments under the Medicare Physician Fee Schedule.
- Many medications and supplies have their costs incorporated in the payment for specific visit level or procedure APCs.
  - Applicable for medications and supplies that cost less than $60 per day
  - Medications and supplies costing $60 or more, a separate payment under a unique APC
  - Drug administration services such as intravenous (IV) lines and intramuscular injections are paid separately

APC facility fee		
Billing option	**CPT billing code**	**Practice setting**
Incident to physician for established patients: Office visit in a hospital-based outpatient clinic	APC code 5012 (was 0634) with HCPCS code G0463	Hospital Outpatient Prospective Payment System

APC, ambulatory payment classification; *CPT*, Current Procedural Technology; *HCPCS*, Healthcare Common Procedural Coding System.

Billing systems

- Healthcare Common Procedural Coding System (HCPCS):
  - A billing increment used for drugs and radiological items
  - Alpha character (C, J, Q, S) followed by four digits
  - Example: J0171—epinephrine 0.1 mg
- Current Procedural Terminology (CPT):
  - Billing unit for procedures or vaccinations
  - Consists of five digits
  - Example: 90686—quadrivalent flu vaccine administration

Transitional care management

- Services following discharge from:
  - Hospital
  - Long-term care (LTC) facility
  - Rehabilitation facility
- Face-to-face visits within 7–14 days by a Medicare Part B eligible provider
- Pharmacist may provide the following:
  - Interactive non-face-to-face service:
    - Communicate with agencies and community services
    - Provide education to the beneficiary, family, guardian, and/or caretaker to support self-management, independent living, and activities of daily living
    - Assess and support treatment regimen adherence and medication management
    - Identify available community and health resources
    - Assist the beneficiary and/or family in accessing needed care and services
    - Medication reconciliation
  - Assist eligible provider in face-to-face visit.
- Incident to rule exception:
  - General supervision—direct oversight relationship, not physical presence relationship, as evidence by sharing a plan of care and documentation
- CPT codes: 99495, 99496

Principle care management

- Principal care management (PCM) services furnish chronic care management (CCM) for patients with a single chronic condition or with multiple chronic conditions but focused on a single high-risk condition.
- Patient must also have had either a recent hospitalization or an acute risk of death, exacerbation or functional decline, or require management that's unusually complex due to comorbidities.
- The goal is to stabilize and return to chronic management.
- PCM is billed as a component of transitional care management.
- PCM services may be expected to last 6 months to 1 year or until patient's death.
- PCM services require 30 minutes before billing.
- The rules are the same as CCM except:
  - For pharmacist services, this may be used for one specific disease state services such as diabetes, heart failure, etc.
- CPT Codes are 99424, 99425, 99426, 99427.

Chronic care management

- CCM is for patients with two or more chronic conditions expected to last 12 months. Examples of conditions include:
  - Alzheimer's disease and related dementia
  - Arthritis (osteoarthritis and rheumatoid)
  - Asthma
  - Atrial fibrillation
  - Cancer
  - Cardiovascular disease
  - Chronic obstructive pulmonary disease
  - Depression
  - Diabetes
  - Hypertension
  - Infectious diseases like HIV and AIDS
- It requires patient consent, which can be either verbal or signed prior to starting CCM.
- An initiating visit must occur for new patients or patients who the billing practitioner has not seen within 1 year upon starting CCM.
- Initiating visit can occur during face-to-face evaluation and management visit, annual wellness visit, or initial preventive physical examination.
- Covered under an annual wellness visit:
  - Health risk assessment to include patient demographics and health status
  - Establish a list of current health care providers
  - Review the patient's potential risk factors for depression
  - Review the patient's functional ability to include safety, such as performing activities of daily living, fall risk, hearing impairment, and home safety
  - Obtain the following measurements: patient height, weight, body mass index, and blood pressure
  - Create a list of risk factors and conditions for which interventions are recommended
  - Provide health advice, referral, counseling and education as needed
- It requires recording patient health information with electronic health record technology, 24-7 access and continuity of care, comprehensive care management, comprehensive care plan, home and community-based care coordination.
- CPT codes are 99439, 99487, 99489, 99490, 99491.
- Complex CCMs:
- Are generally non-face-to-face services provided to Medicare beneficiaries
- Are more complex patients requiring additional staff and assistance
- CPT codes: 99487, 99489

Home health

- Consolidated billing requirements:
  - With the exception of certain covered osteoporosis drugs where the patient meets specific criteria, payment for all services and DME supplies is included in the Home Health Prospective Payment System (HH PPS) episodic rate for individuals under a home health Point-of-Care (POC). The health care provider must deliver the covered home health services with the exception of DME, either directly or under contract.

The provider must bill for such covered home health services, and payment must be made to the facility.
- Osteoporosis medications:
- Osteoporosis drugs are included in a consolidate bill under the home health benefit. The Home Health Agency (HHA) must bill for osteoporosis drugs according to billing instructions.
- Criteria for home health services:
  - Medicare covers home health services when all of the criteria are met:
    - The beneficiary to whom services are furnished is eligible and enrolled in Part A and/or Part B of the Medicare Program;
    - The beneficiary is entitled for home health services;
    - The HHA furnishing the services has a valid agreement in effect to participate in the Medicare program;
    - The services for which payment is claimed are covered under the Medicare home health benefit;
    - Medicare is the appropriate payer; and
    - The services are not otherwise excluded from payment.

Long-term care pharmacies

- Provide medications to patients residing in an LTC facility
- Coordinate with the facility, provider, and payer to review each prescription, verify coverage, comply with packaging and delivery requirements, and provide delivery as needed
- Must comply with Medicare Part D Pharmacy Requirements[1]:
- Comprehensive inventory and inventory capacity
  - Pharmacy operations and prescription orders
  - Special packaging
  - IV medications
  - Custom compounding
  - Pharmacist on-call service (24-7)
  - Delivery service (24-7)
  - Emergency medications (24-7)
  - Emergency log books
  - Miscellaneous reports, forms, and prescription ordering supplies
- Must adhere to Centers for Medicare and Medicaid Services (CMS) LTC requirements for both pharmacy and consultant services[1]:
  - Pharmacy services:
    - Specialized medication carts, emergency drug supplies, and equipment to assist in the storage, control, and dispensing of medications
    - Preparation of computerized medical records for facilities; examples of these records include medication administration records (MARs), physician's monthly order sheets, and treatment records
    - Specialized services such as IV and infusion therapy services
    - Emergency backup systems
    - Pharmacy policies and procedures
    - Facility- and resident-specific reports
  - Consultant pharmacist services:
    - Drug regimen reviews
    - Medication therapy management
    - Counsel patients
    - Present in-services and attend policy meetings

- Pharmacy billing:
  - Billing is based on a drug cost and a professional (dispensing fee).
  - For Medicare Part A services, the skilled nursing facility bills the CMS for the prescription and then pays a negotiated fee-for-service rate to the LTC pharmacy.
  - Medicare Part B may utilize average sale price (ASP) or estimated acquisition cost (EAC).
  - The pharmacy or group purchasing organization (GPO) negotiates with pharmaceutical manufacturers or wholesalers on the price of supplying the drug.
  - For Medicare Part D, LTC pharmacies negotiate reimbursement rates and manufacturer rebates with pharmacy benefit managers (PBMs).
    - Part D plans utilize maximum allowable cost (MAC) pricing for generic drugs, which sets a payer-specific total reimbursement limit for each drug.

Home infusion therapy

- Home infusion therapy (HIT) is the parenteral administration of drugs or biologicals to an individual at home outside the hospital or clinic setting.
  - The infusion drug
  - The external infusion pump and related equipment
  - Supplies other than the drug
  - Professional services
- Home infusion drug is a parenteral drug or biological administered IV or subcutaneously for an administration period of 15 minutes or more, in the home of an individual through a pump that is an item of DME, but does not include insulin pump systems or a self-administered drug or biological on a self-administered drug exclusion list.
- HIT rates with DME
  - DME benefit covers:
    - The infusion drug
    - The external infusion pump and related equipment
    - Supplies other than the drug
    - Pharmacy services, delivery, equipment set up, maintenance of rented equipment, and training and education of the covered items
- Pharmacy services includes drug preparation and dispensing including sterile compounding.
  - New HIT benefit covers professional services (nursing visits)

Benefit categories and codes for home infusion therapy services[2]		
Benefit	**Item/service**	**Codes**
Durable medical equipment	Home infusion drug	J-codes
	External fusion pump	E0779, E0781, E0791, E0780, K0455

(Continued)

Benefit categories and codes for home infusion therapy services[2] —cont'd		
Benefit	**Item/service**	**Codes**
	Medical supplies	A4221, A4222, K0552, A4602, K0604, K0605
Home infusion therapy	In-home professional services ■ Training and education (not included under DME benefit) ■ Professional services including nursing care (e.g., dressing changes and site care) ■ Monitoring and remote monitoring services (bundled into the payment amount for the professional services visit)	G0068 (for other intravenous drugs) G0069 (for subcutaneous drugs) G0070 (for chemotherapy drugs)

DME, durable medical expenses.

Medication therapy management

- Refers to a range of services provided by pharmacists consisting of a medication therapy review, personalized medication record, medication-related action plan, intervention and/or referral, and documentation and follow-up
- Medication therapy management CPT codes:
  - 99605: New patient, face-to-face visit: Initial 15 minutes
  - 99606: Established patient, face-to-face visit: Initial 15 minutes
  - 99607: Face-to-face visit
    - For each additional 15 minutes
    - Used only in addition to 99605 or 99606

Diabetes self-management training

- Covered under Medicare Part B (Medical Insurance)
- Requires:
  - Accreditation from American Association of Diabetes Educators or American Diabetes Association

- Partnership with a Medicare provider who refers the diabetic patient
- Covers outpatient diabetes self-management training once a patient has been diagnosed with diabetes
- Medicare may cover up to 10 hours of initial diabetes self-management training—1 hour of individual training and 9 hours of group training
- An additional 2 hours paid yearly after the first year

Diabetes self-management training		
Medicare code	**Description**	**Available units**
G0108	■ Individual DSMT ■ Medicare allows for 1 h ■ Billable in 30-min increments	2 units = 1 h
G0109	■ Group DSMT ■ Two or more participants ■ Medicare permits 9 h ■ Billable in 30-min increments (1 units)	18 units = 9 h
G0108/ G0109	■ Medicare permits for any combination of 2 h ■ Billable in 30-min increments (1 unit)	4 units = 2 h

DSMT, diabetes self-management training.

Medicare diabetes prevention program[3]

- The goal of Medicare Diabetes Prevention Program is to prevent type 2 diabetes in individuals with an indication of prediabetes.
- Consists of at least 16 intensive "core" sessions of a CMS–approved curriculum furnished over 6 months.
- Furnishes training to include long-term dietary change, increased physical activity, and behavior modification strategies for weight control.
- Primary goal of Medicare Diabetes Prevention Program is at least 5% weight loss by participants.
- CPT codes are G9873-G9879, G9880-G9885, G9890, G9891.

	Core sessions	Core maintenance sessions		Ongoing maintenance sessions			
	16 sessions	Interval 1 (3 sessions)	Interval 2 (3 sessions)	Interval 1 (3 sessions)	Interval 2 (3 sessions)	Interval 3 (3 sessions)	Interval 4 (3 sessions)
	Months 0-6	Months 7–12		Months 13–24			
Attendance only	Attend 1 session (G9873) Attend 4 sessions (G9874) Attend 9 sessions (G9875)	Attend 2 sessions without at least 5% WL (G9876)	Attend 2 sessions without at least 5% WL (G9877)	5% WL and attendance must be achieved to receive payment during ongoing maintenance sessions			
Attendance and WL	5% WL is not required to receive payment	OR Attend 2 sessions with at least 5% (G9878)	OR Attend 2 sessions with at least 5% (G9879)	Attend 2 sessions with at least 5% WL (G9882)	Attend 2 sessions with at least 5% WL (G9883)	Attend 2 sessions with at least 5% WL (G9884)	Attend 2 sessions with at least 5% WL (G9885)

Additional codes

- 5% WL achieved during months 0–12 (G9880).
- 9% WL achieved during months 0–24 (G9881).
- Bridge payment during months 0–24 (G9890).
- Report attendance at sessions that are not associated with a performance goal. Nonpayable codes should be listed (G9891).

W, weight loss.

Remote physiologic monitoring

- Symptoms and conditions that can be tracked through remote patient monitoring, including high blood pressure, diabetes, weight loss or gain, heart conditions, chronic obstructive pulmonary disease, sleep apnea, and asthma
- Collection and interpretation of digitally stored and/or transmitted patient physiologic data (e.g., electrocardiogram, blood pressure, glucose monitoring):
  - Requiring a minimum of 30 minutes of time each 30 days
  - CPT code 99091
- Initial setup and patient education on use of equipment:
  - CPT code 99453
- Management services-based information from remote physiologic monitoring:
  - 20 minutes or more of clinical staff/physician/other qualified health care professional time in a calendar month
  - Requiring interactive communication with the patient/caregiver
  - CPT code 99457Am
- Other pharmacy revenue codes:
- 0250—Drugs and biologicals
- 0636—HCPCS code for drugs requiring detailed coding: radionuclides, vaccines, toxoids, immune globulins, blood factors
- 0637—Self-administrable drugs

Eligibility requirements for federally funded insurance programs

Medicare eligibility

- People aged 65 or older
- Younger people with disabilities
- Individuals with end-stage renal disease (ESRD) (permanent kidney failure requiring dialysis or transplant)

Medicare forms

- Consists of Medicare Part A (Hospital Insurance), Medicare Part B (Medicare Insurance), Medicare Part C (combines Medicare Part A and B), and Medicare Part D (Prescription Drug Coverage)
- Medicare Part A:
  - Is a universal benefit
  - Covers inpatient hospital stays, in patient stays at most skilled nursing facilities, and hospice and home health care
- Medicare Part B:
  - Patient must opt out
  - Covers physician visits, clinical laboratory services, outpatient and preventative care screenings, surgical fees and supplies, physical and occupational therapy, DME, and some prescription medications
- Medicare Part C:
  - Patient may opt in
  - Known as Medicare Advantage
  - Minimum Part A and B services

- Can be combined with Medicare Part D through a Medicare Advantage Prescription Drug
- Patients with MA plans continue to pay Medicare Part B premiums
- Administered by commercial payers
- Medicare Part D:
  - Patient may opt in
  - Covers prescription medications
  - Administered by commercial payers

Medicare eligibility requirements

- Medicare Part A:
  - An individual is eligible for premium free:
    - If they are 65 years of age or older and they or their spouse paid Medicare taxes for at least ten years
    - If they are receiving Social Security or Railroad Retirement Board benefits
    - If they are eligible to Social Security or Railroad benefits but have not filed for them yet
    - If they or their spouse had Medicare-covered government employment
    - If they (or their spouse) did not pay Medicare taxes while they worked, and they are age 65 or older and a citizen or permanent resident of the United States, they may be able to buy Part A; if they are under age 65, they can get Part A without having to pay premiums if:
  - They have been entitled to Social Security or Railroad Retirement Board disability benefits for 24 months. (Note: If they have Lou Gehrig's disease, their Medicare benefits begin the first month they get disability benefits.)
- They are a kidney dialysis or kidney transplant patient.
- Medicare Part B:
  - The eligibility rules for Part B depend on whether a patient is eligible for premium-free Part A or has to pay the premium for Part A coverage
  - Individuals who are eligible for premium-free Part A are also permitted to enroll in Part B.
  - Individuals who are required to pay a premium for Part A must meet the following requirements to enroll in Part B:
    - Be age 65 or older;
    - Be a US resident; *and*
    - Be either a US citizen, *or*
    - Be an alien who has been lawfully admitted for permanent residence and has been residing in the United States for 5 continuous years prior to the month of filing an application for Medicare
- Medicare Part C:
  - Anyone who is enrolled in Original Medicare (Part A and Part B) may be eligible to sign up for a Medicare Advantage (Part C) plan. This includes people under the age of 65 who have qualified for Medicare because of a disability.
  - People who have ESRD are able to enroll in a Medicare Advantage plan. Individuals with ESRD may be able to enroll in a Medicare Special Needs Plan. Special Needs Plans are available for individuals with dependence issues with alcohol or other substances,

autoimmune disorders, cancer, cardiovascular disorders, chronic heart failure, dementia, diabetes mellitus, end-stage liver disease, ESRD that requires dialysis, deVere hematologic disorders, HIV/AIDS, chronic lung disorders, and strokes.

- A Special Needs Plan is a certain type of Medicare Advantage plan that is designed for people with specific health care conditions or circumstances.
- It is not possible for an individual to have a Medicare Advantage plan and Medicare Supplement Insurance (Medigap) policy at the same time.

- Medicare Part D:
  - An individual who is eligible for Medicare coverage is also eligible for Medicare Part D but must be enrolled in Medicare Part A and/or Part B.
  - Medicare Part D Assistance for low-income beneficiaries—low-income subsidy:
  - Administered through the Social Security Administration
  - Must have both Medicare Part A and Part B
  - Based on beneficiary net worth (savings, investments, real estate other than home)
  - Automatically enrolled if on supplemental Security Income or dual eligible
  - Reduction in premiums and Medication copay rates

TRICARE

- TRICARE is a health program for:
  - Uniformed service members and their families
  - National Guard/Reserve members (Army National Guard, Army Reserve, Navy Reserve, Marine Corps Reserve, Air National Guard, Air Force Reserve, and US Coast Guard Reserve) and their families
  - Survivors
  - Former spouses
  - Medal of Honor recipients and their families
  - Others registered in the Defense Enrollment Eligibility Reporting System

TRICARE plans

- TRICARE Prime
- TRICARE Prime Remote
- TRICARE Prime Overseas
- TRICARE Prime Remote Overseas
- TRICARE Select Overseas
- TRICARE for Life
- TRICARE Reserve Select
- TRICARE Retired Reserve
- TRICARE Young Adult
- US Family Health

Comparison between TRICARE plans[4]			
TRICARE plan	Coverage	How it works	Payment
TRICARE Prime[5]	Active-duty service members and their families Retired service members and their families Activated Called or ordered to active-duty service for more than 30 days in a row Guard/Reserve members and their families Nonactivated Guard/Reserve members and their families who qualify for care under the Transitional Assistance Management Program Retired Guard/Reserve members at age 60 and their families Survivors Medal of Honor recipients and their families Qualified former spouses	An assigned PCM who provides most of the patient's care - Military or network provider - Refers you to specialists for care he or she cannot provide - Works with your regional contractor for referrals/authorization - Accepts your copayment - A fixed dollar amount you may pay for a covered health care service or drug and files claims for you	Active-duty service members pay nothing out-of-pocket Active-duty family members pay nothing unless using the point-of-service option All other beneficiaries pay annual enrollment fees and network copayments
TRICARE Prime Remote[6]	Available in designated remote locations in the United States for: Active-duty service members Activated National Guard and Reserve members called or ordered to active-duty service for more than 30 days in a row (Pre-Activation/Pre-Mobilization/Pre-Deployment/TDY orders are not eligible) Active-duty family members who live with TRICARE Prime Remote–enrolled sponsor Activated National Guard/Reserve family members if they live in a designated remote location when the sponsor is activated (and continue to reside at that address)	Primary care manager - Refers patient to specialists for care he or she cannot provide - Works with the regional contractor for referrals/authorization - Helps find a specialist in the network - Files claims for patient	No enrollment fees No out-of-pocket costs for any type of care as long as care is received from your PCM or with a referral Care received without a referral is subject to point-of-service fees

Comparison between TRICARE plans[4]			
TRICARE plan	Coverage	How it works	Payment
TRICARE Prime Overseas[7]	Is a managed care option in overseas areas near military hospitals and clinics for: Active-duty service members Command-sponsored active-duty family members Activated National Guard/Reserve members Command-sponsored family members of activated National Guard/Reserve members	PCM refers patient to a specialist for care they cannot provide and works with International SOS for authorization, when needed	No enrollment fees No copayments for any type of care as long as care is received from your PCM or with a referral Care received without a referral is subject to point-of-service fees
TRICARE Prime Remote Overseas[8]	Is a managed care option in designated remote overseas locations of Eurasia-Africa, Latin America and Canada, and Pacific for: Active-duty service members Command-sponsored active-duty family members Activated National Guard/Reserve members Command-sponsored family members of activated National Guard/Reserve members	PCM refers patient to a specialist for care they cannot provide and works with International SOS for authorization, when needed	No enrollment fees No copayments for any type of care as long as care is received from your PCM or with a referral Care received without a referral is subject to point-of-service fees
TRICARE Select Overseas[9]	Is a self-managed, PPO plan available in the United States for: Active-duty family members Retired service members and their families Family members of activated (called or ordered to active-duty service for more than 30 days in a row) Guard/Reserve members Nonactivated Guard/Reserve members and their families who qualify for care under the Transitional Assistance Management Program, which provides 180 days of premium-free transitional health care benefits after regular TRICARE benefits end Retired Guard/Reserve members at age 60 and their families Survivors Medal of Honor recipients and their families Qualified former spouses	Patient will schedule an appointment with any overseas provider Referrals not required Preauthorization may be required for some types of services	Costs vary based on the sponsor's military status; patient pays: An annual outpatient deductible Cost shares (or percentage) for covered services Group A retirees will have to pay enrollment fees
TRICARE for Life[10]	Is Medicare-wraparound coverage for TRICARE-eligible beneficiaries who have Medicare Part A and B Coverage is automatic if an individual is enrolled in Medicare Part A and B Individual is responsible for paying Medicare Part B premiums	Provider files your claims with Medicare Medicare pays its portion and sends the claim to the TRICARE for Life claims processor TRICARE for Life then pays the provider directly for TRICARE-covered services	There are no out-of-pocket costs for services that both Medicare and TRICARE cover Patient will have out-of-pocket costs for care that is not covered by Medicare and/or TRICARE
TRICARE Reserve Select[11]	Is a premium-based plan available world-wide for qualified Selected Reserve members and their families who are: Not on active-duty orders Not covered under the Transitional Assistance Management Program Not eligible for or enrolled in the FEHB program; it should be noted that survivor coverage is not affected by FEHB eligibility	Schedule an appointment with any TRICARE-authorized provider Request an appointment in a military hospital or clinic Referrals are not required for any type of care	Patient pays Monthly premiums Annual deductibles Cost sharing or percentage for covered services

(Continued)

TRICARE plan	Coverage	How it works	Payment
TRICARE Retired Reserve[12]	Is a premium-based plan available worldwide for qualified Select Reserve members and their families Eligible participants are: Retired Reserve members who are members of the retired Reserve of a Reserve Component who are qualified for non-regular retirement Under age 60 Not eligible for, or enrolled in, the FEHB program Family members of qualified Retired Reserve members Survivors of retired Reserve members if the sponsor was covered by TRICARE Retired Reserve when they died; they are immediate family members of the deceased sponsor (spouses cannot have remarried) TRICARE Retired Reserve coverage would begin before the date the deceased sponsor would have turned 60 years old Survivor coverage is not affected by FEHB eligibility	Schedule an appointment with any TRICARE-authorized provider Request an appointment in a military hospital or clinic Referrals are not required for any type of care	Patient pays Monthly premiums Annual deductibles Cost sharing or percentage for covered services
TRICARE Young Adult[13]	Is a plan that qualified adult children can purchase after eligibility for "regular" TRICARE coverage ends at age 21 (or 23 if enrolled in college) An individual may qualify to purchase TRICARE Young Adult if they are: An unmarried, adult child of an eligible sponsor At least age 21 but not yet 26 years old if enrolled in a full course of study at an approved institution of higher learning and the sponsor provides more than 50% of their financial support, their eligibility may not begin until age 23 or upon graduation, whichever comes first Not eligible to enroll in an employer-sponsored health plan based on your own employment Not otherwise eligible for TRICARE coverage		Monthly premiums Annual deductible Cost sharing
US Family Health[14]	Is an additional TRICARE Prime option available through networks of community-based, not-for-profit health care systems in six areas of the United States Is available to the following beneficiaries: Active-duty family members Retired service members and their families Family members of Activated National Guard/Reserve members Nonactivated National Guard/Reserve members and their families who qualify for care under the Transitional Assistance Management Program Retired National Guard/Reserve members at age 60 and their families Survivors Medal of Honor recipients and their families Qualified former spouses	Patients get all care (including prescription drug coverage) from a primary care provider that they select from the network of private physicians affiliated with one of the not-for-profit health care systems	No enrollment fees and out-of-pocket costs for any type of care as long as care is received from the US Family Health Plan provider

FEHB, Federal Employees Health Benefits; PCM, principal care management.

Medicaid

- Joint federal and state program
- Federal law requires states to cover low-income families, qualified pregnant women and children, and individuals receiving Supplemental Security Income
- Medicaid provides for:
  - Physician services
  - Laboratory and X-ray services
  - Inpatient hospital services
  - Outpatient hospital services
  - Rural health clinic services
  - Home health care
  - Federally qualified health-center services
  - Skilled care at public nursing center
  - Prenatal and nurse-midwife services
  - Early and periodic screening, diagnosis, and treatment
  - Emergency care
- States may provide coverage to other groups, to include individuals receiving home- and community-based services and children in foster care who are not eligible
- State portion of a Medicaid program may pay for:
  - Clinic services
  - Emergency room care
  - Eyeglasses and eye refraction
  - Ambulance services
  - Prescription medications
  - Chiropractic services
  - Prosthetic devices
  - Mental health services
  - Private duty nursing
  - Allergy services
  - Dental care
  - Podiatry services
- Financial eligibility:
  - The Affordable Care Act of 2010 created the opportunity for states to expand Medicaid to cover all low-income Americans under age 65. Eligibility for children was extended to at least 133% of the federal poverty level in every state (most states cover children to higher income levels), and states were given the option to extend eligibility to adults with income at or below 133% of the federal poverty level.
  - Financial eligibility is based on the modified adjusted gross income (MAGI) and is the basis for eligibility for most children, pregnant women, parents, and adults.
  - MAGI examines taxable income and tax filing relationships to determine financial eligibility.
  - Individuals exempt from the MAGI-based income counting rules include those whose eligibility is based on blindness, disability, or age (65 and older).
- Nonfinancial eligibility:
  - Medicaid beneficiaries must be residents of the state in which they are receiving Medicaid. They must be either United States citizens or certain qualified noncitizens. In addition, some eligibility groups are limited by age or by pregnancy or parenting status.
- Effective date of coverage:
  - Is the date of application or the first day of the month of application.
  - Benefits may also be covered retroactively for up to 3 months prior to the month of application, if the individual would have been eligible during that period had they applied.
  - Coverage stops at the end of the month in which a person no longer meets the eligibility requirements.
- Medically needy:
  - States have the option to establish a "medically needy program" for individuals with significant health needs whose income is too high to otherwise qualify for Medicaid under other eligibility groups.
  - Individuals can become eligible by "spending down" the amount of income that is above a state's medically needy income standard.
  - Individuals spend down by incurring expenses for medical and remedial care for which they do not have health insurance.
  - The Medicaid program then pays the cost of services that exceeds the expenses the individual had to incur to become eligible.

Civilian health and medical program of the veterans administration

- The Civilian Health and Medical Program of the Veterans Administration (CHMPVA) is from the Department of Veteran Affairs
- Comprehensive health care benefits program where the VA splits the cost of covered health care services and supplies with eligible beneficiaries
- Eligibility for CHAMPVA:
  - Must be in one of the following categories:
    - "The spouse or child of a Veteran who has been rated permanently and totally disabled for a service-connected disability by a VA regional office **OR**
    - The surviving spouse or child of a Veteran who died from a VA-rated service-connected disability **OR**
    - The surviving spouse or child of a Veteran who was at the time of death rated permanently and totally disabled from a service-connected disability **OR**
    - The surviving spouse or child of a military member who died in the line of duty, not due to misconduct (in most of these cases, these family members are eligible for TRICARE, not CHAMPVA)."[15]
- Services covered under CHAMPVA includes ambulance service, ambulatory surgery, DME, family planning and maternity care, hospice, inpatient services, mental health services, outpatient medical services, prescriptions, skilled nursing care, and transplants.
- Services not covered under CHAMPVA include acupuncture, chiropractic services, dental care, non-FDA-approved drugs, hearing examinations, eye examinations and glasses, laser eye surgery, investigational procedures, and health club memberships.

Worker's compensation

- Is a government-mandated system that pays monetary benefits to workers who become injured or disabled in the course of their employment
- Provides for wage replacement benefits, medical treatment, and vocational rehabilitation
- Criteria for worker's compensation:

- The injured worker must be classified as an employee.
- The employer must have worker's compensation insurance.
- Injury must be work related.
- Employee must meet reporting deadlines.
- The injured worker must attend required medical appointments, treatments, and examinations.
  - Individuals who are not commonly covered under worker's compensation include independent contractors, business owners, volunteers, employees of private homes, farmworkers and farmhands, maritime employees, railroad employees, and casual workers.

Eligibility 340B programs

- The 340B program enables covered entities to stretch scarce federal resources as far as possible, reaching more eligible patients and providing more comprehensive services.
- Manufacturers participating in Medicaid agree to provide outpatient drugs to covered entities at significantly reduced prices.
- Eligible health care organizations/covered entities are defined in statute and include Health Resources and Services Administration (HRSA)-supported health centers and look-alikes, Ryan White clinics and State AIDS Drug Assistance programs, Medicare/Medicaid Disproportionate Share Hospitals (DSHs), children's hospitals, and other safety net providers.
- Eligible organizations/covered entities must register and be enrolled with the 340B program and comply with all 340B program requirements. Once enrolled, covered entities are assigned a 340B identification number that vendors verify before allowing an organization to purchase 340B discounted drugs.
- Section 340B(a)(4) of the Public Health Service Act specifies which covered entities are eligible to participate in the 340B drug program:
  - Federally qualified health centers
    - Health Center Program Award recipients
      - Community-based health care providers that receive funds from the HRSA Health Center Program to provide primary care services in underserved areas
      - Must provide care on a sliding fee scale based on ability to pay
      - Health Center Program Award recipients may be community health centers, migrant health centers, health care for the homeless, and health centers for residents of public housing
    - Health Center Program look-alikes
      - Community-based health care providers that meet the requirements of the HRSA Health Center Program, but do not receive Health Center Program funding
      - Must provide primary care services in underserved areas and provide care on a sliding fee scale based on ability to pay
    - Native Hawaiian Health Centers
      - Receive funding (through the HRSA Health Center Program appropriation) to provide medical and enabling services to Native Hawaiians
      - Native Hawaiian Health Centers improve the health status of Native Hawaiians by providing access to health education, health promotion, and disease prevention services
      - Services provided include nutrition programs, screening and control of hypertension and diabetes, immunizations, and basic primary care services
    - Tribal/urban Indian Health Centers
  - Federally qualified health centers that provide comprehensive primary care and related services to American Indians and Alaska Native
    - Ryan White HIV/AIDS Program grantees
      - Receive federal funding to provide HIV/AIDS treatment and related services to people living with HIV/AIDS who are uninsured or underinsured
      - The funding is used for technical assistance, clinical training, and the development of innovative models of care
    - Hospitals
      - Children's hospitals
  - Children's hospitals must be one of the following classifications:
    - A private nonprofit hospital under contract with state or local government to provide health care services to low-income individuals who are not eligible for Medicare or Medicaid; or
    - Owned or operated by a state or local government; or
    - A public or private nonprofit corporation that is granted governmental powers by a state or local government.
  - To be eligible to participate in the 340B Drug Pricing Program, Children's hospitals must either:
    - Have a disproportionate share adjustment percentage greater than 11.75% for the most recently filed cost report; or
    - Be eligible under a separate indigent care calculation that meets specific criteria including location in an urban area, 100 or more beds, and net inpatient care revenues (excluding Medicare) for indigent care of more than 30% of net during the cost reporting period in which the discharges occur. This indigent care revenue must come from state and local government sources and Medicaid.
  - For-profit hospitals are not eligible to participate in the 340B program.
    - Critical access hospitals
  - Critical access hospitals are designated by the CMS.
    - DSHs
  - To be eligible to participate in the 340B program and purchase outpatient drugs at significantly discounted prices, DSHs must be one of the following classifications:
    - A private nonprofit hospital under contract with state or local government to provide health care services to low-income individuals who are not eligible for Medicare or Medicaid; or
    - Owned or operated by a state or local government; or
    - A public or private nonprofit corporation that is granted governmental powers by a state or local government.

- To be eligible to participate in the 340B Drug Pricing Program, DSHs must:
  - Have a disproportionate share adjustment percentage greater than 11.75%
- For-profit hospitals are not eligible to participate in the 340B program.
  - Freestanding cancer hospitals
- Freestanding Cancer Hospitals must be one of the following classifications:
  - A private nonprofit hospital under contract with state or local government to provide health care services to low-income individuals who are not eligible for Medicare or Medicaid; or
  - Owned or operated by a state or local government; or
  - A public or private nonprofit corporation that is granted governmental powers by a state or local government.
- Freestanding cancer hospitals must either:
  - Have a disproportionate share adjustment percentage greater than 11.75% for the most-recently filed cost report; or
  - Be eligible under a separate indigent care calculation that meets specific criteria including location in an urban area, 100 or more beds, and net inpatient care revenues (excluding Medicare) for indigent care of more than 30% of net during the cost reporting period in which the discharges occur. This indigent care revenue must come from state and local government sources and Medicaid.
- For-profit hospitals are not eligible to participate in the 340B program.
  - Rural referral centers
- Rural referral centers must be one of the following classifications:
  - A private nonprofit hospital under contract with state or local government to provide health care services to low-income individuals who are not eligible for Medicare or Medicaid; or
  - Owned or operated by a state or local government; or
  - A public or private nonprofit corporation that is granted governmental powers by a state or local government.
- Rural referral centers must:
  - Have a disproportionate share adjustment percentage greater than or equal to 8% for the most recently filed cost report
- For-profit hospitals are not eligible to participate in the 340B program.
  - Sole community hospitals
- Sole community hospitals must be one of the following classifications:
  - A private nonprofit hospital under contract with state or local government to provide health care services to low-income individuals who are not eligible for Medicare or Medicaid; or
  - Owned or operated by a state or local government; or
  - A public or private nonprofit corporation that is granted governmental powers by a state or local government.
- Sole community hospitals must:
  - Have a disproportionate share adjustment percentage greater than or equal to 8% for the most-recently filed cost report

- For-profit hospitals are not eligible to participate in the 340B program.
- Covered entities must recertify eligibility yearly.

Claims processing and adjudication

Pharmacy/medical claim processing terminology

Adjudication: The act of processing a pharmacy prescription claim

National Drug Code (NDC): An 11-digit code assigned to all prescription drug products by the labeler or the distributor of the product under FDA regulations; the first five digits identify the drug labeler, the next four numbers identify the product code, and the last two numbers identify the package code

National Provider Identifier (NPI): A number assigned to any health care provider that is used for standardized health data transmissions

Prior authorization (PA): Insurance-required approval for a restricted, nonformulary, or noncovered medication before the prescription can be filled

Real-time claims management system: A program that enables providers to submit electronic pharmacy claims in an online real-time environment

Prescription adjudication process

- When a prescription arrives at the pharmacy, a pharmacy technician or pharmacist is responsible for entering the prescription into the computer system and updating patient information.
- The computer processes the insurance/billing information after the prescription has been entered and submitted.
- If there are no issues with insurance/billing, the prescription is adjudicated with a copay that the patient is responsible for paying at pickup.
- If there are insurance/billing issues, then the claim will not adjudicate, and the technician will receive a rejection code.

Information for pharmacy/medical claims

- Patient information includes the patient's name, date of birth, gender, patient address, patient phone number, relationship to cardholder, pharmacy/prescribers internal patient ID.
- Prescriber information includes prescriber ID (NPI or Drug Enforcement Administration [DEA] number), prescriber's last name, and prescriber's telephone number.
- Pharmacy information consists of identifier (NPI formerly known as the NABP number), pharmacy name, pharmacist name, pharmacy address information, and pharmacy phone number.

General pharmacy claim submission process

Pharmacy billing cycle consists of

- Receipt of prescription
- Patient interview

- Filling of prescription
- Pharmacy claim transmittal
- Payer adjudication
- Point-of-sale patient payment
- Calculation of payer claim balance
- Accounts receivable follow-up
- Payment processing
- Collections and problem resolution

Patient's relationship to cardholder

- The patient's relationship to the cardholder will need to be entered; commonly used relationship codes include:
  - 01: cardholder
  - 02: spouse
  - 03: dependent

Prescription drug benefit card

- A card that contains third-party billing information for prescription drug purchases
- Information contained on a prescription drug benefit card:
  - RxBIN (bank identification number): a six-digit number used to identify the company that will reimburse the pharmacy for the prescription being filled
  - Group code: employer that contracted the insurance company for the policy
  - Issuer: the health insurance company who issued the card
  - ID: may be either numeric or alphanumeric
  - Subscriber (cardholder) name: individual who purchased the policy
  - Primary care provider: optional depending on the plan
  - Copays: may be identified on the card but not required
  - Help-desk telephone number: 24/7 coverage

Dispense as written (DAW) codes[16]

Dispense as written (DAW) codes are a set of National Council for Prescription Drug Programs (NCPDP) codes used to inform third-party provider of the reason for filling a prescription with a brand or generic drug. DAW codes are used to ensure the pharmacy is properly reimbursed by a third-party provider for a prescription being dispensed. These codes are as follows:

- 0 = No product selection indicated
- 1 = Substitution not allowed by provider
- 2 = Substitution allowed; patient requested product dispensed
- 3 = Substitution allowed; pharmacist-selected product dispensed
- 4 = Substitution allowed; generic drug not in stock
- 5 = Substitution allowed; brand drug dispensed as generic
- 6 = Override
- 7 = Substitution not allowed; brand drug mandated by law
- 8 = Substitution allowed; generic drug not available in marketplace
- 9 = Other

Adjudication terminology

- Adjudication: process by which a prescription is submitted electronically to a third-party payer for the pharmacy to be reimbursed for the medication dispensed.
- PBM: company that provides/administer drug benefits
- Switch company: routes the information to correct PBM
- Formulary: a list of drugs approved by the insurance provider in a retail setting
- Drug utilization review (DUR) warning: an alert/message generated by the pharmacy or insurance software to notify the pharmacist of a potential drug safety or payment concern
- Copay: the portion of the medication's price that the patient is responsible for
- Coinsurance: an agreement for cost sharing between the insurer and the covered individual
- Dual copay: copays that have two prices, one for generic and one for brand medications
- Deductible: a set amount that must be paid by the patient or responsible party for each benefit period before the coverage begins

Adjudication process at the pharmacy benefit manager

- Verifies that the claim belongs to an eligible member
- Confirms the drug is on the formulary for the member's plan
- Electronic drug price determined consistent with the sponsor's (i.e., employer) contract
- DUR electronically conducted
- Allowed days' supply and time fills determined
- Payer electronically transmits back to pharmacy fill approval:
  - Amount paid to pharmacy
  - Amount to collect as copay from patient

Drug utilization review process

- Goal: informs the pharmacist of possible problems with the prescription
- Examples of DUR warnings:
  - Medication allergy
  - Drug-drug interaction with the medication
  - Drug-disease interaction with the medication
  - Duplicate medication in the same drug classification
  - Opiate being prescribe from multiple prescribers

Information transmitted during adjudication

- Patient information:
  - Patient name
  - Date of birth
  - Gender
  - Patient's relationship to the cardholder
  - Cardholder/member identification number
  - Group number
  - Prescriber information:
  - Prescriber ID (NPI or DEA number)
  - Prescriber's last name
  - Prescriber's phone number

- Pharmacy information:
  - Pharmacy's NPI number
  - Pharmacy's name
  - Pharmacist's name
  - Pharmacy address information
  - Pharmacy's telephone number
- Prescription information:
  - Date prescription was written
  - Date prescription was dispensed
  - Prescription number
  - New or refill prescription
  - NDC number
  - Quantity dispensed
  - Day's supply
  - Ingredient cost
  - Dispensing fee
  - Total price
  - Deductible or copayment amount
  - Balance due

Third-party claim rejection codes

National council for prescription drug programs rejection codes[17]

Prescription claims that are rejected will have at least one rejection code. The pharmacist or pharmacy technician must correct the prescription claim before resubmitting it to the managed care provider. Listed are some of the more common explanations provided for the rejection of a prescription claim.

Rejection code	Rejection description
1	Missing or invalid BIN
2	Missing or invalid version number
3	Missing or invalid transaction code
4	Missing or invalid processor control number
5	Missing or invalid pharmacy number
6	Missing or invalid group number
7	Missing or invalid cardholder ID number
8	Missing or invalid person code
9	Missing or invalid birth date
10	Missing or invalid gender code
11	Missing or invalid patient relationship code
15	Missing or invalid date of service
16	Missing or invalid prescription/service reference number
19	Missing or invalid day's supply
20	Missing or invalid compound code
22	Missing or invalid dispense as written/product selection code
25	Missing or invalid prescriber ID
26	Missing or invalid unit of measure
28	Missing or invalid date prescription written
29	Missing or invalid number of refills authorized

BIN, bank identification number.

If a prescription has been rejected, it may be resubmitted. Prior to resubmission, all of the rejection codes must be corrected.

Claims submission troubleshooting

- Check all information on prescription and patient information section is correct.
- Check that medication was entered correctly.
- Take steps to change medications that are nonformulary.
- Check quantity and days' supply if plan limits have been exceeded.
- If all information is correct, it is helpful to reach out to the PBM directly.

Drug costs and pricing methods

- Actual acquisition cost (AAC) refers to the state Medicaid agency's determination of pharmacy providers' actual prices paid to acquire drug products marketed or sold by a specific manufacturer,
- Average manufacturer price (AMP) refers to the average price paid to the manufacturer by wholesalers and retail community pharmacies that purchase drugs directly from the manufacturer. It is used to calculate drug rebates under the Medicaid Drug Rebate Program.
- Average wholesale price (AWP) refers to the average price paid by a retailer to buy a drug from a wholesaler. It has been used in the past to determine pricing and reimbursement of prescription drugs to third party providers. The AWP is based on data collected from various manufacturers, distributors, or suppliers.
- Best price is the lowest available price to any wholesaler, retailer, or provider, excluding certain government programs like the 340B Drug Pricing Program and the health program for veterans.
- Dispensing fee is the fee for providing a pharmacy's professional services. The factors affecting the dispensing fee includes staffing, store operations and overhead, prescription preparation, assurance of proper medication use (DUR and patient counseling) and profit.
- EAC is a benchmark previously used by many state Medicaid programs to set payment for drug ingredient cost.
- Federal upper limit sets a reimbursement limit for some generic drugs; calculated as 175% AMP.
- Gross profit refers to the difference between the selling price and the cost of the medication. Gross profit = selling price − cost of the product.
- MAC refers to a payer or PBM-generated list of products that incudes maximum amount that a plan will pay for generic drugs and brand-name drugs that generic versions available.
- National average drug acquisition cost is the national average of the prices at which pharmacies purchase a prescription drug from manufacturers or wholesalers, including some rebates. It can be used to calculate AAC.
- Net profit refers to the actual profit after expenses not included In the calculation of the gross paid have been paid. Net profit = selling price − cost of the product − unaccounted expenses.

- Tier system: a method to differentiate within the formulary encouraged drug products:
  - Tier 1: Generic drugs
  - Tier 2: Preferred brand drugs
  - Tier 3: Nonpreferred brand drugs
  - Tier 4: Preferred specialty drugs
  - Tier 5: Nonpreferred specialty drugs
- Usual and customary refers to the price a provider most frequently charges the general public for a drug.
- Wholesale acquisition cost (WAC) is the manufacturer's list price to wholesalers.

Health care services reimbursement

- Relative value unit (RVU) system:
  What was done (HCPC code) + why it was done (ICD 10) + who did it (NPI number) = coding for service bill

Medicare coding system

- HCPCS:
  - Level 1—CPT codes
    - Five numeric digits (i.e., 99605)
  - Level 2—Codes for product supplies and services not covered under CPT (ambulance, Durable Medical Equipment Prosthetics, Orthotics and Supplies [DMEPOS]):
    - Single alphabetical letter followed by four numeric digits
    - Specific level 2 HCPC codes
- A-codes: Transportation, medical supplies, miscellaneous, and experimental
- B-codes: Enteral and parenteral treatment (tx)
- C-codes: Temporary hospital outpatient prospective payment system
- D-codes: Dental procedures
- E-codes: DME
- G-codes: Temporary procedures and professional services
- H-codes: Rehabilitative services
- J-codes: Drugs administered other than oral method, chemotherapy drugs
- K-codes: Temporary codes for DME regional carriers
- L-codes: Orthotic/prosthetic procedures
- M-codes: Medical services
- P-codes: Pathology and laboratory
- Q-codes: Temporary codes
- R-codes: Diagnostic radiology services
- S-codes: Private payer codes
- T-codes: State Medicaid agency codes
- V-codes: Vision/hearing services

Current procedural terminology codes

- Used in reporting medical services and procedures for payment
- Maintained by the American Medical Association
- Types of CPT codes[18]:
  - Category I: These codes have descriptors that is tied into a procedure or service. Codes range from 00100 to 99499 and are placed into subcategories based on procedure/service type and anatomy.
  - Category II: These alphanumeric tracking codes are auxiliary codes used for performance measurement.

Using them is optional and not required for correct coding.
  - Category III: These are interim alphanumeric codes for new and developing technology, procedures, and services. They were created for data collection, assessment, and in some instances, payment of new services and procedures that currently do not meet the criteria for a category I code.
- Specific CPT codes:
  - Evaluation and management: 99201–99499
    - Example 99211 established patient code to use for "Incident to"
  - Anesthesia: 00100–01999; 99100–99150
  - Surgery: 10000–69990
  - Radiology: 70000–79999
  - Pathology and laboratory: 80000–89398
  - Medicine: 90281–99099; 99151–99199; 99500–99607
    - Example: 99605–99607 medication therapy management services

International classification of diseases codes

- For classifying diagnoses and reason for visits in all health care settings
- Contains three-digit categories for diseases, injuries, and symptoms:
  - Categories are divided into four-digit code categories into subcategories.
  - Subcategories are divided into five-digit subclassifications.
  - Fourth and fifth digits are separated from the first three by a period.
- Codes may be three, four, five, six, or seven alpha/numeric characters.
- Code or codes from A00.0 through T88.9, Z00-Z99.8.

National provider identifier

- NPIs are unique 10-digit identification numbers issued to health care providers.
- Covered health care providers and all health plans and health care clearinghouses must use the NPIs in the administrative and financial transactions adopted under HIPAA.
- NPI numbers do not contain any information regarding the health provider.

Resource-based relative value scale

- A system for describing, quantifying, and reimbursing physician services to one another based upon:
  - Work (time, technical skill and effort, judgement and stress)
  - Practice expense(rent and wages)
  - Professional liability insurance
- Resource-based relative value scales are used by the CMS.
- Includes a conversion factor calculated from the Geographic Practice Cost Index.
- RVU is assigned to each billing code in CPT code book.
- Calculation of RVU:
Work RVU + practice expense RVU + professional liability RVU = total RVU

Total · conversion factor (Geographic Practice Cost Index [GPCI]) = $ added to CPT code

Billing forms

- Physician Fee Schedule[19]:
  - Health care providers and suppliers submit Medicare Professional and Supplier Claims Form 837 P
  - Physicians, practitioners, and suppliers use Health Insurance Claim Form CMS-1500
    - **INSERT SAMPLE CMS-1500**[20]
    - https://www.cms.gov/Medicare/CMS-Forms/CMS-Forms/Downloads/CMS1500.pdf

- Hospital Outpatient Prospective Payment System[21]:
  - Form 8371
    - Is the standard format used by institutional providers to transmit health care claims electronically
    - CMS-1450
    - CMS allows a paper claim, the Form CMS-1450, also known as the UB-04, is the standard claim form to bill Medicare Administrative Contractors

- Medicare Administrative Contractors:
  - Are used by CMS to:
    - Process Medicare fee-for-service (FFS) claims
    - Make and account for Medicare FFS payments
    - Enroll providers in the Medicare FFS program
    - Control provider reimbursement services and audit institutional provider
    - Handle redetermination requests (first-stage appeals process)
    - Respond to provider inquiries
    - Educate providers about Medicare FFS billing requirements
    - Establish local coverage determinations
    - Review medical records for selected claims
    - Coordinate with CMS and other FFS contractors[22]

Coordination of benefits or plan limitations to determine each party's responsibility

- Coordination of benefits refers to a provision ensuring that maximum appropriate benefits are paid to a patient covered under more than one policy without duplication.
- Primary insurance indicates to the first insurance that the patient will use for claims.
- Secondary insurance denotes the insurance used after the primary insurance for any remaining expenses.
- Birthday rule is the method used in deciding a child's primary insurance based on the parent whose date of birth is earlier in the year.

Determining primary coverage

- If patient has one policy, then it is primary.
- If the patient has coverage under two plans, the plan that has been in effect for the patient for the longest period of time is considered primary. However, if an active employee has a plan with the present employer and is still covered by a former employer's plan as a retiree or a laid-off employee, the current plan is primary.
- If the patient is also covered as a dependent under another insurance policy, the patient's plan is primary.

- If an employee patient has coverage under the employer's plan and additional coverage under a government-sponsored plan, such as Medicare, the employer's plan is primary.
- If a retired patient is covered by a spouse's employer's plan and the spouse is still employed, the spouse's plan is primary even if the retired person has Medicare.
- If the patient is a dependent covered by both parents' plans and the parents are not separated or divorced (or if the parents have joint custody of the child), the plan is determined by the birthday.
- If two or more plans cover dependent children of separated or divorced parents who do not have joint custody of their children, the children's primary plan is determined in the following order:
  - The plan of the custodial parent
  - The plan of the spouse of the custodial parent (if the parent has been remarried)
  - The plan of the parent without custody

Plan limitations

- Insurance plans utilize quantity limits to ensure patient safety and control costs.
- Plan limitations may include days' supply, number of permitted refills, and medication cost.
- In most cases community pharmacies will be reimbursed for a 30-day supply of medication from the insurance plan.
- Mail order pharmacies will normally be reimbursed for a 90-day supply of medication from the insurance plan.
- Prescribers will determine the number of refills authorized for a prescription.
- PRN refills indicate a prescription may be refilled up to 1 year from the date the prescription was issued by the prescriber

Reimbursement policies

- AAC: CMS/Health and Human Services determination of the pharmacy providers' actual prices paid to acquire drug products marketed or sold by specific manufacturers.
- AMP: AMP is the average price paid to the manufacturer for the drug in the United States by wholesalers for drugs distributed to retail community pharmacies and retail community pharmacies that purchase drugs directly from the manufacturer.
- ASP: ASP is the weighted average of all nonfederal sales to wholesalers. ASP is net of chargebacks, discounts, rebates, and other benefits tied to the purchase of the drug product, regardless of whether it is paid to the wholesaler or the retailer. Excluded from ASP are sales that are excluded from the best price calculation. ASP is used as a basis of reimbursement for some Medicare Part B covered drugs and biologicals administered in hospital outpatient departments.
- AWP: National average of list prices charged by wholesalers to pharmacies.
- Dispensing fee: The charge for the professional services provided in association with prescription dispensing. Most prescription payers reimburse on the basis of a benchmark of the drug cost (e.g., ASP, AMP, AWP, WAC, AAC) plus a dispensing fee.

- EAC: The estimation of the price typically paid by entities for a particular manufacturer's drug, using the most commonly purchased package size. Some Medicaid agencies use EAC (plus a dispensing fee) as a basis for establishing reimbursement.
- Federal ceiling price: The maximum price that a manufacturer may charge for a covered drug sold to the "big four" federal entities engaged in providing health care services—Veterans Affairs, Department of Defense, Public Health Service (including Indian Health Service), and the Coast Guard.
- WAC: The price paid by a wholesaler (or direct purchaser) in the United States for drugs purchased from the drug's manufacturer or supplier.

Drug formularies

Terminology

- Formulary maintenance: An ongoing process of assuring relative safety and efficacy of mediations available for use within an organization that utilizes new product evaluation, therapeutic class review, formulary changes, and nonformulary drug use review
- Formulary restriction: Limiting the use of specific formulary medications based on specific parameters; may be applied to specific physicians based on theirs areas of expertise, patient disease state, or location
- Formulary: A list of approved prescription medications covered by a prescription drug plan or another insurance plan offering prescription drug benefits
- Medication safety evaluation: A process to review and evaluate drug reaction reports and medication error reports
- Medication use evaluation: A method for evaluating and improving medication-use processes with the intent od improving patient outcomes
- Nonformulary medication: A medication that is not part of a drug formulary
- Pharmacy and Therapeutics (P&T) Committee: A committee consisting of pharmacists, physicians, nurses, and administrators, who are responsible for reviewing and acting on formulation and implementing a health plan's or institutional formulary.
- Therapeutic class review: A review of drug classes by the P&T committee is useful in assuring that optimal drug therapeutic options are available
- Therapeutic equivalent: Drug products with different chemical structures but of the same pharmacologic or therapeutic class and usually having similar therapeutic effects and adverse-reaction profiles when administered to patients in therapeutically equivalent doses
- Therapeutic interchange: Authorized exchange of therapeutic alternatives based upon established and approved written guidelines or protocols within a formulary system

Types of formularies

- Closed formulary: A list of medications that restricts access of a practitioner to some medications; a closed formulary may limit drugs to specific physicians, patient care areas, or disease states
- Open formulary: A list of medications that has no limitation to access to a medication by a practitioner

Role of the P&T committee

- Establishes and maintains the formulary system
- Identifies medications for formulary inclusion by taking into consideration the relative clinical, quality of life, safety, and pharmacoeconomic outcomes
- Evaluates medication use and related outcomes
- Prevents and monitors adverse drug reactions and medications errors
- Evaluates or develops and promotes use of drug therapy guidelines
- Develops policies and procedures for handling medications to include their procurement prescribing, distribution, and administration
- Educates health professionals to the optimal use of medications

340B terminology

- 340B ceiling price: The maximum price drug manufacturers can charge a covered entity for a 340B-purchased covered outpatient drug:
- 340B ceiling price = AMP − unit rebate amount
- 340B-covered entity: A facility/program that is listed in the 340B statute as eligible to purchase drugs through the 340B program and appears on 340B Office of Pharmacy Affairs Information System (OPAIS).
- 340B Drug Pricing Program (340B program): A federal program that requires drug manufacturers participating in the Medicaid drug rebate program to provide covered outpatient drugs to enrolled "covered entities" at or below the statutorily defined ceiling price.
- 340B-eligible patient: A patient of a 340B-covered entity (with the exception of state-operated or -funded AIDS drug purchasing assistance programs) if:
  - The covered entity has established a relationship with the individual, such that the covered entity maintains records of the individual's health care.
  - The individual receives health care services from a health care professional who is either employed by the covered entity or provides health care under contractual or other arrangements (e.g., referral for consultation) such that responsibility for the care provided remains with the covered entity.
  - The individual receives a health care service or range of services from the covered entity that is consistent with the service or range of services for which grant funding or federally qualified health center look-alike status has been provided to the entity. DSHs are exempt from this requirement.
- 340B ID: A unique identification number provided by HRSA to identify a 340B-eligible entity in 340B OPAIS. This 340B ID is used to purchase 340B drugs.
- 340B orphan drug list: HRSA's list of orphan drug designations is used by 340B-covered entities subject to the orphan drug exclusion.
- 340B Prime Vendor Program (PVP): The PVP is managed through an agreement with the HRSA. The PVP serves its participants in these primary roles:
  - Negotiates sub-340B pricing on pharmaceuticals
  - Establishes distribution and networks that improve access to affordable medications
  - Stakeholder education through the 340B university programs

- Providing other value-added products and services
- 340B selling price: The 340B selling price represents the price communicated to the PVP by a supplier or distributor, which may not match the 340B ceiling price as published by HRSA.
- 5i drugs: Drugs that are inhaled, infused, instilled, implanted, or injected.
- Accountable care organizations: Groups of doctors, hospitals, and other health care providers that come together voluntarily to give coordinated high-quality care to their Medicare patients. Coordinated care ensures that patients get the correct care at the right time while avoiding unnecessary duplication of services and preventing medical errors.
- AMP true-up: Occurs when manufacturers restate their reported AMP for a specific time period and then refund any difference to 340B participating entities that had made purchases above the ceiling price.
- Chargeback: The method wholesalers use to request reimbursement from manufacturers for 340B discounts provided to entities for 340B-covered outpatient drugs. Wholesalers purchase drugs from the manufacturer at WAC and sell to 340B entities at the contracted 340B price, which is a lower price. The wholesaler submits a chargeback request to the manufacturer to account for the difference.
- Contract pharmacy: 340B-covered entities may contract with a pharmacy or pharmacies to provide services to the covered entity's patients, including the service of dispensing the entity-owned 340B drugs.
- Covered entity: Refers to a health care provider or organization that is eligible for the 340B program per the 340B statute.
- DSH: Hospitals that serve a significantly disproportionate number of low-income patients; as such, they receive adjustment payments to provide additional help. The primary method of qualification is based on the sum of the percentage of Medicare inpatient days and the percentage of total patient days attributable to patients eligible for Medicaid but not eligible for Medicare Part A.
- DSH inpatient pricing: The voluntary DSH inpatient contracts most GPOs offer their membership; the discount is usually ~2% to 3%. GPOs offer manufacturers this opportunity to put products on the DSH inpatient portfolio at a lower price than what the manufacturer has given the GPO.
- Duplicate discount: Prohibited by the 340B statute, a duplicate discount occurs when a covered entity obtains a 340B discount on a medication and a Medicaid agency obtains a discount in the form of a rebate from the manufacturer for the same medication.
- Electronic handbook: A database that contains grant information for certain HRSA grantees and is used to determine eligibility for certain entities by HRSA.
- Entity-owned pharmacy: A pharmacy that is owned by, and is a legal part of, the 340B entity.
- Federally qualified health center: Community-based health care providers that receive funds from the HRSA Health Center Program to provide primary care services in underserved areas. They must provide care on a sliding fee scale based on ability to pay.
- Federally qualified health center look-alike: Community-based health care providers that meet the requirements of the HRSA Health Center Program but do not receive Health Center Program funding. They provide primary care services in underserved areas.
- GPO: An organization created to influence the purchasing power of entities to obtain discounts from vendors based on the collective buying power of the GPO members. GPOs may set mandatory purchasing participation levels from its members or be completely voluntary. Certain 340B participating hospitals (DSHs), children's hospitals, and freestanding cancer hospitals) are prohibited from purchasing covered outpatient drugs from a GPO or GPO-like arrangement.
- GPO prohibition: 340B participating DSHs, children's hospitals, and freestanding cancer hospitals are prohibited from obtaining covered outpatient drugs through GPOs.
- Medicaid best price: Medicaid best price is the lowest manufacturer price paid for a prescription drug, regardless of package size, by any purchaser. Best price is reported to CMS and states, but otherwise is confidential. Included in best price are cash discounts, free goods that are contingent upon purchase, volume discounts, and rebates. Excluded from best price are prices paid by the federal government (e.g., prices to the "big four," 340B-covered entities, federal supply schedule, state pharmaceutical assistance programs, depot prices, and nominal pricing to covered entities).
- Medicaid carve-in: 340B entities may elect to bill Medicaid for drugs purchased at 340B prices. The site must also provide each Medicaid state it plans to bill, and the billing number(s) it will list on the bill to the state. Billing number(s) may include the billing provider's NPI only, state-assigned Medicaid number only, or both NPI and state-assigned Medicaid number.
- Medicaid carve-out: A covered entity site does not provide drugs purchased at the 340B price to Medicaid patients.
- Medicaid rebate net price: The price for covered outpatient drugs paid by state Medicaid programs, including the manufacturer rebates received by the states.
- Medicare DSH adjustment percentage: An adjustment applied to hospitals that treat a high percentage of low-income patients. This adjustment results in an additional payment to these hospitals. Factors included in this adjustment are the sum of the ratios of Medicare Part A Supplemental Security Income patient days to total Medicare patient days and Medicaid patient days to total patient days in the hospital.
- Nonfederal AMP: The average price paid to a manufacturer by wholesalers for drugs distributed to nonfederal purchasers. Nonfederal AMP is not publicly available. 340B and prime vendor subceiling prices are excluded from a manufacturer's nonfederal AMP calculations.
- Pharmaceutical pricing agreement (PPA): The 340B statute requires that the Secretary of Health and Human Services enter into a PPA with each manufacturer of covered outpatient drugs in which the manufacturer agrees to charge a price for covered outpatient drugs that will not exceed an amount determined under the statute (340B ceiling price).

- The PPA, and the subsequent PPA addendum, must be signed by a manufacturer as a condition for participating in the Medicaid program. Signing the PPA does not prohibit a manufacturer from charging a price for a covered outpatient drug that is lower than the 340B ceiling price.
- PVP sub-340B pricing: Pricing below the statutory 340B ceiling price that is negotiated by the prime vendor.
- Replenishment (340B outpatient drug): 340B drug replenishment occurs when a non-340B drug is dispensed to a 340B-eligible patient, and the entity later replaces the non-340B dispensed drug with a 340B purchased drug because of patient eligibility.
- Start date: Refers to an entity's start date in the 340B program and are updated quarterly.
- Sub-340B price: Represents the contracted pricing available to PVP participants that is below the statutory 340B ceiling price. Pricing has been arranged by the prime vendor with the manufacturer for 340B-covered entities.
- Termination date: Indicates the date that the 340B entity is terminated from the 340B program. The covered entity is no longer eligible to participate in the 340B program on the day is terminated from the 340B program or the day it becomes ineligible. The covered entity must stop purchasing, using, and administering 340B drugs once it is terminated from the 340B program.
- Unit rebate amount: Unit rebate amount is used in the 340B ceiling price calculation. Unit rebate amount is calculated:
  - Brand: Greater of (23.1% of AMP or AMP − best price) plus Consumer Price Index-Urban (CPI-U) adjustment
  - Generic/over the counter: 13% of AMP plus CPI-U adjustment
  - Blood factors/pediatric-only indications: Greater of (17.1% of AMP or AMP − best price) plus CPI-U adjustment
- WAC: The price paid by a wholesaler (or direct purchaser) in the United States for drugs purchased from the drug's manufacturer or supplier.[23]

Prior authorization

Prior authorization terminology

- Prior authorization (PA) in pharmacy is a requirement from your health insurance company that your doctor obtain approval from your plan before it will cover the costs of a specific medicine, medical device, or procedure.
- Established to assure appropriate use of medications and to assure the use of the most cost-effective therapy
- Utilization management method for high-risk, low-value or expensive medications and is used to discourage stockpiling
- Types of PAs:
  - Requests for restricted medication:
    - Drugs that may be unsafe when combined with other medications, or at certain doses
    - Prescribed only for exclusive health conditions or reasons
    - Medications that are often misused or abused
    - Medications that have a lower cost, equally effective alternative that is available

  - Drugs often used for cosmetic purposes
  - Drugs deemed low value from evidence-based literature.
  - Request for an override on established restricted limitations such as:
    - Quantity for a medication to be dispensed
    - Brand versus generic
    - Early refill
    - Age or sex restrictions
    - Brand medication quantity limit
    - 72-hour emergency supply
- Medication types that normally need a PA:
  - Medications that may be unsafe when taken with other medications or at certain doses
  - Medications that are prescribed only for excusive health conditions or reasons
  - Medications that have a lower-cost, equally effective alternative that is offered
  - Medications used for cosmetic purposes
  - Medications that are often misused or abused
  - Medications considered low value from evidence-based literature
- Step therapy:
  - A tool used by payers in the prior approval process for more expensive medications in a therapeutic class.
  - The provider (physician or pharmacist) must provide documentation that cheaper and/or safer or evidence suggesting mor optimal medications were tried initially.
  - Evidence must be provided why the considered optimal choice of therapy did not work for a patient.
  - The steps usually follow the medication tier level in a formulary.

Prior authorization information

Role of prior authorization

- Addresses the need for additional clinical patient information
- Promotes appropriate drug use and to prevent misuse
- Administration of step therapy
- Administration of quality management rules

Required prior authorization information

- Patient information:
  - Name, insurance(s) ID number, date of birth, address, phone number
  - Weight and height information
  - Allergies
  - Clinical diagnosis
  - Laboratory results
  - Over-the-counter medication use
  - Nondrug therapy use
- Required prescriber information:
  - Provider name, specialty
  - Office phone/fax number, address, e-mail
  - NPI number, DEA number
  - Office contact person
- Required medication information:
  - Drug name generic and brand, dose, formulation, directions

- New or ongoing therapy
- Location it will be administered
- Duration of therapy
- Diagnosis and corresponding ICD-10 number:
  - For which the medication is being requested
  - Other patient diagnoses
- Other required information:
  - What medications have been tried for the diagnosis in the past and why they were discontinued
  - What medications does the patient have a contraindication or intolerance to and why or what happened
  - Supporting laboratory or test results for the requested medication
  - Other information to justify the use of the medication
  - If the request is different from established quantity limits, the reason for the increased amount of medication
  - Signatures
  - Ordering provider
  - Sometimes signature of the patient is required

Prior authorization process

- The prescriber's office is responsible for obtaining the PA.
- The pharmacy can request the process to be started and resubmit the claims when they are approved.
- Ultimate approval is obtained from the prescriber's office.
- Pharmacy approval is obtained from the physician's office within 16 hours to 2 days.

Formulary exception process

- Each insurance plan develops its own policies and guidelines
- Evaluation of medical necessity by clinical staff in the plan:
  - Medically necessary—services or supplies that are proper and needed for the diagnosis or treatment of a medical condition and are provided for the diagnosis, direct care, and treatment of the medical condition, meet the standards of good medical practice in the local area, and are not for the convenience of the patient or the provider[24]
- Determination if adequate step therapy has been attempted for patient
- Assess scientific evidence to support the exception for use
- Evaluate appropriateness of requesting provider to manage and monitor the medication (The payer may determine only a specialist may manage the medication.)

Electronic prior authorization

- Permits individualized information for a drug that is needed for determination
- May be determined by algorithm or (auto scores) versus clinical review cutting the time to determinations
- Turnaround time ranges from seconds to less than 4 hours

Prior authorization rejections

- Missing information
- Insufficient information
- Incorrect information

- Step therapy not attempted or other established guidelines for approval set by the payer
- Therapy approved but dose, duration, or quantity not within guidelines and not justified
- Therapy determined not medically necessary
- Therapy not within the provider's scope
- Therapy considered experimental

Third-party prior authorization rejections

- Reasons for PA rejections:
  - Missing information
  - Insufficient information
  - Incorrect information
  - Step therapy not attempted or other established guidelines for approval set by the payer
  - Therapy approved but dose, duration, or quantity not within guidelines and not justified
  - Therapy determined not medically necessary
  - Therapy not within the provider's scope
  - Therapy considered experimental
- Reject error codes[25]

Reject error category	Reject error code	Reject description
Beneficiary	58	Date of birth is missing or invalid
Beneficiary	65	First and/or last name is/are blank
Beneficiary	66	Gender code is missing or invalid
Beneficiary	65	HIC number and name combination—invalid
Beneficiary	64	HIC number is missing or invalid
Beneficiary	95	Not eligible for service
Facility	97	An address component is missing or invalid
Facility	44	Name is missing
Facility	35	Not a pilot participant state
Facility	44	NPI does not match the name of the physician
Facility	43	NPI is missing or invalid
Medical info	AF	Diagnosis code qualifier is missing or invalid
Medical info	AF	Diagnosis code is missing or invalid
Medical info	AF	Diagnosis code qualifier is missing or invalid
Medical info	AG	Incorrect modifier for the procedure code
Medical info	15	Number of units is missing or invalid
Medical info	33	Place of service code is missing or invalid
Medical info	AG	Procedure code is invalid

(Continued)

Reject error category	Reject error code	Reject description
Medical info	AG	Procedure code is missing
Medical info	AG	Procedure code qualifier is missing or invalid
Ordering physician	97	An address component is missing or invalid
Ordering physician	44	First and/or last name is missing
Ordering physician	35	Not a pilot participant state
Ordering physician	44	NPI does not match the name of the physician
Ordering physician	43	NPI does not match the name of the physician
Rendering MD/ supplier	97	An address component is missing or invalid
Rendering MD/ supplier	44	First and/or last name is missing
Rendering MD/ supplier	35	Not a pilot participant state
Rendering MD/ supplier	44	NPI does not match the name of the physician
Rendering MD/ supplier	43	NPI does not match the name of the physician
Requester	97	An address component is missing or invalid
Requester	44	First and/or last name is/ are missing
Requester	35	Not a pilot participant state
Requester	44	NPI does not match the name of the physician
Requester	43	NPI does not match the Name of the Physician

AF and *AG* are rejection codes assigned by NCPDP; *HIC*, Health Insurance Claim; *NPI*, National Provider Identifier.

Prior authorizations issues

- Prescriber says PA was approved but claim is still not adjudicating.
  - Resolution: Call prescriber for confirmation documentation of approval, then contact processor.
- The claim adjudicates but the copay is too high for patient to afford.
  - Resolution: Contact prescriber for confirmation documentation of approval, then contact processor.
- The PA was approved but the claim rejects stating days' supply limitations are exceeded.
  - Resolution: Confirm day supply information on prescription is correct and resubmit once corrected. If day supply is accurate, contact processor.
- PA was denied.
  - Resolution: Contact prescriber to discuss medication or therapy change or have patient and prescriber file an appeal.

Denial and appeal process

- Review the reason for the PA denial provided in an explanation of benefits.
- Write an appeal letter:
  - First level of appeal—reviewed by a medical reviewer
  - Second level of appeal—reviewed by a medical (physician) director
  - Third level of appeal—external review
- File a complaint to the state insurance commissioner.

Audits and compliance

- Audits occur as a result of fraud, waste, and abuse.
- Medicare Recovery Audit Contractor Program (RAC) goal is identified and correct Medicare improper payments through the efficient detection and collection of overpayments made on claims of health care services provided to Medicare beneficiaries and the identification of underpayments to providers so that the CMS can implement actions that will prevent future improper payments in all 50 states.
  - 2003: Medicare Modernization Act enacted.
  - 2009: FFS RAC implemented.
  - 2010: Affordable Care Act expands RAC to include Medicare Parts C and D.
  - 2012: First Part D RAC audits conducted.
  - Medicare Recovery Audit Contractors review claims on a postpayment basis. The RACs detect and correct past improper payments and have the authority to perform audits as needed.
- Audits can be prevented by maintaining proper documentation that illustrates:
  - Service is medically necessary.
  - Service met any prior approval requirements.
  - Therapy is necessary according to accepted standards of care.
  - Medication is found in the formulary.
- Examples of actions that may lead to an audit:
  - Billing for unnecessary services (not medically necessary)
  - Overcharging for services or supplies
  - Billing for services or supplies not provided
  - Misusing billing codes to increase reimbursement
  - Pay for referrals

Audit and compliance terminology

- Audit: Formal review of compliance with a particular set of standards (e.g., policies and procedures, laws and regulations used as a base measures); performed by both the government and commercial payers
- Fraud: Knowingly submitting, or causing to be submitted, false claims or making misrepresentations of fact to obtain payment for which no entitlement would otherwise exist or knowingly soliciting, receiving, offering or paying remuneration (e.g., kickbacks, bribes, or rebates) to induce or reward referrals for items or services reimbursed by Federal Health programs

- Waste: Practices that directly or indirectly result in unnecessary cost to the Medicare program to include overusing services or misuse of resources
- FWA: Fraud, waste and abuse
- Compliance: Refers to complying with all Medicare laws and regulations
- Compliance officer: An organization's employee responsible for ensuring overall compliance with all laws, regulations and contracts
- Inspector General in the Office of the Inspector General: Responsible for scheduling audits, evaluations, investigations, and law enforcement efforts related to the Medicare program

340B audits

340B Drug Pricing Program-covered entities must ensure program integrity and maintain accurate records documenting compliance with all 340B program requirements. Covered entities are subject to audit by the manufacturer or the federal government. Failure to adhere may make the 340B-covered entity responsible to manufacturers for refunds of discounts or cause the covered entity to be removed from the 340B program

- Types of 340B audits:
  - Field/on-site audits
  - Purchase verification
  - Investigational audit
  - Desk/mail audit
  - Prescriber/member audits
  - Telephone audits

340B audit process

Preaudit

- Human Resources and Services Administration (HRSA) conducts both onsite and remote audits.
- Covered entities identified for an audit receive a letter explaining what to expect and how to appropriately prepare.
- Auditors oversee an introductory teleconference with the organization to ask for and obtain specified documents, including policies, procedures, and internal controls.
- Auditors work with the entity to schedule a meeting and to discuss expectations of the onsite audit.

Onsite or remote audit

- HRSA conducts both onsite and remote audits.
- Auditors collect and examine select 340B program data and internal controls.
- Audit procedures include, at a minimum:
  - Review of relevant policies and procedures
  - Verification of eligibility, to include GPO prohibition, maintaining auditable records, and outpatient clinic eligibility
  - Verification of internal controls to prevent diversion and duplicate discounts, including how the covered entity defines whether a patient is considered inpatient or outpatient, HRSA Medicaid Exclusion File designations, and accuracy of covered entity's 340B OPAIS record

- Review of 340B program compliance at covered entity, to include outpatient facilities, and contract pharmacies
- Testing of 340B drug transaction records on a sample or judgmental basis
- The same audits are used for remote audits except the use of secure workspaces, secured emails, and Zoom. Communication with the auditor and the entity are encrypted and secure. Zoom is the preferred method to review sample items and patient records. Secure workspaces and secured email are scanning paper documents.
- Auditors finding are reported to the Office of Pharmacy Affairs (OPA) and must undergo OPA review.

Postaudit

- Auditors forward a preliminary report to OPA for review.[26]
- OPA reviews the preliminary report, drafts a Final Report, and issues the report to the entity, with a request for a corrective action plan (CAP), if applicable.

Notice and hearing

- An entity has 30 calendar days from the date of the receipt of the HRSA Final Report to review the findings of the report and the request for a CAP.
- If a covered entity agrees with the Final Report, a covered entity must submit a CAP to HRSA within 60 calendar days for HRSA's approval. If a covered entity is submitting disagreement with the audit findings, the covered entity should not submit a CAP until HRSA review of the disagreement is complete. When HRSA review of the disagreement is complete, HRSA will request a CAP at that time if one is still required.
- If a covered entity disagrees with the Final Report, they will notify HRSA in writing within 30 calendar days with supporting documentation. OPA reviews the covered entity's response and may reissue the Final Report.
- If an entity fails to submit a CAP, an entity may be removed from the 340B program.
- Once an audit report is finalized by OPA, the findings and any associated sanctions will be summarized on the OPA public website.

Corrective action plan implementation and repayment

- Full CAP implementation and settlement with manufacturers is expected to be complete within 6 months of the CAP approval date. Covered entities who fail to meet this requirement may be terminated from the 340B program.
- HRSA will post a notice on its website to alert manufacturers of violations that have occurred. This notice will identify the findings of the audit requiring repayment and entity contact information for manufacturers to utilize.
- The covered entity may be required to provide additional documentation, as outlined by HRSA, to include repayment to manufacturers.
- HRSA may reaudit a covered entity to ensure compliance with 340B program requirements has occurred.

■ Covered entities with a reaudit that identifies the issue has not been resolved may experience additional audits. A finding of noncompliance with the diversion prohibition in two or more audits may be considered systematic, serious, and intentional, which may result in termination from the 340B program.

HRSA 340B audit data requests[27]

■ 340B policies and procedures
■ Documentation of a covered entity's eligibility: Includes notice of grant award or contract
■ Data request for sample period: Includes medications dispensing information for a specific time period
■ List of eligible providers: Includes provider's name NPI number and evidence whether individual is employed or under contract with the covered entity
■ Purchasing documentation: List of wholesalers and 340B drug purchase orders during the selected timeframe
■ Contract pharmacy documentation: Includes copies of contract agreements, lists of participating pharmacies, and policies/procedures governing the contract relationship
■ Documentation of self-disclosures: Includes copies of any self-disclosure of noncompliance with OPA
■ Medicaid billing documentation: Includes Medicaid fee-for-service billing documentation

Contract documentation for claims billed to specific insurance plans

During a pharmacy audit the following items will be checked:

■ Prescription requirements:
  • Date of issuance
  • Prescribers signature
  • Prescriber's authority
  • Drug name
  • Drug strength
  • Drug dosage form
  • Quantity of drug prescribed
  • Directions for use
  • Number of refills authorized by the prescriber (if any)
  • "Brand name medically necessary" if no generic substitution is allowed
  • If handwritten, controlled substance prescription must be in ink or pencil that cannot be erased
  • Prescribers must manually sign controlled substance prescriptions on the date issued
■ Days supply of medication is accurately calculated
■ Whether the NDC number submitted the same as the NDC number dispensed
■ Whether the number of doses exceed FDA labeling
■ Use-as-directed sig codes exceed more than one billing per month:
  • Shampoos—document frequency of use and size of area to be treated
  • Creams and ointments—document frequency of use and size of area to be treated
  • Migraine medications—document number of headaches treated per month

  • Insulin—document exact regular dosage and maximum daily dosage for any sliding scale directions
  • Diabetic syringes, test strips, or lancets—document the maximum use per day
■ Refill practices-do not bill or auto refill without consent or request from patient
■ Patient-driven inappropriate refill practices:
  • Stockpiling of medication by patient
  • Red flags indicating drug diversion
■ Overrides during point of sale
  • Submit claims with vacation supply override codes only if the patient is on vacation.
  • Submit claims with known PA override codes only if the patient meets the PA criteria.
■ Prescription origin checks:
  • Do not alter prescription origin codes.
    • Prescription origin codes

Code	Appropriate use
1	Written—Prescription is presented to the pharmacy on a prescription pad.
2	Telephone—Prescription is conveyed to the pharmacy verbally by telephone call, voicemail, or other electronically recorded verbal message.
3	Electronic—Prescription is transmitted to the pharmacy by the National Council Drug Programs' SCRIPT Standard or Health Level Standard transactions.
4	Facsimile—Prescription is transmitted to the pharmacy by facsimile machine.
5	Pharmacy—A origin code is used when a pharmacy staff member must create a new prescription number from an existing prescription.

  • Verify the prescriber DEA number and office telephone number for all controlled substance prescriptions received by telephone. If the caller or prescriber is unknown, confirm the contact information with a secondary source.
■ Appropriate use of DAW Codes:
  • 0 = No product selection indicated
  • 1 = Substitution not allowed by provider
    • Appropriate only when the prescriber indicated verbally or on the prescription that substitution is not allowed—"substitution is not allowed," "dispense as written," or "brand name medically necessary"
  • 2 = Substitution allowed; patient requested product dispensed
    • Appropriate only when the patient indicated the patient requests the brand-name version of the drug prescribed
  • 3 = Substitution allowed; pharmacist-selected product dispensed
  • 4 = Substitution allowed, generic drug not in stock
  • 5 = Substitution allowed; brand drug dispensed as generic
    • The pharmacist opted to dispense the brand-name drug and elected to be reimbursed for the generic drug
  • 6 = Override
    • Appropriate when an override DAW code is required

- 7 = Substitution not allowed; brand drug mandated by state law
  - May occur if state law requires drug testing of generic drugs that has not been completed
- 8 = Substitution allowed; generic drug not available in marketplace
  - May occur if the generic drug has been approved by the FDA but not yet manufactured and distributed
- 9 = Other
- Partial fill procedures:
  - Adjudicate partial fills appropriately. Do not "owe patient" any drug quantity if the fill quantity to be dispensed has been filled.
  - Only use partial fill functionality of the billing system when unable to fill the full quantity to be dispensed.
  - Do not bill the payer for the full amount of a partial refill.
  - Do not bill the provider for a second dispensing fee when completing a partial refill.
- Selection of package sizes:
  - Select the smallest commercially available package size to address the prescription requirements.
  - Ensure the NDC dispensed matches the NDC billed, particularly for generic and compounded medications.
- Document beneficiary receipt of prescription:
  - Always obtain signatures from patients or their agent at the time of prescription pickup.
  - Do the following if Medicaid payment occurs:
  - Reverse any claim within the past year.
  - Submit a check and explanation for any older claim.
  - Pharmacy must report overpayment within 60 days from the date the overpayment is identified.

Federal laws/regulations

- False Claims Act:
  - Forbids submitting a fraudulent claim or making a false statement or representation in connection with a claim
  - Encourages submitting suspected fraud and abuse against the government by protecting and rewarding individuals in whistleblower cases
  - Protects the relator (individual who makes an accusation) from employer retaliation
- Antikickback statute:
  - Makes it illegal to knowingly offer incentives to induce referral for services that are paid by government health care programs
  - Financial actions are often considered to be incentives, which include illegal direct payments to physicians
- Physician self-referral law (Stark Law):
  - Makes it illegal for physicians and members of their immediate family to have financial relationships with clinics to which they refer their patients
- Sarbanes-Oxley Act:
  - A comprehensive reform of financial practices for businesses focused on publicly held corporations, financial reporting, audit procedures, and their internal financial controls
- Social Security Act that includes the Exclusion Statute (removes provider from Medicare eligibility) and the Civil Monetary Penalties Law (allows Medicare to not pay claim or demand paid money returned)

- United States Criminal Code—Offenses may include fines, imprisonment, or both

Accrediting bodies and surveys

- Accreditation: Acknowledgment from accrediting body certifying that an organization or individual has met specific standards
- Function of accreditation agencies:
  - Establishing the minimum level of care
  - Deciding on the best programs and procedures to achieve the minimum level of care
  - Determining how to monitor success or failure
  - Establishing standards for quality and safety
- Purpose of accreditation:
  - To select those health care entities they wish to do business with either as sole or preferred providers
  - May incentivize providers by offering additional payment to entities who have achieved accreditation or certain levels of accreditation

The Joint Commission

- Accredits and certifies hospitals and health care organizations that provide ambulatory and office-based surgery, behavioral health, home health care, laboratory, and nursing care center services
- Accreditation evaluates the pharmacy's:
  - Controlled substance security and diversion mitigation
  - High-risk medication processes:
    - Sterile compounding and USP 797 compliance
    - Chemotherapy safety
    - Pediatric medication processes
  - Hazardous drug management and USP readiness
  - Alignment with The Joint Commission requirements for complex medication orders
  - Medication-related technologies including computerized order entry, bar code medication administration, smart pump technology, and in-pharmacy technology
  - Specialty pharmacy and home infusion pharmacy under the home care accreditation
- Has been granted "deemed" tatus" for participation in Medicare (This status states that the institution has met the Medicare Conditions of Participation and is eligible for Medicare funding. The institution does not need to meet the requirements for annual Medicare surveys by state inspectors.)
- Provides certification for disease-specific and advanced disease-specific care, palliative care, and home care staffing
- Establishes national patient safety goals and universal protocols for those accredited or certified; the 2022 goals include:
  - Ambulatory
  - Assisted living community
  - Behavioral health care and human services
  - Critical access hospital
  - Home care
  - Hospital
  - Laboratory
  - Nursing care center
  - Office-based surgery

- Examples of national patient safety goals:
  - Identify patients correctly.
  - Use medicines safely.
  - Prevent infection.
  - Prevent patients from falling.
  - Prevent mistakes in surgery.
  - Identify individuals serves safety risk.
  - Improve patient safety risks.
  - Improve staff communication.
  - Prevent bed sores.

Centers for Medicare and Medicaid Services

- Department of Health and Human Services: Responsible for improving the health and well-being of individuals by providing for productive health and human services and by providing sound, advances in medicine, public health, and social services
- Oversees:
  - Medicare: A federal health insurance program for:
    - People who are 65 or older
    - Certain younger people with disabilities
    - People with ESRD requiring dialysis or a transplant
  - Medicaid: A state and federal program that provides health coverage if you have a very low income. Federal government matches states funding at an average of 53%.
  - Children's Health and Insurance Program (CHIP): Provides low-cost health coverage to children in families that earn too much money to qualify for Medicaid. In some states, CHIP covers pregnant women. Each state offers CHIP coverage and works closely with its state Medicaid program.

Utilization review accreditation commission

- Utilization Review Accreditation Commission (URAC) standards address risk management, consumer protection and empowerment, operations and infrastructure, performance monitoring and improvement, pharmacy dispensing, pharmacy product handing and security, patient service and communication, and reporting performance measures to URAC.
- Accreditation is available in the following areas:
  - Specialty pharmacy accreditation
  - Mail order service pharmacy accreditation
  - Pharmacy services accreditation
  - Rare disease designation
  - Specialty pharmacy services accreditation
  - Specialty pharmacy accreditation for small business
  - Mail service pharmacy accreditation for small business
  - Infusion pharmacy accreditation
  - Medicare HIT supplier accreditation
  - Pharmacy benefit management accreditation

Opioid stewardship designation

- Developed by URAC
- Promote patient safety and the appropriate use of opioid medication, as well as to encourage innovation in managing opioid use and decreasing the risk of substance abuse disorder

Human resources and services administration

- An agency of the US Department of Health and Human Services responsible for improving health care to people who are geographically isolated, economically, or medically vulnerable
- Goals:
  - Take workable steps to attain health equity and improve public health.
  - Improve access to quality health services.
  - Promote a health workforce and health infrastructure able to deal with current and emerging needs.
  - Optimize HRSA operations and strengthen program engagement.
- Responsible for oversight of the 340B drug rebate program

Det norske veritas (DNV) health care

- Accredits and certifies health care facilities worldwide
- Certifies the following facilities:
  - Stroke care
  - Infection prevention
  - Sterile processing
  - Orthopedic center of excellence
  - Foot and ankle surgery
  - Hip and knee replacement
  - Shoulder surgery
  - Spine surgery
  - Cardiac center of excellence
  - Chest pain
  - Extracorporeal
  - Heart failure
  - VAD facility
  - Palliative care

CHAPTER REVIEW QUESTIONS

1. Which type of health plan requires a patient to use network providers only?
   a. HMO
   b. Point of service
   c. PPO
   d. Both b and c
2. Which is a program created by pharmaceutical and medical supply manufacturers to assist financially needy patient purchase necessary medications and supplies?
   a. Drug discount card
   b. Health savings account
   c. Manufacturer discount card
   d. Patient assistance program
3. Which form of Medicare covers physician visits, clinical laboratory services, and outpatient and preventative care screenings?
   a. Medicare Part A
   b. Medicare Part B
   c. Medicare Part C
   d. Medicare Part D

4. To be eligible for Medicare Part D assistance for low-income beneficiaries, which Medicare programs must an individual be enrolled?
   a. Medicare Parts A and B
   b. Medicare Parts A and C
   c. Medicare Parts B and C
   d. Medicare Parts A, B, and C

5. Medicaid is a joint program between which programs?
   a. County and federal programs
   b. County and state programs
   c. Federal and state programs
   d. County, state, and federal programs

6. Which term refers to the amount of a prescription bill the patient is responsible?
   a. Copayment
   b. Deductible
   c. EAC
   d. Usual/customary/reasonable

7. Which relationship holder code is assigned to the cardholder of the insurance for a prescription?
   a. 01
   b. 02
   c. 03
   d. 04

8. Which term refers to a six-digit number used to identify the company that will reimburse the pharmacy for the prescription being filled
   a. Group code
   b. RxPCN
   c. RxBIN
   d. Subscriber

9. Which DAW code should be assigned to a prescription claim if the prescriber does not permit the pharmacy to dispense a generic medication?
   a. DAW 0
   b. DAW 1
   c. DAW 2
   d. DAW 3

10. All of the following patient information is transmitted during adjudication *except* for which one?
    a. Patient's birthdate
    b. Patient's gender
    c. Patient's NPI number
    d. Patient's relationship to the cardholder

11. A pharmacy technician adjudicates a prescription for a patient and receives a rejection code 9. What must be corrected?
    a. Date the prescription was filled
    b. Days' supply of medication dispensed
    c. Patient's birthdate
    d. Patient's gender

12. In a tier system of medications, which tier indicates generic drugs?
    a. 1
    b. 2
    c. 3
    d. 4

13. How many digits are found in a CPT code?
    a. 3
    b. 4
    c. 5
    d. 6

14. An NPI number is assigned to health care providers. How many digits are in a NPI number?
    a. 6
    b. 8
    c. 10
    d. 12

15. Maya is the daughter of parents who are divorced and is the covered under both parent's plans. How is the Maya's primary plan determined?
    a. Following the birth rule of the parents
    b. Using the plan of the custodial parent
    c. Using the plan of the spouse of the custodial parent
    d. Using the plan of the parent without custody

16. Which acronym refers to the national average of list prices charged by wholesalers to pharmacies?
    a. AAC
    b. AMP
    c. ASP
    d. AWP

17. Under which situation would a pharmacy need to request an override for a medication with established restricted limitations?
    a. Age or sex restrictions
    b. Early refill on a medication
    c. Quantity for a medication to be dispensed
    d. All the above

18. Which party is responsible for initiating a PA for medication for a patient?
    a. Patient
    b. Pharmacy
    c. Prescriber's office
    d. All of the above

19. Which of the following actions may lead to an audit of a pharmacy?
    a. Using a CPT code G0108 for individual diabetes self-management training
    b. Using a DAW code of 0 when dispensing a generic medication
    c. Using a CPT code of 99607 for a new patient, face-to-face visit
    d. All the above

20. Which organization oversees CHIP?
    a. CMS
    b. HRSA
    c. The Joint Commission
    d. URAC

21. Which organization established national patent safety goals for ambulatory care, assisted living communities, behavioral health care and human services, critical access hospital, home care, laboratory, nursing care centers, and office-based surgery?
    a. CMS
    b. HRSA
    c. The Joint Commission
    d. URAC

22. Who developed the Opioid Stewardship designation?
    a. CMS
    b. HRSA
    c. The Joint Commission
    d. URAC

23. Which form of Medicare utilizes the STAR rating system to assess the quality of health and drug services received by consumers?
    a. Medicare Part A
    b. Medicare Part B
    c. Medicare Part C
    d. Medicare Part D
24. Which piece of legislation encourages submitting suspected fraud and abuse against the government by protecting and rewarding individuals in whistleblower cases?
    a. Anti-Kickback Statute
    b. False Claims Act
    c. Physician Self-Referral Law
    d. Sarbanes-Oxley Act
25. Which of the following health care facilities is *not* eligible to participate in the 340B program?
    a. Children's hospital
    b. DSH
    c. For-profit hospitals
    d. Freestanding cancer hospitals

REFERENCES

1. Long-term care pharmacy: the evolving marketplace and emerging policy issues. Avalere Health. 2015. Accessed September 7, 2022. https://www.mhainc.com/uploadedfiles/content/resources/avalere_ltc%20pharmacy%20the%20evolving%20marketplace%20and%20emerging%20policy%20issues....pdf
2. Medicare Part B home infusion therapy services with the use of durable medical equipment. 2019. Accessed September 7, 2022. https://www.cms.gov/files/document/se19029.pdf
3. Medicare Diabetes Prevention Program (MDPP) expanded. CMS. Published March 30, 2022. Accessed September 7, 2022. https://innovation.cms.gov/innovation-models/medicare-diabetes-prevention-program
4. Enroll or purchase a plan. TRICARE. Published March 18, 2021. Accessed September 21, 2022. https://www.tricare.mil/Plans/Enroll
5. TRICARE prime. TRICARE. Published February 15, 2002. Accessed September 21, 2022. https://www.tricare.mil/Plans/HealthPlans/Prime/
6. TRICARE prime remote. TRICARE. Published August 18, 2021. Accessed September 21, 2022. https://www.tricare.mil/Plans/HealthPlans/TPR
7. TRICARE prime overseas. TRICARE. Published October 19, 2020. Accessed September 21, 2022. https://www.tricare.mil/Plans/HealthPlans/TPO.
8. TRICARE select overseas. TRICARE. Accessed September 21, 2022. https://www.tricare.mil/Plans/HealthPlans/TSO
9. TRICARE select overseas. TRICARE. Published August 3, 2022. Accessed September 21, 2022. https://www.tricare.mil/Plans/HealthPlans/TSO
10. TRICARE for life. TRICARE. Published June 5, 2018. Accessed September 21, 2022. https://www.tricare.mil/Plans/HealthPlans/TFL
11. TRICARE reserve select. TRICARE. Published December 10, 2018. Accessed September 30, 2022. https://www.tricare.mil/Plans/HealthPlans/TRS/UsingTRS
12. TRICARE retired reserve. TRICARE. Published December 15, 2020. Accessed September 30, 2022. https://www.tricare.mil/Plans/HealthPlans/TRR
13. TRICARE young adult. TRICARE. Published October 11, 2022. Accessed September 30, 2022. https://www.tricare.mil/Plans/HealthPlans/TYA
14. US family health plan. TRICARE. Published March 17, 2022. Accessed September 30, 2022. https://www.tricare.mil/Plans/HealthPlans/USFHP
15. Health care benefits for dependents (CHAMPVA). Published March 5, 2022. Accessed September 30, 2022. https://www.benefits.gov/benefit/318
16. Dispense as written (DAW) product selection code. Research Data Assistance Center. 2022. Accessed October 2, 2022. https://resdac.org/cms-data/variables/dispense-written-daw-product-selection-code
17. Reject codes. Published June 1, 2019. Accessed October 2, 2022. https://www.caremark.com/portal/asset/CVSCaremarkPayerSheetRejectCodes.pdf
18. CPT overview and code approval. AMA. 2022. Accessed October 2, 2022. https://www.ama-assn.org/practice-management/cpt/cpt-overview-and-code-approval
19. Medicare billing: 837P and form CMS-1500. Medicare Learning Network. Published June 2022. Accessed October 2, 2022. https://www.cms.gov/Outreach-and-Education/Medicare-Learning-Network-MLN/MLNProducts/Downloads/837P-CMS-1500.pdf
20. CMS1500. CMS.gov. Accessed October 2, 2022. https://www.cms.gov/Medicare/CMS-Forms/CMS-Forms/Downloads/CMS1500.pdf
21. Medicare billing: 871 & form cms-1450. Medicare Learning Network. Published July 2022. Accessed October 2, 2022. https://www.cms.gov/files/document/837I-Form-CMS-1450-MLN006926.pdf
22. What's a mac. CMS.gov. Published January 12, 2022. Accessed October 2, 2022. https://www.cms.gov/Medicare/Medicare-Contracting/Medicare-Administrative-Contractors/What-is-a-MAC
23. 340B glossary of terms. Apexus 340B Prime Vendor Program. Published July 26, 2022. Accessed October 5, 2022. https://www.340Bpvp.com/Documents/Public/340B%20Tools/340B-glossary-of-terms.pdf
24. Medically necessary. CMS.gov. Published May 14, 2006. Accessed October 6, 2022. https://www.cms.gov/apps/glossary/search.asp?Term=medically+necessary&Language=English&Submit-TermSrch=Search
25. Reject error codes. CMS.gov. Accessed October 6, 2022. https://www.cms.gov/files/document/prior-authorization-reject-codes.pdf
26. Audits of covered entities. HRSA. Published October 2022. Accessed October 8, 2022. https://www.hrsa.gov/opa/program-integrity
27. 340B HRSA audit overview and checklist. National Coalition of STD Directors. Published October 12, 2021. Accessed October 8, 2022. https://www.ncsddc.org/wp-content/uploads/2021/10/HRSA-Audit-Overview-and-Checklist-10.12.21-1.pdf

10

Technician Product Verification Certificate

Technician product verification certificate domains

Identifying the correct product name, strength, and dosage form
- Identify commonly prescribed medications, their strength and dosage forms
- Distinguish medications with multiple formulations
- Identify appropriate quantities for common medications
- Identify the different routes of medication administration
- Recognize common medication dosage forms
- Recognize-look-a-like medications
- Identify appropriate auxiliary label(s) and when to use them
- Recognize medication guides and when to provide them to patients

Calculating the amount of product to dispense based on prescribed dosage and frequency
- Recognize commonly mistaken signa codes and "do not use" abbreviations that may still be used in prescribing practices
- Prescription processing
  - Prescription components
  - Drug Enforcement Administration numbers
  - Prescription label requirements
  - Medication order requirements
  - Medication order label requirements
  - Sterile product label requirements
  - Unit dose label requirements
  - Repackaged drug label requirements
  - Dispense as written codes

- Perform calculations that involve conversion of units in the metric system
- Calculate the amount of product to dispense based on pre-scribed dosage and frequency
- Calculate basic pharmacy problems using ratios and proportions
- Calculate percent strength of a medication expressed as weight/weight, volume/volume and/or weight/volume
- Perform calculations that allow a compounded prescription to be reduced or enlarged
- Perform dilution calculations
- Perform allegation calculations
- Calculate accurate days' supply for medications

Evaluating the integrity of product characteristics (e.g., Intact packaging and expiration dates)
- Differentiate between expiration and beyond-use dates
- Identify signs of product instability
- List best practices to identify product tampering

Identifying the correct product name, strength, and dosage form

Commonly dispensed medications[i]

Pharmacies dispense hundreds of medications every day. When reviewing a new prescription for a patient, it is extremely important the pharmacy technician is familiar with both the medication's brand and generic name, its indication, and its available dosage forms and strengths. By knowing this information, the pharmacy technician is able to determine the appropriateness of the prescription. If the medication is

---

[i]The top 300 of 2020. ClinCalc. Accessed August 4, 2022. https://clincalc.com/DrugStats/Top300Drugs.aspx.

not indicated for the prescribed condition or the dose is sub-therapeutic or excessive for the patient's age or weight it is the pharmacy technician's responsibility to notify the pharmacist of this immediately to prevent a medication mishap.

Generic name	Brand name	Drug classification	Indication(s)	Recommended daily dosage	Commonly dispensed quantities (community pharmacy-30-day supply)	Generic dosage forms and strengths
atorvastatin	Lipitor	HMG-CoA Reductase Inhibitor	Dyslipidemia, hyper-cholesterolemia, and hypertriglyceridemia	10–80 mg PO qd	30 tablets	TAB: 10 mg, 20 mg, 40 mg, 80 mg
levothyroxine	Synthroid	Hormone	Hypothyroidism	50–200 mcg PO qd	30 tablets	CAP: 13 mcg, 25 mcg, 50 mcg, 75 mcg, 88 mcg, 100 mcg, 112 mcg, 125 mcg, 137 mcg, 150 mcg, 175 mcg, 200 mcg; TAB: 25 mcg, 50 mcg, 75 mcg, 88 mcg, 100 mcg, 112 mcg, 125 mcg, 137 mcg, 150 mcg, 175 mcg, 200 mcg, 300 mcg; INJ: various
lisinopril	Zestril, Prinivil	ACE Inhibitor	HTN, myocardial infarction, and congestive failure	5–40 mg PO qd	30 tablets	TAB: 2.5 mg, 5 mg, 10 mg, 20 mg, 30 mg, 40 mg
metformin	Glucophage, Glucophage XR	Biguanide	Diabetes mellitus type 2	IR: 850–1000 mg PO bid ER: 1000–2000 mg ER PO qpm	60 tablets 60 tablets	TAB: 500 mg, 850 mg, 1000 mg; ER TAB: 500 mg, 750 mg, 1000 mg; SOL: 500 mg per 5 mL
metoprolol	Lopressor (metoprolol tartrate), Toprol-XL (metoprolol succinate)	Beta blocker	HTN, angina, and myocardial infarction	Metoprolol tartrate: 50–200 mg PO bid Metoprolol succinate: 50–400 mg PO qd	30 tablets 30 tablets	Metoprolol tartrate: TAB: 25 mg, 37.5 mg, 50 mg, 75 mg, 100 mg; INJ: various Metoprolol succinate: ER TAB: 25 mg, 50 mg, 100 mg, 200 mg
amlodipine	Norvasc	Calcium channel blocker	HTN and coronary artery disease	5–10 mg PO qd	30 tablets	TAB: 2.5 mg, 5 mg, 10 mg
albuterol (inhaled)	Proventil HFA, Ventolin HFA	Short-acting beta agonists	Bronchospasms	MDI: 2 puffs inhaled q4–6 h prn; Alt: 1 puff inhaled q4 h prn NEB: 2.5–5 mg NEB q20 min ×3, then 2.5–10 mg NEB q1–4 h prn; Alt: 10–15 mg/h continuous NEB	1 inhaler	MDI: 90 mcg per actuation; NEB (0.083%): 2.5 mg per 3 mL; NEB (0.5%): 5 mg per mL
omeprazole	Prilosec, Prilosec OTC	Proton pump inhibitor	GERD, gastric ulcer, duodenal ulcer and Helicobacter pylori infection	20 mg PO qd	30 tablets	DR CAP: 10 mg, 20 mg, 40 mg; DR TAB: 20 mg; DR ODT: 20 mg

(Continued)

Generic name	Brand name	Drug classification	Indication(s)	Recommended daily dosage	Commonly dispensed quantities (community pharmacy-30-day supply)	Generic dosage forms and strengths
losartan	Cozaar	Angiotensin receptor blocker	HTN, stroke prevention, and diabetic nephropathy	50–100 mg/day PO divided qd or bid	30–60 tablets	TAB: 25 mg, 50 mg, 100 mg
gabapentin	Neurontin	Anticonvulsant	Seizures	300–1200 mg PO tid	90 capsules	CAP: 100 mg, 300 mg, 400 mg; TAB: 600 mg, 800 mg; SOL: 50 mg per mL
hydrochlorothiazide	a	Thiazide diuretic	HTN and peripheral edema	HTN: 12.5–50 mg PO qd Edema: 25–200 mg PO qd	30 tablets (capsules)	CAP: 12.5 mg; TAB: 12.5 mg, 25 mg, 50 mg
sertraline	Zoloft	Selective serotonin reuptake inhibitor	Major depressive disorder, obsessive-compulsive disorder, panic disorder, posttraumatic stress disorder, and premenstrual dysphoric disorders	50–200 mg PO qd	30 tablets	TAB: 25 mg, 50 mg, 100 mg; SOL: 20 mg per mL
simvastatin	Zocor	HMG-CoA reductase inhibitor	Dyslipidemia, hypercholesterolemia, and hypertriglyceridemia	20–40 mg PO qpm	30 tablets	TAB: 5 mg, 10 mg, 20 mg, 40 mg, 80 mg
montelukast	Singulair	Leukotriene inhibitor	Bronchospasms and allergic rhinitis	10 mg PO qpm	30 tablets	TAB: 10 mg
hydrocodone/ acetaminophen	a	Opioid	Mild to moderate pain	2.5–10 mg hydrocodone PO q4–6 h prn	20 tablets	2.5 mg/325 mg, 5 mg/300 mg, 5 mg/325 mg, 7.5 mg/300 mg, 7.5 mg 325 mg, 10 mg/300 mg, 10 mg/325 mg; SOL: 7.5 mg/320 mg per 15 mL, 10 mg/325 mg per 15 mL
pantoprazole	Protonix	Proton pump inhibitor	GERD	20–40 mg PO qd	30 tablets	DR TAB: 20 mg, 40 mg; INJ: various
furosemide	Lasix	Loop diuretic	HTN and edema	HTN: 10–40 mg PO bid Edema: 40–120 mg/day	60 tablets 30 tablets	TAB: 20 mg, 40 mg, 80 mg; SOL: 10 mg per mL, 40 mg per 5 mL; INJ: various
fluticasone	Flovent HFA, Flovent Diskus, Flonase Allergy Relief	Corticosteroid	Asthma and respiratory allergies	Flovent HFA: 2–4 puffs inhaled bidFlovent Diskus: 2 puffs (100 mcg or 250 mcg per blister) inhaled bid	1 inhaler 1 inhaler	MDI: 44 mcg per actuation, 110 mcg per actuation, 220 mcg per actuation
escitalopram	Lexapro	Selective serotonin reuptake inhibitor	Major depressive disorder and generalized anxiety disorder	10 mg PO qd	30 tablets	TAB: 5 mg, 10 mg, 20 mg; SOL: 5 mg per 5 mL
fluoxetine	Prozac	Selective serotonin reuptake inhibitor	Major depressive disorder, obsessive-compulsive disorder, panic disorder, and bipolar disorder	20–80 mg PO qam	30 capsules	CAP: 10 mg, 20 mg, 40 mg; DR CAP: 90 mg; TAB: 10 mg, 20 mg, 60 mg; SOL: 20 mg per 5 mL

(Continued)

Generic name	Brand name	Drug classification	Indication(s)	Recommended daily dosage	Commonly dispensed quantities (community pharmacy-30-day supply)	Generic dosage forms and strengths
rosuvastatin	Crestor	HMG-CoA reductase inhibitor	Dyslipidemia, hypercholesterolemia, hypertriglyceridemia, atherosclerotic cardiovascular disease, and cardiovascular event prevention	5–40 mg PO qd	30 tablets	TAB: 5 mg, 10 mg, 20 mg, 40 mg
bupropion	Wellbutrin XL, Wellbutrin SR	Norepinephrine-dopamine reuptake inhibitor	Major depressive disorder, smoking cessation, and ADHD	IR: 100 mg PO tid 12 h ER: 150 mg ER PO bid 24 h ER: 300 mg ER PO qam	90 tablets 60 tablets	TAB: 75 mg, 100 mg; ER TAB (12 h): 100 mg, 150 mg, 200 mg; ER TAB (24 h): 150 mg, 300 mg
amoxicillin	a	Penicillin	Bacterial infections, pharyngitis, otitis media, sinusitis, and *H. pylori* infection	Bacterial: 500–875 mg PO q12 h Pharyngitis: 1000 mg PO q24 h Otitis media: 1 g PO q8 h ×5–10 days Sinusitis: 1 g PO q8 h ×5–10 days *H pylori*: 1 g PO bid ×5–14 days	20 capsules (tablets) 20 capsules (tablets) 60 capsules (tablets) 60 capsules (tablets) 56 capsules (tablets)	CAP: 250 mg, 500 mg; TAB: 500 mg, 875 mg; ER TAB: 775 mg; CHEWABLE: 125 mg, 250 mg; SUSP: 125 mg per 5 mL, 200 mg per 5 mL, 250 mg per 5 mL, 400 mg per 5 mL
dextroamphetamine/amphetamine	Adderall, Adderall XR	Norepinephrine-dopamine reuptake inhibitor	ADHD	5–40 mg/day PO divided qd to tid	30–90 capsules (tablets)	ER CAP: 5 mg, 10 mg, 15 mg, 20 mg, 25 mg, 30 mg; TAB: 5 mg, 7.5 mg, 10 mg, 12.5 mg, 15 mg, 20 mg, 30 mg
trazodone	a	Serotonin modulator	Major depressive disorder, insomnia	50–100 mg PO bid to tid	60–90 tablets	TAB: 50 mg, 100 mg, 150 mg, 300 mg
duloxetine	Cymbalta	Serotonin-norepinephrine reuptake inhibitor	Major depressive disorder, generalized anxiety disorder, neuropathic pain, and fibromyalgia	60 mg PO qd	30 capsules	DR CAP: 20 mg, 30 mg, 40 mg, 60 mg
prednisone	a	Corticosteroid	Adrenal insufficiency, asthma, corticosteroid-responsive conditions, and gout	5–60 mg PO qd	30 tablets	TAB: 1 mg, 2.5 mg, 5 mg, 10 mg, 20 mg, 50 mg; SOL: 5 mg per 5 mL, 5 mg per mL
tamsulosin	Flomax	Alpha-1 blocker	Benign prostatic hyperplasia	0.4 mg PO qd	30 capsules	CAP: 0.4 mg
ibuprofen	Motrin IB (OTC), Advil (OTC)	NSAID	Mild to moderate pain, fever, inflammation, osteoarthritis, rheumatoid arthritis, and dysmenorrhea	300–800 mg PO tid to qid	90 tablets	CAP: 200 mg; TAB: 100 mg, 200 mg, 400 mg, 600 mg, 800 mg; CHEWABLE: 50 mg, 100 mg; SUSP: 100 mg per 5 mL, 50 mg per 1.25 mL

(Continued)

Generic name	Brand name	Drug classification	Indication(s)	Recommended daily dosage	Commonly dispensed quantities (community pharmacy-30-day supply)	Generic dosage forms and strengths
citalopram	Celexa	Selective serotonin reuptake inhibitor	Major depressive disorder and obsessive-compulsive disorder	20–60 mg PO qd	30 tablets	TAB: 10 mg, 20 mg, 40 mg; SOL: 10 mg per 5 mL
meloxicam	Mobic	NSAID	Osteoarthritis, rheumatoid arthritis and moderate-severe pain	5–15 mg PO qd	30 capsules (tablets)	CAP: 5 mg, 10 mg; TAB: 7.5 mg, 15 mg
pravastatin	[a]	HMF-CoA reductase inhibitor	Dyslipidemia, hypercholesterolemia, hypertriglyceridemia, and atherosclerotic cardiovascular disease	10–80 mg PO qd	30 tablets	TAB: 10 mg, 20 mg, 40 mg, 80 mg
carvedilol	Coreg, Coreg CR	Beta blocker	HTN, heart failure with reduced ejection fraction, and left ventricular dysfunction	IR: 6.25–25 mg PO bid ER: 20–80 mg ER PO qam	60 tablets 30 capsules	TAB: 3.125 mg, 6.25 mg, 12.5 mg, 25 mg; ER CAP: 10 mg, 20 mg, 40 mg, 80 mg
potassium chloride	Klor-con, Micro-K	Electrolyte	Hypokalemia	40–100 mEq/day PO in 2–5 divided dose	60 capsules (10 mEq BID)	ER CAP: 8 mEq, 10 mEq; ER TAB: 8 mEq, 10 mEq, 15 mEq, 20 mEq; PWDR: 20 mEq per pkt, 25 mEq per pkt; SOL: 20 mEq per 15 mL, 40 mEq per 15 mL; INJ: various
tramadol	[a]	Opioid	Moderate to moderate severe chronic pain	50–100 mg PO q4–6 h prn	40 tablets (10-day supply	TAB: 50 mg, 100 mg; ER TAB: 100 mg, 200 mg, 300 mg
clopidogrel	Plavix	Antiplatelet	Acute coronary syndrome and thrombotic event prevention	75 mg PO qd	30 tablets	TAB: 75 mg, 300 mg
insulin glargine	Lantus, Basaglar, Semglee, Toujeo	Insulin	Diabetes mellitus type 1 and diabetes mellitus type 2	Individualize dose SC/IV bid to qid	Varies based on daily dose	Pen: 100 units/mL, vial: 100 units/mL
atenolol	Tenormin	Beta blocker	HTN, angina, cardiovascular event prevention (postmyocardial infarction), and migraine headache prophylaxis	25–100 mg PO qd	30 tablets	TAB: 25 mg, 50 mg, 100 mg
venlafaxine	Effexor XR	Serotonin-norepinephrine reuptake inhibitor	Major depressive order, generalized anxiety disorder, panic disorder, and migraine headache prophylaxis	IR: 75–225 mg/day PO divided bid to tid ER: 75–225 mg ER PO qd	60–90 tablets 30 tablets	ER CAP: 37.5 mg, 75 mg, 150 mg; TAB: 25 mg, 37.5 mg, 50 mg, 75 mg, 100 mg; ER TAB: 37.5 mg, 75 mg, 150 mg, 225 mg

(Continued)

Generic name	Brand name	Drug classification	Indication(s)	Recommended daily dosage	Commonly dispensed quantities (community pharmacy-30-day supply)	Generic dosage forms and strengths
alprazolam	Xanax, Xanax XR	Benzodiazepine	Generalized anxiety disorder and panic disorder	0.25–0.5 mg PO tid ER: 3–6 mg PO qd	90 tablets 30 tablets	TAB: 0.25 mg, 0.5 mg, 1 mg, 2 mg; ER TAB: 0.5 mg, 1 mg, 2 mg, 3 mg; ODT: 0.25 mg, 0.5 mg, 1 mg, 2 mg; SOL: 1 mg per mL
norethindrone/ethinyl estradiol	Junel, Lo Loestrin FE Loestrin	Estrogen/progesterone oral contraceptive	Contraception, dysmenorrhea, and endometriosis	1 tablet daily	1 package	TAB: 0.5 mg/2.5 mcg, 1 mg/5 mcg
allopurinol	Zyloprim	Xanthine oxidase inhibitor	Gout prophylaxis and hyperuricemia	200–600 mg/day PO divided qd to qid	30–120 tablets	TAB: 100 mg, 300 mg; INJ: various
lisinopril/hydrochlorothiazide	Zestoretic	ACE inhibitor/thiazide diuretic	HTN	1–2 tabs PO qd	30–60 tablets	TAB: 10 mg/12.5 mg, 20 mg/12.5 mg, 20 mg/25 mg
cyclobenzaprine	[a]	Skeletal muscle relaxant	Muscle spasms and fibromyalgia	IR: 1–2 tabs PO qd ER: 15 mg ER PO qd up to 3 weeks	30–60 tablets 21 capsules	TAB: 5 mg, 7.5 mg, 10 mg; ER CAP: 15 mg, 30 mg
clonazepam	Klonopin	Benzodiazepine	Seizure disorder, panic disorder, anxiety, and sleepless legs syndrome	0.5–5 mg PO tid	90 tablets	TAB: 0.5 mg, 1 mg, 2 mg; ODT: 0.125 mg, 0.25 mg, 0.5 mg, 1 mg, 2 mg
zolpidem	Ambien, Ambien CR	Sedative/hypnotic	Insomnia	5–12.5 mg qhs ER 6.25–12.5 mg PO qhs	30 tablets 30 capsules	TAB: 5 mg, 10 mg; ER TAB: 6.25 mg, 12.5 mg; SL TAB: 1.75 mg, 3.5 mg
azithromycin	Zithromax	Macrolide	Bacterial infection, pharyngitis/tonsillitis, pneumonia, acute bacterial COPD exacerbation, and chlamydial infection	500 mg PO ×1 on day 1, then 250 mg PO q24 h ×4 days	6 tablets	TAB: 250 mg, 500 mg, 600 mg; PWDR: 1 g per pkt; SUSP: 100 mg per 5 mL, 200 mg per 5 mL; INJ: various
oxycodone	OxyContin	Opioid	Severe chronic pain	IR: Individualize dose q4–6 h ER: individualize dose q12 h	40 capsules (tablets) (10-day supply) 20 tablets (10-day supply)	CAP: 5 mg; TAB: 5 mg, 10 mg, 15 mg, 20 mg, 30 mg; ER TAB: 10 mg, 20 mg, 40 mg, 80 mg; SOL: 5 mg per 5 mL, 100 mg per 5 mL
warfarin	Jantoven	Anticoagulant	Deep vein thrombosis/pulmonary embolism	Dose dependent on INR reading	30 tablets	TAB: 1 mg, 2 mg, 2.5 mg, 3 mg, 4 mg, 5 mg, 6 mg, 7.5 mg, 10 mg

(Continued)

Generic name	Brand name	Drug classification	Indication(s)	Recommended daily dosage	Commonly dispensed quantities (community pharmacy-30-day supply)	Generic dosage forms and strengths
methylphenidate	Ritalin, Ritalin LA, Concerta	Norepinephrine-dopamine reuptake inhibitor	ADHD	IR: 5–15 mg PO bid to tid ER: 10–20 mg ER PO qd to bid	60–90 tablets 30–60 tablets (capsules)	ER CAP (qd, 50% IR/50% DR): 10 mg, 20 mg, 30 mg, 40 mg, 60 mg; ER CAP (qd, 30% IR/70% ER): 10 mg, 20 mg, 30 mg, 40 mg, 50 mg, 60 mg; TAB: 5 mg, 10 mg, 20 mg; ER TAB (qd-bid): 10 mg, 20 mg; ER TAB (qd): 18 mg, 27 mg, 36 mg, 54 mg, 72 mg; CHEWABLE: 2.5 mg, 5 mg, 15 mg; SOL: 5 mg per 5 mL, 10 mg per 5 mL
apixaban	Eliquis	Anticoagulant	Thromboembolism/stroke prophylaxis, deep vein thrombosis, and deep vein thrombosis/pulmonary embolism prophylaxis	5 mg PO bid	60 tablets	TAB: 2.5 mg, 5 mg
glipizide	Glucotrol and Glucotrol XL	Sulfonylureas	Diabetes mellitus type 2	2.5–20 mg PO qd to bid	30–60 tablets	TAB: 5 mg, 10 mg; ER TAB: 2.5 mg, 5 mg, 10 mg
ergocalciferol (vitamin D$_2$)	Drisdol	Vitamin	Hypoparathyroidism, vitamin D deficiency, osteomalacia, and dietary supplement	1500–2000 units PO qd	1 capsule	CAP: 50,000 units; TAB: 400 units, 2000 units; SOL: 8000 units per mL
quetiapine	Seroquel and Seroquel XR	Antipsychotic	Schizophrenia, bipolar disorder, major depressive disorder, and generalized anxiety disorder	IR: 150–750 mg/day PO divided bid to tid ER: 400–800 mg ER PO qpm	60–90 tablets 30 tablets	TAB: 25 mg, 50 mg, 100 mg, 200 mg, 300 mg, 400 mg; ER TAB: 50 mg, 150 mg, 200 mg, 300 mg, 400 mg
budesonide/formoterol	Symbicort	Long-acting beta-2 agonist/corticosteroid	Asthma and COPD	2 puffs (160 mcg/4.5 mcg per actuation) inhaled bid	1 inhaler	MDI: 80 mcg/4.5 mcg per actuation, 160 mcg/4.5 mcg per actuation
estradiol	Estrace	Estrogen	Moderate to severe menopausal vasomotor symptoms, menopausal vulvovaginal atrophy, osteoporosis, and hypoestrogenism	1–2 mg PO qd	30 tablets	TAB: 0.5 mg, 1 mg, 2 mg
oxycodone/acetaminophen	Percocet	Opioid	Moderate to moderate severe pain	IR: Individualize dose PO q4–6 h	40 tablets (10-day supply)	TAB: 2.5 mg/325 mg, 5 mg/325 mg, 7.5 mg/325 mg, 10 mg/325 mg; SOL: 5 mg/325 mg per 5 mL

(Continued)

Generic name	Brand name	Drug classification	Indication(s)	Recommended daily dosage	Commonly dispensed quantities (community pharmacy-30-day supply)	Generic dosage forms and strengths
ondansetron	Zofran	5-HT3 receptor antagonist	Nausea/vomiting prevention	8 mg PO/IV q8 h prn	21 tablets (1-week supply)	TAB: 4 mg, 8 mg, 16 mg, 24 mg; ODT: 4 mg, 8 mg; SOL: 4 mg per 5 mL; INJ (prefilled syringe): 4 mg per 2 mL; INJ (vial): 2 mg per mL
naproxen	Naprosyn	NSAID	Mild to moderate pain, osteoarthritis, rheumatoid arthritis, acute gout, and dysmenorrhea	250–500 mg PO q12 h	60 tablets	TAB: 250 mg, 375 mg, 500 mg; DR TAB: 375 mg, 500 mg; SUSP: 125 mg per 5 mL
glimepiride	Amaryl	Sulfonylurea	Diabetes mellitus type 2	1–4 mg PO qd	30 tablets	TAB: 1 mg, 2 mg, 4 mg
spironolactone	Aldactone	Potassium sparing diuretic	HTN, edema, heart failure, hyperaldosteronism, hypokalemia, and hirsutism	25–200 mg/day PO divided qd to bid	30 tablets	TAB: 25 mg, 50 mg, 100 mg
clonidine	a	Alpha agonists	HTN and Tourette syndrome	0.1–0.4 mg PO bid	60 tablets	TAB: 0.1 mg, 0.2 mg, 0.3 mg; INJ: various
insulin lispro	Humalog, Admelog, Lyumjev	Insulin	Diabetes mellitus	Individualize dose SC/IV bid to qid	Varies based on daily dose	INJ (KwikPen U-100 pen, Junior KwikPen U-100 pen): 100 units per mL; INJ (U-100 vial): 100 units per mL
loratadine	Claritin	Antihistamine	Allergic rhinitis, sneezing, itchy/watery eyes, and itchy nose/throat	10 mg PO qd prn	30 tablets	TAB: 10 mg; ODT: 10 mg; SOL: 1 mg per mL
cetirizine	Zyrtec Allergy	Antihistamine	Allergy symptoms and chronic idiopathic urticaria	5–10 mg PO qd prn	30 tablets	CAP: 10 mg; TAB: 5 mg, 10 mg; ODT: 10 mg; CHEWABLE: 5 mg, 10 mg; SOL: 1 mg per mL
topiramate	Topamax	Anticonvulsant	Seizures and migraine headache prophylaxis	IR: 200 mg PO bid ER: 200–400 mg ER PO qd;	60 capsules 30 capsules	ER CAP: 25 mg, 50 mg, 100 mg, 200 mg; ER SPRINKLE CAP: 25 mg, 50 mg, 100 mg, 150 mg, 200 mg; SPRINKLE CAP: 15 mg, 25 mg; TAB: 25 mg, 50 mg, 100 mg, 200 mg
lorazepam	Ativan	Benzodiazepine	Anxiety, insomnia, status epilepticus, and chemo-related nausea/vomiting	2–6 mg/day PO/IM/IV divided bid to tid	60–90 tablets	TAB: 0.5 mg, 1 mg, 2 mg; SOL: 2 mg per mL; INJ: 2 mg per mL, 4 mg per mL
norgestimate/ethinyl estradiol	Sprintec, Tri-Sprintec	Estrogen/progestin oral contraceptive	Contraception, dysmenorrhea and endometriosis	1 tab PO qd	1 packet	Monophasic pack; 25 mcg EE triphasic pack; 35 mcg EE triphasic pack

(Continued)

Generic name	Brand name	Drug classification	Indication(s)	Recommended daily dosage	Commonly dispensed quantities (community pharmacy-30-day supply)	Generic dosage forms and strengths
lamotrigine	Lamictal, Lamictal XR	Anticonvulsant	Bipolar disorder, partial seizures, primary generalized tonic-clonic seizures, neuropathic pain, and migraine prophylaxis	200 mg PO qd	30 tablets	TAB: 25 mg, 100 mg, 150 mg, 200 mg; ER TAB: 25 mg, 50 mg, 100 mg, 200 mg, 250 mg, 300 mg; ODT: 25 mg, 50 mg, 100 mg, 200 mg; CHEWABLE: 5 mg, 25 mg; blue convenience pack; green convenience pack; orange convenience pack
diltiazem	Cardizem, Cardizem CD, Cardizem LA	Calcium channel blocker	HTN and angina	IR: 180–360 mg/day PO divided q6–8 h 12-h ER: 120–180 mg ER PO bid 24-h ER: 180–360 mg/day PO divided q6–8 h	90–120 tablets 60 capsules 90–120 capsules	ER CAP (12 h): 60 mg, 90 mg, 120 mg; ER CAP (24 h): 120 mg, 180 mg, 240 mg, 300 mg, 360 mg, 420 mg; TAB: 30 mg, 60 mg, 90 mg, 120 mg; ER TAB (24 h): 180 mg, 240 mg, 300 mg, 360 mg, 420 mg; INJ: various
losartan/hydrochlorothiazide	Hyzaar	Angiotensin receptor blocker/thiazide diuretic	HTN and stroke prevention	1 tab PO qd	30 tablets	TAB: 50 mg/12.5 mg, 100 mg/12.5 mg, 100 mg/25 mg
hydroxyzine	Vistaril	Antihistamine	Anxiety, pruritis/urticaria, nausea/vomiting, and insomnia	50–100 mg PO q6 h prn	120 capsules	CAP: 25 mg, 50 mg, 100 mg; TAB: 10 mg, 25 mg, 50 mg; SOL: 10 mg per 5 mL; INJ: 25 mg per mL, 50 mg per m
buspirone	a	Nonbenzodiazepine anxiolytic	Anxiety and adjunct for depression	20–60 mg/day PO divided bid to tid	60–90 tablets	TAB: 5 mg, 7.5 mg, 10 mg, 15 mg, 30 mg
latanoprost	Xalatan	Prostaglandin analog	Intraocular pressure	1 gtt in eye(s) qpm	1 bottle	SOL: 0.005%
paroxetine	Paxil, Paxil CR	Selective serotonin reuptake inhibitor	Depressive disorder, panic disorder, and social anxiety disorder	20–50 mg PO qam ER: 25–62.5 mg PO qam	30 tablets 30 tablets	CAP: 7.5 mg; TAB: 10 mg, 20 mg, 30 mg, 40 mg; ER TAB: 12.5 mg, 25 mg, 37.5 mg; SUSP: 10 mg per 5 mL
lisdexamfetamine	Vyvanase	Norepinephrine-dopamine reuptake inhibitor	ADHD	30–70 mg PO qam	30 capsules	CAP: 10 mg, 20 mg, 30 mg, 40 mg, 50 mg, 60 mg, 70 mg; CHEWABLE: 10 mg, 20 mg, 30 mg, 40 mg, 50 mg, 60 mg

(Continued)

Generic name	Brand name	Drug classification	Indication(s)	Recommended daily dosage	Commonly dispensed quantities (community pharmacy-30-day supply)	Generic dosage forms and strengths
fluticasone/salmeterol	Advair HFA, Advair Diskus	Long-acting beta 2-agonists/corticosteroid	Asthma	Advair HFA: 2 puffs inhaled q12 hAdvair Diskus: 1 puff inhaled q12 h	I canister	Advair HFA: MDI: 45 mcg/21 mcg per actuation, 115 mcg/21 mcg per actuation, 230 mcg/21 mcg per actuation Advair Diskus: DPI: 100 mcg/50 mcg per blister, 250 mcg/50 mcg per blister, 500 mcg/50 mcg per blister
pregabalin	Lyrica and Lyrica CR	Anticonvulsant	Diabetic neuropathic pain, neuralgia, partial seizures, and fibromyalgia	Lyrica: 50–100 mg PO tid Lyrica CR: 165–330 mg PO qd	90 capsules 30 capsules	Lyrica: CAP: 25 mg, 50 mg, 75 mg, 100 mg, 150 mg, 200 mg, 225 mg, 300 mg; SOL: 20 mg per mL Lyrica CR: ER TAB: 82.5 mg, 165 mg, 330 mg
propranolol	[a]	Beta blocker	HTN, angina, post-myocardial infarction cardiovascular prevention, atrial flutter/fibrillation, supraventricular arrhythmias, and migraine headache prophylaxis	80–240 mg/day PO divided bid to tid	60–90 tablets (capsules)	ER CAP: 60 mg, 80 mg, 120 mg, 160 mg; TAB: 10 mg, 20 mg, 40 mg, 60 mg, 80 mg; SOL: 20 mg per 5 mL, 40 mg per 5 mL; INJ: various
cephalexin	Keflex	Cephalosporin	Bacterial infection, streptococcal pharyngitis, urinary tract infection, bacterial skin infection, and endocarditis[a]	1000–4000 mg/day PO divided q6–12 h	20–40 capsules (10-day supply)	CAP: 250 mg, 500 mg, 750 mg; TAB: 250 mg, 500 mg; SUSP: 125 mg per 5 mL, 250 mg per 5 mL
cholecalciferol (vitamin D$_3$)	[a]	Vitamin	Vitamin D deficiency and osteoporosis	800–2000 units PO qd	30 capsules	CAP: 400 units, 1000 units, 2000 units, 5000 units, 10,000 units, 50,000 units; TAB: 400 units, 1000 units, 2000 units, 3000 units, 5000 units, ODT: 1000 units; CHEWABLE: 400 units, 1000 units; SOL: 400 units per mL, 5000 units per mL, 2000 units per 0.16 mL; SPRAY: 1000 units per actuation

(Continued)

Generic name	Brand name	Drug classification	Indication(s)	Recommended daily dosage	Commonly dispensed quantities (community pharmacy- 30-day supply)	Generic dosage forms and strengths
insulin aspart	NovoLog, Fiasp	Insulin	Diabetes mellitus	Individualize dose SC/IV bid-qi	Varies based on daily dose	NJ (PenFill U-100 cartridge): 100 units per mL; INJ (FlexPen U-100 pen, FlexPen ReliOn U-100 pen): 100 units per mL; INJ (U-100 vial, ReliOn U-100 vial): 100 units per mL
finasteride	Proscar, Propecia	5-alpha reductase inhibitors	Proscar: benign prostatic hypertrophy Propecia: male pattern baldness	Proscar: 5 mg Propecia: 1 mg	30 tablets 30 tablets	TAB: 1 mg, 5 mg
fenofibrate	Tricor	Fibrate	Dyslipidemia, hypertriglyceridemia, and hypercholesterolemia	40–160 mg PO qd	30 tablets	CAP: 50 mg, 150 mg; TAB: 40 mg, 48 mg, 54 mg, 120 mg, 145 mg, 160 mg
sitagliptin	Januvia	DPP-4- inhibitor	Diabetes mellitus type 2	100 mg PO qd	30 tablets	TAB: 25 mg, 50 mg, 100 mg
folic acid (vitamin B$_9$)	[a]	Vitamin	Dietary supplement and megaloblastic anemia	0.4 mg PO qd	30 tablets	TAB: 0.4 mg, 0.8 mg, 1 mg; INJ: various
doxycycline	Vibramycin	Tetracycline	Mild to moderate to severe bacterial infections, acne, pneumonia, and sinusitis	100 mg PO/IV qd	10 capsules	CAP: 50 mg, 75 mg, 100 mg, 150 mg; DR CAP (75% IR/ 25% DR): 40 mg; TAB: 20 mg, 50 mg, 75 mg, 100 mg, 150 mg; DR TAB: 50 mg, 75 mg, 100 mg, 150 mg, 200 mg; SUSP: 25 mg per 5 mL; INJ: various
rivaroxaban	Xarelto	Anticoagulant	Thromboembolism/ stroke prophylaxis and deep vein thrombosis/pulmonary embolism	20 mg PO qd	30 tablets	TAB: 2.5 mg, 10 mg, 15 mg, 20 mg; SUSP: 1 mg per mL
tizanidine	Zanaflex	Muscle relaxant	Spasticity	Individualize dose PO q6–8 h prn	30 tablets (10-day supply)	CAP: 2 mg, 4 mg, 6 mg; TAB: 2 mg, 4 mg
amoxicillin/clavulanate	Augmentin, Augmentin XR	Penicillin	Bacterial infections, sinusitis, urinary tract infection, pneumonia, and diverticulitis	500 mg/125 mg– 875 mg/125 mg PO q12 h ER: 2000 mg PO q12h × 7–10 days	20 tablets (10-day supply) 20 tablets (10-day supply)	TAB: 250 mg/ 125 mg, 500 mg/ 125 mg, 875 mg/ 125 mg; ER TAB: 1000 mg/62.5 mg; SUSP: 125 mg/ 31.25 mg per 5 mL, 200 mg/28.5 mg per 5 mL, 250 mg/62.5 mg per 5 mL, 400 mg/57 mg per 5 mL

(Continued)

Generic name	Brand name	Drug classification	Indication(s)	Recommended daily dosage	Commonly dispensed quantities (community pharmacy-30-day supply)	Generic dosage forms and strengths
amitriptyline	a	Tricyclic antidepressant	Depression, neuropathic pain, fibromyalgia and migraine prophylaxis	25–150 mg PO qhs	30 tablets	TAB: 10 mg, 25 mg, 50 mg, 75 mg, 100 mg, 150 mg
lovastatin	a	HMG CoA reductase inhibitor	Hypercholesterolemia, dyslipidemia, atherosclerotic cardiovascular dizziness, and cardiovascular event prevention	10–80 mg PO qpm	30 tablets	TAB: 10 mg, 20 mg, 40 mg
alendronate	Fosamax	Bisphosphonates	Osteoporosis	70 mg PO qwk	4 tablets	TAB: 5 mg, 10 mg, 35 mg, 40 mg, 70 mg; SOL: 70 mg per 75 mL
levetiracetam	Keppra, Keppra XR	Anticonvulsant	Seizures	500–1500 mg PO/ IV q12 h ER: 1000–3000 mg PO qd	60 tablets 30 tablets	TAB: 250 mg, 500 mg, 750 mg, 1000 mg; ER TAB: 500 mg, 750 mg; DISPERSE TAB: 250 mg, 500 mg, 750 mg, 1000 mg; SOL: 100 mg per mL; INJ: various
sumatriptan	Imitrex	Selective serotonin receptor agonists	Migraine and cluster headache	25–100 mg PO ×1; max 200 mg/24 h; may repeat dose once after 2 h	12 tablets	TAB: 25 mg, 50 mg, 100 mg; INJ (autoinjector): 6 mg; INJ (vial): 6 mg per 0.5 mL
hydralazine	a	Vasodilator	HTN and congestive heart failure	10–50 mg PO qid	120 tablets	TAB: 10 mg, 25 mg, 50 mg, 100 mg; INJ: 20 mg per mL
sulfamethoxazole/ trimethoprim	Bactrim, Bactrim DS	Sulfonamide	Bacterial infection, urinary tract infection, and bacterial meningitis	160 mg TMP PO bid	20 tablets (10-day supply)	TAB: 400 mg/80 mg, 800 mg/160 mg; SUSP: 200 mg/ 40 mg per 5 mL; INJ: various
aripiprazole	Abilify	Antipsychotic	Schizophrenia, bipolar disorder, and major depressive disorder	10–15 mg PO qd	30 tablets	TAB: 2 mg, 5 mg, 10 mg, 15 mg, 20 mg, 30 mg; ODT: 10 mg, 15 mg, 20 mg, 30 mg; SOL: 1 mg per mL
celecoxib	Celebrex	NSAID	Osteoarthritis, rheumatoid arthritis, dysmenorrhea and acute pain	200 mg PO qd	30 capsules	CAP: 50 mg, 100 mg, 200 mg, 400 mg

aBrand name discontinued in United States according to Epocrates.

A complete listing of the Top 300 medications prescribed based upon prescriptions filled can be accessed at https://clincalc.com/DrugStats/Top300Drugs.aspx. 5-HT3, 5-hydroxytryptamine; ACE, angiotensin converting enzyme; ADHD, attention deficit hyperactivity disorder; ALT, alternate; bid, twice a day; CAP, capsule; COPD, chronic obstructive pulmonary disease; CR, controlled release; DPP-4, dipeptidyl-peptidase 4; DR, delayed release; EE, ethinyl estradiol; ER, extended release; GERD, gastroesophageal reflux disease; gtt, drops; HFA, hydrofluoroalkane; HMG-CoA; HTN, hypertension; IB, ibuprofen; INJ, injection; INR, international normalized ratio; IR, immediate release; IV, intravenous; max, maximum; MDI, metered dose inhaler; NEB, nebulizer; NSAID, nonsteroidal antiinflmammatory drug; ODT, oral disintegrating tablet; pkt, packet; PO, by mouth; prn, as needed; PWDR, powder; q, every; qam, every morning; qd, every day; qhs, at bedtime; qi, qid; qid, four times a day; qpm, every evening; qwk, every week; SC, subcutaneous; SL, sublingual; SOL, solution; SUSP, suspension; TAB, tablet; tid, three times a day; TMP, trimethoprim; XR, extended release.

Common dosage forms

Enteral dosage forms

- Tablet: A hard formulation in which the drugs and other ingredients are machine compressed into a shape. They vary in size, weight, hardness, thickness, and disintegration and dissolution rates. Tablets may be film coated, sugar coated, compressed, and effervescent. Other forms of tablets include:
  - Chewable tablet: An oral dosage form intended to be chewed and then swallowed by the patient rather than swallowed whole (e.g., carbamazepine).

- Delayed-release tablet: The dosage form is formulated so that the drug is released slowly over time; (e.g., pantoprazole).
- Enteric-coated tablets: A tablet coated with a material that permits transit through the stomach to the small intestine before the medication is released.
- Sublingual tablet: A tablet that dissolves when placed beneath the tongue and absorbs into the blood through tissue there. Sublingual dosage form are used when results must occur quickly (e.g., nitroglycerin).
- Troche: A tablet is administered buccally between the gums and the inner lining of the mouth cheek (e.g., clotrimazole oropharyngeal).
- Capsule: A solid dosage form in which the drug is enclosed in a hard or soft soluble container, usually of a form of gelatin. They range in sizes from a 000 (largest) to 5 (smallest). The gelatin shell dissolves in the stomach and releases the medication from the capsule. Many capsules are intended to be swallowed; however, sprinkles are capsules where the contents are sprinkled over food. Fluoxetine is an example of a capsule and Depakote is available as a sprinkle dosage form.
- Caplet: A smooth, coated, oval-shaped medicinal tablet in the general shape of a capsule (e.g., acetaminophen)
- Lozenge: Various-shaped solid dosage forms, usually containing a medicinal agent and a flavoring substance, that are intended to be dissolved slowly in the oral cavity for localized or systemic effects.
- Bulk powders: Contain the active ingredient in a small powder paper or foil envelope. The patient empties the envelope into a glass of water or juice and drinks it. Examples include cholestyramine and psyllium.
- Solution: A clear liquid made up of one or more ingredients dissolved in a solvent.
  - Aqueous solution: Water is used as the solvent.
  - Nonaqueous solution: A solution that predominantly contain solvents other water.
- Syrup: A concentrated solution of sugar in water or other aqueous liquid. They are more viscous than water and contain less than 10% alcohol.
- Elixir: A sweetened hydroalcoholic (water and alcohol) liquids for oral use. They are less viscous than a syrup and an alcohol content of 5% to 40%.
- Emulsion: An emulsion is a two-phase system in which one liquid is dispersed in the form of small globules throughout another liquid. The dispersed liquid is known as the internal phase, whereas the dispersion medium as the external or continuous phase. Emulsions contain a stabilizing agent known as an emulsifier.
  - Oil-in-water: Oil is the dispersed phase, and an aqueous solution is the continuous phase.
  - Water-in-oil: Water is the dispersed phase, and oil is the continuous phase.
- Suspension: A coarse dispersion containing finely divided insoluble material suspended in a liquid medium. Oral suspensions are flavored and sweetened. Some oral suspensions are packaged as a lyophilized powder and are reconstituted with water.

Parenteral dosage forms

- Sprays: A collection of drops dispersed in a gas.

- Inhalant solution: A solution of a drug or combination of drugs for administration as a nebulized mist intended to reach the respiratory tree.
- Enemas: A liquid injected into the rectum for therapeutic or diagnostic purposes.
- Aerosol: Suspension of tiny particles or droplets in the air, such as dusts, mists, or fumes, which may be inhaled or absorbed by the skin.
- Spray: A jet of liquid in fine drops, coarser than a vapor; it is produced by forcing the liquid from the minute opening of an atomizer, mixing it with air.
- Creams: An emulsion of oil and water in approximately equal proportions.
- Lotions: A liquid for topical application that contains insoluble solids or liquids.
- Ointments: A homogenous, viscous, semisolid preparation that is most commonly a greasy, thick oil (oil 80% and water 20%) with a high viscosity that is intended for external application to the skin or mucus membranes.
- Gel: A two-phase system containing an extremely fine solid particle that, when mixed, is difficult to distinguish between the two phases and is considered a semisolid form. Gels contain a gelling agent to increase the viscosity of the compound.
- Pastes: A semisolid dosage forms that contain a large proportion of solid component. They differ from ointments in their consistency, as they contain larger amounts of solids and consequently are thicker and stiffer.
- Transdermal patch: A medicated patch applied to the skin.
- Lotion: A low- to medium-viscosity medicated or non-medicated topical preparation, intended for application to unbroken skin.
- Tincture: A dilute solution consisting of a medicinal substance in alcohol or in alcohol and water, usually 10% to 20% by volume.
- Liniment: A solutions or mixture of various substances in oil, alcoholic solution of soap, or emulsions, intended for external application.
- Implant: A drug delivery system that provides controlled delivery of a drug over a period of time at the site of implantation.
- Suppository: A form of medicine contained in a small piece of solid material, such as cocoa butter or glycerin, that melts at body temperature. A suppository is inserted into the rectum, vagina, or urethra, and the medicine is absorbed into the bloodstream.
- Solutions, suspensions, emulsions are available as parenteral dosage forms but have been specifically formulated based upon their route of administration.

Look-a-like medications

FDA-approved list of generic drug names with tall man letters

The FDA issued a list of approved generic drug names using tall man lettering (TML). TML is a method that utilizes lettering to distinguish look-alike drug names. Beginning on the left side of the drug name, TML emphasizes the differences between similar drug names by capitalizing unlike letters. In addition TML can be utilized with color or boldfacing to draw awareness to the similarities between look-alike drug names.

FDA-approved list of generic drug names with tall man letters[ii]	
Drug Name With Tall Man Letters	**Confused With**
acetaZOLAMIDE	acetoHEXAMIDE
acetoHEXAMIDE	acetaZOLAMIDE
buPROPion	busPIRone
busPIRone	buPROPion
chlorproMAZINE	chlorproPAMIDE
chlorproPAMIDE	chlorproMAZINE
clomiPHENE	clomiPRAMINE
clomiPRAMINE	clomiPHENE
cycloSERINE	cycloSPORINE
cycloSPORINE	cycloSERINE
DAUNOrubicin	DOXOrubicin
dimenhyDRINATE	diphenhydrAMINE
diphenhydrAMINE	dimenhyDRINATE
DOBUTamine	DOPamine
DOPamine	DOBUTamine
DOXOrubicin	DAUNOrubicin
glipiZIDE	glyBURIDE
glyBURIDE	glipiZIDE
hydrALAZINE	hydrOXYzine—HYDROmorphone
HYDROmorphone	hydrOXYzine—hydrALAZINE
hydrOXYzine	hydrALAZINE—HYDROmorphone
medroxyPROGESTERone	methylPREDNISolone—methylTESTOSTERone
methylPREDNISolone	medroxyPROGESTERone—methylTESTOSTERone
methylTESTOSTERone	medroxyPROGESTERone—methylPREDNISolone
mitoXANTRONE	Not specified
niCARdipine	NIFEdipine
NIFEdipine	niCARdipine
prednisoLONE	predniSONE
predniSONE	prednisoLONE
risperiDONE	rOPINIRole
rOPINIRole	risperiDONE
sulfADIAZINE	sulfiSOXAZOLE
sulfiSOXAZOLE	sulfADIAZINE
TOLAZamide	TOLBUTamide
TOLBUTamide	TOLAZamide
vinBLAStine	vinCRIStine
vinCRIStine	vinBLAStine

[ii]US Food and Drug Administration (FDA) and Institute for Safe Medication Practices (ISMP). FDA and ISMP lists of look-alike drug names with recommended tall man letters. ISMP. Published 2016. Accessed July 28, 2022. https://www.ismp.org/recommendations/tall-man-letters-list.

From FDA Name Differential Project: FDA list of established drug names recommended to use tall man lettering (TML). US Food and Drug Administration.

Institute for Safe Medication Practices list of additional drug names with tall man letters

The Institute for Safe Medication Practices (ISMP) provides a list of additional drug names with recommendations of the placement of tall man letters. The ISMP follows the CD3 rule. The methodology recommends working from the left of the drug name first by capitalizing all the characters to the right once two or more different letters are observed, and then, working from the right, returning two or more letters common to both words to lowercase letters. When the rule cannot be used because there are no common letters on the right side of the name, the procedure proposes capitalizing the central part of the word only. When use of this rule fails to lead to the best tall man lettering option (e.g., makes names appear too similar, makes names hard to read based on pronunciation), an alternative option is considered. It should be noted that this list is not approved by the FDA.

Drug name	Confused drug name[iii]
Aciphex	Accupril, Aricept
Actos	Actonel
Adderall	Adderall XR, Inderal
ALPRAZolam	clonazePAM, LORazepam
amiodarone	amantadine
amLODIPine	aMILopride
ARIPiprazole	proton pump inhibitors, RABEprazole
atorvastatin	atomoxetine
buPROPion	busPIRone
Cardizem	Cardene
CeleBREX	CeleXA, Cerebyx
cetirizine	sertraline, stavudine
clonazePAM	ALPRAZolam, clobazam, clonidine, clozapine, LORazepam
Cozaar	Colace, Zocor
Depakote	Depakote ER
DULoxetine	Dexilant, FLUoxetine, Paroxetine
gabapentin	gemfibrozil
glipiZIDE	glyBURIDE
HumaLOG	HumuLIN, NovoLOG
hydroCHLOROthiazide	hydrALAZINE, hydrOXYzine
HYDROcodone	oxyCODONE
Jantoven	Janumet, Januvia
Lantus	Latuda, Lente
Levothyroxine	lamotrigine, Lanoxin, liothyronine
Lotronex	Protonix
medroxyPROGESTERone	HYDROXYprogesterone, methylPREDNISolone, methylTESTOSTERone
metFORMIN	metroNIDAZOLE
metoprolol succinate	metoprolol tartrate

(Continued)

Drug name	Confused drug name[iii]
NIFEdipine	niCARdipine, niMODipine
oxyCODONE	HYDROcodone, oxybutynin, OxyCONTIN, oxyMORphone
Paxil	Doxil, Plavix, Taxol
Plavix	Paxil, Pradaxa
Prandin	Avandia
prednisoLONE	predniSONE
propylthiouracil	Purinethol
PROzac	Prograf, PriLOSEC, Provera
SandIMMUNE	SandoSTATIN
SEROquel	Desyrel, SEROquel XR, Serzone, SINEquan
SINEquan	saquinavir, SEROquel, Singulair, Zonegran
SITagliptin	sAXagliptin, SUMAtriptan
SOLU-Medrol	DEPO-Medrol, Solu-CORTEF
Spiriva	Apidra, Inspra
sulfADIAZINE	sulfasalazine, sulfiSOXAZOLE
tacrolimus	tamsulosin
TEGretol	TEGretol XR, Tequin, TRENtal
Toujeo	Tradjenta, Tresiba, Trulicity
Tresiba	Tanzeum, Tarceva, Toujeo, Tradjenta
Trulicity	Tanzeum, Toujeo, Tradjenta, Tresiba
Zebeta	Diabeta, Zetia
Zestril	Zegerid, Zetia, ZyPREXA
Zetia	Bextra, Zebeta, Zestril
Zocor	Cozaar, ZyrTEC
Zyloprim	zolpidem
ZyPREXA	CeleXA, Reprexain, Zestril, ZyrTEC
ZyrTEC	Lipitor, Zerit, Zocor, ZyPREXA, ZyrTEC-D

A complete listing of the ISMP List of Look-Alike Drug Names with Recommended Tall Man Letters can be found in Appendix A or be accessed at https://www.ismp.org/sites/default/files/attachments/2017-11/tallmanletters.pdf.

A health care organization should implement processes to reduce the risk of potential errors involving look-alike and sound-alike medications. Examples of strategies used include using both the brand and generic names on prescriptions and labels; including the purpose of the medication on prescriptions; configuring computer selection screens to prevent look-alike names from appearing consecutively; and changing the appearance of look-alike product names to draw attention to their dissimilarities.

Medication guides

Medication guides are paper handouts that come with many prescription medicines. The guides address issues that are specific to particular drugs and drug classes, and they contain FDA-approved information that can help patients avoid serious adverse events. The FDA requires that medication guides be issued with certain prescribed drugs and biological products when the agency determines that:

- Certain information is necessary to prevent serious adverse effects,
- Patient decision making should be informed by information about a known serious side effect with a product, or
- Patient adherence to directions for the use of a product are essential to its effectiveness.

A medication guide must be provided to the patient or the patient's agent:

- When the patient or the patient's agent requests a medication guide
- When a drug is dispensed in an outpatient setting (e.g., retail pharmacy, hospital ambulatory care pharmacy), and the product will then be used by the patient without direct supervision by a health care professional
- The first time a drug is dispensed to a health care professional for administration to a patient in an outpatient setting, such as in a clinic or dialysis or infusion center
- The first time a drug is dispensed in an outpatient setting of any kind, after a medication guide is materially changed (e.g., after addition of a new indication, new safety information)
- When a drug is subject to a risk evaluation and mitigation strategy (REMS) that includes specific requirements for reviewing or providing a medication guide as part of an element to assure safe use (possibly in conjunction with distribution), the medication guide must be provided in accordance with the terms of the REMS

Examples of medications requiring a medication guide be provided			
Abilify (aripiprazole)	Humira (adalimumab)	Plavix (clopidogrel)	Victoza (liraglutide)
Aciphex (rabeprazole)	Invokana (canagliflozin)	Prevacid (lansoprazole)	Viibryd (Vilazodone)
Advair HFA or Diskus (fluticasone/ salmeterol)	Jantoven (warfarin)	Prilosec (omeprazole)	Viramune (nevirapine)
Ambien (zolpidem)	Janumet (metformin)	Protonix (pantoprazole)	Vraylar (cariprazine)
Celebrex (celecoxib)	Januvia (sitagliptin)	Prozac (fluoxetine)	Vyvanase (lisdexam-fetamine

(Continued)

Examples of medications requiring a medication guide be provided —cont'd			
Cipro (ciprofloxacin)	Jardiance (empagliflozin)	Serevent (salmeterol)	Wellbutrin (bupropion)
Cymbalta (duloxetine hydrochloride)	Keppra (levetiracetam)	Seroquel (quetiapine)	Xanax (alprazolam)
Depakote (divalproex sodium)	Mobic (meloxicam)	Singulair (montelukast)	Xarelto (Rivaroxaban)
Desyrel (trazodone)	Motrin (ibuprofen)	Suboxone (buprenor-phine)	Zoloft (sertraline)
Dilantin (phenytoin)	Neurontin (gabapentin)	Tegretol (car-bamazepine)	Zyprexa (olanzapine)
Eliquis (Apixaban)	Nexium (esomepra-zole)	Topamax (topiramate)	
Enbrel (etanercept)	Pacerone (amiodarone)	Tradjenta (linagliptin)	
Fosamax (alendronate)	Paxil (paroxetine)	Trulicity (dulaglutide)	
From US Food and Drug Medication Guides https://www.accessdata.fda.gov/scripts/cder/daf/index.cfm?event=medguide.page			

A complete listing of medications requiring a Medication Guide can be accessed at https://www.accessdata.fda.gov/scripts/cder/daf/index.cfm?event=medguide.page

Calculating the amount of product to dispense based on prescribed dosage and frequency

Commonly used abbreviations				
	Abbreviation	**Meaning**	**Abbreviation**	**Meaning**
Route of administration				
	BUC, buc	Buccally (in the cheek)	PO, po	By mouth
	IA	Intraarterial	PR, pr	By rectum
	ID	Intradermal	PV, pv	By vagina
	IM	Intra-muscularly	SL	Sublingual (under tongue)
	IT	Intrathecally	TOP, top	Topical (on the skin)
	IV	Intravenously	Vag	Vaginal
Dosage form	**Abbreviation**	**Meaning**	**Abbreviation**	**Meaning**
	amp	Ampule	MDI	Metered dose inhaler
	cap	Capsule	oint	Ointment

Commonly used abbreviations —cont'd				
Dosage form	**Abbreviation**	**Meaning**	**Abbreviation**	**Meaning**
	DPI	Dry powder inhaler	sol	Solution
	ECT	Enteric-coated tablet	supp	Suppository
	elix	Elixir	susp	Suspension
	inj	Injection	syr	Syrup
	IV	Intravenous	tab	Tablet
	IVP	Intravenous push	TDS	Transdermal delivery system
	IVPB	Intravenous piggyback	TPN	Total parenteral nutrition
	ODT	Oral disinte-grating tablet	ung	ointment
Types of solutions	**Abbreviation**	**Meaning**	**Abbreviation**	**Meaning**
	D5LR	5% dextrose in lactated Ringer's Solution	NS	Normal saline solution (0.9%)
	D5NS	5% dextrose in normal saline solution	½ NS	½ Normal saline solution (0.45%)
	D5W	5% dextrose in water	RL or R/L	Ringer's lactate solution
	D10W	10% dextrose in water	SWFI	Sterile water for injection
	D20W	20% dextrose in water		
	DW	Distilled water		
Time of administration	**Abbreviation**	**Meaning**	**Abbreviation**	**Meaning**
	AC, ac	Before meals	q	Each, every
	AM, am	Morning	Q4h	Every 4 h
	ATC	Around the clock	Q6h	Every 6 h
	BID, bid	Twice a day	Q8h	Every 8 h
	h, hr	Hour	Qh	Every hour
	hs	At bedtime	QID, qid	Four times a day
	PC, pc	After meals	Stat, stat	Immediately
	PM, pm	Afternoon	TID	Three times a day
	PRN, prn	As needed	Wk	Week

(Continued)

Commonly used abbreviations —cont'd				
Time of adminis- tration	**Abbre- viation**	**Meaning**	**Abbre- viation**	**Meaning**
Measure- ments	**Abbre- viation**	**Meaning**	**Abbre- viation**	**Meaning**
	cc	Cubic centimeter	mg/kg	Milligram/ kilogram
	g	Gram	mL	Milliliter
	gal	Gallon	mOsm	Milliosmole
	gr	Grain	#	Number or pound
	gtt(s)	Drop(s)	pt	Pint or patient
	kg	Kilogram	qt	Quart
	L	Liter	s̄s̄	One half
	lb	Pound	TBSP, tbsp	Tablespoon
	mcg	Microgram	TSP, tsp	Teaspoon
	mg	Milligram		
Miscella- neous pharmacy abbre- viations	**Abbre- viation**	**Meaning**	**Abbre- viation**	**Meaning**
	aa	Of each		
	aaa	Apply to affected area	non rep	Do not repeat
	ad	Up to, so as to make	NR	No refill
	c̄	with	RX	Take this drug
	DAW	Dispense as Written	s̄	Without
	dtd	Give of such doses	Sig, Signa	Write on label
	Disp	Dispense	Ut dict or ud	As directed
	IPA	Isopropyl alcohol	w	With
	m ft	Mix and make	w/o	Without
	non rep	Do not repeat	VO	Verbal order
	NKA	No known allergies		
	NKDA	No known drug allergies		

Do not use	**Potential problem**	**Use instead**
U, u (unit)	Mistaken for "0" (zero), the number "4" (four) or "cc"	Write "unit"
IU (International Unit)	Mistaken for IV (intravenous) or the number "10" (ten)	Write "International Unit"
Q.D., QD, q.d., qd (daily) Q.O.D., QOD, q.o.d., qod (every other day)	Mistaken for each other Period after the "Q" mistaken for "I" and the "O" mistaken for "I"	Write "daily" Write "every other day"
Trailing zero (X.0 mg)[b] Lack of leading zero (.X mg)	Decimal point is missed	Write X mg Write 0.X mg
MS MSO$_4$ and MgSO$_4$	Can mean morphine sulfate or magnesium sulfate Confused for one another	Write "morphine sulfate" Write "magnesium sulfate"

[a]Applies to all orders and all medication-related documentation that are hand-written (including free-text computer entry) or on preprinted forms.

[b]Exception: A "trailing zero" may be used only where required to demonstrate the level of precision of the value being reported, such as for laboratory results, imaging studies that report size of lesions, or catheter/tube sizes. It may not be used in medication orders or other medication-related documentation.

(From: The Joint Commission. Do not use list fact sheet. All Rights Reserved. https://www.jointcommission.org/resources/news-and-multimedia/fact-sheets/facts-about-do-not-use-list.)

Institute of Safe Medication Practices list of error-prone abbreviations

Many pharmacy abbreviations have been misinterpreted and involved in medication errors that have resulted in harmful and sometimes deadly results to patients. These errors have been reported to the Institute of Safe Medication Practices (ISMP) through the ISMP National Medication Errors Reporting Program. The ISMP has compiled a list of abbreviations and has organized it into the following categories:

- Abbreviations for doses/measurement units
- Abbreviations for route of administration
- Abbreviations for frequency/instructions for use
- Miscellaneous abbreviations associated with medication use
- Drug name abbreviations
- Stemmed/coined drug names
- Dose designations and other information
- Symbols
- Apothecary or household abbreviations

The ISMP strongly advocates that these abbreviations, symbols, and dose designations should **never** be used in communicating medical information that includes telephone or verbal prescription, computer-generated labels, labels for drug storage bins, medication administration records, or pharmacy and prescriber computer order entry screens.

Joint Commission "Do Not Use" list

Joint Commission "Do Not Use" list

Any health care institution accredited by The Joint Commission (TJC) must include the TJC's "Do Not Use" list in their formulary and adhere to the list to reduce medication errors.

Institute of Safe Medication Practices' list of error-prone abbreviations			
Abbreviations for doses/measurement units[iv]			
Error-prone abbreviation, symbols, and dose designations	**Intended meaning**	**Misinterpretation**	**Best practice**
cc	Cubic centimeters	Mistaken as u (units)	Use mL
IU	International unit(s)	Mistaken as IV (intravenous) or the number 10	Use unit(s) (international units can be expressed as units alone)
l	Liter	Lowercase letter l mistaken as the number 1	Use L (UPPERCASE) for liter
mL	Milliliter	Lowercase letter l mistaken as the number 1	Use mL (lowercase m, UPPERCASE L) for milliliter
MM or M	Million	Mistaken as thousand M has been used to abbreviate both million and thousand (M is the Roman numeral for thousand)	Use million
M or K	Thousand	Mistaken as million M has been used to abbreviate both million and thousand (M is the Roman numeral for thousand)	Use thousand
Ng or ng	Nanogram	Mistaken as mg Mistaken as nasogastric	Use nanogram or nanog
U or u	Units	Mistaken as zero or the number 4, causing a 10-fold overdose or greater (e.g., 4U seen as 40 or 4u seen as 44) Mistaken as cc, leading to administering volume instead of units (e.g., 4u seen as 4cc)	Use unit(s)
μg	Microgram	Mistaken as mg	Use mcg
Abbreviations for route of administration			
Error-prone abbreviations, symbols, and dose designations	**Intended meaning**	**Misinterpretation**	**Best practice**
AD, AS, AU	Right ear, left ear, each ear	Mistaken as OD, OS, OU (right eye, left eye, each eye)	Use right ear, left ear, or each ear
IN	Intranasal	Mistaken as IM or IV	Use NAS (all UPPERCASE letters) or intranasal
IT	Intrathecal	Mistaken as intratracheal, intratumor, intratympanic, or inhalation therapy	Use intrathecal
OD, OS, OU	Right eye, left eye, each eye	Mistaken as AD, AS, AU (right ear, left ear, each ear)	Use right eye, left eye, or each eye
Per os	By mouth, orally	The os was mistaken as left eye (OS, oculus sinister)	Use PO, by mouth, or orally
SC, SQ, sq, or sub q	Subcutaneous(ly)	SC and sc mistaken as SL or sl (sublingual) SQ mistaken as "5 every" The q in sub q has been mistaken as "every"	Use SUBQ (all UPPERCASE letters, without spaces or periods between letters) or subcutaneous(ly)

Prescription requirements (Figure 10.1)

- Prescriber information:
  - Name of physician or prescriber
  - Address of physician (prescriber), including the street number, street name (office or suite number if applicable), city, state, and zip code
- Drug Enforcement Administration (DEA) number for controlled substances
- National Provider Identifier number (depending on state regulations)
- Medicare/Medicaid number (depending on state regulations)
- State license (depending on state regulations)

```
┌─────────────────────────────────────────────────────────────────────┐
│                                                                       │
│  Dr. Tracy Crum                              11287 E Villanova Drive  │
│  DEA#AC1243170                               Aurora, CO 30358         │
│  LIC#44550                                   Phone: 303-555-1212      │
│                                                                       │
│                                                                       │
│  Date: 12/12/18                                                       │
│                                                                       │
│                                                                       │
│  Patient's name:  Billie Jones          Age: 83 yrs                   │
│  Address: 125 Grand Canyon Drive, Tucson, Arizona  85707             │
│                                                                       │
│                                                                       │
│  Rx:                                                                   │
│                        KCl 10 mEq tab                                 │
│                        1 daily     #30                                │
│                                                                       │
│                                                                       │
│                                                                       │
│                                                                       │
│  Substitution permitted Ⓨ N                                          │
│  Refills 1 2 3 4 5 ⑥ 7 8 9          Signature____Tracy L Crum, MD    │
│                                                                       │
└─────────────────────────────────────────────────────────────────────┘
```

Fig. 10.1. Sample of the information required on a physician's prescription order. (From Davis K, Guerra A: *Mosby's pharmacy technician: principles and practice*, 5th ed. Elsevier; 2019.)

- Date the prescription was written
- Patient information:
  - Patient's name
  - Patient's home address, including the number, street, city, state, and zip code
- Inscription:
  - Name of medication (may be either brand or generic)
  - Strength of medication (if applicable)
  - Dosage form
  - Quantity of medication to be dispensed
- Subscription: Instructions to the pharmacist
- Signa: Directions to the patient
- Refill information
- Physician's signature: must be in ink (handwritten prescriptions); stamped signatures are illegal

Drug Enforcement Administration numbers

A DEA number is required for all controlled substance prescriptions and can be validated manually by remembering the following:

- New DEA registration numbers issued before 1985 to physicians, dentists, veterinarians, and other health care prescribers began with the letter A.
- New DEA registration numbers issued after 1985 began with either the letter B or F.

- A DEA number beginning with the letter M indicates the practitioner is a midlevel practitioner (physician assistant or nurse practitioner).
- Prescribers employed by a Drug Addiction Treatment facility will have the letter X as the first letter of their DEA number.
- The letter G is assigned to prescribers under the Department of Defense.
- The second letter of the DEA registration number begins with the first letter of practitioner's last name.
- The first two letters are followed by a sequence of seven numbers. To determine if the DEA number is valid:
  - Add the first, third, and fifth numbers together.
  - Next add the second, fourth, and sixth numbers together. Multiply this sum by two.
  - Add the first and second sets of numbers together. The number farthest from the left (one's column) should be same as seventh number in the DEA number.
    - Example: What should the seventh number in Dr. Andrew Shed's DEA number if his DEA number begins with BS452589?
    Add 4 +2 + 8, which totals 14.
    Add 5 +5 + 9, which totals 19; multiply 19 by 2 and the product is 38.
    Add 14 + 38, which totals 52. The last number should be a 2.
    A valid DEA number for Dr. Andrew Shed would be BS4525892.

Medication order requirements

- Prescriber's information, including the physician's name, DEA number (controlled substances only), and hospital-assigned ID
- Date of the medication order
- Patient information, including the room number, bed number, and ID number assigned to the patient
- Name, strength, and dosage form of medication
- When to be administered (frequency); in some hospitals, the frequency is assigned a specific time
- Duration of therapy
- Prescriber's signature

Steps in prescription processing

- Intake:
- Receipt of prescription:
  - Presented by patient or patient representative
  - Telephoned in from the prescriber's office by a designated individual from the practice
  - Faxed by the prescriber's office or the patient
  - Submitted electronically by the prescriber's office
- Data input:
  - Patient information:
    - Patient full name
    - Patient home address (number, street, city, state, zip code)
    - Telephone number to include area code (home, mobile, and work)
    - Birth date
    - Sex
    - Allergies
    - Generic preference
    - Request for non-child-resistant container
  - Prescription drug benefits:
    - Prescription drug card information:
- Complete electronic transaction routing information (RxPCN)
- Group number, which identifies the prescription coverage for a group of individuals under contract
- Subscriber number, which identifies individual who pays the premiuk
- Person code:
  - 01 = Cardholder
  - 02 = Spouse
  - 03 = Dependent
- Bank identification number, which is a six-digit number assigned by National Council for Prescription Drug Programs (NCPDP) required to process a prescription claim
- Help desk number, which is a 24-hour telephone number to assist pharmacies
  - Prescriber information
    - Prescriber name
    - Office address (street number, street, city, state, and zip code)
    - DEA number for controlled substances
    - National Provider Identifier depending on state regulations
    - Medical license depending on state regulations
  - Medication:
    - Name
    - Strength

- Quantity (expressed in metric units)
- Refills
- Calculating days' supply:
  - Days' supply for oral solids (e.g., tablets, capsules)

Days' Supply

$$= \text{Total quantity dispensed} \div (\text{Number of tablets dispensed per dose} \times \text{number of doses per day})$$

- Days' supply for oral liquids

Days' Supply

$$= \text{Total volume dispensed (mL)} \div (\text{Number of mL administered per dose} \times \text{number of doses per day})$$

- Days' supply for inhalers

Days' Supply

$$= \text{Number of sprays or inhalations per container} \div (\text{Number of inhalations per dose} \times \text{number of doses per day})$$

- Days' supply for insulin:
  - 1 mL = 100 international units.
  - Insulin vials contain 10 mL of insulin.
  - Insulin pens contain 3 mL of insulin.

Days' Supply

$$= \text{Number of international units per container} \div (\text{Number of international units per dose} \times \text{number of doses per day})$$

- Days' supply for ophthalmic solutions or suspensions
- 1 mL is equal to 20 drops

Days' Supply

$$= \text{Number of drops per container} \div (\text{Number of drops per dose} \times \text{number of doses per day})$$

- Directions for use:
  - Prescriber may write directions for use on the prescription using abbreviation. When inputting the directions for use, the pharmacy will need to input them using a format the system is able to understand, which may include "shortcuts."
  - Best practices:
- Begin with a verb.
- Do not use abbreviations.
- Identify dosage form.
- Indicate route of administration.
- Use everyday language; avoid medical or pharmacy terminology.
  - Prescription refills:
    - Must include number of approved refills.
    - If no refills are indicated, then zero should be entered.
    - The pharmacy technician must be aware of a state's definition of "prn" refills.
  - Generic substitution:
    - If a prescriber permits a generic medication to be dispensed, the generic must be dispensed.

- The pharmacy technician must be familiar with state regulations regarding the dispensing of brand name medications. States may require that the prescriber write in their own handwriting "dispense as written" or "brand name medically necessary."
- Some states may permit the prescriber to check a box on the prescription requiring the brand name drug to be dispensed.
  - Dispense as written codes:
    - Dispense as written codes are used to ensure the pharmacy is properly reimbursed by a third-party provider for a prescription being dispensed. These codes are as follows:
- 0 = No product selection indicated.
- 1 = Substitution not allowed by provider.
- 2 = Substitution allowed; patient requested product dispensed.
- 3 = Substitution allowed; pharmacist-selected product dispensed.
- 4 = Substitution allowed; generic drug not in stock.
- 5 = Substitution allowed; brand drug dispensed as generic.
- 6 = Override.
- 7 = Substitution not allowed; brand drug mandated by law.
- 8 = Substitution allowed; generic drug not available in marketplace.
- 9 = Other.
  - Prescription adjudication:
    - Process by which a prescription is submitted electronically for reimbursement
    - The prescription claim maybe be rejected for reimbursement for a variety of reasons; rejection codes used:

Rejection code	Rejection description
1	Missing or invalid bank identification number
2	Missing or invalid version number
3	Missing or invalid transaction code
4	Missing or invalid processor control number
5	Missing or invalid pharmacy number
6	Missing or invalid group number
7	Missing or invalid cardholder ID number
8	Missing or invalid person code
9	Missing or invalid birth date
10	Missing or invalid gender code
11	Missing or invalid patient relationship code
15	Missing or invalid date of service
16	Missing or invalid prescription/service reference number
19	Missing or invalid day's supply
20	Missing or invalid compound code
22	Missing or invalid dispense as written/product selection code

Rejection code	Rejection description
25	Missing or invalid prescriber ID
26	Missing or invalid unit of measure
28	Missing or invalid date prescription written
29	Missing or invalid number of refills authorized
54	Nonmatched National Drug Code number
60	Drug not covered for patient
75	Prior authorization required
79	Refill too soon

- Correction must be made to the claim before the claim will be reimbursed
- Drug utilization evaluation
  - Is a requirement of Omnibus Budget Reconciliation Act of 1990 (OBRA'90) whereby a patient profile is created for each patient which is used by the pharmacist when reviewing a patient's medication therapy
  - Pharmacist is responsible for conducting the drug utilization evaluation, which is used to identify:
    - Clinical abuse or misuse
    - Drug allergy problems
    - Drug overutilization
    - Drug underutilization
    - Drug-disease contraindications
    - Drug-drug interactions
    - Incorrect dosages
    - Incorrect duration of drug treatment
    - Therapeutic duplication
- Scanning the prescription:
  - Many pharmacies scan the original prescription resulting in a digital copy of the prescription being stored in the pharmacy information system
  - Used as a quality assurance tool to reduce medication errors
- Prescription labeling:
  - Prescription labeling requirements:
    - Date when prescription was filled
    - Serial (prescription) number of the prescription
    - Name and address of the pharmacy
    - Name of the patient
    - Name of the prescribing physician
    - All directions for use of the prescription
    - Generic or brand name of the prescription
    - Strength of the medication
    - Name of the drug manufacturer
    - Quantity of the drug
    - Expiration date of the prescription
    - Initials of the licensed pharmacist
    - Number of refills allowed
  - Medication order labeling requirements:
    - Name and location of the patient
    - Trade or generic name of drug
    - Strength of drug
    - Quantity of drug for the outpatient prescription labels
    - Expiration date of medication
    - Lot number of medication

- Sterile product label requirements:
  - Pharmacy name
  - Patient name
  - Date of filling
  - Ingredients (strength and quantity of each)
  - Total volume
  - Directions for use
  - Infusion rate
  - Beyond-use date (BUD)
- Unit dose label requirements:
  - Trade or generic name of drug
  - Drug manufacturer
  - Strength of drug
  - BUD
  - Lot number of medication

- Repackaged drug label requirements:
  - Name of medication
  - Drug manufacturer's name
  - Dosage form
  - Strength of drug
  - BUD
  - Lot number (batch number) of medication
- Auxiliary labels
  - Auxiliary labels provide specific instructions such as when to take a medication (e.g., before or after a meal); warnings to avoid specific foods, beverages, or other medications; side effects (e.g., drowsiness, dizziness or photosensitivity); storage conditions (e.g., refrigerator or freezer); or other cautionary warnings regarding a medication.

Commonly used auxiliary labels

Auxiliary label	Common drug classifications and examples
Caution: Federal law prohibits the transfer of this drug to any person other than the patient for whom it was prescribed.	All controlled substance prescriptions must have this auxiliary label
Avoid exposure to sunlight.	Tetracycline antibiotics (e.g., tetracycline and doxycycline), fluoroquinolone antibiotics (e.g., ciprofloxacin), sulfonamide antibiotics (sulfasalazine and sulfamethoxazole/trimethoprim), antifungals, antiarrhythmics (e.g., amiodarone), nonsteroidal antiinflammatory drugs (e.g., ibuprofen, celecoxib and meloxicam), loop diuretics (e.g., furosemide and torsemide), thiazide diuretics (e.g., hydrochlorothiazide), potassium-sparing diuretics (spironolactone), and serotonin modulators (e.g., trazodone)
Discolor urine or feces.	Ferrous sulfate, phenazopyridine, and nitrofurantoin
Do not drink alcohol when taking medications.	Selective serotonin reuptake inhibitors (e.g., citalopram, escitalopram, paroxetine, and sertraline), tricyclic antidepressants (e.g., amitriptyline), monoamine oxidase inhibitors (e.g., tranylcypromine and phenelzine), antipsychotics (e.g., risperidone and aripiprazole), benzodiazepines (e.g., alprazolam, lorazepam, clonazepam, and diazepam), nonbenzodiazepine hypnotic (e.g., zolpidem), nonsteroidal antiinflammatory drug (e.g., ibuprofen, celecoxib, and meloxicam), hydantoins (e.g., phenytoin), sulfonylureas (e.g., glipizide, glyburide, and glimepiride), opioid analgesics (e.g., oxycodone, acetaminophen/codeine, and acetaminophen/hydrocodone), nitroimidazoles (e.g., metronidazole), and disulfiram
Do not take if pregnant, nursing, trying to conceive.	Tetracycline antibiotics (e.g., tetracycline, doxycycline, and minocycline), isotretinoin, and finasteride
Do not take with dairy products, antacids, or iron preparations.	Tetracycline antibiotics (e.g., tetracycline and doxycycline), fluoroquinolone antibiotics (e.g., ciprofloxacin), levothyroxine, and gabapentin
Do not take with grapefruit.	HMG-CoA reductase inhibitors (e.g., atorvastatin, simvastatin, and lovastatin), calcium channel blockers (e.g., nifedipine), amiodarone, and buspirone
Do not smoke when taking medications.	Oral contraceptives (e.g., ethinyl estradiol/norethindrone, ethinyl estradiol/norgestimate, ethinyl estradiol/levonorgestrel, desogestrel/ethinyl estradiol, drospirenone/ethinyl estradiol and etonogestrel/ethinyl estradiol)
Take on an empty stomach.	Levothyroxine and penicillin
Finish all medication as prescribed.	All antibiotics and antifungal and antiviral medications
May interfere with contraceptives.	Antibiotics (e.g., doxycycline); examples of other medications include carbamazepine, felbamate, oxcarbazepine, phenobarbital, phenytoin, primidone, and topiramate
May cause dizziness.	First-generation antihistamines, anticonvulsants (e.g., phenytoin, topiramate, and carbamazepine), benzodiazepines (e.g., alprazolam, lorazepam, and diazepam), nonbenzodiazepine hypnotics (e.g., zolpidem), nonsteroidal antiinflammatory drugs (e.g., ibuprofen, celecoxib, and meloxicam), tricyclic antidepressants (e.g., amitriptyline), selective serotonin reuptake inhibitors (paroxetine and sertraline), antipsychotics (e.g., risperidone and aripiprazole), opioid analgesics (e.g., oxycodone, acetaminophen/oxycodone, acetaminophen/hydrocodone, and tramadol), beta blockers (e.g., metoprolol, propranolol, and atenolol), calcium channel blockers (e.g., amlodipine and diltiazem), angiotensin-converting enzyme inhibitors (e.g., lisinopril and enalapril), and angiotensin II receptor antagonists (e.g., losartan and valsartan)

(Continued)

Commonly used auxiliary labels —cont'd	
Auxiliary label	**Common drug classifications and examples**
May cause drowsiness.	First-generation antihistamines (e.g., diphenhydramine), benzodiazepines (e.g., alprazolam, lorazepam, and diazepam), nonbenzodiazepine hypnotics (e.g., zolpidem), barbiturates (e.g., phenobarbital), nonsteroidal antiinflammatory drugs (e.g., ibuprofen, celecoxib, and meloxicam), tricyclic antidepressants (e.g., amitriptyline), monoamine oxidase inhibitors (e.g., phenelzine), antipsychotics (e.g., risperidone and aripiprazole), muscle relaxants (e.g., cyclobenzaprine and carisoprodol), opioid analgesics (e.g., oxycodone, acetaminophen/oxycodone, acetaminophen/hydrocodone, and tramadol), anticonvulsants (e.g., phenytoin, topiramate, and carbamazepine), beta blockers (e.g., metoprolol, propranolol, and atenolol), calcium channel blockers (e.g., amlodipine and diltiazem), angiotensin-converting enzyme inhibitors (e.g., lisinopril and enalapril), and angiotensin II receptor antagonists (e.g., losartan and valsartan)
Take at bedtime.	Alpha blockers (e.g., terazosin and doxazosin)
Take on an empty stomach 1 h before meals or 2 h after a meal.	Tetracycline antibiotics (e.g., tetracycline and doxycycline)
Take with food.	Macrolide antibiotics (e.g., azithromycin and erythromycin), corticosteroids (e.g., prednisone), nonsteroidal antiinflammatory drugs (e.g., ibuprofen, celecoxib, and meloxicam)
Take with a full glass of orange juice or eat a banana.	Loop diuretics (e.g., furosemide and torsemide), thiazide diuretics (e.g., hydrochlorothiazide)
Take with water.	Sulfonamide antibiotics (e.g., sulfasalazine and sulfamethoxazole/trimethoprim), nonsteroidal antiinflammatory drugs (e.g., ibuprofen, celecoxib, and meloxicam), bisphosphonates (e.g., alendronate and ibandronate)
Refrigerate.	Insulin (e.g., Lantus Solostar and Humalog KwikPen, Glucagon-like peptide 1 (GLP-1) agonists (e.g., dulaglutide and semaglutide), tumor necrosis factor inhibitor (e.g., adalimumab and etanercept), prostaglandin analogs (e.g., latanoprost)
Do not crush, chew, or cut the dose.	AcipHex, Ambien Controlled release (CR), Avodart, Cardizem Controlled delivery (CD), Coreg Controlled release (CR), Depakote Extended release (ER), Fosamax Plus D, Lovaza, Minocin, Paxil, Pradaxa, Prevacid, and Tegretol Extra release (XR)

- Patient product information (PPI) sheets:
  - FDA requires PPIs to be provided to the patient when receiving select medication drug classifications to include oral contraceptives and estrogens.
  - Information contained on a PPI includes:
    - Clinical pharmacology
    - Indications and use
    - Contraindications
    - Warnings
    - Precautions
    - Adverse reactions
    - Drug abuse
    - Overdosage
    - Dosage and administration
    - How supplied

Pharmacy conversions

The metric system is the official system of measurement in the United States. The metric system is based upon multiples of 10. To convert from a larger unit of measurement to a smaller unit of measurement, multiply by a multiple of 10. To convert from a smaller unit of measurement to a larger unit of measurement, divide by a multiple of 10. Pharmacy technicians must be able to calculate doses of medication in any of these systems and convert them from one system to another system. It is essential that technicians memorize the basic conversions.

Metric prefixes

Nano-: One-billionth of the basic unit (meter, gram, or liter)
Micro-: One-millionth of the basic unit
Milli-: One-thousandth of the basic unit
Centi-: One-hundredth of the basic unit
Deci-: One-tenth of the basic unit
Deka-: 10 times the basic unit
Hecto-: 100 times the basic unit
Kilo-: 1000 times the basic unit

Metric units of measurement

Weight (gram): The gram is the basic unit of measurement of weight in the metric system. Other commonly used measurements in the practice of pharmacy are microgram (mcg), milligram (mg), gram (g), and kilogram (kg).

1000 micrograms (mcg) = 1 milligram (mg)

1000 milligrams (mg) = 1 gram (g)

1000 grams (g) = 1 kilogram (kg)

Volume (liter): The liter (L) is the basic unit of measurement of volume in the metric system. In addition to the liter, the milliliter (mL) is commonly used in the practice of pharmacy.

1000 milliliters (mL) = 1 liter (L)

Length (meter): The meter is the basic unit of measurement of length in the metric system. Other commonly used measurements in the practice of pharmacy are the millimeter (mm), centimeter (cm), and meter (m).

$$1000 \text{ millimeters (mm)} = 100 \text{ centimeters (cm)}$$

$$100 \text{ centimeters (cm)} = 1 \text{ meter (m)}$$

Household system of measurement
The metric system can be converted to the household system
Weight (household to metric):

$$1 \text{ pound (lb)} = 16 \text{ oz}$$

$$2.2 \text{ lb} = 1 \text{ kg}$$

Volume (household to metric)

$$5 \text{ milliliters (mL)} = 1 \text{ teaspoon (tsp)}$$

$$15 \text{ mL} = 3 \text{ tsp} = 1 \text{ tablespoon (tbsp)}$$

$$2 \text{ tbsp} = 1 \text{ fluid ounce (fl oz)}$$

$$8 \text{ fl oz} = 1 \text{ cup (c)}$$

$$2 \text{ cups} = 1 \text{ pint (pt)}$$

$$2 \text{ pt} = 1 \text{ quart (qt)}$$

$$4 \text{ qt} = 1 \text{ gallon (gal)}$$

Apothecary system
Currently, the only units of measurements that appear on prescriptions are the grain (gr), dram (3), ounce. When using the apothecary system, place the unit of measurement before the amount and use lower case Roman numerals.

Weight (apothecary to metric):

$$\text{gr i} = 60 \text{ mg, } 64.8 \text{ mg or } 65 \text{ mg}$$

Volume (apothecary to metric)

$$1 \text{ fluid dram (fl 3 or fl dr)} = 3.7 \text{ mL}$$

$$8 \text{ fl dr} = 1 \text{ fl oz}$$

Weight (avoirdupois to metric):

$$1 \text{ lb} = 454 \text{ g}$$

$$1 \text{ oz} = 30 \text{ g}$$

$$1 \text{ gr} = 64.8 \text{ g}$$

Volume (avoirdupois to metric):

$$1 \text{ fl oz} = 30 \text{ mL}$$

$$1 \text{ pt} = 473 \text{ mL}$$

$$1 \text{ gal} = 3785 \text{ mL}$$

Differences between the systems of measurement
The metric system is the approved system of measurement in pharmacy. Differences exist between manufacturer's products and their weights. For example, a manufacturer may indicate that 1 pint is equal to 473 mL but others may indicate that a pint is equal to 480 mL. The rule is to follow the metric system since it is the approved system of measurement.

Calculating the quantity to be dispensed

- Prescribers normally will indicate the number of tablets, milliliters of solution, or grams of a solid to dispense.
- In situations where a day's supply is indicated, do the following:
  - Oral dosage form: Determine the quantity of oral dosage forms to be dispensed/dose multiplied by the number of doses/day multiplied by the number of days.
  - Liquid oral dosage form: Determine the volume (mL) to be dispensed/dose multiplied by the number of doses/day multiplied by the number of days.

Calculate basic pharmacy problems using ratios and proportions

- A ratio expresses a relationship between two quantities or two measurements. For example 3:4 is a ratio and is read "3 is to 4" where the first number is the numerator in a fraction and the second number is the denominator in the fraction.
- To convert a ratio to a percent:
  - Write the ratio as a fraction (e.g., 3:4 = ¾).
  - Convert the fraction to a decimal (e.g., ¾ = 0.75).
  - Multiply the decimal by 100 (e.g., 0.75 × 100 = 0.75%).
- A proportion is an equivalent relationship of two ratios. For example, $\frac{3}{4} = \frac{6}{8}$ is a proportion.
- To solve a proportion problem, calculate by cross multiplying and dividing or by "means and extremes."

Cross-multiply method:

- $2/10 = 4/x$
- Cross multiply: $2x = (10)(4)$
- Divide both sides of equation by 2: $(2x)/2 = (10)(4)/2$ where $x = 20$

Means and extremes method:

- Set up 2:10::4:x where $(2)(x)$ equals $(10)(4)$.
- Divide both sides of proportion by 2: $(2x)/2 = (10)(4)/2$ where $x = 20$.

Calculate percent strength of a medication expressed as weight/weight, volume/volume, and/or weight/volume

- Percent weight in weight (w/w) is equal to the number of grams of ingredient dissolved in 100 g of the compound.
- Percent weight in volume (w/v) is equal to the number of grams of ingredient dissolved in 100 mL of solution.
- Percent volume in volume (v/v) is equal to the number of milliliters of a substance dissolved in 100 mL of solution.

Dilution calculations

A concentration is a strength that shows the quantity of drug dissolved in either a solid or a liquid. It can be expressed as a fraction (e.g., mg/mL, mEq/mL, or units/mL), as a ratio (e.g., 1:100, 1:1000, or 1:10,000), or as a percentage (e.g., 10%, 25%, or 50%). Percents are found in solids (%w/w) and in solutions (%w/v or %v/v); %w/w is the number of grams per 100 g, %w/v is the number of grams per 100 mL, and %v/v is the number of milliliters per 100 mL.

Most problems involving concentrations result in a dilution of a substance. In a daily application, a pharmacist receives an order to prepare a product of a given strength and volume (weight). These are known as the final strength and final volume. The pharmacist must go to the shelf, choose the product at a given strength (initial strength), and determine the amount (initial volume) needed to prepare the compound. The same process would be done in preparing solids, except initial weight and final weight would be substituted for initial and final volumes.

Use the following equation for this type of situation:

Initial volume × Initial strength = Final volume × Final strength

Hints to prevent errors in solving dilution problems:

- Initial strength must be larger than final strength.
- Initial volume must be less than final volume.
- Final volume minus initial volume equals amount of diluent (inert substance) to be added to make the final volume.

Alligation calculations

Alligations are used in pharmacy when a pharmacist or pharmacy technician is compounding either a solution or a solid. The strength being prepared is different from the strength of the substance on the shelf. In this situation, there are substances of at least two different concentrations on the shelf— one that is greater than the desired concentration and one that is less than the desired concentration.

For example, a pharmacist receives an order to prepare 4 ounces of a 10% solution using a 25% and 5% solution. How much of each these should the pharmacist use?

Step 1: Draw a tic-tac-toe table.

Step 2: Place the highest concentration in the upper left corner, the lowest concentration in the lower left corner, and the desired concentration in the middle.

25%		
	10%	
5%		

Step 3: Subtract the desired concentration from the highest concentration and place that number in the lower right corner and express the answer as parts. Then subtract the lowest concentration from the desired concentration and place that number in the upper right corner and label it as parts.

25%		5 parts
	10%	
5%		15 parts

Step 4: Total the number of parts: 5 + 15 parts = 20 parts.

Step 5: Set up a proportion using the parts of the highest and lowest concentration and the total quantity to be prepared.

25%: (5 parts/20 parts) × 4 oz = 1 oz of 25% required
5%: (15 parts/20 parts) × 4 oz = 3 oz of 5% required

Enlarging/reducing a formula

- When a formula specifies a specific total quantity, and you are asked to determine a different total quantity the following formula may be used:

  Total quantity of formula (as specified)
  ÷ Total quantity of formula (as desired)
  = Quantity of ingredient (as specified) in formula ÷ X

- To determine the amounts of each ingredient to be used to prepare a specified amount of the formula, the following formula can be used:

  Total number of parts in formula (as specified)
  ÷ Number of parts of an ingredient (as specified)
  = Total quantity of formula (as desired) ÷ X (quantity of an ingredient)

Evaluating the integrity of product characteristics

Expiration and beyond-use-dates

- An expiration date identifies the time during which a manufactured drug product, active ingredient, or added substance can be expected to meet the requirements of a monograph. The expiration date limits the time during which a conventionally manufactured product, active pharmaceutical ingredient, or added substance may be dispensed or used.
- A BUD is the date or time in which a compounded non-sterile preparation or a compounded sterile preparation (CSP) cannot be used, stored, or transported. The date is determined from the date or time the preparation was compounded.

- BUD for compounded nonsterile preparation:

Type of preparation	BUD (days)	Storage temperature
Aqueous dosage forms		
Nonpreserved aqueous dosage form	14	Refrigerator
Preserved aqueous dosage form	35	Controlled room temperature or refrigerator
Nonaqueous dosage forms		
Oral liquids (nonaqueous)	90	Controlled room temperature or refrigerator
Other nonaqueous dosage forms	180	Controlled room temperature or refrigerator

BUD, beyond-use date.

- BUD for CSP:
  - Category 1 CSPs BUD:
- A shorter BUD must be assigned when the stability of the CSP or its components is less than the hours or days stated in the previous table. The BUD must not exceed the shortest remaining expiration date or BUD of any of the starting components, regardless of the source. The table establishes the longest permitted BUDs for Category 1 CSPs. Category 1 CSPs may be prepared in an **segregated compounding area** or cleanroom suite.

	Controlled room temperature (20°C-25°C)	Refrigerator (2°C–8°C)
BUD	≤12h	≤24h

BUD, beyond-use date.

  - Category 2 CSPs BUD:
- The tables establishes the longest permitted BUDs for Category 2 CSPs. Category 2 CSPs must be prepared in a cleanroom suite.

Compounding method	Sterility testing performed and passed	Controlled room temperature (20°C–25°C)	Refrigerator (2°C–8°C)	Freezer (−25°C–10°C)
Aseptically processed CSPs	No	Prepared from one or more nonsterile starting component(s): 1 day	Prepared from one or more nonsterile starting component(s): 4 days	Prepared from one or more nonsterile starting component(s): 45 days
Aseptically processed CSPs	No	Prepared from only sterile starting components: 4 days	Prepared from only sterile starting components: 10 days	Prepared from only sterile starting components: 45 days
Aseptically processed CSPs	Yes	30 days	45 days	60 days
CSP Terminally sterilized CSPs	No	14 days	28 days	45 days
Terminally sterilized CSPs	Yes	45 days	60 days	90 days

CSP, compounded sterile preparation.

Identify signs of product instability

Signs of preparation instability	
Dosage form	**Signs of instability**
Capsules	Change in the physical appearance or consistency of the capsule or the contents, such as hardening, brittleness, or softening of the shell; discoloration or expansion/distortion of the gelatin capsule
Powders	Not free-flowing; caking or discoloration, nonuniform color; uncharacteristic odor; a release of pressure upon opening the container may indicate a release of carbon dioxide resulting from bacteria or other degradation
Solutions, elixirs, and syrups	Precipitates, discoloration, haziness, gas formation and microbial growth; unclear and inappropriate color and/or odor
Emulsions	Nonuniform globule size distribution and viscosity; breaking, creaming, gas formation, discoloration, and/or microbial growth
Suspensions	Caking, difficulty in resuspending, crystal growth, discoloration, and/or microbial growth; nonuniform particle size distribution and viscosity
Ointments	Nonuniform appearance and uncharacteristic odor; change in consistency of a separation of liquid; formation of granules or grittiness or dryness
Creams	Nonuniform appearance and/or uncharacteristic odor: emulsion breakage, crystal growth, shrinking due to evaporation; water; gross microbial contamination; discoloration
Suppositories	Nonuniform appearance; excessive softening, drying, hardening, or shriveling evidence of oil stains on the packaging
Gels	Nonuniform appearance and/or uncharacteristic odor; shrinkage, separation of liquid from the gel, discoloration, and/or microbial contamination

Signs of medication tampering

- Medication tampering is the inappropriate or illegal adulteration of a drug formulated under specified conditions, which may occur either during manufacturing or at the pharmacy before distributing to the patient or consumer.
- Sign of medication tampering:
  - Medication packaging:
    - Breaks, cracks, or holes are apparent in the outer or inner wrapping or protective cover or seal.
    - Outer or inner covering appears to have been disturbed, unwrapped, or replaced.
    - A plastic or tight-fitting wrap around the top of the bottle appears distorted or stretched, as though it had been rolled down and then put back into place
    - The bottom of the cap is not intact.
    - The cap is not on tight.

- Bits of paper or glue are stuck on the rim of the container, making it seem as if the container once had a bottle seal.
- The cotton plug or filler in the bottle is torn, sticky, or stained.
- The expiration date, lot number, and other information are not the same on both the container and its outer wrapping or box.
  - Tablets:
    - Tablets look different than they usually do.
    - Tablets are not all the same size and thickness.
    - Tablets have a strange or different odor or taste.
    - Tablets are broken.
  - Capsules:
    - Capsules look different than they usually do.
    - Capsules are cracked or dented.
    - Capsules are not all the same size and color.
    - Capsules are not all the same length.
  - Intravenous liquids:
    - Metal crimp is damaged.
    - Flip top is missing.
    - Product is discolored or cloudy or contains flakes or other foreign matter.
- Transaction patterns associated with medication tampering include:
  - Repeated canceled removals of a specific drug
  - Repeated returns of a specific drug
  - Frequent inventory counts that permit access to the drug supply without registering a transaction
  - Excessively frequent access to patient-controlled analgesia (PCA) keys, or access to PCA keys for patients not under the care of the staff member
- Methods to detect tampering:
  - Verifying the drug packaging is intact
  - Ensuring that the medication does not appear to be adulterated
  - Monitoring for canceled transactions and returns
  - Monitoring for patterns for a specific drug
- Warning signs of potential tampering by employees:
  - Missing, manipulated, or broken tamper-evident seals
  - Patient complaints of ineffective pain medication
  - Higher-than-average narcotic waste by a specific employee
  - Large number of cancellations on dispensing machines by one employee
  - Employee wearing long sleeves in warm weather
  - Employee taking frequent trips to the bathroom
  - Use of a multidose vial when a single-dose vial is available
  - Treating a patient with a narcotic when other drugs are more appropriate
  - Employee being in areas where they do not belong or volunteering to do tasks near narcotic supplies
  - Employee disappearing for long periods of time
  - Lethargic behavior of the employee
  - Exhibition of opioid withdrawal symptoms, including anxiety, agitation, nausea, vomiting, or abdominal pain
  - Uncharacteristic emotional outburst or verbal response

- Recommended actions to be taken in situations of tampering:
  - Documenting fully the tampering incident to include photographing the tampered medication
  - Securing the medication and having it analyzed
  - Determining if a patient has been harmed as a result of the tampering
  - Reporting tampering to the FDA Office of Criminal Investigations, professional and pharmacy boards, and law enforcement and local public health officials upon confirmation of the tampering incident

Best practices to prevent product tampering

- Ensuring medications are kept secure at all times
- Maintaining a regular schedule of controlled substance counts
- Requiring a witness be present for all inventory counts
- Limiting the number of PCA keys available to health care workers
- Storing PCA keys in a single-access compartment in an automated drug cabinet
- Ensuring that all returns are placed in a specified return bin instead of returning directly to patient stock
- Witnessing and documenting narcotic waste
- Installing surveillance cameras near automated dispensing machines
- Placing surveillance cameras in areas to monitor sterile supply items and noncontrolled medications
- Conducting regular, facility-wide audits of narcotic use
- Providing access to peer assistance programs

CHAPTER REVIEW QUESTIONS

1. A physician has prescribed amlodipine for a patient to be taken once a day for hypertension. Which strength is not available?
   a. 2.5 mg
   b. 5 mg
   c. 7.5 mg
   d. 10 mg
2. The pharmacy technician is reviewing a patient's prescription for atorvastatin and observes the prescriber failed to indicate a strength. The pharmacy technician contacts the physician's office asking which strength is to be given to the patient. The physician's office asks which is the lowest dose for atorvastatin. How should the pharmacy technician respond?
   a. 0.4 mg
   b. 1 mg
   c. 2 mg
   d. 10 mg
3. A physician prescribes gabapentin 400 mg PO TID for a patient. Which dosage form should the pharmacy technician select from its inventory?
   a. Capsule
   b. Oral solution
   c. Oral tablet
   d. Sublingual tablet

4. A physician has prescribed Cymbalta for a patient for depression. The patient requests that the generic be dispensed. Which medication should the pharmacy technician select from the shelf?
   a. Bupropion
   b. Citalopram
   c. Duloxetine
   d. Fluoxetine
5. A physician prescribes the following prescription:
   Levothyroxine 100 mcg 3 months' supply
   1 tab PO QD
   How many tablets should be dispensed?
   a. 30
   b. 60
   c. 90
   d. 120
6. Which auxiliary label should be affixed to a prescription bottle of ferrous sulfate?
   a. Avoid exposure to sunlight
   b. Caution: Federal law prohibits the transfer of this drug to any person other than the patient for whom it was prescribed
   c. Discolors urine or feces
   d. Do not drink alcohol when taking medications
7. A patient presents this prescription to the pharmacy:
   Coreg CR 20 mg #60
   I cap PO BID for hypertension
   Refill × 2
   What error did the pharmacy technician discover?
   a. Coreg CR is not indicated for hypertension
   b. Coreg CR is not taken twice a day
   c. Coreg CR is not available as a capsule
   d. Coreg CR is a not a brand drug name
8. The pharmacy technician receives the following prescription:
   Latanoprost 0.005% 2.5 mL
   i gtt os q pm
   How should the directions to the patient appear on the prescription label?
   a. Instill one drop in left ear each evening.
   b. Instill one drop in left eye each evening.
   c. Instill one drop in the right ear each evening.
   d. Instill one drop in left ear each evening.
9. The pharmacy technician receives the following prescription from a patient:
   Alprazolam 0.5 mg 30 tablets
   1 tab PO tid
   Refill 1 time
   Which auxiliary label should be affixed to the prescription bottle?
   a. Avoid exposure to sunlight.
   b. Caution: Federal law prohibits the transfer of this drug to any person other than the patient for whom it was prescribed.
   c. Discolors urine or feces.
   d. Do not take with dairy products, antacids, or iron preparations.
10. A patient presents the following prescription to the pharmacy technician today:
    Joan Ritter

2921 11th St S
Arlington, VA 22204

Amber Wells January 4, 2022
11608 Brandon Hill Way
Reston, VA 20194-1215

Acetaminophen with codeine 30 mg #30
1 tab PO q 4-6 h prn pain

Refill × 1 Joan Ritter AR 4525892
Why would the pharmacy technician not fill this prescription?
a. Acetaminophen with codeine cannot be refilled.
b. Acetaminophen with codeine directions are incorrect.
c. DEA number is invalid.
d. Prescription has expired.

11. The pharmacy technician is presented the following prescription from the patient:
Albuterol MDI 90 mcg/inhalation 200 inhalations
2 puffs inhaled q 6 h for bronchospasms
How many days will the prescription last?
a. 16 days
b. 25 days
c. 50 days
d. 100 days

12. The patient presents the following prescription to the pharmacy technician:
Losartan 50 mg #60
1 tab PO BID
Refill × 2
Which DAW code should the pharmacy technician input into the computer?
a. 0
b. 1
c. 2
d. 3

13. A patient presents a prescription for Magic Mouthwash 16 fl oz. How many mL should the pharmacy technician dispense?
a. 120
b. 240
c. 480
d. 720

14. The pharmacy technician receives a prescription to compound an ointment for psoriasis. Using the following formula
Coal tar, 2 g
Precipitated sulfur, 3 g
Salicylic acid, 1 g
Fluocinonide ointment, 24 g
Aquabase, 70 g
How many grams of coal tar should be used to compound 1 pound of the ointment?
a. 2
b. 4.54
c. 6.81
d. 9.08

15. A pharmacy technician receives the following prescription order to compound:
Liquified phenol 2.5%
Calamine lotion ad 240 mL

Sig: Apply to affected area as directed 4 times a day.
a. 2.4 mL
b. 3.6 mL
c. 4.8 mL
d. 6 mL

16. The pharmacy technician receives the following prescription from a patient:
Timolol ophthalmic solution 0.25% 5 mL
1 gtt each eye twice a day
How many days will the prescription last?
a. 20 days
b. 25 days
c. 30 days
d. 50 days

17. Which patient code should the pharmacy technician input for the spouse of the cardholder of a prescription plan?
a. 00
b. 01
c. 02
d. 03

18. Which auxiliary label should be affixed to a prescription bottle of furosemide?
a. Do not crush, chew, or cut the dose.
b. Refrigerate.
c. Take at bedtime.
d. Take with a full glass of orange juice or eat a banana.

19. When must a pharmacy distribute a medication guide to the patient or the patient's agent?
a. When a drug is dispensed in an outpatient setting
b. When a drug is subject to an REMS that includes specific requirements for reviewing or providing a medication guide as part of an element to assure safe use
c. When the patient or the patient's agent requests a medication guide
d. All of the above

20. Which medication(s) require a medication guide be distributed to the patient?
a. Amoxicillin
b. Ciprofloxacin
c. Tetracycline
d. All the above

21. Which of the following pharmacy abbreviations appears on TJC's "Do Not Use" list?
a. AC
b. BID
c. PO
d. QOD

22. Which of the following should be done if medication tampering is suspected?
a. Report it to FDA Office of Criminal Investigations.
b. Report it to law enforcement.
c. Report it to the state board of pharmacy.
d. All of the above.

23. The pharmacist is checking a solution the pharmacy technician has compounded and observes instability in the preparation. Which is a sign of instability in a solution?
a. Creaming
b. Difficulty in resuspending
c. Discoloration
d. Emulsion breakage

24. The pharmacy technician is checking a suspension the pharmacy technician has compounded and observes instability in the preparation. Which is a sign of instability in a suspension?
    a. Creaming
    b. Difficulty in resuspending
    c. Emulsion breakage
    d. Nonuniform appearance

25. The pharmacy technician receives the following prescription:
    Amoxicillin 250 mg/mL 150 mL
    5 mL PO tid
    What is the BUD for this prescription?
    a. 7 days
    b. 14 days
    c. 21 days
    d. 35 days

A APPENDIX

ISMP list of look-alike drug names with recommended tall man letters

Drug name with tall man letters	Confused with
ALfentanil	fenta**NYL**—**SUF**entanil
ALPRAZolam	clonaze**PAM**—**LOR**azepam
a**MIL**oride	am**LODIP**ine
am**LODIP**ine	a**MIL**oride
ARIPiprazole	**RABE**prazole
aza**CITID**ine	aza**THIO**prine
aza**THIO**prine	aza**CITID**ine
BUPivacaine	**ROP**ivacaine
car**BAM**azepine	**OX**carbazepine
CARBOplatin[b]	**CIS**platin[b]
ce**FAZ**olin	cefo**TE**tan—cef**OX**itin—cef**TAZ**idime—cef**TRIAX**one
cefo**TE**tan	ce**FAZ**olin—cef**OX**itin—cef**TAZ**idime—cef**TRIAX**one
cef**OX**itin	ce**FAZ**olin—cefo**TE**tan—cef**TAZ**idime—cef**TRIAX**one
cef**TAZ**idime	ce**FAZ**olin—cefo**TE**tan—cef**OX**itin—cef**TRIAX**one
cef**TRIAX**one	ce**FAZ**olin—cefo**TE**tan—cef**OX**itin—cef**TAZ**idime
Cele**BREX**[c]	Cele**XA**[c]
Cele**XA**[c]	Cele**BREX**[c]
chlordiaze**POXIDE**	chlorpro**MAZINE**[b]
chlorpro**MAZINE**[b]	chlordiaze**POXIDE**
CISplatin[b]	**CARBO**platin[b]
clo**BAZ**am	clonaze**PAM**
clonaze**PAM**	**ALPRAZ**olam—clo**BAZ**am—clo**NID**ine—clo**ZAP**ine—**LOR**azepam
clo**NID**ine	clonaze**PAM**—clo**ZAP**ine—Klono**PIN**[c]

Drug name with tall man letters	Confused with
clo**ZAP**ine	clonaze**PAM**—clo**NID**ine
cyclo**PHOS**phamide	cyclo**SERINE**[b]—cyclo**SPORINE**[b]
cyclo**SERINE**[b]	cyclo**PHOS**phamide—cyclo**SPORINE**[b]
cyclo**SPORINE**[b]	cyclo**PHOS**phamide—cyclo**SERINE**[b]
DACTINomycin	**DAPTO**mycin
DAPTOmycin	**DACTIN**omycin
DEPO-Medrol[c]	**SOLU**-Medrol[c]
dex**AMETH**asone	dexmede**TOMID**ine
dexmede**TOMID**ine	dex**AMETH**asone
diaze**PAM**	dil**TIAZ**em
dil**TIAZ**em	diaze**PAM**
DOCEtaxel	**PACL**itaxel
DOXOrubicin[b]	**IDA**rubicin
dro**NAB**inol	dro**PER**idol
dro**PER**idol	dro**NAB**inol
DULoxetine	**FLU**oxetine—**PAR**oxetine
e**PHED**rine	**EPINEPH**rine
EPINEPHrine	e**PHED**rine
epi**RUB**icin	eri**BUL**in
eri**BUL**in	epi**RUB**icin
fenta**NYL**	**AL**fentanil—**SUF**entanil
flavox**ATE**	fluvoxa**MINE**
FLUoxetine	**DUL**oxetine—**PAR**oxetine
flu**PHENAZ**ine	fluvoxa**MINE**
fluvoxa**MINE**	flavox**ATE**—flu**PHENAZ**ine
guai**FEN**esin	guan**FACINE**

(Continued)

Drug name with tall man letters	Confused with
guan**FACINE**	guai**FEN**esin
Huma**LOG**c	Humu**LIN**c
Humu**LIN**c	Huma**LOG**c
hydr**ALAZINE**b	hydro**CHLORO**thiazide —hydr**OXY**zineb
hydro**CHLORO**-thiazide	hydr**ALAZINE**b—hydr**OXY**zineb
HYDROcodone	oxy**CODONE**
HYDROmorphoneb	morphine—oxy**MOR**phone
HYDROXYpro-gesterone	medroxy**PROGESTER**oneb
hydr**OXY**zineb	hydr**ALAZINE**b—hydro**CHLORO**thiazide
IDArubicin	**DOXO**rubicinb—idaru**CIZU**mab
idaru**CIZU**mab	**IDA**rubicin
in**FLIX**imab	ri**TUX**imab
ISOtretinoin	tretinoin
Klono**PIN**c	clo**NID**ine
La**MIC**talc	Lam**ISIL**c
Lam**ISIL**c	La**MIC**talc
lami**VUD**ine	lamo**TRI**gine
lamo**TRI**gine	lami**VUD**ine
lev**ETIRA**cetam	lev**OCARN**itine—levo**FLOX**acin
lev**OCARN**itine	lev**ETIRA**cetam
levo**FLOX**acin	lev**ETIRA**cetam
LEVOleucovorin	leucovorin
LORazepam	**ALPRAZ**olam—clonaze**PAM**
medroxy-**PROGESTER**oneb	**HYDROXY**progesterone
met**FORMIN**	metro**NIDAZOLE**
methazol**AMIDE**	meth**IMA**zole—met**OL**azone
meth**IMA**zole	methazol**AMIDE**—met**OL**azone
met**OL**azone	methazol**AMIDE**—meth**IMA**zole
metro**NIDAZOLE**	met**FORMIN**
metyra**PONE**	metyro**SINE**
metyro**SINE**	metyra**PONE**
mi**FEPRIS**tone	mi**SOPROS**tol
mig**ALA**statb	mig**LU**statb
mig**LU**statb	mig**ALA**statb
mi**SOPROS**tol	mi**FEPRIS**tone
mito**MY**cin	mito**XANTRONE**b
mito**XANTRONE**b	mito**MY**cin
Nex**AVAR**c	Nex**IUM**c
Nex**IUM**c	Nex**AVAR**c
ni**CAR**dipineb	**NIFE**dipineb—ni**MOD**ipine
NIFEdipineb	ni**CAR**dipineb—ni**MOD**ipine
ni**MOD**ipine	ni**CAR**dipineb—**NIFE**dipineb
Novo**LIN**c	Novo**LOG**c
Novo**LOG**c	Novo**LIN**c

Drug name with tall man letters	Confused with
OLANZapine	**QUE**tiapine
OXcarbazepine	car**BAM**azepine
oxy**BUTY**nin	oxy**CODONE**—Oxy**CONTIN**c—oxy**MOR**phone
oxy**CODONE**	**HYDRO**codone—oxy**BUTY**nin—Oxy**CONTIN**c—oxy**MOR**phone
Oxy**CONTIN**c	oxy**BUTY**nin—oxy**CODONE**—oxy**MOR**phone
oxy**MOR**phone	**HYDRO**morphoneb—oxy**BUTY**nin—oxy**CODONE**—Oxy**CONTIN**c
PACLitaxel	**DOCE**taxel
PARoxetine	**DUL**oxetine—**FLU**oxetine
PAZOPanib	**PONAT**inib
PEMEtrexed	**PRALA**trexate
penicill**AMINE**	penicillin
PENTobarbital	**PHEN**obarbital
PHENobarbital	**PENT**obarbital
PHYSostigmine	py**RID**ostigmine
PONATinib	**PAZOP**anib
PRALAtrexate	**PEME**trexed
Pri**LOSEC**c	**PRO**zacc
PROzacc	Pri**LOSEC**c
py**RID**ostigmine	**PHYS**ostigmine
QUEtiapine	**OLANZ**apine
qui**NID**ine	qui**NINE**
qui**NINE**	qui**NID**ine
RABEprazole	**ARIP**iprazole
ra**NITI**dinea	ri**MANTA**dine
rif**AMP**in	rif**AXIM**in
rif**AXIM**in	rif**AMP**in
ri**MANTA**dine	ra**NITI**dinea
Risper**DAL**c	r**OPINIR**oleb
risperi**DONE**b	r**OPINIR**oleb
ri**TUX**imab	in**FLIX**imab
romi**DEP**sin	romi**PLOS**tim
romi**PLOS**tim	romi**DEP**sin
r**OPINIR**oleb	Risper**DAL**c—risperi**DONE**b
ROPivacaine	**BUP**ivacaine
Sand**IMMUNE**c	Sando**STATIN**c
Sando**STATIN**c	Sand**IMMUNE**c
s**AX**agliptin	**SIT**agliptin
SITagliptin	s**AX**agliptin—**SUMA**triptan
Solu-**CORTEF**c	**SOLU**-Medrolc
SOLU-Medrolc	**DEPO**-Medrolc—Solu-**CORTEF**c
SORAfenib	**SUNI**tinib
SUFentanil	**AL**fentanil—fenta**NYL**

(Continued)

Drug name with tall man letters	Confused with
sulf**ADIAZINE**[b]	sulfa**SALA**zine
sulfa**SALA**zine	sulf**ADIAZINE**[b]
SUMAtriptan	**SIT**agliptin—**ZOLM**itriptan
SUNItinib	**SORA**fenib
tia**GAB**ine	ti**ZAN**idine
ti**ZAN**idine	tia**GAB**ine
tra**MAD**ol[b]	tra**ZOD**one[b]
tra**ZOD**one[b]	tra**MAD**ol[b]
val**ACY**clovir	val**GAN**ciclovir
val**GAN**ciclovir	val**ACY**clovir

Drug name with tall man letters	Confused with
ZOLMitriptan	**SUMA**triptan
Zy**PREXA**[c]	Zyr**TEC**[c]
Zyr**TEC**[c]	Zy**PREXA**[c]

[a]These drugs have been discontinued and are not marketed in the United States.

[b]These drug names are also on the FDA list.

[c]Brand names always start with an uppercase letter. Some brand names incorporate tall man letters in initial characters and may not be readily recognized as brand names. A double dagger follows all brand names on the ISMP list.

APPENDIX B

ISMP list of error-prone abbreviations

Error-prone abbreviations, symbols, and dose designations	Intended meaning	Misinterpretation	Best practice
Abbreviations for doses/measurement units			
cc	Cubic centimeters	Mistaken as u (units)	Use mL
IU[a]	International unit(s)	Mistaken as IV (intravenous) or the number 10	Use unit(s) (international units can be expressed as units alone)
l	Liter	Lowercase letter l mistaken as the number 1	Use L (UPPERCASE) for liter
ml	Milliliter	Lowercase letter l mistaken as the number 1	Use mL (lowercase m, UPPERCASE L) for milliliter
MM or M	Million	Mistaken as thousand	Use million
M or K	Thousand	Mistaken as million M has been used to abbreviate both million and thousand (M is the Roman numeral for thousand)	Use thousand
Ng or ng	Nanogram	Mistaken as mg Mistaken as nasogastric	Use nanogram or nanog
U or u[a]	Unit(s)	Mistaken as zero or the number 4, causing a 10-fold overdose or greater (e.g., 4U seen as 40 or 4u seen as 44) Mistaken as cc, leading to administering volume instead of units (e.g., 4u seen as 4cc)	Use unit(s)
μg	Microgram	Mistaken as mg	Use mcg
Abbreviations for route of administration			
AD, AS, AU	Right ear, left ear, each ear	Mistaken as OD, OS, OU (right eye, left eye, each eye)	Use right ear, left ear, or each ear
IN	Intranasal	Mistaken as IM or IV	Use NAS (all UPPERCASE letters) or intranasal

(Continued)

Error-prone abbreviations, symbols, and dose designations	Intended meaning	Misinterpretation	Best practice
IT	Intrathecal	Mistaken as intratracheal, intratumor, intratympanic, or inhalation therapy	Use intrathecal
OD, OS, OU	Right eye, left eye, each eye	Mistaken as AD, AS, AU (right ear, left ear, each ear)	Use right eye, left eye, or each eye
Per os	By mouth, orally	The os was mistaken as left eye (OS, oculus sinister)	Use PO, by mouth, or orally
SC, SQ, sq, or sub q	Subcutaneous(ly)	SC and sc mistaken as SL or sl (sublingual) SQ mistaken as "5 every" The q in sub q has been mistaken as "every"	Use SUBQ (all UPPERCASE letters, without spaces or periods between letters) or subcutaneous(ly)
Abbreviations for frequency/instructions for use			
HS	Half-strength	Mistaken as bedtime	Use half-strength
hs	At bedtime, hours of sleep	Mistaken as half-strength	Use HS (all UPPERCASE letters) for bedtime
o.d. or OD	Once daily	Mistaken as right eye (OD, oculus dexter), leading to oral liquid medications administered in the eye	Use daily
Q.D., QD, q.d., or qd[a]	Every day	Mistaken as q.i.d., especially if the period after the q or the tail of a handwritten q is misunderstood as the letter i	Use daily
Qhs	Nightly at bedtime	Mistaken as qhr (every hour)	Use nightly or HS for bedtime
Qn	Nightly or at bedtime	Mistaken as qh (every hour)	Use nightly or HS for bedtime
Q.O.D., QOD, q.o.d., or qod[a]	Every other day	Mistaken as qd (daily) or qid (four times daily), especially if the o is poorly written	Use every other day
q1d	Daily	Mistaken as qid (four times daily)	Use daily
q6PM, etc.	Every evening at 6 p.m.	Mistaken as every 6 hours	Use daily at 6 p.m. or 6 p.m. daily
SSRI	Sliding scale regular insulin	Mistaken as selective-serotonin reuptake inhibitor	Use sliding scale (insulin)
SSI	Sliding scale insulin	Mistaken as strong solution of iodine (Lugol's)	Use sliding scale (insulin)
TIW or tiw	3 times a week	Mistaken as 3 times a day or twice in a week	Use 3 times weekly
BIW or biw	2 times a week	Mistaken as 2 times a day	Use 2 times weekly
UD	As directed (ut dictum)	Mistaken as unit dose (e.g., an order for "dil**TIAZ**em infusion UD" was mistakenly administered as a unit [bolus] dose)	Use as directed
Miscellaneous abbreviations associated with medication use			
BBA, BGB	Baby boy A (twin), baby girl B (twin)	B in BBA mistaken as twin B rather than gender (boy) B at end of BGB mistaken as gender (boy) not twin B	When assigning identifiers to newborns, use the mother's last name, the baby's gender (boy or girl), and a distinguishing identifier for all multiples (e.g., Smith girl A, Smith girl B)
D/C	Discharge or discontinue	Premature discontinuation of medications when D/C (intended to mean discharge) on a medication list was misinterpreted as discontinued	Use discharge and discontinue or stop

(Continued)

Error-prone abbreviations, symbols, and dose designations	Intended meaning	Misinterpretation	Best practice
IJ	Injection	Mistaken as IV or intrajugular	Use injection
OJ	Orange juice	Mistaken as OD or OS (right or left eye); drugs meant to be diluted in orange juice may be given in the eye	Use orange juice
Period following abbreviations (e.g., mg., mL.)[b]	mg or mL	Unnecessary period mistaken as the number 1, especially if written poorly	Use mg, mL, etc., without a terminal period

Drug name abbreviations

To prevent confusion, avoid abbreviating drug names entirely. Exceptions may be made for multiingredient drug formulations, including vitamins, when there are electronic drug name field space constraints; however, drug name abbreviations should *never* be used for any medications on the ISMP List of High-Alert Medications (in <u>Acute Care Settings, Community/Ambulatory Settings,</u> and <u>Long-Term Care Settings</u>). Examples of drug name abbreviations involved in serious medication errors include:

Antiretroviral medications (e.g., DOR, TAF, TDF)	DOR: doravirine TAF: tenofovir alafenamide TDF: tenofovir disoproxil fumarate	DOR: Dovato (dolutegravir and lami**VUD**ine) TAF: tenofovir disoproxil fumarate TDF: tenofovir alafenamide	Use complete drug names
APAP	acetaminophen	Not recognized as acetaminophen	Use complete drug name
ARA A	vidarabine	Mistaken as cytarabine ("ARA C")	Use complete drug name
AT II and AT III	AT II: angiotensin II (Giapreza) AT III: antithrombin III (Thrombate III)	AT II (angiotensin II) mistaken as AT III (antithrombin III) AT III (antithrombin III) mistaken as AT II (angiotensin II)	Use complete drug names
AZT	zidovudine (Retrovir)	Mistaken as azithromycin, aza**THIO**prine, or aztreonam	Use complete drug name
CPZ	Compazine (prochlorperazine)	Mistaken as chlorpro**MAZINE**	Use complete drug name
DTO	diluted tincture of opium or deodorized tincture of opium (Paregoric)	Mistaken as tincture of opium	Use complete drug name
HCT	hydrocortisone	Mistaken as hydro**CHLORO**thiazide	Use complete drug name
HCTZ	hydro**CHLORO**thiazide	Mistaken as hydrocortisone (e.g., seen as HCT250 mg)	Use complete drug name
MgSO4[a]	magnesium sulfate	Mistaken as morphine sulfate	Use complete drug name
MS, MSO4[a]	morphine sulfate	Mistaken as magnesium sulfate	Use complete drug name
MTX	methotrexate	Mistaken as mito**XANTRONE**	Use complete drug name
Na at the beginning of a drug name (e.g., Na bicarbonate)	Sodium bicarbonate	Mistaken as no bicarbonate	Use complete drug name
NoAC	novel/new oral anticoagulant	Mistaken as no anticoagulant	Use complete drug name
OXY	oxytocin	Mistaken as oxy**CODONE**, Oxy**CONTIN**	Use complete drug name
PCA	procainamide	Mistaken as patient-controlled analgesia	Use complete drug name
PIT	Pitocin (oxytocin)	Mistaken as Pitressin, a discontinued brand of vasopressin still referred to as PIT	Use complete drug name
PNV	prenatal vitamins	Mistaken as penicillin VK	Use complete drug name
PTU	propylthiouracil	Mistaken as Purinethol (mercaptopurine)	Use complete drug name
T3	Tylenol with codeine No. 3	Mistaken as liothyronine, which is sometimes referred to as T3	Use complete drug name

(Continued)

Error-prone abbreviations, symbols, and dose designations	Intended meaning	Misinterpretation	Best practice
TAC or tac	triamcinolone or tacrolimus	Mistaken as tetracaine, Adrenalin, and cocaine; or as Taxotere, Adriamycin, and cyclophosphamide	Use complete drug names Avoid drug regimen or protocol acronyms that may have a dual meaning or may be confused with other common acronyms, even if defined in an order set
TNK	TNKase	Mistaken as TPA	Use complete drug name
TPA or tPA	tissue plasminogen activator, Activase (alteplase)	Mistaken as TNK (TNKase, tenecteplase), TXA (tranexamic acid), or less often as another tissue plasminogen activator, Retavase (retaplase)	Use complete drug name
TXA	tranexamic acid	Mistaken as TPA (tissue plasminogen activator)	Use complete drug name
ZnSO4	zinc sulfate	Mistaken as morphine sulfate	Use complete drug name
Stemmed/coined drug names			
Nitro drip	nitroglycerin infusion	Mistaken as nitroprusside infusion	Use complete drug name
IV vanc	Intravenous vancomycin	Mistaken as Invanz	Use complete drug name
Levo	levofloxacin	Mistaken as Levophed (norepinephrine)	Use complete drug name
Neo	Neo-Synephrine, a well known but discontinued brand of phenylephrine	Mistaken as neostigmine	Use complete drug name
Coined names for compounded products (e.g., magic mouthwash, banana bag, GI cocktail, half and half, pink lady)	Specific ingredients compounded together	Mistaken ingredients	Use complete drug/product names for all ingredients Coined names for compounded products should only be used if the contents are standardized and readily available for reference to prescribers, pharmacists, and nurses
Number embedded in drug name (not part of the official name) (e.g., 5-fluorouracil, 6-mercaptopurine)	fluorouracil mercaptopurine	Embedded number mistaken as the dose or number of tablets/capsules to be administered	Use complete drug names, without an embedded number if the number is not part of the official drug name
Dose designations and other information			
1/2 tablet	Half tablet	1 or 2 tablets	Use text (half tablet) or reduced font-size fractions (½ tablet)
Doses expressed as Roman numerals (e.g., V)	5	Mistaken as the designated letter (e.g., the letter V) or the wrong numeral (e.g., 10 instead of 5)	Use only Arabic numerals (e.g., 1, 2, 3) to express doses
Lack of a leading zero before a decimal point (e.g., .5 mg)[a]	0.5 mg	Mistaken as 5 mg if the decimal point is not seen	Use a leading zero before a decimal point when the dose is less than one measurement unit
Trailing zero after a decimal point (e.g., 1.0 mg)[a]	1 mg	Mistaken as 10 mg if the decimal point is not seen	Do not use trailing zeros for doses expressed in whole numbers
Ratio expression of a strength of a single-entity injectable drug product (e.g., **EPINEPH**rine 1:1,000; 1:10,000; 1:100,000)	1:1,000: contains 1 mg/mL 1:10,000: contains 0.1 mg/mL 1:100,000: contains 0.01 mg/mL	Mistaken as the wrong strength	Express the strength in terms of quantity per total volume (e.g., **EPINEPH**rine 1 mg per 10 mL) **Exception:** combination local anesthetics (e.g., lidocaine 1% and **EPINEPH**rine 1:100,000)

(Continued)

Error-prone abbreviations, symbols, and dose designations	Intended meaning	Misinterpretation	Best practice
Drug name and dose run together (problematic for drug names that end in the letter l [e.g., propranolol20 mg; **TEG**retol300 mg])	propranolol 20 mg **TEG**retol 300 mg	Mistaken as propranolol 120 mg Mistaken as **TEG**retol 1300 mg	Place adequate space between the drug name, dose, and unit of measure
Numerical dose and unit of measure run together (e.g., 10 mg, 10Units)	10 mg 10 mL	The m in mg, or U in Units, has been mistaken as one or two zeros when flush against the dose (e.g., 10 mg, 10Units), risking a 10- to 100-fold overdose	Place adequate space between the dose and unit of measure
Large doses without properly placed commas (e.g., 100000 units; 1000000 units)	100,000 units 1,000,000 units	100000 has been mistaken as 10,000 or 1,000,000 1000000 has been mistaken as 100,000	Use commas for dosing units at or above 1,000 or use words such as 100 thousand or 1 million to improve readability **Note**: Use commas to separate digits only in the United States; commas are used in place of decimal points in some other countries
Symbols			
ʒ or ℥[b]	Dram Minim	Symbol for dram mistaken as the number 3 Symbol for minim mistaken as mL	Use the metric system
x1	Administer once	Administer for 1 day	Use explicit words (e.g., for 1 dose)
> and <	More than and less than	Mistaken as opposite of intended Mistakenly have used the incorrect symbol < mistaken as the number 4 when handwritten (e.g., <10 misread as 40)	Use more than or less than
↑ and ↓[b]	Increase and decrease	Mistaken as opposite of intended Mistakenly have used the incorrect symbol ↑ mistaken as the letter T, leading to misinterpretation as the start of a drug name, or mistaken as the numbers 4 or 7	Use increase and decrease
/ (slash mark)[b]	Separates two doses or indicates per	Mistaken as the number 1 (e.g., 25 units/10 units misread as 25 units and 110 units)	Use per rather than a slash mark to separate doses
@[b]	At	Mistaken as the number 2	Use at
&[b]	And	Mistaken as the number 2	Use and
+[b]	Plus or and	Mistaken as the number 4	Use plus, and, or in addition to
°	Hour	Mistaken as a zero (e.g., q2° seen as q20)	Use hr, h, or hour
Φ or ⌀[b]	Zero, null sign	Mistaken as the numbers 4, 6, 8, and 9	Use 0 or zero, or describe intent using whole words
#	Pound(s)	Mistaken as a number sign	Use the metric system (kg or g) rather than pounds Use lb if referring to pounds
Apothecary or household abbreviations			

Explicit apothecary or household measurements may *only* be safely used to express the directions for mixing dry ingredients to prepare topical products (e.g., dissolve 2 capfuls of granules per gallon of warm water to prepare a magnesium sulfate soaking aid). Otherwise, metric system measurements should be used.

(Continued)

Error-prone abbreviations, symbols, and dose designations	Intended meaning	Misinterpretation	Best practice
gr	Grain(s)	Mistaken as gram	Use the metric system (e.g., mcg, g)
dr	Dram(s)	Mistaken as doctor	Use the metric system (e.g., mL)
min	Minim(s)	Mistaken as minutes	Use the metric system (e.g., mL)
oz	Ounce(s)	Mistaken as zero or 0_2	Use the metric system (e.g., mL)
tsp	Teaspoon(s)	Mistaken as tablespoon(s)	Use the metric system (e.g., mL)
tbsp or Tbsp	Tablespoon(s)	Mistaken as teaspoon(s)	Use the metric system (e.g., mL)
Common abbreviations with contradictory meanings	**Contradictory meanings**		**Correction**
B	Breast, brain, or bladder		Use breast, brain, or bladder
C	Cerebral, coronary, or carotid		Use cerebral, coronary, or carotid
D or d	Day or dose (e.g., parameter-based dosing formulas using D or d [mg/kg/d] could be interpreted as either day or dose [mg/kg/day or mg/kg/dose]; or x3d could be interpreted as either 3 days or 3 doses)		Use day or dose
H	Hand or hip		Use hand or hip
I	Impaired or improvement		Use impaired or improvement
L	Liver or lung		Use liver or lung
N	No or normal		Use no or normal
P	Pancreas, prostate, preeclampsia, or psychosis		Use pancreas, prostate, preeclampsia, or psychosis
S	Special or standard		Use special or standard
SS or ss	Single strength, sliding scale (insulin), signs and symptoms, or ½ (apothecary) SS has also been mistaken as the number 55		Use single strength, sliding scale, signs and symptoms, or one-half or ½

[a]On The Joint Commission's "Do Not Use" lis.t

[b]Relevant mostly in handwritten medication information

APPENDIX C

Practice exams

Chapter 1 Sterile Compounding

1. Which is an indication Humira (adalimumab)?
   a. Acute myocardial infarction
   b. Chronic obstructive pulmonary disease
   c. Rheumatoid arthritis
   d. Ventricular arrhythmias
2. Which is the route of administration for enoxaparin?
   a. Intramuscularly
   b. Intravenously
   c. Intrathecal
   d. Subcutaneously
3. Which is the generic name for Lantus insulin?
   a. Insulin aspart
   b. Insulin detemir
   c. Insulin glargine
   d. Insulin isophane
4. Which medication is indicated for kidney, heart, and liver transplant prophylaxis?
   a. Mycophenolate mofetil
   b. Naloxone
   c. Ondansetron
   d. Phytonadione
5. A patient is diagnosed with Crohn's disease. Which medication is an appropriate treatment?
   a. Cisplatin injection
   b. Infliximab injection
   c. Labetalol HCl injection
   d. Lidocaine HCl injection
6. Which is an example of a narrow therapeutic index injectable medication?
   a. Amiodarone
   b. Ciprofloxacin
   c. Isoniazid
   d. Vancomycin
7. When filling prescriptions for narrow therapeutic index injectable medications, which medication must a pharmacy technician pay close attention?
   a. Acyclovir
   b. Ampicillin
   c. Ciprofloxacin
   d. Heparin
8. Which form of water possesses an antimicrobial agent?
   a. Bacteriostatic water for injection USP
   b. Purified water USP
   c. Sterile water for irrigation USP
   d. Water for injection USP
9. Which is a measurement of concentration of heparin?
   a. g/mL
   b. mg/mL
   c. mOs/mL
   d. units/mL
10. Which medication is indicated for deep vein thrombosis prophylaxis?
    a. Dopamine HCl injection
    b. Enoxaparin
    c. Epoprostenol sodium injection
    d. Flumazenil injection
11. A patient has been diagnosed with cytomegalovirus retinitis. Which medication may be prescribed for this condition?
    a. Fluphenazine injection
    b. Folic acid injection
    c. Foscarnet sodium injection
    d. Interferon alfa-2b
12. Which is the brand name for mannitol injection?
    a. CellCept
    b. Oncaspar
    c. Osmitrol
    d. Tysabri

13. Which is the concentration for phenytoin sodium injection?
    a. 10 mg/mL
    b. 50 mg/mL
    c. 65 mg/mL
    d. 100 mg/mL

14. How long must a Class I, Class II, or Class III biological safety cabinet be turned on prior to compounding?
    a. At least 10 minutes
    b. At least 15 minutes
    c. At least 20 minutes
    d. At least 30 minutes

15. How many types of Class II biological safety cabinets are used in working with materials contaminated with (or potentially contaminated with) pathogens requiring a defined biosafety level?
    a. 2
    b. 3
    c. 4
    d. 6

16. What type of International Organization for Standardization (ISO) class environment does a primary engineering control provide?
    a. Class 5
    b. Class 6
    c. Class 7
    d. Class 8

17. What is the minimum airflow differential between the buffer and ante area?
    a. 10 feet/min
    b. 20 feet/min
    c. 30 feet/min
    d. 40 feet/min

18. Which ISO Class has a maximum of 3520 particles per cubic meter?
    a. ISO Class 5
    b. ISO Class 6
    c. ISO Class 7
    d. ISO Class 8

19. What is the maximum temperature for compounding sterile preparations?
    a. 68°F or cooler
    b. 70°F or cooler
    c. 72°F or cooler
    d. 74°F or cooler

20. A pharmacy technician is compounding a sterile preparation. What is the maximum humidity of the compounding area to prevent microbial growth?
    a. Less than 60%
    b. Less than 65%
    c. Less than 70%
    d. Less than 75%

21. How often must sterile compounding equipment be recertified?
    a. Every 3 months
    b. Every 4 months
    c. Every 6 months
    d. Every 12 months

22. Under which ISO Class condition must viable air sampling be performed?
    a. ISO Class 3
    b. ISO Class 4

    c. ISO Class 5
    d. All the above

23. What is the minimum inflow velocity of a Class II biological cabinet?
    a. 50 feet/min
    b. 75 feet/min
    c. 100 feet/min
    d. 150 feet/min

24. What is the in-use time for a single-dose container prepared in an ISO-5 environment?
    a. 6 hours
    b. 12 hours
    c. 24 hours
    d. 28 days

25. How many categories of compounded sterile preparations (CSPs) have been established under USP <797>?
    a. 2 categories of CSPs
    b. 3 categories of CSPs
    c. 4 categories of CSPs
    d. 6 categories of CSPs

26. What is the minimum number of times a day a controlled temperature area used for compounding sterile products must be monitored?
    a. Once a day
    b. Twice a day
    c. Three times a day
    d. Four times a day

27. What is the minimum frequency that environmental monitoring of temperature be conducted in a sterile compounding area?
    a. Daily
    b. Every 6 hours
    c. Every 12 hours
    d. Weekly

28. How long must hands and forearms be washed with soap and water?
    a. 10 seconds
    b. 15 seconds
    c. 20 seconds
    d. 30 seconds

29. How long must a Class II biological safety cabinet be turned on prior to compounding a sterile preparation?
    a. 10 minutes
    b. 15 minutes
    c. 30 minutes
    d. 45 minutes

30. Prior to entering the buffer area what must be applied to the hands before sterile gloves are donned?
    a. Antiseptic hand cleanser
    b. 70% isopropyl alcohol
    c. Hydrogen peroxide
    d. Povidone iodine solution

31. After being initially evaluated for aseptic manipulation, what frequency must compounding personnel be reassessed for Category 2 CSPs?
    a. Every 3 months
    b. Every 6 months
    c. Every 9 months
    d. Every 12 months

32. How often must compounding personnel demonstrate their aseptic technique?
    a. Every 3 months
    b. Every 6 months
    c. Every 9 months
    d. Every 12 months
33. A patient is to receive 1 L of normal saline solution at a rate of 125 mL/hour. How long will it take to infuse the liter of normal saline solution?
    a. 0.125 hours
    b. 0.8 hours
    c. 8 hours
    d. 10 hours
34. A patient has been prescribed 1 L of total parenteral nutrition (TPN) to be infused over 10 hours. What is the flow rate for the TPN?
    a. 10 mL/hour
    b. 50 mL/hour
    c. 100 mL/hour
    d. 1000 mL/hour
35. You receive an order to add 44 mEq of sodium chloride to an IV bag. Sodium chloride is available as 4 mEq/mL solution. How many milliliters of sodium chloride will need to be added to IV bag?
    a. 10 mL
    b. 11 mL
    c. 12 mL
    d. 15 mL
36. The physician orders 10 mEq of a medication in 1000 mL of D5W to be infused at 125 mL/hour. If the first bag is hung at 7 a.m., when should the second bag be hung?
    a. 12 p.m.
    b. 3 p.m.
    c. 5 p.m.
    d. 7 p.m.
37. A patient is to receive 1 L of IV 20% fat emulsion over 10 hours using a 15 gtt/mL infusion set. What should the flow rate be set to in the infusion pump in drops per minute?
    a. 2 drops/min
    b. 25 drops/min
    c. 75 drops/min
    d. 1500 drops/min
38. A 1 liter bag of solution containing 20 mEq of KCl is piggybacked into a continuous D10W solution. The infusion rate is 3 mL/min. How many bags will need to be supplied for 24 hours?
    a. 2 bags
    b. 3 bags
    c. 4 bags
    d. 6 bags
39. A patient is to receive 1 L of lactated Ringer's solution over 12 hours. What is the flow rate in milliliters per minute?
    a. 1.38 mL/min
    b. 16.66 mL/min
    c. 33.33 mL/min
    d. 83.33 mL/min
40. What substance is used to sanitize the gloves prior to compounding a sterile preparation?
    a. 70% isopropyl alcohol
    b. 70% rubbing alcohol

c. Hydrogen peroxide
d. Any of the above
41. Which is the proper sequence in removing personal protective equipment after compounding a sterile preparation?
    a. Gloves, goggles/face shield, gown, mask/respirator
    b. Goggles/face shield, mask/respirator, gloves, gown
    c. Gown, gloves, goggles/face shield, mask/respirator
    d. Mask/respirator, goggles/face shield, gown. gloves
42. When cleaning a horizontal laminar airflow workbench how should the flat work surface be cleaned?
    a. Wipe side to side (left to right) from the back to the front
    b. Wipe side to side (right to left) from the back to the front
    c. Wipe side to side (left to right) from the front to the back
    d. Wipe side to side (right to the left) from the back to the front
43. Prior to compounding a sterile preparation using a vertical laminar flow workbench, which is the minimum amount of time that 70% isopropyl alcohol remain on the disinfected areas?
    a. 15 seconds
    b. 30 seconds
    c. 45 seconds
    d. 60 seconds
44. Which of the following is considered a critical site?
    a. Needle
    b. Needle hub
    c. Syringe plunger
    d. All the above
45. Which substance should be used to clean the critical site of a vial?
    a. Alcohol-based hand rub
    b. 70% isopropyl alcohol swab
    c. 70% rubbing alcohol swab
    d. Soap and water
46. The pharmacy technician is performing a straight draw into a vial. At what angle should the bevel of the needle be inserted into the center of the rubber stopper?
    a. 30°
    b. 45°
    c. 60°
    d. 75°
47. Under which ISO Class environment should the pharmacy technician withdraw fluid from an ampule?
    a. Class 5
    b. Class 6
    c. Class 7
    d. Class 8
48. At what point should a sharps container be disposed?
    a. Sharps container should be disposed of when it is 50% full.
    b. Sharps container should be disposed of when it is 60% full.
    c. Sharps container should be disposed of when it is 75% full.
    d. Sharps container should be disposed of when it is 90% full.

49. What is the minimum time a pharmacy must maintain a compounding record of a medication?
    a. 1 year from the date the medication was prepared
    b. 2 years from the date the medication was prepared
    c. 3 years from the date the medication was prepared
    d. 4 years from the date the medication was prepared
50. Which information is required on a Medication Formulation Record?
    a. Assigned internal identification number (e.g., prescription or order number)
    b. Beyond-use date and storage requirements
    c. Date and time of preparation
    d. All the above
51. What information is required on a compounding record?
    a. Information to describe the compounding process and to ensure it is repeatable
    b. Reference source to support the stability of CSP
    c. Vendor, lot number, and expiration date for each component for the CSP
    d. All the above
52. Which component of a total parenteral nutrition provides nitrogen, which is necessary to using proteins in the body?
    a. Amino acids
    b. Dextrose
    c. Fats
    d. All the above
53. Which of the following concentrations of dextrose is available to compound a TPN?
    a. 10%
    b. 20%
    c. 30%
    d. 50%
54. Which TPN additive maintains the appropriate pH of body fluids in the body?
    a. Calcium
    b. Chloride
    c. Magnesium
    d. Phosphate
55. Which is the last component to be added to a TPN?
    a. Additives
    b. Amino acids
    c. Dextrose
    d. Fats
56. Which additive should be added first to a TPN admixture?
    a. Calcium
    b. Chloride
    c. Phosphate
    d. Potassium
57. A pharmacy has received an order to compound an ophthalmic solution. What should the pH be of the ophthalmic solution?
    a. 5.4
    b. 6.4
    c. 7.4
    d. 8.4
58. When compounding a sterile product from a nonsterile component, which sterilization method may be used?
    a. Dry heat
    b. Filtration
    c. Steam
    d. All the above
59. Which is an example of TPN additive?
    a. Ca gluconate
    b. Multivitamins parenteral
    c. Multiple trace elements
    d. All the above
60. The pharmacy technician is compounding a TPN for an adult patient. How much dextrose should the TPN contain?
    a. 10 to 30 kcal/kg per day
    b. 30 to 45 kcal/kg per day
    c. 45 to 60 kcal/kg per day
    d. 60 to 75 kcal/kg per day
61. For a pharmacy to be compliant with USP <797>, what written documentation must be maintained by the facility?
    a. Biennial inventory documentation
    b. Master Formulation Records and Compounding Records
    c. State Board of Pharmacy inspections
    d. All the above
62. By what means may a pharmacy dispose of a sharps container?
    a. Dispose of the sharps container with regular pharmacy trash.
    b. Drop off the sharps container at a supervised collection site.
    c. Utilize a sharps container mail back program.
    d. All the above
63. Which is a characteristic of a sharps disposal container?
    a. Able to close with a loose-fitting, puncture-resistant lid
    b. Made of glass
    c. Properly labeled to warn of hazardous waste inside the container
    d. All the above
64. What is the maximum number of particles per cubic meter of air in an ISO Class 7 environment?
    a. 3520
    b. 35,200
    c. 352,000
    d. 3,520,000
65. What is the tonicity of an ophthalmic solution?
    a. Between 0.6% and 2%
    b. Between 2% and 4%
    c. Between 4% and 6%
    d. Between 6% and 7.4
66. Which compounded sterile preparation is administered intrathecally?
    a. Epidural
    b. Irrigation solution
    c. Nasal solution
    d. Ophthalmic solution
67. Which term refers to the absorption process where there is a separation of oil in water in an emulsion?
    a. Aggregation
    b. Cracking
    c. Creaming
    d. Separation

68. Which is the maximum batch size for CSPs requiring a sterility test?
    a. 100 units
    b. 150 units
    c. 200 units
    d. 250 units
69. Which standards must be followed when compounding a hazardous nonsterile preparation?
    a. USP <795>
    b. USP <797>
    c. USP <800>
    d. Both a and c
70. Which of the following is a classification of a hazardous drug?
    a. Antineoplastic drug
    b. Drugs with reproductive risks for men or women
    c. Nonantineoplastic drugs
    d. All the above
71. How often must chemotherapy gloves be changed by individuals receiving or stocking hazardous drugs?
    a. Every 30 minutes
    b. Every hour
    c. Every 2 hours
    d. Every 4 hours
72. How often must an individual handling hazardous drugs change their gown?
    a. Every 30 minutes
    b. Every hour

c. Every 2–3 hours
d. Every 3–4 hours
73. How often must an individual be assessed on their handling of hazardous drugs?
    a. At least every 6 months
    b. At least every 12 months
    c. At least every 2 years
    d. At least every 3 years
74. Which of the following must be contained in a spill kit?
    a. National Institute for Occupational Safety and Health-approved respirator
    b. Shoe covers
    c. Sterile gloves
    d. All the above
75. A facility must maintain a list of all hazardous drugs and must include any items on the current list published by the National Institute of Occupational Safety and Health. How often must a facility review this list?
    a. Quarterly
    b. Semiannually
    c. Annually
    d. Biennially

Chapter 2 Hazardous Drug Management

1. An antineoplastic hazardous drug must be stored in an externally ventilated, negative pressure room with a minimum of how many air changes per hour (ACPH)?
   a. 12
   b. 14
   c. 16
   d. 18

2. Under which condition(s) must a pharmacy technician unpack antineoplastic hazardous drugs (HDs) and all hazardous drug active pharmaceutical ingredients?
   a. Neutral/normal pressure areas relative to the surrounding areas
   b. Negative pressure areas relative to the surrounding areas
   c. Positive pressure areas relative to the surrounding areas
   d. Both a and b

3. What is the minimum inflow velocity for either a Class II Type B1 or Class II Type B2 biological safety cabinets?
   a. 75 feet/min
   b. 100 feet/min
   c. 125 feet/min
   d. 150 feet/min

4. What is the minimum inflow velocity for a Class I biological safety cabinet?
   a. 75 feet/min
   b. 100 feet/min
   c. 125 feet/min
   d. 150 feet/min

5. Which Class II biological safety cabinet (BSC) may be used in compounding both volatile toxic chemicals and radionucleotides under no special conditions?
   a. Type A1
   b. Type A2
   c. Type B1
   d. Type B2

6. A pharmacy technician is working with infectious microbiological agents. Under which BSC should the work be performed?
   a. Class I BSC
   b. Class II Type B1 BSC
   c. Class II Type B2 BSC
   d. Class III BSC

7. Which of the following is a requirement for a containment secondary engineering control used in compounding sterile and nonsterile hazardous preparations?
   a. Be internally vented
   b. Have a minimum of 20 air changes per hour
   c. Have a negative pressure
   d. The washing sink must be at least 2 meters from the containment primary engineering control (C-PEC)

8. Which standard address handling hazardous drugs?
   a. USP <795>
   b. USP <797>
   c. USP <800>
   d. USP <1160>

9. What is the minimum number of ACPH of high-efficiency particulate air-filtered air for a buffer room in an ISO Class 7 environment?
   a. 10 ACPH
   b. 12 ACPH
   c. 20 ACPH
   d. 30 ACPH

10. When manipulating nonsterile hazardous drugs which USP standards must be followed?
    a. USP <795>
    b. USP <797>
    c. USP <798>
    d. USP <800>

11. Which Class II biological safety cabinet is NOT suitable when using toxic chemicals and volatile radionucleotides?
    a. Type A1
    b. Type A2
    c. Type B1
    d. Type B2

12. Which process results in the inhibition or destruction of microorganisms?
    a. Cleaning
    b. Deactivation
    c. Decontamination
    d. Disinfection

13. Which is an example C-PEC used in nonsterile compounding of hazardous drugs?
    a. Class I BSC
    b. Containment ventilated enclosure
    c. Compounding aseptic containment isolator (CACI)
    d. All the above

14. A pharmacy technician has been asked to deactivate a hazardous drug contaminant by decontaminating the surface. Which substance should be used?
    a. Sterile alcohol
    b. Sodium hypochlorite
    c. Sodium thiosulfate
    d. Sterile water

15. How often must decontamination be performed?
    a. Daily
    b. Every other day
    c. Weekly
    d. Biweekly

16. Which substance should be used when disinfecting an area?
    a. Sterile alcohol
    b. Sodium hypochlorite
    c. Sodium thiosulfate
    d. Sterile water

17. Which personal protective equipment must be worn when using cleaning agents where splashing may occur?
    a. Disposable gown
    b. Double chemotherapy gloves
    c. Eye protection
    d. All the above

18. An individual has been exposed to a hazardous drug. Which of the following will affect the severity of the exposure?
    a. Drug's potency
    b. Drug's toxicity
    c. Route of exposure
    d. All the above

19. Which of the following does the National Institute for Occupational Safety and Health (NIOSH) recommend for preventing health care worker exposure to hazardous drugs?
    a. Conduct weekly training reviews with all potentially exposed workers in workplaces where hazardous drugs are used.
    b. Establish procedures and provide training for handling hazardous drugs safely, cleaning up spills, and using all equipment and personal protective equipment (PPE) properly.
    c. Implement a program for safely handling hazardous drugs at work and review this program every week on the basis of the workplace evaluation.
    d. All the above

20. Which of the following can be done to prevent employee exposure to hazardous drugs?
    a. Use open-system drug transfer devices.
    b. Use unventilated cabinets.
    c. Wear PPEs.
    d. All the above.

21. Which of the following should be done after an individual has been exposed to hazardous medications?
    a. Have the individual undergo a psychological examination.
    b. Have the individual visit their family doctor to document and confirm complete documentation.
    c. Obtain urine samples for baseline counts after exposure.
    d. Refer to the hazardous medication's safety data sheet and decontaminate according to instructions.

22. What is the first thing one should do when a hazardous drug spill occurs?
    a. Assess the size and scope of the spill.
    b. Don appropriate PPEs to include gloves and respirator.
    c. Obtain the spill kit and respirator.
    d. Post signs to limit access to spill area.

23. How often must reusable PPEs be decontaminated and cleaned?
    a. After being used one time
    b. After being used two times
    c. After being used three times
    d. After being used four times

24. When should double chemotherapy gloves be worn?
    a. Double chemotherapy gloves should be worn when handling shipping drug cartons or drug vials of hazardous drugs.
    b. Double chemotherapy gloves should be worn when handling hazardous drug waste.
    c. Double chemotherapy gloves should be worn when handling waste from patients recently treated with hazardous drugs.
    d. All the above.

25. How often should a gown be changed when handling hazardous drugs assuming a spill or splash has not occurred, and no permeation information is provided?
    a. Every 30 minutes
    b. Every 2–3 hours
    c. Every 4–5 hours
    d. Every 6–8 hours

26. Which is appropriate protective outerwear to wear when handling a hazardous drug?
    a. Cloth laboratory coat
    b. Disposable gown
    c. Isolation gown
    d. Surgical scrubs

27. All of the following provide respiratory protection from drug exposure *except* which one?
    a. Full facepiece, chemical cartridge-type respirator
    b. NIOSH-certified respirator
    c. Surgical N95 respirator
    d. Surgical mask

28. The pharmacy technician is withdrawing a subcutaneous injection from a vial in a controlled device. Which personal protective equipment must be worn?
    a. Double chemotherapy gloves
    b. Eye/face protection
    c. Protective gown
    d. Both a and c

29. Which form of respiratory protection provides a barrier to splashes, droplets, and sprays around the nose and mouth?
    a. An appropriate full-facepiece, chemical cartridge-type respirator or powered air-purifying respirator
    b. A NIOSH-certified N95 respirator
    c. A surgical mask
    d. A surgical N95 respirator

30. Which regulation(s) determine the disposal of personal protective equipment?
    a. Local regulations
    b. State regulations
    c. Federal regulations
    d. All the above

31. What type of environment must antineoplastic hazardous drugs on the current NIOSH hazardous drug list be unpacked?
    a. Negative pressure relative to the surrounding area
    b. Negative pressure or neutral/normal pressure relative to the surrounding areas
    c. Neutral/normal pressure relative to the surrounding areas
    d. Positive pressure relative to the surrounding areas

32. What type of training must an individual undergo prior to transporting a hazardous drug for the first time?
    a. Cardiopulmonary resuscitation training
    b. First aid training
    c. Spill control training
    d. All the above

33. What information must appear on a hazardous drug label/accessory labeling for when transporting a hazardous drug?
    a. Disposal instructions
    b. Hazardous drug category information
    c. Storage instructions
    d. All the above

34. Which regulations must be followed when transporting a hazardous drug?
    a. Local regulations
    b. State regulations
    c. Federal regulations
    d. All the above

35. If a shipping container of hazardous drugs appears damaged, which action(s) should be done?
    a. Seal the container without opening and contact the supplier.
    b. Enclose the unopened package of hazardous drugs in a pervious container and label the outer container as "Hazardous."
    c. If the supplier will not accept the return, contact NIOSH.
    d. All the above.
36. What type of environment must hazardous drug waiting to be returned be stored?
    a. Negative pressure environment
    b. Neutral pressure environment
    c. Positive pressure environment
    d. Any of the above
37. How many criteria must a drug meet to be identified as hazardous or potentially hazardous?
    a. One
    b. Two
    c. Three
    d. Six
38. Which pharmacy activity requires pharmacy personnel to wear a double pair of chemotherapy gloves?
    a. Preparing and dispensing a hazardous drug in a BSC or CACI
    b. Receiving/unpacking a hazardous drug
    c. Storing a hazardous drug
    d. Transporting a hazardous drug
39. Which PPEs must an individual wear when withdrawing and/or mixing an intravenous solution from a vial or ampule?
    a. Only double chemotherapy gloves
    b. Only double chemotherapy gloves and protective gown
    c. Only double chemotherapy gloves, protective gown and eye/face protection
    d. Double chemotherapy gloves, protective gown, eye/face protection, and respiratory protection
40. Which medication contains manufacturer's special handling information (MSHI) in the package insert and/or meets the NIOSH definition of hazardous drug and are classified by the National Toxicology Program (NTP) as a "human carcinogen" and /or classified by the International Agency for Research on Cancer (IARC) as "carcinogenic" or "probably carcinogenic"?
    a. Abacavir
    b. Estrogen
    c. Fluorouracil
    d. Methimazole
41. Which dosage form requires a nurse to wear double chemotherapy gloves when administering the medication to a patient?
    a. Capsule
    b. Prefilled syringe
    c. Topical medication
    d. All the above
42. Which dosage form requires the administrator to wear a protective gown when being administered to the patient?
    a. Capsule
    b. Injector
    c. Oral liquid drug
    d. Tablet

43. Which drug meets the NIOSH definition of a hazardous drug but are not drugs that have MSHI or are classified by the NTP or classified by the IARC?
    a. Azathioprine
    b. Conjugated estrogens
    c. Tamoxifen
    d. Warfarin
44. Which medication contains MSHI in the package insert and/or meets the NIOSH definition of a hazardous drug and are classified by the NTP or classified by the IARC?
    a. Anastrozole
    b. Clomiphene
    c. Cyclophosphamide
    d. Divalproex
45. According to the NIOSH, which term refers to fertility impairment in humans?
    a. Carcinogenicity
    b. Genotoxicity
    c. Reproductive toxicity
    d. Teratogenicity
46. Which organization is responsible for enforcing the Resource Conservation and Recovery Act regulations?
    a. Drug Enforcement Administration
    b. Environmental Protection Agency
    c. FDA
    d. USP
47. According to USP <800> how often should environmental wipe sampling be conducted?
    a. At least every 3 months
    b. At least every 6 months
    c. At least every 9 months
    d. At least every 12 months
48. Which medication is included on the P list of hazardous waste?
    a. Cyclophosphamide
    b. Lindane
    c. Nitroglycerin
    d. Selenium sulfide
49. A facility that handles hazardous drugs must have a Hazard Communication Program. Which is a requirement of a Hazard Communication Plan?
    a. Access to areas where hazardous drugs/substances are being handled must be unrestricted.
    b. Each hazardous drug/substance used in the facility must have a safety data sheet for the drug/chemical.
    c. Hazardous drug/substance handling areas must be located close to patient area.
    d. Personnel of reproductive capability must undergo a pregnancy test prior to handling hazardous drugs or substances.
50. When compounding hazardous drugs how often should gloves be changed under normal conditions?
    a. Every 15 minutes
    b. Every 30 minutes
    c. Every 45 minutes
    d. Every 60 minutes
51. Which of the following is (are) involved in a medical surveillance program for a comprehensive control program?
    a. Assessing and documenting a health care worker's symptoms associated with a hazardous drug
    b. Assessing and documenting a health care worker's physical findings associated with a hazardous drug

c. Assessing and documenting a health care worker's laboratory values associated with a hazardous drug
d. All the above

52. Which USP standard(s) defines the criteria for a medication surveillance program?
a. USP <795>
b. USP <797>
c. USP <800>
d. All the above

53. What color chemotherapy waste bags should be used for soft trace items such as needles, empty vials and syringes, gloves, gowns, and tubing be disposed?
a. Blue
b. Green
c. Red
d. Yellow

54. Which of the following must be contained in a hazardous drug spill kit?
a. Adsorbent chemotherapy pads and towels
b. Metal scraper
c. NIOSH-approved respirator mask
d. All the above

55. Which topic(s) must be addressed during hazardous drug training?
a. Known or suspected HD exposure
b. Proper use of PPEs
c. Spill management procedures
d. All the above

Chapter 3 Regulatory Compliance

1. Which regulatory agency is responsible for protecting the public health by guaranteeing the safety, efficacy and security of our drug supply?
   a. Centers of Medicare and Medicaid Services (CMS)
   b. Drug Enforcement Administration (DEA)
   c. Environmental Protection Agency (EPA)
   d. FDA

2. Which form of Medicare provides for prescription medications, biologicals, insulin, vaccines, and select medical supplies?
   a. Medicare Part A
   b. Medicare Part B
   c. Medicare Part C
   d. Medicare Part D

3. A pharmacy technician has a question regarding sterile compounding standard. Which USP standard should they refer?
   a. USP <795>
   b. USP <797>
   c. USP <800>
   d. USP <825>

4. Which governmental agency is responsible for developing Patient Package Inserts (PPIs)?
   a. CMS
   b. DEA
   c. EPA
   d. FDA

5. Which term(s) refers to practices that, directly or indirectly, result in unnecessary costs to the Medicare program?
   a. Abuse
   b. Fraud
   c. Waste
   d. Both a and c

6. Which government organization(s) is responsible for issuing specific conditions regarding the storage and transportation of hazardous waste?
   a. Department of Transportation
   b. EPA
   c. FDA
   d. Both a and b

7. Who may use a hospital's DEA registration number in prescribing controlled substances?
   a. Hospital resident
   b. Physician's assistant
   c. Staff physician
   d. All the above

8. Which is an example of a Schedule IV controlled substance medication?
   a. Alprazolam
   b. Benzphetamine
   c. Diphenoxylate/atropine
   d. Meperidine

9. Which of the following controlled substance schedules has no accepted medical use in the United States?
   a. Schedule I
   b. Schedule II
   c. Schedule III
   d. Schedule IV

10. Which DEA Form is known as a Certificate of Registration?
    a. DEA Form 222
    b. DEA Form 223
    c. DEA Form 224
    d. DEA Form 224a

11. Which government agency is responsible for overseeing standards of the Health Insurance Portability and Accountability Act standards?
    a. CMS
    b. DEA
    c. FDA
    d. EPA

12. Which federal legislation defined adulteration?
    a. Controlled Substance Act (CSA) of 1970
    b. Food, Drug and Cosmetic Act (FDCA 1938)
    c. Title I Compounding Quality Act
    d. Title II Drug Supply Chain Security Act (DSCSA)

13. Which organization accredits and certifies hospitals and health care organizations that provide ambulatory and office-based surgery, behavioral health, home health care, laboratory, and nursing care center services?
    a. Accreditation Commission for Health Care
    b. Center for Pharmacy Practice Accreditation
    c. The Joint Commission
    d. Utilization Review Accreditation Commission

14. Which is an element of pharmacy accreditation?
    a. Examining generic usage
    b. Examining medication error rates
    c. Examining policies and procedures
    d. All the above

15. Which component(s) of the Health Insurance Portability and Accountability Act (HIPAA) addresses protected health information PHI?
    a. HIPAA Privacy Rule
    b. HIPAA Security Rule
    c. HIPAA Electronic Health Care Transactions and Code Setting Standards
    d. Both a and c

16. Which is an example of protected health information PHI?
    a. Patient's name
    b. Patient's address
    c. Patient's e-mail address
    d. All the above

17. Which of the following would be an example of health care fraud?
    a. Billing for nonexistent prescriptions
    b. Prescribing unnecessary prescriptions
    c. Unknowingly billing for brand name drugs when generics are dispensed
    d. Both b and c

18. Which of the following is a labeling requirement that must appears on a prescription medication's packaging?
    a. Inactive ingredients
    b. National Drug Code number
    c. "Use" or "Uses," followed by the medication's indication(s)
    d. "Warning" or "Warnings" and "Do not use" followed by all contraindications for use with the product

19. Which legislation requires a drug manufacturer and repackagers to put a unique product identifier on certain prescription drug packages, such as a bar code that can be easily read electronically?
    a. CSA of 1970
    b. FDCA 1938
    c. HIPAA
    d. Title II DSCSA
20. Which of the following are eligible to receive Medicare benefits?
    a. Adult patients over the age of 60 years of age
    b. Adult patients with end-stage renal disease
    c. Patients with disabilities
    d. All the above
21. Which form of Medicare is also known as Medicare Advantage?
    a. Medicare Part A
    b. Medicare Part B
    c. Medicare Part C
    d. Medicare Part D
22. Which organization is responsible for responsible for overseeing pharmacy security requirements?
    a. CMS
    b. Drug Enforcement Administration (DEA)
    c. EPA
    d. FDA
23. Which organization is responsible for overseeing the handling of substances which may be ignitable, corrosive, reactive, or toxic?
    a. CMS
    b. DEA
    c. EPA
    d. FDA
24. Which drug recall is classified when a product that might cause a temporary health problem or pose slight threat of a serious nature?
    a. Class I
    b. Class II
    c. Class III
    d. Class IV
25. Which term is synonymous to "black box warning"?
    a. Boxed Warning
    b. Instructions for Use
    c. Medication Guide
    d. PPI
26. Which organization is responsible for the use and disposal or radioactive materials?
    a. DEA
    b. EPA
    c. FDA
    d. Nuclear Regulatory Commission
27. Which term refers to a label which draws attention to serious or life-threatening risks?
    a. Boxed Warning
    b. Drug Monograph
    c. Instructions for Use
    d. Medication Guides
28. Which organization is responsible for supervising Risk Evaluation and Mitigation Strategy?
    a. CMS
    b. DEA
    c. FDA
    d. EPA

29. Which is established by an authority as a point of reference?
    a. Law
    b. Regulation
    c. Standard
    d. Statute
30. Which term is synonymous for statute?
    a. Act
    b. Law
    c. Regulation
    d. Standard
Rationale: a. An act is also known as a statute. A law or regulation is not synonymous with statute.
31. Which organization certifies pharmacy technicians?
    a. American Pharmacists Association
    b. American Society of Health System Pharmacists
    c. Pharmacy Technician Certification Board
    d. Both a and c
32. Which term refers to a legal document attesting that an individual meets certain objectives standards usually provided by a neutral professional organization?
    a. Certification
    b. Licensure
    c. Registration
    d. Reciprocation
33. Which legislation changed the federal legend on a prescription to "Rx" only?
    a. Pure Food and Drug Act of 1906
    b. Durham-Humphrey Amendment to FDCA of 1951
    c. Kefauver-Harris Amendment to FDCA of 1962
    d. FDA Modernization Act of 2003
34. Which legislation assigned an 11-digit to each medication?
    a. Drug Listing Act of 1972
    b. Medicare Modernization Act of 2003
    c. FDA Modernization Act of 2003
    d. Patient Protection and Affordable Care Act of 2010
35. Which form is issued by a reverse distributor when a pharmacy transfers schedule II controlled to the reverse distributor?
    a. DEA Form 41
    b. DEA Form 106
    c. DEA Form 107
    d. DEA Form 222
36. What is the maximum day supply of isotretinoin that may be dispensed at one time?
    a. 30 days
    b. 45 days
    c. 60 days
    d. 90 days
37. A patient is diagnosed with multiple myeloma. What is the maximum number of days' supply of Thalomid that may be prescribed?
    a. 14 days
    b. 28 days
    c. 42 days
    d. 56 days
38. When must a Medication Guide be provided to a patient?
    a. When the patient or the patient's agent requests a Medication Guide
    b. Whenever a drug is dispensed to a health care professional for administration to a patient in an outpatient setting

c. Whenever a drug is dispensed in an outpatient setting of any kind and the medication will them be used by the patient with direct supervision by a health care professional

d. All the above

39. Which of the following medications requires a Medication Guide be given to a patient?
a. Alendronate
b. Amoxicillin
c. Furosemide
d. Losartan

40. Which legislation requires Medication Guides be provided to patients?
a. Food, Drug and Cosmetic Act of 1938
b. Occupational Safety and Health Act of 1970
c. Poison Prevention Packaging Act of 1970
d. Omnibus Budget Reconciliation Act of 1990

41. Which of the following drug classifications require a patient product insert be provided to a patient?
a. Angiotensin-converting enzyme inhibitors
b. Loop diuretics
c. Macrolide antibiotics
d. Oral contraceptives

42. How often must a pharmacy technician who performs nonsterile compounding demonstrate their knowledge competency in hand hygiene, garbing, cleaning/sanitizing and documenting Master Formulation Records and compounding records (CR)?
a. Every 6 months
b. Every 12 months
c. Every 2 years
d. Every 3 years

43. How often must a pharmacy technician who compounds both Category 1 and 2 sterile products must demonstrate their competency in aseptic technique?
a. Every 6 months
b. Every 12 months
c. Every 2 years
d. Every 3 years

44. How often must a pharmacy technician demonstrate their competency in handling hazardous drugs?
a. Every 6 months
b. Every 12 months
c. Every 2 years
d. Every 3 years

45. A pharmacy is being audited for an administrative inspection by the DEA. Which pharmacy record(s) may be reviewed?
a. Dispensing records
b. Drug destruction records
c. Drug receiving records
d. All the above

46. How often must pharmacy personnel who compound Category 3 compounded sterile preparations (CSPs) undergo aseptic manipulation competency testing?
a. Every 3 months
b. Every 6 months
c. Every 9 months
d. Every 12 months

47. Which of the following is (are) a common finding(s) among an administrative inspection by the DEA of a pharmacy?
a. Adhering to "red flags" when dispensing controlled substances
b. Failing to maintain complete and accurate records
c. Running prescription drug monitoring program reports
d. All the above

48. How long must a pharmacy retain the Master Formulation Record and CR be retained for a compounded nonsterile preparation (CNSP)?
a. 1 year
b. 2 years
c. 3 years
d. 7 years

49. Which of the following is only required on the compounding record but not on the master formulation record of a CNSP?
a. Assigned beyond-use date (BUD) and storage requirements
b. Date and time of preparation of the CNSP
c. If applicable, calculations to determine and verify quantities and/or concentrations of components and strength or activity of the API(s)
d. Name, strength or activity, and dosage form of the CNSP

50. Which category of compounded sterile preparation (CSP) requires endotoxin testing?
a. Category 1
b. Category 2
c. Category 3
d. Both b and c

51. Which BUD should be assigned to a Category 3 compounded sterile preparation which has been aseptically processed, sterility tested and stored at controlled room temperature?
a. 30 days
b. 60 days
c. 90 days
d. 120 days

52. How long must an individual wash their hands and forearms up to their elbows with soap and water before compounding a nonsterile preparation?
a. 15 seconds
b. 30 seconds
c. 45 seconds
d. 60 seconds

53. When compounding nonsterile preparations, how often must the work surface be cleaned?
a. At the beginning of each shift
b. At the end of each shift
c. After spills
d. All the above

54. Which of the following factors can affect a CNSP's stability?
a. Drug classification
b. Temperature
c. Time of the year
d. All the above

55. Which BUD should be assigned to an oral suspension of amoxicillin that has been reconstituted?
    a. 14 days
    b. 35 days
    c. 90 days
    d. 180 days
56. Which form of Medicare requires participating pharmacies to implement a continuous quality improvement program?
    a. Medicare Part A
    b. Medicare Part B
    c. Medicare Part C
    d. Medicare Part D
57. Which is the first step in the continuous quality improvement process?
    a. Analyze the problem
    b. Define the current situation
    c. Develop an action plan
    d. Identify a need/issue/problem and develop a problem statement
58. In a "just culture," which term indicates that a mistake was not intended?
    a. Adverse event
    b. At-risk behavior
    c. Human behavior
    d. Reckless behavior
59. Which of the following is (are) an example(s) of a root cause of a medication error?
    a. Human
    b. Manufacturing
    c. Organizational
    d. All the above
60. What type of dispensing error occurs when the pharmacy technician does not provide a medication guide to a patient?
    a. Compliance error
    b. Documentation error
    c. Medication education error
    d. Wrong formulation error
61. The pharmacy technician fails to bring to the attention of the pharmacist that a patient's internationalized normalized ratio has fallen below the therapeutic range identified for the patient by their physician. Which type of medication has occurred?
    a. Adverse drug error
    b. Deteriorated drug error
    c. Monitoring error
    d. Wrong drug preparation error
62. Which organization sponsors National Prescription Drug Take Back events?
    a. Board of Pharmacy
    b. DEA
    c. FDA
    d. Joint Commission
63. The pharmacy technician is taking the temperature of the refrigerator and reads 47 °F. Which term defines this temperature?
    a. Freezer
    b. Cold
    c. Cool
    d. Room temperature

64. Which medication(s) may be flushed down the toilet?
    a. Hydromorphone
    b. Meperidine
    c. Oxycodone
    d. All the above
65. A patient informs the pharmacy technician they suspect they have experienced an adverse event as a result of a medication that they have just been prescribed and have taken. Which form should the pharmacy technician inform the patient to use?
    a. FDA Form 3000
    b. FDA Form 3000B
    c. FDA Form 3500
    d. FDA Form 3500B
66. Which organization has identified and published High-Alert Medications and Classes/Categories of medications that have shown an added risk of substantial harm in error in an acute care setting, community/ambulatory care setting, and long-term care setting?
    a. Board of Pharmacy
    b. FDA
    c. Institute of Safe Medication Practices
    d. Office of Inspector General
67. Under which health care setting(s) have anti-coagulants been identified as a High Alert Drug Class/Category?
    a. Acute care
    b. Community/ambulatory care
    c. Long-term care
    d. All the above
68. Which term refers to a systematic process to identify the causal factors that contributed to the occurrence of a sentinel event that is an unexpected occurrence involving death or serious physical or psychological injury or risk?
    a. Continuous quality improvement
    b. Failure mode effects analysis
    c. Quality assurance
    d. Root cause analysis
69. Which of the following is an example of a wrong drug preparation?
    a. Dispensing a medication that exceeded its BUD
    b. Dispensing atomoxetine 40 mg instead of atorvastatin 40 mg
    c. Dispensing metoprolol tartrate instead of metoprolol succinate when metoprolol succinate was ordered
    d. Using the incorrect diluent when preparing a sterile preparation
70. Which of the following is (are) an effect of dispensing error?
    a. The medication dispensed is contraindicated with other prescription medications prescribed or over-the-counter medications the patient is taking.
    b. The medication has no effect on the patients hepatic function.
    c. The patient receives a therapeutic dose of the prescribed medication.
    d. All the above.

71. A patient demonstrates low health literacy. Which of the following may contribute to an individual's health literacy?
    a. Patient earned a college degree.
    b. Patient has English as a second language.
    c. Patient possesses a high socioeconomic status.
    d. All the above.

72. Levothyroxine should be stored at room temperature. According to the USP, which temperature range is considered room temperature?
    a. 40°F and 48°F
    b. 46°F and 59°F
    c. 56°F and 66°F
    d. 59°F and 86°F

73. Which of the following substance(s) should be mixed with a medication that is to be disposed of in the trash?
    a. Dirt
    b. Cat litter
    c. Coffee grounds
    d. All the above

74. Which is considered a "best practice" when compounding a sterile preparation in a hospital setting?
    a. Follow USP standards for sterile compounding.
    b. Master formulation records are verified by a third individual.
    c. Pharmacy technicians possess a Pharmacy Technician Certification Board certification (Certified Pharmacy Technician).
    d. All the above.

75. Which organization(s) have issued a list of approved generic drug names only using Tall Man Lettering?
    a. DEA
    b. FDA
    c. Institute of Safe Medication Practices
    d. Both b and c

Chapter 4 Controlled Substances Diversion

1. Which of the following may be the result of controlled substance diversion?
   a. Employment opportunities
   b. Financial gains for employers
   c. Positive publicity
   d. Professional licensing/certification suspension or revocation
2. Felix is suspected of being under the influence of a controlled substance at work in the pharmacy. Which of the following is an example of a behavioral sign of a drug impairment?
   a. Blood-shot eyes
   b. Dilated pupils
   c. Mood swings
   d. Significant weight loss
3. Patrice is thought to be under the influence of marijuana. Which of the following is an example of a physical sign of impairment?
   a. Confusion and memory loss
   b. Deterioration in physical appearance
   c. Drowsiness
   d. Relationship problems with coworkers
4. According to the Drug Enforcement Administration (DEA), which of the following is a commonly abused drug classification?
   a. Anabolic steroids
   b. Angiotensin converting enzyme inhibitors
   c. Bronchodilators
   d. Phosphodiesterase 5 inhibitors
5. Which stage of the drug use process would involve removing expired controlled substances from the holding area of the pharmacy?
   a. Administration
   b. Preparation and dispensing
   c. Prescribing
   d. Waste and removal
6. Which of the following is an example of a chain of custody control used by a provider?
   a. Ensuring a valid prescription/medication order exists from an authorized prescriber for all controlled substances prescribed
   b. Transporting controlled substances only by properly trained employees
   c. Using barcode scanning when refilling automated dispensing devices
   d. Utilizing key controls and passwords to access controlled substances
7. Which of the following is an example of drug diversion occurring the procurement of a controlled substance?
   a. Pharmacy staff accepts a verbal order for a controlled substance but does not confirm it with prescriber.
   b. Pharmacy staff diverts the overfill of a multidose vial.
   c. Pharmacy staff removes a controlled substance invoice from their pharmacy records.
   d. Pharmacy staff removes an expired controlled substance from the holding area of the pharmacy awaiting its disposal.

8. Pharmacy personnel are dispensing a controlled setting in a long-term care pharmacy setting. Which of the following is an example of diversion?
   a. Pharmacy staff removes controlled substance waste from an unsecure waste container.
   b. Pharmacy staff removes controlled substances from an automated distribution device for a discharged patient.
   c. Pharmacy staff replaces a controlled substance with another medication while repackaging the medication for a patient.
   d. An unauthorized pharmacy staff orders schedule II-controlled substances on a stolen DEA Form 222.
9. A nurse administers a controlled substance to a patient in the hospital. Which of the following would be an example of diversion during the administration process?
   a. Nurse documents the administration of hydrocodone/acetaminophen to the patient but does not administer it.
   b. Nurse replaces controlled substance waste in a syringe with saline.
   c. Nurse self-prescribes acetaminophen with codeine for themself.
   d. Nurse compromises the product container of a controlled substance.
10. Which of the following is a component of a Controlled Substance Diversion Prevention Program (CSDPP)?
    a. Administrative controls
    b. Core-level controls
    c. Provider-level controls
    d. All the above
11. Institutional policy and procedures should indicate current legal and regulatory requirements involving controlled substances. Which of the following should be addressed under an institution's policies and procedures?
    a. Maintaining controlled substance procurement and disposition records and inventories
    b. Policies and procedures for reporting controlled substance diversion
    c. Self-monitoring practices to prevent, identify, and correct potential fraud, waste, or abuse of controlled substances within the organization
    d. All the above
12. Which of the following is a function performed by CSDPP?
    a. Creating a diversion response team to respond to suspected controlled substance diversion
    b. Developing and implementing polices/procedures addressing access to controlled substances
    c. Providing findings to the respective individuals
    d. Providing training on institutional policies, procedures and regulatory requirements for controlled substances
13. Which of the following is an example of a method used to ensure chain of custody is maintained in a health care facility?
    a. Permitting all health care workers working in a health care facility authorization to access controlled substances
    b. Providing passcodes to enter the pharmacy or opening an automated dispensing device to all employees employed at the health care facility

c. Removing a health care worker's access to controlled substances immediately upon termination from the institution

d. Using non-tamper-proof packaging to permit an individual to access a medication.

14. Which pharmacy practice would minimize controlled substance diversion in a high-risk pharmacy area?
    a. Conducting a physical inventory of all controlled substances to include outdated and unusable at least every 3 months
    b. Ensuring the pharmacist is responsible for all drugs and controlled substances dispensed and distributed in the health care setting
    c. Increasing controlled drug inventory in surgical suites when a health care pharmacy has a satellite pharmacy
    d. Minimizing satellite pharmacy staffing whenever surgery and procedural areas are staffed

15. Which practice could be implemented in a retail pharmacy to prevent diversion of controlled substances?
    a. Dispersing Schedule II, III, IV, and V controlled substances throughout the pharmacy with noncontrolled substances
    b. Maintaining a perpetual inventory of all scheduled controlled substances and auditing them quarterly
    c. Maximizing the use of temporary user and patient identifiers
    d. Screening potential employees by verifying reference checks and performing drug screening

16. To prevent diversion of controlled substances in a hospital pharmacy, which process could be initiated?
    a. Requiring employee belongings be permitted to be stored in the controlled substance storage area
    b. Utilizing biometric authentication instead of using passwords
    c. Utilizing manufacturer's default code for electronic or keypad locks on cabinets or carts
    d. Verifying controlled substance inventory counts are conducted by two rotating, licensed, or otherwise authorized pharmacy personnel quarterly

17. To make sure that controlled substance returns, and waste are not diverted from the pharmacy which is a best practice to use?
    a. Ensuring a procedure exists for wasting fentanyl and that it adheres to only DEA, FDA, and state-specific guidelines
    b. Involve three witnesses to observe the wasting and documentation of all controlled substances
    c. Requiring controlled substances be wasted within 24 hours to the time of administration of the controlled substance
    d. Segregating expired and unusable controlled substances from other medications and are being monitored until they are returned by a reverse distributor or disposed of properly

18. Which piece of information is required on a controlled substance administration record?
    a. Amount wastes with cosignature
    b. Expiration date
    c. National Drug Code number
    d. Prescriber's name

19. How many individual(s) should count and sign for receipt of controlled substances?
    a. 1
    b. 2
    c. 3
    d. 4

20. Which of the following is an example of a high-risk area in a health care facility?
    a. Anesthesia areas
    b. Emergency departments
    c. Operating areas
    d. All the above

21. Which monitoring and surveillance practice should be implemented to prevent diversion of controlled substances?
    a. Ensure the pharmacy is involved in settling controlled substance discrepancies.
    b. Minimize the number of staff in assisting the pharmacist in surveillance monitoring.
    c. Review automated dispensing device reports every 6 months.
    d. Verify perpetual inventories on a yearly basis.

22. Which of the following practices will help ensure the proper chain of custody of controlled substances?
    a. Transport controlled substances by properly trained employees.
    b. Use administrative personnel to validate the dispensing and receipt of controlled substances.
    c. Utilize generic passcodes in the pharmacy.
    d. Utilize pneumatic tube systems to deliver controlled substances.

23. Best practices utilized to ensure controlled substances are securely stored in a pharmacy should include which of the following?
    a. An employee's access to controlled substances is removed within 1 month upon being terminated and is documented.
    b. Controlled substances should be stored in a locked and secured location and only available to authorized individuals.
    c. Passwords should be used instead of identification and biometric authentication methods.
    d. Pharmacy Technician Certification Board-certified pharmacy technicians should be used to verify monthly controlled substances counts.

24. Which of the following is an appropriate security control measure for a retail pharmacy?
    a. Ensuring the pharmacy department is responsible for approving access to controlled substances and for adding/removing users access to automated dispensing devices
    b. Limiting access to controlled substances in automated dispensing devices to authorized individuals, and an existing process to withdraw their access privileges
    c. Using e-prescribing to remove the opportunity of prescriptions pads being stolen, altered, or forged from a physician's office and being presented at the pharmacy
    d. Verifying controlled substance inventory counts are conducted by two rotating, licensed, or otherwise authorized pharmacy personnel monthly

25. Which of the following is considered a best practice when ordering controlled substances?
   a. A pharmacy technician should reconcile controlled substances received against what is indicated on the invoice and documents receipt.
   b. DEA Controlled Substance Ordering System (CSOS) orders should be acknowledged as being received within 72 hours of placing the order.
   c. Invoices should be reconciled to statements from the wholesaler to ensure all quantities have been received and accounted for.
   d. Ordering and receiving duties should be done by the same individual.

26. It is suspected that controlled substances are being diverted from a high-risk area in a health care facility. Which action should be taken?
   a. Establishing a process for providing an after-hours supply of medications if the satellite pharmacy is not open
   b. Manually inventorying controlled substances located in the automated dispensing device vault monthly by two unlicensed or authorized pharmacy employees
   c. Minimize the staffing of the satellite pharmacy whenever surgery and procedural areas are staffed to minimize payroll expenses.
   d. The lead pharmacy technician being responsible for all drugs and controlled substances dispensed and distributed in the health care setting

27. A pharmacy must be registered with the DEA and possess a state license in order to dispense controlled substances. Which form must be submitted by the pharmacy to register with the DEA?
   a. DEA Form 222
   b. DEA Form 223
   c. DEA Form 224
   d. DEA Form 224a

28. How many numbers does a DEA number contain?
   a. 5
   b. 6
   c. 7
   d. 9

29. What does the letter *F* indicate when it is the first letter of a DEA number?
   a. A practitioner who received their DEA registration number prior to 1985
   b. A practitioner who received their DEA registration number after 1985
   c. A prescriber working under the Department of Defense
   d. A prescriber employed by a Drug Addiction Treatment facility

30. Which of the following DEA numbers is a valid DEA number for a nurse practitioner whose last name is Smith?
   a. AS3525894
   b. MS4525892
   c. NS4525893
   d. PS4525882

31. According to the Controlled Substance Act, how long must a copy of the completed DEA Form 222 be maintained by the pharmacy?
   a. 1 year
   b. 2 years
   c. 5 years
   d. 7 years

32. Upon discovery the pharmacy has been broken into and listed chemicals have been taken. Which document should be used to report the theft of listed chemicals?
   a. DEA Form 41
   b. DEA Form 106
   c. DEA Form 107
   d. DEA Form 222

33. Which is an advantage of the CSOS?
   a. Has a maximum number of 20 line items per order
   b. Has different identification information than what is found a paper DEA Form 222 to avoid confusion between the two systems
   c. Lower transaction costs for the pharmacy due to order accuracy and no paperwork
   d. Permits just-in-time ordering resulting in smaller pharmacy inventories

34. Within how many day(s) after the discovery of the theft or loss of controlled substances does the DEA need to be notified electronically?
   a. 1 day
   b. 2 days
   c. 5 days
   d. 7 days

35. Which controlled substance schedule has the lowest potential of abuse?
   a. Schedule II
   b. Schedule III
   c. Schedule IV
   d. Schedule V

36. Which medication is an example of a Schedule III controlled substance?
   a. Buprenorphine
   b. Lorazepam
   c. Pregabalin
   d. Tramadol

37. The pharmacy is conducting a DEA physical inventory. Which drug schedule requires an actual physical count if the bottle contains less than 1000 tablets or capsules?
   a. Schedule II
   b. Schedule III
   c. Schedule IV
   d. Schedule V

38. What type of inventory indicates the actual quantity of a specific medication on hand at a specific time?
   a. Biennial inventory
   b. Initial inventory
   c. Inventory for damaged substances
   d. Perpetual inventory

39. When must an inventory for newly scheduled control substance be conducted?
   a. On the first day of the month after it has been classified as a controlled substance
   b. On the last day of the month after it has been classified as a controlled substance
   c. On the medication's effective date as a controlled substance
   d. On the date the state board of pharmacy announces the medication is a controlled substance

40. Which of the following is classified as a Schedule Listed Chemical Product (SLCP) according to the Combat Methamphetamine Epidemic Act of 2005 (CMEA)?
    a. Dextromethorphan
    b. Loperamide
    c. Pseudoephedrine
    d. All the above

41. What is the minimum age for an individual to purchase an SLCP?
    a. 16 years of age
    b. 18 years of age
    c. 20 years of age
    d. 21 years of age

42. What is the maximum amount of an SLCP that may be sold in 1 day?
    a. 2.4 g
    b. 3.6 g
    c. 7.5 g
    d. 9 g

43. The letter *M* would be the first letter of a DEA number assigned to which practitioner?
    a. Dentist
    b. Physician
    c. Physician assistant
    d. Psychiatrist

44. Which DEA form is used to record spillage of a controlled substance?
    a. DEA Form 41
    b. DEA Form 106
    c. DEA Form 107
    d. DEA Form 222

45. Which controlled substance schedule is assigned to diphenoxylate/atropine?
    a. Schedule II
    b. Schedule III
    c. Schedule IV
    d. Schedule V

46. Which medication is an example of schedule II-controlled substance?
    a. Acetaminophen with codeine
    b. Hydrocodone with acetaminophen
    c. Tramadol
    d. Zolpidem

47. When does a newly controlled substance need to be inventoried?
    a. On its effective date as a controlled substance
    b. When it has been classified as a controlled substance
    c. When it has been ordered by the pharmacy
    d. All the above

48. Upon discovery of a pharmacy burglary of controlled substances how soon must the local DEA office be notified?
    a. 12 hours
    b. 1 business day
    c. 2 business days
    d. 1 week

49. Which of the following medications is considered an SLCP?
    a. Cetirizine
    b. Diphenhydramine
    c. Ibuprofen
    d. Pseudoephedrine

50. Which is an approved federal document presented by an individual to purchase an SLCP?
    a. Driver's license with photograph
    b. United States passport
    c. Voter's registration card
    d. All the above

51. What is the maximum amount of an SLCP a pharmacy may sell to an individual in 30 days?
    a. 3.6 g
    b. 5 g
    c. 7.5 g
    d. 9 g

52. According to the CMEA of 2005, how long must a pharmacy retain either a paper or electronic log of all purchasers of SLCPs?
    a. 6 months
    b. 1 year
    c. 2 years
    d. 7 years

53. How often must self-certification of all sellers of SLCPs take place?
    a. Every 6 months
    b. Every year
    c. Every 2 years
    d. Every 7 years

54. Where must a pharmacy store SLCPs?
    a. Behind the counter
    b. In a locked cabinet
    c. With the over-the-counter medications
    d. Either a or b

55. Which is a method by which a controlled substance could be diverted?
    a. Documenting waste
    b. Documenting of medications on time
    c. Having associates sign off on wasting medications
    d. Self-prescribing controlled substances by the prescriber

56. Which of the following observation(s) by the pharmacy technician might indicate drug diversion?
    a. Pharmacy staff frequently disappear during their shift.
    b. Pharmacy staff volunteering for overtime or coming to work on their day's off.
    c. Written prescriptions are altered.
    d. All the above.

57. Which surveillance method should the human resources department perform to prevent controlled substance diversion?
    a. Conducting background checks
    b. Documenting training and competency requirements for authorized staff
    c. Ensuring compliance of random drug testing is performed according to institution's policy and procedure manual
    d. All the above

58. In a hospital pharmacy, which of the actions observed by the pharmacy technician might indicate a controlled substance is being diverted?
    a. Creating a verbal order for a controlled substance after it has been verified with the physician
    b. Observing expired controlled substances are accounted for in a secure pharmacy location
    c. Observing no overrides on drug dispensing machines
    d. Replacing controlled substance waste in a syringe with saline

59. Controlled substances can be diverted from a pharmacy's purchase history. Which practice(s) can be implemented to identify diversion based upon changes in purchases?
    a. Comparing noncontrolled substance purchase invoices to noncontrolled substance purchase orders and receipt into the pharmacy's perpetual inventory
    b. Identifying usual peaks in quantity or frequency of controlled substance purchases
    c. Reconciling invoices to statements or wholesale purchase history reports to detect missing invoices
    d. All the above

60. Which practice will help maintain a perpetual inventory of controlled substances on a consistent basis?
    a. Conducting a complete inventory for controlled substances in automated dispensing devices every other week by two authorized health care workers
    b. Counting controlled substance inventory in the pharmacy narcotic vault every other month
    c. Delivering, replenishing, and stocking of controlled substances in patient care areas are performed by authorized pharmacy personnel and require an auditable verification of delivery and receipt
    d. All the above

61. How often should reports be reviewed to monitor controlled substance use in patient care areas?
    a. Monthly
    b. Every 2 months
    c. Quarterly
    d. Biannually

62. Which of the following should be included in surveillance processes of controlled substances?
    a. Defining monitoring and surveillance measures
    b. Establishing threshold of variance requiring action
    c. Establishing surveillance procedures
    d. All the above

63. Which of the following may indicate someone has tampered with a medication?
    a. The flip top of the medication container is present.
    b. The lot numbers on the vial and its box containing the product match.
    c. The metal crimp on the vial is intact.
    d. The product color appears discolored.

64. Which action(s) taken by the pharmacy might prevent medication tampering?
    a. Ensuring medications are kept secure at all times
    b. Monitoring cancelled transactions and returns
    c. Verifying the drug packaging is intact
    d. All the above

65. What action(s) may a pharmacy take to prevent medication tampering in a health care facility?
    a. Ensuring medications are kept secure at all times
    b. Requiring a witness to be present for all inventory counts

c. Storing patient-controlled analgesia keys in a single access compartment in an automated drug cabinet
    d. All the above

66. What action(s) should a pharmacy take if medication tampering has occurred?
    a. Determine if the patient has been harmed as a result of the tampering.
    b. Report the tampering incident to American Society of Health System Pharmacists.
    c. Secure the medication and have it analyzed by the CMS.
    d. All the above.

67. Which of the following patient action(s) may lead the pharmacy staff to suspect the prescription is fraudulent?
    a. A patient alters the original prescription.
    b. A patient engages in "doctor shopping."
    c. A patient using a computer to create prescriptions for nonexistent prescribers.
    d. All the above.

68. Which of the following practices may indicate prescriptions being presented are out of the scope of the practitioner?
    a. A patient receives a 30-day zolpidem 5 mg, and the patient returns 29 days after receiving the initial prescription for a refill.
    b. A prescriber is writing fewer controlled substance prescriptions compared with other practitioners in the community.
    c. Multiple individuals appearing simultaneously with prescriptions from different prescribers,
    d. Noncommunity residents presenting prescriptions from the same prescriber.

69. A prescription for a controlled substance is presented at the pharmacy. Which of the following may cause the pharmacy technician to suspect it may be fraudulent?
    a. The prescription contains quantities consistent with approved medical usage.
    b. The prescription is written using conventional pharmacy abbreviations.
    c. The prescription is written with a dosage consistent with approved medical usage.
    d. The prescription is written using different color inks.

70. Which action(s) may a pharmacy take to prevent fraudulent prescriptions from being presented there?
    a. Checking the date on the prescription to determine if it has been presented within 24 hours of being issued by the prescriber
    b. Contacting the prescriber for verification of all controlled substance prescriptions
    c. Requiring proper identification when a prescription is being picked up
    d. All the above

Chapter 5 Medication History

1. Which term refers to a situation in which a medication should not be given a patient because it may have adverse effects on the patient?
   a. Adverse drug event
   b. Contraindication
   c. Drug allergy
   d. Idiosyncratic reaction

2. Which term refers to a group of substances that are needed for normal cell function, growth, and development?
   a. Dietary supplement
   b. Herbal supplement
   c. Medication
   d. Vitamin

3. Which term refers to the amount of medicine taken at one time?
   a. Dosage form
   b. Dose
   c. Frequency
   d. Route of administration

4. The pharmacy technician is collecting a patient's social history; what would it consist of?
   a. A compilation of filled prescription information to include medication name, dosage, quantity and date filled
   b. A disease, illness, or injury; any physiologic, mental, or psychological condition or disorder the patient experienced
   c. A record of the relationships among family members along with their medical histories
   d. A summary of life-style practices and habits that may have a direct or indirect effect on their health. Life-style practices includes diet, exercise, sexual orientation, level of sexual activity, and occupation. Habits take into consideration use of tobacco, alcohol, and other substances.

5. Which term is synonymous with high blood sugar?
   a. Hyperglycemia
   b. Hyperlipidemia
   c. Hypertension
   d. Hyperthyroidism

6. A patient is reviewing the physician's notes on "My Chart" observes the physician has indicated they are experiencing tachycardia. The patient asks the pharmacy technician what tachycardia is. How should the technician respond?
   a. Temporary failure to breathe
   b. Rapid heart rate
   c. Slow breathing
   d. Slow heart rate

7. A patient asks the pharmacy technician the meaning of *neuralgia*, which appears on the prescription's directions. How should the technician respond?
   a. Neuralgia means bone pain.
   b. Neuralgia means severe pain along a nerve.
   c. Neuralgia means kidney pain.
   d. Neuralgia means painful urination.

8. What is the meaning of dermatitis?
   a. Inflammation of the bronchial membranes
   b. Inflammation of the ear
   c. Joint pain
   d. Skin inflammation

9. The patient asks the pharmacy technician the meaning of the term *rhinitis*, which appears on the prescription's direction. Which is an appropriate response?
   a. *Rhinitis* means intense itching.
   b. *Rhinitis* means inflammation of the tendon.
   c. *Rhinitis* means inflammation of the bladder.
   d. *Rhinitis* means runny nose.

10. Which medical term refers to painful urination?
    a. Anuresis
    b. Dysuria
    c. Glycosuria
    d. Polyuria

11. Which drug classification prevents an irregular heartrate?
    a. Antianginal
    b. Antiarrhythmic
    c. Antispasmodic
    d. Vasodilator

12. Which medical term refers to the inflammation of the eyelids?
    a. Arthritis
    b. Blepharitis
    c. Conjunctivitis
    d. Encephalitis

13. Which term refers to an inflammation of the heart muscle?
    a. Bradycardia
    b. Cardiomyopathy
    c. Endocarditis
    d. Tachycardia

14. Which of the following is harm experienced by a patient as a result of exposure to a medication?
    a. Adverse drug event
    b. Drug intolerance
    c. Idiosyncratic reaction
    d. Medication allergy

15. Which medical term refers to the condition of indigestion?
    a. Diplopia
    b. Dyslexia
    c. Dyspepsia
    d. Dyspnea

16. What type of nonadherence occurs when a new prescription is prescribed for a patient, but the patient fails to obtain the medication?
    a. Intentional medication nonadherence
    b. Primary nonadherence
    c. Secondary nonadherence
    d. Unintentional nonadherence

17. What type of nonadherence occurs when a patient discontinues their therapy early without consulting their physician?
    a. Intentional nonadherence
    b. Primary nonadherence
    c. Secondary nonadherence
    d. Unintentional nonadherence

18. For a patient to be considered adherent, what percent of their prescribed doses must a patient take?
    a. 80%
    b. 85%
    c. 90%
    d. 95%
19. Which of the following is a barrier to medication adherence?
    a. Ability to pay for a patient's medication
    b. Adverse side effects of a medication
    c. Limited health literacy
    d. All the above
20. Which of the following may result from medication non-adherence?
    a. Decreased morbidity
    b. Increased mortality
    c. Unavoidable health care costs
    d. All the above
21. When should a child be administered the *Haemophilus influenzae* (ActHIB) type b vaccine?
    a. At 0, 1–2 months, 6–18 months
    b. At 2, 4, 12–15 months
    c. At 2, 4, 6, 12–15 months
    d. At 2, 4, 6, and 15–18 months, 4–6 years
22. How many dose(s) of Heplisav-B would a 23-year-old patient receive?
    a. 1 dose
    b. 2 doses
    c. 3 doses
    d. 4 doses
23. A 52-year-old adult is to receive the Zoster recombinant (Shingrix) vaccine. How many dose(s) should they receive?
    a. 1 dose
    b. 2 doses
    c. 3 doses
    d. 4 doses
24. The pharmacy technician has been asked to retrieve Hepatitis B from the pharmacy's inventory. Which vaccine should be selected?
    a. ActHIB
    b. Engerix-B
    c. Havrix
    d. Trumenba
25. A 16-year-old patient is scheduled to receive Gardasil 9. How many doses should the patient receive?
    a. 1 dose
    b. 2 doses
    c. 3 doses
    d. 4 doses
26. When should an adult receive their next dose of their tetanus, diphtheria, and pertussis vaccine?
    a. Every year
    b. Every 2 years
    c. Every 5 years
    d. Every 10 years
27. Which vaccine should be administered annually to a patient?
    a. Influenza
    b. Measles, mumps, and rubella
    c. Varicella
    d. Zoster (recombinant)
28. A pediatric patient is to receive a two-dose series of the Bexsero (Meningococcal serotype B) vaccine. When is it the soonest the patient may receive the second dose?
    a. 1 month after the first dose
    b. 2 months after the first dose
    c. 3 months after the first dose
    d. 6 months after the first dose
29. What is the minimum age for a patient to receive the pneumococcal (PCV13) vaccine?
    a. 6 weeks of age
    b. 1 year of age
    c. 2 years of age
    d. 5 years of age
30. After receiving the first dose of the zoster recombinant vaccine for shingles, how long must an adult wait to receive their second dose of this vaccine?
    a. 14 days
    b. 28 days
    c. 1–2 months
    d. 2–6 months
31. How many dose(s) of the varicella vaccine should an adult receive?
    a. 1 dose
    b. 2 doses
    c. 3 doses
    d. 4 doses
32. What is the minimum age for a child to receive their diphtheria, tetanus, and acellular pertussis vaccine?
    a. 2 weeks
    b. 4 weeks
    c. 6 weeks
    d. 8 weeks
33. What type of medication error occurs as a result of the pharmacy scale is not calibrated properly?
    a. Human
    b. Manufacturing
    c. Organizational
    d. Technical
34. Which type of medication error occurs when the pharmacy technician fails to provide to a patient receiving a nonsteroidal anitiinflammatory drug proper educational materials?
    a. Compliance error
    b. Documentation error
    c. Medication education error
    d. Monitoring error
35. Which type of dispensing error occurs as a result of interruptions during critical phase during the dispensing process?
    a. Distraction error
    b. Fear error
    c. Rushed error
    d. Selection error
36. What type of dispensing error occurs when the pharmacy technician does not match the National Drug Code (NDC) number on the manufacturer's bottle with the NDC number on the prescription label?
    a. Capture/habit error
    b. Distraction error
    c. Fear error
    d. Rushed error

37. According to the National Coordinating Council for Medication Error Reporting and Prevention Index for Categorizing Medication Errors, which category is assigned when circumstances have a potential for causing errors?
    a. Category A
    b. Category B
    c. Category C
    d. Category D
38. Which category of medication error results in an error occurring but did not produce harm to the patient?
    a. Category A
    b. Category D
    c. Category H
    d. Category I
39. The pharmacy technician catches an error when the patient is picking up their prescription. Which category of medication error would this be classified as?
    a. Category B
    b. Category C
    c. Category E
    d. Category H
40. Which of the following is (are) a "Right of Patient Safety"?
    a. Drug
    b. Dose
    c. Dosage form
    d. All the above
41. According to the Institute of Safe Medication Practices (ISMP), which abbreviation should never used on a verbal, handwritten or electronic abbreviation?
    a. am
    b. cc
    c. mg
    d. TID
42. Which organization issued an approved list of generic drug names *only* using Tall Man Letters?
    a. FDA
    b. Institute of Safe Medication Practices
    c. The Joint Commission
    d. Both a and b
43. Which pharmacy abbreviation appears on *both* the ISMP "List of Error-Prone Abbreviations, Symbols, and Dose Designations" and the Joint Commission's "Do Not Use" list?
    a. OJ
    b. OS
    c. QOD
    d. UD
44. Which drug name abbreviation appears on both the ISMP "List of Error-Prone Abbreviations, Symbols, and Dose Designations" and the Joint Commission's "Do Not Use" list?
    a. APAP
    b. CPZ
    c. HCTZ
    d. MgSO4
45. According to the ISMP, which abbreviation has a contradictory abbreviation?
    a. A
    b. B
    c. J
    d. O

46. Which of the following processes may a health care organization to reduce the potential errors involving look-alike and sound-alike medications?
    a. Configure computer selection screens to prevent look-alike names from appearing consecutively.
    b. Include the purpose of the medication on prescriptions.
    c. Use both brand and generic drug names on prescriptions and labels.
    d. All the above.
47. Which of the following is a patient requirement to follow their medication regimen?
    a. Being able to read medication literature provided by the pharmacy and understand the literature
    b. Being able to listen to the pharmacist or pharmacy technician attentively when picking up their prescription
    c. Being able to communicate to the pharmacist or pharmacy technician when picking up their prescription
    d. All the above
48. Which of the following patient actions might alert the pharmacy technician the patient may have low health literacy?
    a. The patient fills out completely medical and pharmacy forms.
    b. The patient refills their chronic medications on time.
    c. The patient refers to their medications by shapes and colors.
    d. All the above.
49. Which of the following might indicate the patient lacks health literacy skills?
    a. The patient avoids reading printed medication materials when in front of a pharmacist.
    b. The patient mispronounces words.
    c. The patient uses a child to interpret what the pharmacist is saying when counseling the patient.
    d. All the above.
50. Which of the following may be the result patient nonadherence?
    a. Avoidable health care costs
    b. Decreased morbidity
    c. Decreased mortality
    d. All the above
51. Polypharmacy refers to a patient being prescribed a minimum of how many medications?
    a. 3 medications
    b. 5 medications
    c. 7 medications
    d. 10 medications
52. The pharmacist is discussing the various types of polypharmacy with their pharmacy technician. What is the maximum number of medications a patient would be taking to be classified as "no polypharmacy"?
    a. 0 medications
    b. 1 medication
    c. 3 medications
    d. 4 medications
53. What is the minimum number of medications a patient would be taking concurrently for the term "excessive polypharmacy" to be applicable?
    a. 8 medications
    b. 10 medications
    c. 12 medications
    d. 15 medications

54. Which of the following is a risk factor for polypharmacy?
   a. A patient experiencing being treated for one condition by one physician
   b. A 21-year-old patient being treated for influenza symptoms
   c. A patient using multiple pharmacies to fill their prescriptions
   d. All the above
55. One of the concerns of polypharmacy is the development of adverse drug effects ADEs. Which drug classification is associated with preventable ADEs?
   a. Angiotensin-converting enzyme inhibitors
   b. Biguanides
   c. Thiazide diuretics
   d. All the above
56. Which of the following situations may contribute to polypharmacy for a patient?
   a. A patient being treated for chronic mental health conditions
   b. A patient being treated for multiple conditions by the same physician
   c. A patient using the same pharmacy location to fill all of their medications
   d. All the above
57. Which patient action may occur as a result of high medication costs?
   a. Patients may skip doses.
   b. Patients may not refill their prescriptions.
   c. Patients may seek low-cost alternative therapies.
   d. All the above
58. As a patient ages, the risk of adverse drug reactions increase as a changes in which of the following?
   a. Pharmacognosy
   b. Pharmacokinetics
   c. Pharmacogenomics
   d. Pharmacodynamics
59. Which of the following can affect a patient's health literacy?
   a. Access to health care
   b. Differences in a patient's education
   c. Medication cost
   d. Patient's gender
60. Which is a strategy a health care organization can implement to reduce the risk of potential medication errors involving look-alike and sound-alike medications?
   a. Configure computer screens to prevent looking-alike names from appearing consecutively.
   b. Ensure the appearance of look-alike medication names are consistent in appearance.
   c. Include the three primary indications of the medication on the prescription.
   d. Utilize generic names only on prescription labels only.
61. Which organization has developed a list additional drug names with recommendations of the placement of tall man letters and is not approved by the FDA?
   a. American Pharmacists Association
   b. American Society of Health System Pharmacists
   c. ISMP
   d. TJC

62. Which of the following are strategies the FDA utilizes in distinguishing look-alike drug names?
   a. Adhere to CD3 rule.
   b. Capitalize like letters of similar drug names.
   c. Utilize boldfacing to draw awareness to similarities between look-alike drug names.
   d. All the above.
63. Which of the following are practices employed by the ISMP to distinguish similar medication names?
   a. Brand names start with a lowercase letter.
   b. Generic names stat with an uppercase letter.
   c. Brand names appear in black and generic names/ other products appear in red.
   d. All the above.
64. Which system of measurement should be used with liquid volumes?
   a. Apothecary
   b. Avoirdupois
   c. Household
   d. Metric
65. Which organization established the "do not use" list of abbreviations?
   a. FDA
   b. ISMP
   c. TJC
   d. All the above
66. A pharmacy technician pulls a bottle of lisinopril 20 mg instead of lisinopril 10 mg for a patient's prescription. Which type of error is this?
   a. Human
   b. Manufacturing
   c. Organizational
   d. Technical
67. Which abbreviation appears *only* on the ISMP's Error-Prone Abbreviations, Symbols and Dose Designation List?
   a. AD, AS, AU
   b. Q.O.D., QOD, q.o.d., or qod
   c. IU
   d. U
68. A pillbox can hold up to how many days of medication doses?
   a. 14 days
   b. 21 days
   c. 28 days
   d. 35 days
69. According to the TJC, what is the minimum number of identifiers that should be provided by the patient prior to administering point of care testing?
   a. 2
   b. 3
   c. 4
   d. 5
70. According to the TJC, all the following are acceptable patient identifiers *except* which one?
   a. The individual's medical record number
   b. The individual's name
   c. The individual's social security number
   d. The individual's telephone number

Chapter 6 Medication Therapy Management

1. A patient is diagnosed with a cardiovascular condition. Which drug classification might be prescribed by their physician?
   a. Angiotensin II receptor antagonists
   b. Antihistamine
   c. Bronchodilator
   d. Proton pump inhibitor

2. Which body system would an anticoagulant be prescribed to treat?
   a. Cardiovascular
   b. Circulatory
   c. Endocrine
   d. Respiratory

3. What unit of measurement will be used in administering lantus insulin?
   a. IU/mL
   b. mcg/mL
   c. mg/mL
   d. mOsm/mL

4. Which of the following dosage forms is classified as an enteral dosage form?
   a. Aerosol
   b. Cream
   c. Elixir
   d. Suppository

5. How is enoxaparin administered to a patient?
   a. Intradermally
   b. Intramuscularly
   c. Intravenously
   d. Subcutaneously

6. Which term refers to a storage temperature of 20°C–25°C?
   a. Cool storage temperature
   b. Freezer storage
   c. Refrigerator storage
   d. Room temperature

7. Which vaccine requires to be stored in a freezer?
   a. diphtheria, tetanus, and acellular pertussis
   b. Havrix
   c. Measles, mumps, and rubella
   d. Zostavax

8. Which beyond-use-date should be assigned to a nonsterile water-containing topical/dermal preparation?
   a. No more than 7 days
   b. No more than 14 days
   c. No more than 30 days
   d. No more than 6 months

9. At what angle should a subcutaneous injection be injected?
   a. 5–15 degrees
   b. 15–35 degrees
   c. 45–90 degrees
   d. 90 degrees

10. A patient has read the drug literature for one of their medications and wants to know what *neuralgia* means. How would you explain the meaning of neuralgia to the patient?
    a. *Neuralgia* means bone pain.
    b. *Neuralgia* means ear pain.
    c. *Neuralgia* means kidney pain.
    d. *Neuralgia* means nerve pain.

11. A patient's medical history consists of many components. Which term refers to a summary of their lifestyle practices?
    a. Family history
    b. Medication history
    c. Social history
    d. Surgical history

12. Which term refers to a severe mental disorder in which a person loses the ability to recognize reality or relate to others?
    a. Alzheimer disease
    b. Bipolar disorder
    c. Depression
    d. Psychosis

13. A patient complains of a buildup of fluid in the body tissues. Which term describes this condition?
    a. Angina
    b. Edema
    c. Osteoporosis
    d. Urinary incontinence

14. What type of nonadherence occurs when the patient chooses not to follow their medication regimen?
    a. Intentional medication nonadherence
    b. Primary nonadherence
    c. Secondary nonadherence
    d. Unintentional medication nonadherence

15. Which is a risk factor for polypharmacy?
    a. Filling one's prescriptions at the same pharmacy
    b. Multiple medical conditions being managed by multiple physicians
    c. Patients having acute mental health conditions
    d. Patent's age, especially in patients 30 years of age and older

16. Which drug classification has been shown to contribute to preventable adverse drug effects (ADEs) in older patients?
    a. Cephalosporins
    b. Oral hypoglycemics
    c. Topical corticosteroids
    d. All the above

17. Polypharmacy refers to taking multiple medications to treat the same medical condition. There are multiple types of polypharmacy, and they include no polypharmacy, polypharmacy, and excessive polypharmacy. How many different medications does a patient need to be taking for the term polypharmacy to be used ?
    a. 0 medications
    b. <4 medications
    c. 5–9 medications
    d. 10 medications or greater

18. Which type of diabetes is a result of a defect in the beta cells of the pancreas?
    a. Gestational diabetes mellitus
    b. Type 1 diabetes mellitus
    c. Type 2 diabetes mellitus
    d. Both b and c

19. The pharmacy technician is reviewing a patient's medical history and observes they have a complaint of dysuria. What is dysuria?
    a. Excessive urination
    b. Inability to urinate
    c. Involuntary urination
    d. Painful urination

20. A patient has been told by their physician they have been prescribed an antipruritic. They ask the pharmacy technician what an antipruritic does. Which would be an appropriate response to the patient?
    a. An antipruritic blocks the effects of histamine.
    b. An antipruritic prevents nausea and vomiting.
    c. An antipruritic relieves itching.
    d. An antipruritic reduces inflammation.
21. Which disease state occurs as blockage of blood flow to the heart muscle?
    a. Atherosclerosis
    b. Hyperlipidemia
    c. Myocardial infarction
    d. Stroke
22. What period of time is used in determining an individual's average blood glucose or blood sugar level when performing an A1C or HbA1c test?
    a. 1 month
    b. 2 months
    c. 3 months
    d. 6 months
23. A patient has a fasting plasma glucose level of 92 mg/dL. How would the patient be classified?
    a. Normal
    b. Prediabetes
    c. Diabetes
    d. Extreme diabetes
24. Which form of hyperlipidemia would find low-density lipoprotein elevated, serum cholesterol moderately increased, and serum triglyceride levels in a normal range?
    a. Type I
    b. Type IIa
    c. Type IIb
    d. Type III
25. Which is considered a normal A1C level in a patient?
    a. <5.7%
    b. 5.9%
    c. 6.1%
    d. 6.5%
26. The pharmacy technician is taking a patient's blood pressure at the pharmacy, and the patient's blood pressure measures 131/86. How would the patient's blood pressure be classified?
    a. Normal
    b. Elevated
    c. Stage 1 hypertension
    d. Stage 2 hypertension
27. According to the American Medical Association, a patient must take a minimum of what percent of their medication to be considered adherent?
    a. 75%
    b. 80%
    c. 85%
    d. 90%
28. Which term is also known as a therapeutic action plan?
    a. Medication-related action plan
    b. Medication therapy review
    c. Personal medication list
    d. Personal medication record

29. Which of the following tasks may a pharmacy technician perform when participating in the patient medication record (PMR) process?
    a. Explaining to the patient how to use the PMR
    b. Participating in the initial patient interview
    c. Updating the patient's PMR
    d. All the above
30. Which type of medication error occurs if an illegible prescription leads to an error that reaches the patient?
    a. Improper dose error
    b. Prescribing error
    c. Unauthorized drug error
    d. Wrong time error
31. The pharmacist fails to review a prescribed regimen for its appropriateness; which type of medication error is this?
    a. Compliance error
    b. Deteriorated drug error
    c. Monitoring error
    d. Omission error
32. Which is an effect of inappropriate prescribing?
    a. Patient adherence
    b. Patient injury
    c. Patient receives the appropriate treatment
    d. All the above
33. Which of the following would a pharmacy technician find in a PMR?
    a. Action steps for the patient to take
    b. Appointment information
    c. Notes for the patient
    d. Patient allergies
34. The pharmacy dispenses a prescription for atorvastatin 20 mg, which expired last month. What type of medication error would this be classified?
    a. Deteriorated drug error
    b. Improper dose error
    c. Wrong dosage form error
    d. Wrong drug preparation error
35. The physician prescribed levothyroxine 100 mcg; however the pharmacist dispensed levothyroxine 150 mcg. What type of medication is this?
    a. Improper dose error
    b. Omission error
    c. Wrong administration technique error
    d. Wrong dosage form error
36. A patient is hospitalized and is scheduled to receive metformin 500 mg orally twice a day. The nursing staff failed to administer the patient's first dose of metformin in the morning, but the patient did receive the evening dose. What type of medication error is this?
    a. Compliance error
    b. Monitoring error
    c. Omission error
    d. Unauthorized drug error
37. A patient has been prescribed Lantus Solostar insulin. The pharmacy technician instructs the patient to administer the Lantus Solostar intramuscularly. Which type of medication error was committed?
    a. Compliance error
    b. Improper dose error
    c. Wrong administration technique error
    d. Wrong time error

38. A patient has called in a refill for 90 tablets of simvastatin 20 mg. Upon reviewing the patient's profile, the pharmacy technician observes the last time the prescription was filled was 6 months ago. What type of medication is this?
    a. Compliance error
    b. Improper dose error
    c. Monitoring error
    d. Unauthorized drug error

39. The pharmacy technician dispenses tetracycline to a patient, which expired last month. What type of medication error would this be classified?
    a. Compliance error
    b. Deteriorated drug error
    c. Wrong administration error
    d. Wrong drug preparation error

40. A patient takes their nitroglycerin sublingual tablets orally. What type of medication error would this be considered?
    a. Compliance error
    b. Wrong administration technique error
    c. Wrong dosage form error
    d. Wrong drug preparation error

41. The pharmacy technician reconstitutes amoxicillin with 108 mL of distilled water instead of using 88 mL of distilled water. Which type of medication error would this be?
    a. Deteriorated drug error
    b. Wrong dosage form error
    c. Wrong drug preparation error
    d. Unauthorized drug error

42. A patient has been prescribed timolol ophthalmic 0.5% solution to be administered one drop in left eye once a day for open angle glaucoma. The patient administers one drop to their right eye. Which type of medication error is this?
    a. Compliance error
    b. Improper dose error
    c. Wrong administration technique error
    d. Wrong drug preparation error

43. Which category of medication error occurs that may have contributed to or resulted in temporary harm to patient and patient required intervention?
    a. Category E
    b. Category F
    c. Category G
    d. Category I

44. What is the effect of a Category I medication error?
    a. No error
    b. Error, no harm
    c. Error, harm
    d. Error, death

45. Which category of medication error is assigned when a medication error occurred but did not reach the patient?
    a. Category A
    b. Category B
    c. Category C
    d. Category D

46. Which category of medication error is assigned when an error occurs that may have contributed to or resulted in temporary harm to patient and resulted in hospitalization?
    a. Category E
    b. Category F

    c. Category G
    d. Category H

47. What is the effect of a Category H medication error?
    a. No error
    b. Error, no harm
    c. Error, harm
    d. Error, death

48. Which of the following is a medication therapy management (MTM) service that may be provided to a patient?
    a. Administering medication to a patient
    b. Offering support services to a patient to improve their adherence to their medication
    c. Offering training to patients to help them understand the proper use of their medications
    d. All the above

49. The pharmacy technician has been asked to identify patients who would benefit from MTM services. Which patient would benefit from these services?
    a. A patient who is under the care of one prescriber
    b. A patient who is taking diphenhydramine for an allergic reaction
    c. A patient who adheres to their medication regimen
    d. A patient who has experienced a transition of care and their medication regimen has changed

50. According to the Centers for Medicare and Medicaid Services (CMS), which is a requirement for MTM programs?
    a. MTM provides the therapeutic outcomes for targeted beneficiaries through reduced medication use.
    b. MTM is coordinated with any care management plan established for a targeted individual under an acute care improvement program.
    c. MTM is developed in cooperation with licensed and practicing pharmacists, pharmacy technicians, and physicians.
    d. MTM may be furnished by pharmacists or other qualified providers.

51. A pharmacy technician is recording MTM services for billing/reimbursement. Which component of MTM would this fall?
    a. Documentation and follow-up
    b. Intervention/referral
    c. Medication therapy review
    d. Personal medication record

52. How long must a pharmacy maintain documentation for MTM services to comply with CMS?
    a. 2 years
    b. 5 years
    c. 7 years
    d. 10 years

53. Under which category of a patient's record would a pharmacy technician find a patient's laboratory results?
    a. Assessment
    b. Collaboration
    c. Objective observations
    d. Patient demographics

54. Which of the following is an example of a chronic condition covered under MTM?
    a. Acne
    b. Diabetes
    c. Gastroesophageal reflux disease
    d. Influenza

55. During a medication therapy review (MTR), which task may a pharmacy technician perform?
    a. Assess patient symptoms.
    b. Collect data from patient profiles.
    c. Design a plan to address each identified medication-related problem.
    d. Evaluate patient clinical information.

56. Which of the following medications that a patient is taking may require a referral?
    a. Albuterol
    b. Azithromycin
    c. Lisinopril
    d. Methotrexate

57. Which is a goal of the pharmacy team when conducting a medication therapy review?
    a. Establish practical steps for both the patient and health care team to follow.
    b. Identify ways to improve patient adherence.
    c. Improve a patient's knowledge of their medications.
    d. Recognize and remedy problems or errors related to medication safety.

58. Which term is defined as is a process of collecting patient-specific information, evaluating their medication therapies to identify medication-related problems, developing a list of medication-related problems, and creating a plan to resolve them?
    a. Medication-related Action Plan (MAP)
    b. MTM
    c. MTR
    d. PMR

59. Which of the following should be included in the ideal MTM program?
    a. Face-to-face interaction between the nurse and the pharmacist
    b. Individualized services provided directly by a pharmacy technician to the patient
    c. Opportunities for pharmacists to identify patients who should receive MTM services
    d. Payment for MTM services based on the complexity of the patient's medical condition and the time necessary to educate the patient

60. One of the goals of MTM is to reduce the potential risks associated with polypharmacy. What can a pharmacy technician do reduce this risk?
    a. Counsel the patient on the risks of polypharmacy.
    b. Develop a personal medication record for the patient.
    c. Encourage physicians to consider "deprescribing" a patient's medications.
    d. Refer the patient to a health care professional for disease-management education.

61. Which of the following tasks would a pharmacy technician perform during an MTR?
    a. Assess all relevant patient clinical information.
    b. Interview the patient to collect demographic and general health information.
    c. Review the patient's medications for any potential medication-related problems.
    d. Work with the patient and their physician to resolve any medication-related issues.

62. What criteria would a pharmacy technician use to identify a patient for MTM services?
    a. Have at least two "acute disease states" and take both multiple prescriptions for chronic and acute conditions and are likely to incur high annual costs
    b. Have at least two "core chronic disease states," take multiple chronic or maintenance prescription medications, and are likely to incur high annual drug costs
    c. Have at least four "acute disease states" and take both multiple prescriptions for chronic and acute conditions and household income is below the national poverty level
    d. Have at least four "core chronic disease states," take multiple chronic or maintenance prescription medications, and household income is below the national poverty level

63. Which MTM process would a pharmacy technician collect a patient's immunization?
    a. Intervention/referral
    b. MAP
    c. MTR
    d. PMR

64. When during the medication therapy management process would a pharmacy technician observe the patient is not adhering to their medication regimen?
    a. Intervention and/or referral
    b. MAP
    c. MTR
    d. PMR

65. The pharmacy technician is calling a patient to remind them of their upcoming MTM appointment with the pharmacist. The patient informs the technician they have a list of all of the medications they are taking. How should the technician respond?
    a. "Thank you, but that won't be needed, since the pharmacy computer has a record of your current medications."
    b. "Thank you. Bring the list with you for appointment, since will save us time."
    c. "Thank you. If you remember, bring your pill containers with you to your appointment."
    d. " Thank you. In addition to the list, please bring your pill bottles, any over-the-counter medications, vitamins, topical medications, and lab reports."

Chapter 7 Immunization Administration

1. Which act was amended that permitted pharmacy technicians to administer immunizations if they met specific requirements?
   a. Food, Drug and Cosmetic Act
   b. Health Insurance Portability and Accountability Act
   c. Omnibus Reconciliation Act
   d. Public Readiness and Emergency Preparedness Act
2. How many dose(s) of the diphtheria, tetanus, and acellular pertussis vaccine are administered to a child?
   a. 2
   b. 3
   c. 4
   d. 5
3. Which vaccine is administered intranasally?
   a. FluMist Quadravalent
   b. Gardasil 9
   c. Pneumovax
   d. Varivax
4. Up to what age may a patient receive the human papillomavirus vaccine?
   a. 9 years of age
   b. 9 years of age
   c. 26 years of age
   d. 50 years of age
5. What is the minimum age for child to receive the diphtheria, tetanus, and acellular pertussis (DTaP)?
   a. 6 weeks of age
   b. 6 months of age
   c. 12 months of age
   d. 10 years of age
6. Which is (are) pharmacy technician requirement(s) to administer immunizations?
   a. Must complete an American Society of Health System Pharmacists-approved training for administering immunizations
   b. Must have completed a basic cardiopulmonary resuscitation course
   c. Must complete a minimum of 2 hours of ACPE-approved, immunization-related continuing pharmacy education during the state licensing period(s)
   d. All the above
7. Which form of immunity occurs as a result of a patient being administered antibodies to a disease rather than producing them through their own immune system?
   a. Active immunity
   b. Humoral immunity
   c. Passive immunity
   d. Vaccine-induced immunity
8. Which of the following is a substance used to keep a vaccine effective after it is manufactured?
   a. Adjuvant
   b. Antigen
   c. Preservative
   d. Stabilizer
9. How many measles, mumps, and rubella (MMR) doses should a child receive?
   a. 1 dose
   b. 2 doses
   c. 3 doses
   d. 4 doses
10. How long should an adult wait to receive the second dose of the Comirnaty vaccine?
    a. 14 days
    b. 21 days
    c. 28 days
    d. 48 days
11. What is the minimum age for child to receive the varicella vaccine?
    a. Birth
    b. 6 weeks of age
    c. 6 months of age
    d. 12 months of age
12. What is the minimum age for a child to receive the measles, mumps, and varicella vaccine?
    a. Birth
    b. 6 weeks of age
    c. 6 months of age
    d. 12 months of age
13. Which is the brand name for the zoster recombinant vaccine?
    a. Havrix
    b. Shingrix
    c. Trumenba
    d. Varivax
14. What is the minimum age for an adult to receive the recombinant zoster vaccine?
    a. 19 years of age
    b. 21 years of age
    c. 50 years of age
    d. 65 years of age
15. Which is the brand name for the measles, mumps, rubella, and varicella vaccine (MMRV)?
    a. Pediarix
    b. Pentacel
    c. ProQuad
    d. Quadracel
16. The pharmacy has received an order for the pneumococcal 13-valent conjugate vaccine. Which vaccine should be selected?
    a. Engerix-B
    b. Havrix
    c. Pneumovax 23
    d. Prevnar 13
17. How often should the influenza vaccine be administered to a patient?
    a. Annually
    b. Every 2 years
    c. Every 5 years
    d. Every 7 years
18. Which vaccine is administered subcutaneously?
    a. Haemophilus influenzae type b (Hib)
    b. Inactivated influenza (IIV)
    c. Pneumococcal conjugate (PCV13)
    d. Zoster, live
19. Which angle should Zoster, recombinant (RZV) vaccine be administered?
    a. 30 degrees
    b. 45 degrees
    c. 60 degrees
    d. 90 degrees

20. Which diluent should be used to mix with M-M-R II (MMR)?
    a. 0.45% sodium chloride
    b. 0.9% sodium chloride
    c. Distilled water
    d. Sterile water
21. Which vaccine may be stored either in the refrigerator or room temperature?
    a. Imovax (RABHDCV)
    b. Menveo (MenACWY)
    c. Pentacel (DTaP-IPV/Hib)
    d. ProQuad (MMRV)
22. How much time is permitted between reconstitution and administration as stated in the package insert for Shingrix (RZV)?
    a. 30 minutes
    b. 60 minutes
    c. 6 hours
    d. 8 hours
23. Which needle size and gauge should be used to administer a vaccine to a 13-year-old child in the anterolateral thigh muscle?
    a. $\frac{5}{8}''$ needle; 22–25 gauge
    b. 1″ needle; 22–25 gauge
    c. 1–1¼″ needle; 22–25 gauge
    d. 1–1 ½″ needle; 22–25 gauge
24. When administering an intramuscular vaccine to the deltoid muscle of either a child or adult, how many inches below the acromion process should the vaccine be administered?
    a. 1 inch
    b. 2 inches
    c. 3 inches
    d. 4 inches
25. Which diluent should be used when preparing Shingrix?
    a. 0.4% sodium chloride
    b. 0.9% sodium chloride
    c. AS01B adjuvant suspension
    d. Sterile water
26. Under which environment may 0.9% sodium chloride be stored?
    a. Freezer
    b. Refrigerator
    c. Room temperature
    d. Both b and c
27. After reconstituting Varivax with sterile water, what is the maximum amount of time that may pass before administering it to the patient?
    a. Immediately
    b. 30 minutes
    c. 6 hours
    d. 24 hours
28. Which vaccine must be administered subcutaneously?
    a. Diphtheria-tetanus-pertussis (DTaP, Tdap)
    b. Measles, mumps and rubella (MMR)
    c. Meningococcal serogroups A, C, W, Y (MenACWY)
    d. Pneumococcal conjugate (PCV13)

29. What length needle and gauge should be used in administering human papillomavirus (HPV) vaccine to a 19-year-old female patient weighing 115 pounds in their deltoid muscle?
    a. $\frac{5}{8}''$ needle; 22–25 gauge
    b. 1″ needle; 22–25 gauge
    c. 1–1¼″ needle; 22–25 gauge
    d. 1–1.5″ needle; 22–25 gauge
30. Which factor(s) affect the selection of a specific needle to administer a vaccine?
    a. Patient's age
    b. Patient's gender
    c. Route of administration
    d. All the above
31. At what angle should a vaccine be injected subcutaneously into the fatty tissue of the anterolateral thigh of a patient?
    a. 30 degrees
    b. 45 degrees
    c. 60 degrees
    d. 90 degrees
32. A child is being administered the DTaP vaccine. At what angle should the vaccine be administered intramuscularly?
    a. 30 degrees
    b. 45 degrees
    c. 60 degrees
    d. 90 degrees
33. A patient is receiving multiple vaccines at the same time. How far apart should the injection sites be from one another?
    a. 1 inch or more
    b. 2 inches or more
    c. 3 inches or more
    d. 4 inches or more
34. Which of the following may be discarded in a sharps disposal container?
    a. Used alcohol pads
    b. Used gloves
    c. Used needles
    d. All the above
35. At what point should a sharps disposal container be disposed?
    a. One-quarter full if it does not have a marked line
    b. One-half full if it does not have a marked line
    c. Two-thirds full if it does not have a marked line
    d. Three-quarters /completely full if it does not have a marked line
36. After reconstituting a vaccine which temperature must it be maintained if it is not used immediately?
    a. Below 2°C
    b. Between 2°C and 8°C
    c. Between 8°C and 12°C
    d. Between 12°C and 16°C
37. Prior to reconstituting a vaccine and after removing the protective cap, which should be used to clean the vial's stopper?
    a. Alcohol swab
    b. Betadine swab
    c. Hot water
    d. Hydrogen peroxide

38. Which diluent should be used when reconstituting Menveo (MenACWY)?
    a. 0.4% sodium chloride
    b. 0.9% sodium chloride
    c. MenCWY
    d. Sterile water
39. After Shingrix is reconstituted, what is the maximum time permitted between reconstitution and use?
    a. Immediately
    b. 6 hours
    c. 8 hours
    d. 24 hours
40. Which vaccine is administered subcutaneously?
    a. Diphtheria-tetanus (DT, Td)
    b. Hepatis A
    c. IIV
    d. Varicella
41. Where would an infant receive a subcutaneous injection?
    a. In the anterolateral thigh muscle
    b. In the deltoid muscle
    c. In the fatty tissue over the triceps
    d. Both b and c
42. What size need would be used in administering an intramuscular injection in the anterolateral thigh muscle of a child?
    a. 5/8″
    b. 1″
    c. 1–1¼″
    d. 1–1½″
43. What size needle should be used in administering an intramuscular immunization in a 201-lb woman?
    a. 1″ needle
    b. 1–1.5″ needle
    c. 1.5″ needle
    d. 2″ needle
44. At what angle should a needle be inserted in an adult for a subcutaneous injection?
    a. 30 degrees
    b. 45 degrees
    c. 75 degrees
    d. 90 degrees
45. Which vaccine is administered via inhalation?
    a. FluMist
    b. Gardasil
    c. Shingrix
    d. Tenivac
46. Which vaccine is administered orally?
    a. M-M-R-II
    b. Rotateq
    c. Shingrix
    d. Varivax
47. Which of the following should be done when a temperature excursion occurs?
    a. Document the details of the incident.
    b. Label the exposed vaccines "Do Not Use."
    c. Notify the vaccine coordinator immediately.
    d. All the above.
48. Which of the following practices should be done when storing vaccines?
    a. Place vaccines and diluents with the latest expiration dates in front of those with earlier expiration dates.
    b. Store vaccines and diluents with similar packaging or names on different shelves.

c. Position vaccines and diluents in rows with no space between them.
    d. All the above.
49. Which of the following vaccines requires a Vaccine Information Statement (VIS) be dispensed prior to the administration of the vaccine?
    a. HPV
    b. Influenza
    c. Varicella
    d. All the above
50. Under the National Childhood Vaccine Injury Act, which of the following vaccines does not require the health care provider to provide a VIS unless the vaccine has been purchased under a Centers for Disease Control contract?
    a. Adenovirus
    b. Pneumococcal polysaccharide
    c. Rabies
    d. All of them
51. Who is responsible for ordering vaccines for a health care facility?
    a. Medical doctor
    b. Nursing supervisor
    c. Pharmacist-in-charge
    d. Vaccine coordinator/alternate vaccine coordinator
52. The vaccines for children require the use of a continuous monitoring and recording device known as a "digital data logger." How often must the temperature be recorded?
    a. At least every 15 minutes
    b. At least every 30 minutes
    c. At least every 45 minutes
    d. At least every 60 minutes
53. The pharmacy is required to maintain a temperature monitoring log. What information should be recorded on the temperature monitoring log?
    a. Date
    b. Minimum/maximum temperature
    c. Name of individual who checked and recorded the temperature
    d. All the above
54. Who is responsible for ensuring that vaccines are being rotated properly and expired vaccines are removed?
    a. Medical director
    b. Nursing supervisor
    c. Pharmacist n-charge
    d. Vaccine coordinator/alternate vaccine coordinator
55. What is the minimum number of times vaccines should be inventoried?
    a. Once a month
    b. Twice a month
    c. Three times a month
    d. Four times a month
56. What is the maximum number of doses of a vaccine that may be drawn up at one time?
    a. 5 doses
    b. 10 doses
    c. 15 doses
    d. 20 doses
57. Where should the temperature monitoring device be placed in the storage unit?
    a. On the top shelf of the storage unit and surrounded by the vaccines
    b. On the bottom shelf of the storage unit and surrounded by the vaccines

c. On the center shelf of the storage unit and
   surrounded by the vaccines
d. Any of the above

58. A 5-year-old patient weighing 45 pounds is experiencing hives after receiving an immunization. How much diphenhydramine should be administered to the patient?
   a. 10–15 mg/dose
   b. 15–20 mg/dose
   c. 20–25 mg/dose
   d. 25–50 mg/dose

59. Which is the minimum dose of epinephrine (1 mg/mL) that should be administered to a patient experiencing anaphylaxis?
   a. 0.05 mL
   b. 0.1 mL
   c. 0.15 mL
   d. 0.2 mL

60. Which program should be used to report an adverse reaction associated with the administration of a vaccine?
   a. FAERS
   b. Vaccine Error Reporting Program
   c. Vaccine Adverse Event Reporting System
   d. Any of the above

Chapter 8 Point of Care Testing

1. Which task may a pharmacy technician *not* perform in point of care testing?
   a. Collect patient consent forms for the test.
   b. Collect patient specimen(s) according to manufacturer's instructions, including storage and handling of specimen.
   c. Identify qualified patients for a point of care test.
   d. Interpret test results according to the manufacturer's instructions.

2. Which organization is responsible for enforcing the Bloodborne Pathogen Standard?
   a. Environmental Protection Agency (EPA)
   b. FDA
   c. Department of Health and Human Services
   d. Occupational Safety and Health Administration

3. How often does an institution's exposure control plan need to be reviewed and updated?
   a. Quarterly
   b. Biannually
   c. Annually
   d. Biennially

4. Under the Bloodborne Pathogen Standard, which vaccination is addressed?
   a. Hepatitis A
   b. Hepatitis B
   c. Hepatitis C
   d. Hepatitis D

5. How often must employees be trained according to the Bloodborne Pathogen Standard?
   a. Quarterly
   b. Biannually
   c. Annually
   d. Biennially

6. Which action can reduce the risk of bloodborne exposure during point of care testing?
   a. Obtaining a hepatitis C vaccine
   b. Recapping needles properly
   c. Reporting all occupational exposures within a month of the occurrence
   d. Wearing required personal protective equipment (PPE)

7. Which color container is assigned to indicate biohazardous waste?
   a. Black
   b. Red
   c. White with blue lid
   d. Yellow

8. What is the minimum number of patient identifiers be provided by the patient prior to administering the point of care testing according to The Joint Commission?
   a. 2
   b. 3
   c. 4
   d. 5

9. Which of the following is (are) appropriate PPE to be used when there is a possibility of exposure to infectious material?
   a. Eye protection
   b. Gloves
   c. Lab coat or gown
   d. All the above

10. Which of the following is considered a physical assessment?
    a. Auditory inspection
    b. Diastolic and systolic blood pressure
    c. Olfactory inspection
    d. All the above

11. A patient assessment consist of which of the following?
    a. Body temperature
    b. Heart rate
    c. Oxygen saturation
    d. Visual inspection

12. Which is considered a normal heart rate for a patient?
    a. <50 beats per minute
    b. 50–60 beats per minute
    c. 60–100 beats per minute
    d. >110 beats per minute

13. Which of the following may slow a patient's heart rate?
    a. Beta blockers
    b. Dehydration
    c. Stress
    d. Thyroid medication

14. Which of the following is a normal respiration rate for a patient?
    a. <10 breaths per minute
    b. 12–20 breaths per minute
    c. 22–30 breaths per minute
    d. >30 breaths per minute

15. Which of the following is used to measure a patient's oxygen saturation?
    a. CENTOR Score
    b. Glucometer
    c. Oximeter
    d. Sphygmomanometer

16. Which is considered as a common specimen for waived and nonwaived testing?
    a. Throat swab samples
    b. Urine sample
    c. Whole blood sample
    d. All the above

17. A patient is informed they have been diagnosed with elevated hypertension. Which blood pressure reading is associated with this category of hypertension?
    a. 120–129/<80
    b. 130–139/80–89
    c. $\geq 140/\geq 90$
    d. >180/>120

18. Which of the following is a symptom associated with diabetes?
    a. Polydipsia
    b. Polyphagia
    c. Polyuria
    d. All the above

19. Which of the following fasting plasma glucose levels may indicate the patient is prediabetic?
    a. <80 mg/dL
    b. 80–100 mg/dL
    c. 100–125 mg/dL
    d. >125 mg/dL

20. Which of the following may lower a patient's heart rate?
    a. Anxiety
    b. Dehydration
    c. Infection
    d. Regular exercise

21. Which of the following drug classifications is indicated in treating diabetes?
    a. Beta adrenergic antagonists
    b. Biguanides
    c. Fibrates
    d. Omega-3 acid ethyl esters
22. Which of the following diagnostic tests is used in diagnosing diabetes?
    a. Fasting plasma glucose
    b. Glycosylated hemoglobin
    c. Oral glucose tolerance
    d. All the above
23. Which drug classification could be prescribed to treat dyslipidemia?
    a. Angiotensin II receptor blockers
    b. Biguanides
    c. Loop diuretics
    d. 3-hydroxy-3-methylglutaryl coenzyme A reductase inhibitors
24. A patient complains of experiencing sore throat, fever, headache, swelling of the tonsils, the presence of creamy white patches on the tonsils, redness at the back of the throat, tender lymph nodes, nausea, and vomiting. Which condition may the patient be experiencing?
    a. Acute pharyngitis
    b. COVID-19
    c. Influenza
    d. Influenza-like-symptoms
25. Which condition can be detected by performing a rapid tests such as a nucleic acid amplification test (NAAT), antigen, or antibody tests?
    a. COVID-19
    b. Gonorrhea
    c. Influenza
    d. Syphilis
26. Which of the following components of a patients medical history may indicate their genetic predisposition to disease such as cardiac diseases?
    a. Chief complaint
    b. Family history
    c. Surgical history
    d. Symptoms
27. A patient provides the pharmacy technician with a list of medications they are currently taking. Which term refers to this list?
    a. Family history
    b. Immunization history
    c. Medication history
    d. Social history
28. Which condition is the CENTOR Score used as a screening tool?
    a. Chlamydia
    b. COVID-19
    c. Group A Streptococcus pharyngitis
    d. Influenza
29. If a patient receives a CENTOR Score of 2 or 3 points, which course of action should be taken?
    a. An antibiotic or throat culture is necessary.
    b. Patient should receive a throat culture and treat with an antibiotic if culture is positive.
    c. Rapid strep testing and/or culture should be considered.
    d. Patient should be hospitalized.

30. Which organization is responsible for developing, implementing, and publishing Clinical Laboratory Improvement Amendments (CLIA) rules and regulations?
    a. Centers for Medicare and Medicaid Services (CMS)
    b. Centers for Disease Control and Prevention (CDC)
    c. EPA
    d. FDA
31. Which organization is responsible for enforcing CLIA regulatory compliance?
    a. CMS
    b. CDC
    c. Drug Enforcement Administration (DEA)
    d. FDA
32. Which organization is responsible for conducting CLIA laboratory inspections?
    a. CMS
    b. CDC
    c. DEA
    d. FDA
33. Which organization is responsible for developing CLIA Categorization rules and providing guidance?
    a. CMS
    b. CDC
    c. DEA
    d. FDA
34. Which organization is responsible for issuing lab certificates under the CLIA?
    a. CMS
    b. CDC
    c. DEA
    d. FDA
35. Which of the following is an example of waived test?
    a. Hematocrit
    b. Hemoglobin
    c. Pregnancy test
    d. All the above
36. How long is a Certificate of Waiver CoW) valid?
    a. 1 year
    b. 2 years
    c. 4 years
    d. 5 years
37. Which document permits a lab to administer tests the FDA categorizes as waived tests?
    a. Certificate of Accreditation (CoA)
    b. Certificate of Compliance (CoC)
    c. Certificate of Registration (CoR)
    d. CoW
38. Which document is awarded to a lab that performs moderate and highly complex tests and comply with the standards of a private nonprofit accreditation organization approved by the CMS?
    a. CoA
    b. CoC
    c. CoR
    d. CoW
39. Which is a disadvantage of using NAAT?
    a. Can be self-administered at home
    b. Capable of detecting low levels of pathogens
    c. Expensive reagents
    d. High sensitivity and specificity

40. Which is an advantage of using lateral flow technology?
   a. It is able to detect proteins, haptens, and nucleic acids.
   b. Good antibody preparation is required.
   c. Inaccurate sample volume reduces precision.
   d. Restriction on test volume provides a limit of sensitivity of the test.

41. Which piece of equipment would be used to perform tests on whole blood, serum, plasma, or urine samples to determine concentrations of analytes such as cholesterol, electrolytes, and glucose?
   a. Glucometer
   b. HgbA1C analyzers
   c. Internationalized normalized ratio (INR) analyzer
   d. Serum chemistry analyzers

42. Which of the following is a quantitative test?
   a. HIV
   b. Home pregnancy test
   c. Prothrombin time (PT)/INR
   d. All the above

43. Which of the following is a qualitative test?
   a. A1C
   b. COVID-19 test
   c. Lipid panel
   d. All the above

44. Which test is used to assess a patient's warfarin therapy?
   a. A1C
   b. HIV
   c. Lipid panel
   d. PT/INR

45. Which point-of care test measures the presence of human chorionic gonadotropin in urine?
   a. A1C
   b. COVID-19
   c. Hepatitis C
   d. Home pregnancy

46. Where would an individual find information in the manufacturer instructions information regarding the use of reagents beyond their expiration date?
   a. Precautions
   b. Reagents and materials supplied
   c. Storage and stability
   d. Test procedure

47. What effect on point-of-care testing may occur if current instructions are not followed during the testing?
   a. Delay in appropriate treatment
   b. Inaccurate results
   c. Misdiagnosis of the patient
   d. All the above

48. Where on the manufacturer's instructions would you find the purpose of the test?
   a. Intended use
   b. Sample collection and preparation
   c. Summary
   d. Test principle

49. Which of the following tests is (are) considered to be quantitative?
   a. A1C test
   b. COVID-19 test
   c. Pregnancy test
   d. All the above

50. Which term refers to the proportion of patients that do not have the disease that test negative?
   a. Negative predictive value
   b. Positive predictive value
   c. Sensitivity
   d. Specificity

51. Which is the sensitivity of a test if there are 75 true positives and 5 true negatives?
   a. 6.25%
   b. 12.5%
   c. 87.5%
   d. 93.75%

52. What is the positive predictive value if there were 95 true-positive cases and 10 false-positive cases?
   a. 9.53%
   b. 89.47%
   c. 90.47%
   d. 110.52%

53. Which of the following should be used in recording the results of a quantitative test?
   a. Positive
   b. Reactive
   c. Units of measurement
   d. All the above

54. Unlike the results of a qualitative test, which of the following must appear on the results of a quantitative test?
   a. Date of the test
   b. Lot number of the test
   c. Reportable range for the test
   d. Test results

55. Under which condition(s) should a test be repeated?
   a. Quantitative (numerical) results have values beyond the measuring range of the instrument.
   b. Test results are confirmed with the patient's clinical information.
   c. The test system provides a valid test result.
   d. All the above.

56. What information should appear on the label of the sample?
   a. Date and time the sample was analyzed
   b. Individual who analyzed the sample results
   c. Unique patient identifier
   d. All the above

57. When recording a refrigerator or freezer's temperatures, which information must be recorded?
   a. Date of the reading
   b. Individual who took the reading
   c. Temperature
   d. All the above

58. Which of the following records must be maintained by a pharmacy performing point of care testing?
   a. Daily temperature checks
   b. Lot numbers, dates used and received, and expiration dates of reagents
   c. Personnel training/competency assessments
   d. All the above

59. According to the clinical Laboratory Improvement Amendment of 1988, which temperature range should a freezer for sample storage be maintained?
   a. −25°C and −15°C
   b. −15°C and −5°C
   c. −5°C and +2°C
   d. +2°C and +8°C

60. Which of the following is a benefit of quality assessment in a pharmacy performing quality control assessment?
   a. Better patient outcomes
   b. Increased costs
   c. Increased errors
   d. All the above

Chapter 9 Billing and Reimbursement

1. Which reimbursement program is created by pharmaceutical and medical supply manufacturers to help financially needy patients purchase necessary medications and supplies?
   a. Drug discount card
   b. Health savings account
   c. Manufacturer-sponsored prescription coupon
   d. Patient assistance program

2. Which health plan requires a beneficiary to use only network providers?
   a. Health maintenance organization (HMO)
   b. Point-of-service (POS)
   c. Preferred provider organization
   d. All the above

3. Which of the following is (are) an example(s) of cost containment strategies utilized by health plans?
   a. Capitation reimbursement
   b. Preauthorization
   c. Referral
   d. All the above

4. Which form of health care provides preventative care for beneficiaries?
   a. HMO
   b. Indemnity
   c. POS
   d. Both a and b

5. What are GoodRx and SingleCare an example of?
   a. Drug discount card
   b. Manufacture discount program
   c. Manufacture-sponsored prescription coupon
   d. Patient assistance programs

6. Which of the following may a health savings account be used to pay?
   a. Durable medical expenses
   b. Insulin without a prescription
   c. Over-the-counter medications accompanied by a physician's prescription.
   d. Prescription copayments

7. The Healthcare Common Procedural Coding System (HCPCS) consists of one alphabetical character followed by four digits. Which of the following alphabetical characters may be used?
   a. A
   b. J
   c. L
   d. T

8. Which Current Procedural Technology (CPT) code would be used in medication therapy management for an established, face-to-face visit for 15 minutes?
   a. 99424
   b. 99439
   c. 99495
   d. 99606

9. Which is an eligibility requirement for Medicare?
   a. Age 65 or older
   b. Younger individuals with disabilities
   c. Individuals with end-stage renal disease
   d. All the above

10. Who is eligible to participate in TRICARE?
    a. Medal of Honor recipients and their families
    b. National Guard/Reserve members and their families
    c. Uniformed service members and their families
    d. All the above

11. Manuel Gonzalez has a dependent child who is covered under their commercial insurance plan. Until what age will the dependent child be covered under his insurance plan?
    a. 18 years of age
    b. 21 years of age
    c. 26 years of age
    d. 30 years of age

12. Which method of reimbursement is defined as the maximum amount of payment for a given prescription determined by the insurer?
    a. Ambulatory payment classification
    b. Capitation
    c. Reasonable and customary
    d. Usual and customary

13. A long-term care pharmacy provides medications to patients in a long-term care facility. Which Medicare requirements must the pharmacy comply?
    a. Medicare Part A
    b. Medicare Part B
    c. Medicare Part C
    d. Medicare Part D

14. How many hours does Medicare B permit for a group diabetes self-management training?
    a. 1 hour
    b. 2 hours
    c. 9 hours
    d. 10 hours

15. Which patient relationship code is assigned to the spouse of the cardholder when billing for a prescription claim?
    a. 00
    b. 01
    c. 02
    d. 03

16. Which term refers to a six-digit number used to identify the company that will reimburse the pharmacy for the prescription being filled?
    a. Group code
    b. Issuer
    c. RxBIN
    d. Subscriber

17. Which dispense as written (DAW) code is assigned when the prescriber does not indicate a brand medication?
    a. 0
    b. 1
    c. 2
    d. 3

18. Which term refers to the portion of the medication's price that the patient is responsible for?
    a. Copay
    b. Coinsurance
    c. Dual copay
    d. Deductible

19. Which of the following processes occurs during the adjudication process by the pharmacy benefit manager?
    a. Drug price is determined based upon its average wholesale price.
    b. DUR is conducted manually by the pharmacist.
    c. It is verified that the claim belongs to an eligible member.
    d. All the above.
20. Which of the following may be discovered during a drug utilization review?
    a. Drug-drug interaction
    b. Early refill of medication
    c. Prescription filled at another location
    d. All the above
21. What information is transmitted during the adjudication of a prescription claim?
    a. Patient's telephone number
    b. Pharmacy's National Provider Identifier (NPI) number
    c. Universal product code of the medication
    d. All the above
22. What prescription information is transmitted during the adjudication of a prescription?
    a. Date the prescription was written
    b. Prescription number
    c. Quantity dispensed
    d. All the above
23. What does a prescription rejection code "8" indicate?
    a. Missing or invalid group number
    b. Missing or invalid cardholder ID number
    c. Missing or invalid person code
    d. Missing or invalid birthdate
24. What does a prescription rejection code "19" indicate?
    a. Missing or invalid gender code
    b. Missing or invalid day's supply
    c. Missing or invalid prescriber ID
    d. Missing or invalid number of refills authorized
25. What can be done to ensure a prescription claim is not rejected?
    a. Ensure the medication is on the formulary.
    b. Ensure the day's supply has not been exceeded.
    c. Verify patient information is correct.
    d. All the above.
26. If all patient, prescription, and provider information is correct, who should the pharmacy staff contact?
    a. Patient
    b. Patient's employer
    c. Prescriber
    d. Pharmacy benefit manager
27. Tier systems are used in formulary systems to encourage the use of specific drug products. Which type of drug is classified as a Tier 1 drug?
    a. Generic drugs
    b. Nonpreferred brand drugs
    c. Preferred brand drugs
    d. Preferred specialty drugs
28. Which tier of drugs is nonpreferred specialty drugs?
    a. Tier 4
    b. Tier 5
    c. Tier 6
    d. Tier 7

29. Which term refers to the price a pharmacy actually pays for a medication sold by the manufacturer?
    a. Actual acquisition cost
    b. Average manufacturer's price
    c. Average wholesale price
    d. Best price
30. Which price is used to calculate drug rebates under the Medicaid Drug Rebate Program?
    a. Actual acquisition cost
    b. Average manufacturer's price
    c. Average wholesale price
    d. Best price
31. Which is a factor used in determining the dispensing fee for providing a pharmacy's dispensing fee?
    a. Actual acquisition cost
    b. Drug utilization review
    c. Federal upper limit
    d. Maximum allowable cost
32. Which formula is used in calculating gross profit?
    a. Gross profit = Selling price − Average manufacturer price
    b. Gross profit = Selling price − Estimated acquisition cost
    c. Gross profit = Selling price − Cost of the product
    d. Gross profit = Selling price − Cost of the product-unaccounted expenses
33. Which cost is used in determining the reimbursement of a generic drug to the pharmacy by a pharmacy benefit manager?
    a. Average manufacturer price (AMP)
    b. Estimated acquisition cost (EAC)
    c. Maximum allowable cost
    d. National average drug acquisition cost
34. Which type of code is used for billing medication therapy management services provided by the pharmacy?
    a. CPT codes
    b. HCPCS codes
    c. International Classification of Diseases-10 codes
    d. NPI number
35. Which rule is used in deciding a child's primary insurance?
    a. Birthday rule
    b. Clark's rule
    c. Health Insurance Portability and Accountability Act (HIPAA) privacy rule
    d. HIPAA security rule
36. If two or more plans cover dependent children of separated or divorced parents who do not have joint custody of their children, which plan is considered the primary plan?
    a. The plan of the custodial parent
    b. The plan of the spouse of the custodial parent (if the parent has been remarried)
    c. The plan of the parent without custody
    d. As decided by the court system
37. Which of the following may be used in determining a prescription plan's limitations?
    a. Day's supply
    b. Medication cost
    c. Number of permitted refills
    d. All the above

38. What period of time is a "PRN" refill valid?
    a. 1 year from the date the prescription was picked up by the patient or their caregiver
    b. 1 year from the date the prescription was presented by the patient
    c. 1 year from the date the prescription was written
    d. 1 year from the date the prescription was filled
39. The price of a prescription medication is calculated by adding the drug cost to the prescription's dispensing fee. Which drug cost may be used in determining the price of a prescription?
    a. Actual acquisition cost (AAC)
    b. AMP
    c. Average wholesale price (AWP)
    d. Any of the above
40. Which pricing method is the basis of reimbursement for some Medicare Part B covered drugs and biologicals administered in hospital outpatient departments?
    a. AAC
    b. Utilize average sale price
    c. AWP
    d. All the above
41. Which price is used in calculating the price for a covered drug by the Department of Defense?
    a. EAC
    b. Federal ceiling price
    c. Wholesale acquisition cost
    d. All the above
42. Which term refers to a list of approved medications covered by a prescription plan?
    a. Formulary
    b. Formulary maintenance
    c. Formulary restriction
    d. Nonformulary medication
43. Which action should be performed to prevent a prescription from being rejected during adjudication?
    a. Ensure the days' supply does not exceed plan limitations.
    b. Ensure medication was entered correctly.
    c. Ensure patient information is correct.
    d. All the above
44. Which term refers to the authorized exchange of therapeutic alternatives based upon established and approved written guidelines or protocols within a formulary system?
    a. Formulary restriction
    b. Therapeutic class review
    c. Therapeutic equivalent
    d. Therapeutic interchange
45. Which is a function of the Pharmacy and Therapeutics Committee?
    a. Educates health professionals to the optimal use of medications
    b. Establishes and maintains the formulary system
    c. Evaluates or develops and promotes use of drug therapy guidelines
    d. All the above
46. Who oversees a 340B Drug Pricing Program?
    a. Local government
    b. State government
    c. Federal government
    d. All the above
47. Which of the following would *not* qualify as a 340B-eligible patient?
    a. A patient is covered under a state-operated or -funded AIDS drug purchasing assistance program.
    b. The individual receives health care services from a health care professional who is either employed by the covered entity or provides health care under contractual or other arrangements (e.g., referral for consultation) such that responsibility for the care provided remains with the covered entity.
    c. The covered entity has established a relationship with the individual, such that the covered entity maintains records of the individual's health care.
    d. The individual receives a health care service or range of services from the covered entity that is consistent with the service or range of services for which grant funding or federally qualified health center look-alike status has been provided to the entity.
48. Which of the following is considered a 5i drug?
    a. An injectable drug
    b. An oral drug
    c. A topical dru
    d. All the above.
49. Under which condition would a medication require prior authorization for a restricted medication?
    a. Age or sex restrictions for the medication
    b. Early refill of medication
    c. Medication prescribed for exclusive health conditions
    d. Quantity of the medication being prescribed
50. Which of the following medications would require prior authorization?
    a. Amoxicillin
    b. Hydrochlorothiazide
    c. Naproxen
    d. Retin-A Micro
51. Under which condition would an override be requested by the pharmacy?
    a. Generic medication is being dispensed.
    b. Medication is being refilled on time.
    c. 72-hour emergency supply of the medication is requested.
    d. All the above.
52. Who is responsible for obtaining the prior authorization?
    a. Nurse
    b. Patient
    c. Pharmacy
    d. Prescriber
53. Why might a prior authorization be rejected?
    a. Duration of therapy is not consistent with its guidelines.
    b. Step therapy has been attempted.
    c. Therapy is medically necessary.
    d. Therapy is within the provider's scope of practice.
54. Which information must be collected for a prior authorization to be submitted?
    a. Medication information
    b. Patient information
    c. Prescriber information
    d. All the above

55. A prior authorization for a prescription medication has been rejected. Which of the following may explain why it was rejected?
    a. Incorrect information has been submitted.
    b. Therapy is medically necessary.
    c. Therapy is approved, and dose, duration, and quantity fall within the guidelines.
    d. All the above.

56. The pharmacy receives prior authorization rejection error code 58. Why was the prior authorization rejected?
    a. Date of birth is missing or invalid.
    b. First and/or last name is/are blank.
    c. Gender code is missing or invalid.
    d. Not eligible for service.

57. Why may prior authorization be required prior to the filling of a specific medication?
    a. Assure the appropriate use of medications
    b. Encourage stockpiling of medications
    c. Utilization management method for low-risk and inexpensive medications
    d. All the above

58. What role does prior authorization play in prescription processing?
    a. Discourages the need of step therapy in the medication use process
    b. Prevents medication misuse
    c. Reduces the need for additional clinical patient information
    d. All the above

59. Who establishes the formulary exception process in the practice of pharmacy?
    a. Insurance plans
    b. Pharmacies
    c. Physicians
    d. All of the above

60. Which of the following is an example of fraud?
    a. The pharmacy is billing for a brand-name medication when the generic drug is dispensed.
    b. The pharmacy is billing for nonexistent prescriptions.
    c. The physician is prescribing more medications than necessary to treat a specific condition.
    d. All the above.

61. Which of the following can be done by a pharmacy to prevent an audit?
    a. Maintain documentation that the service is medically necessary.
    b. Maintain documentation that the therapy is necessary according to accepted standards of care.
    c. Maintain documentation that the medication is found in the pharmacy formulary.
    d. All the above.

62. Which form of Medicare is a universal benefit?
    a. Medicare Part A
    b. Medicare Part B
    c. Medicare Part C
    d. Medicare Part D

63. Under which condition may a pharmacy audit be performed?
    a. Abuse
    b. Fraud
    c. Waste
    d. All the above

64. Which of the following situations may precipitate a pharmacy audit?
    a. Billing for medically necessary pharmacy services
    b. Paying for pharmacy referrals
    c. Using appropriate billing codes
    d. All the above

65. 340B Drug Pricing Program–covered entities must ensure program integrity and maintain accurate records documenting compliance with all 340B Program requirements. Which of the following is (are) an example(s) of 340B audit?
    a. Field on-site audits
    b. Purchase verification
    c. Prescriber/member audits
    d. All the above

66. Which organization performs 340B audits?
    a. Centers of Medicare and Medicaid Services (CMS)
    b. FDA
    c. Health Resources and Services Administration (HRSA)
    d. The Joint Commission (TJC)

67. During a pharmacy audit by a pharmacy benefit manager, which of the following may indicate pharmacy impropriety?
    a. The patient signature is absent upon receipt of a prescription medication.
    b. Appropriate DAW codes are used.
    c. Number of doses dispensed meets FDA labeling.
    d. National Drug Code (NDC) numbers submitted is the same as NDC number dispensed.

68. Which legislation may remove Medicare provider's eligibility?
    a. Anti-Kickback Statute
    b. False Claims Act
    c. Sarbanes-Oxley Act
    d. Social Security Act

69. During a TJC inspection of an accredited facility's pharmacy, which of the following are evaluated?
    a. Controlled substance security
    b. Hazardous drug management
    c. USP <797> compliance
    d. All the above

70. Which organization oversees the Children's Health and Insurance Program?
    a. CMS
    b. HRSA
    c. TJC
    d. Utilization Review Accreditation Commission

Chapter 10

1. A patient presents the following prescription to be filled at the community pharmacy:
Joan Ritter
2921 N 11th St
Arlington, VA 22204
703-979-1400

Jose Gonzalez   May 18, 202X
1300 Key Blvd   Arlington, VA 22209

Pantoprazole 60 mg   #30
1 TAB PO every day for GERD

Refill × 2   Joan Ritter

The pharmacy technician is reviewing the prescription for completeness. What does the pharmacy technician observe?
a. Frequency of taking the medication is incorrect.
b. Medication dosage is incorrect.
c. Medication indication is incorrect.
d. There is nothing incorrect with the prescription.

2. The following prescription is presented at the pharmacy:
Terry McManus N.P.
2921 N 11th St
Arlington, VA 22204
703-979-1400

Ed Tarboosch   April 1, 222X
1021 Arlington Blvd   Arlington VA 22209

Lisinopril 10 mg   #90
1 tab PO q am

Refill ×3   Terry McManus

The directions on the pharmacy prescription label read as follows:
"Take 1 tablet by mouth every evening."
What error exists in the directions on the prescription label?
a. Quantity to take
b. Route of administration
c. When to take the medication
d. No errors appear in the directions for use on the prescription label

3. The following prescription is presented at the pharmacy:
Dr. Martha Livingston
11400 South Lakes Drive
Reston, VA 20194
703-435-8163

Olivia Baker   June 30, 20XX
11606 Brandon Hill Way   Reston, VA 20194

Amoxicillin 500 mg   10 days' supply
1 cap PO TID

Refill 0   Dr. Martha Livingston

How many capsules should be dispensed?
a. 10 capsules
b. 20 capsules
c. 30 capsules
d. 40 capsules

4. The following prescription is presented at the pharmacy:
Andrew Shedlock
2610 Cates Avenue
Raleigh, NC 27606
919-470-3130

Rocky Mizner   July 28, 202X
1912 Hidden Knoll Place Apt 208 Raleigh, NC 27606

Lorazepam   1 mg   #30
1 Tab PO QD

Refill ×1   Andrew Shedlock

What is wrong with the prescription preventing it from being filled?
a. Physician's DEA number is missing.
b. The directions for use are incorrect for the medication.
c. The medication dosage is incorrect.
d. Nothing is wrong with the prescription.

5. The following prescription is presented at the pharmacy:
Dr. Michael Silverstein
381 Elden Street Suite 100
Herndon, VA 20170
703-481-1505

Louisa Damico   June 29, 202X
1514 Coat Ridge Court   Herndon, VA 20171

Levothyroxine 100 mcg #60
I Tab PO QD 30 minutes before first meal of the day

Refill ×3   Dr. Michael Silverstein

The patient requested that Synthroid be dispensed. Which DAW code should the pharmacy technician enter into the pharmacy computer?
a. DAW 0
b. DAW 1
c. DAW 2
d. DAW 3

6. The following information appears on a prescription:
Ibuprofen 600 mg   #60
1 tab PO q 6–8 hr prn dysmenorrhea

Refill ×1

How should the directions appear on the prescription label?
a. Take 600 mg by mouth every 6–8 hours prn dysmenorrhea.
b. Take 1 tablet every 6–8 hours as needed for dysmenorrhea.
c. Take 1 tablet by mouth 3–4 times a day for dysmenorrhea.
d. Take 1 tablet by mouth every 6–8 hours as needed for dysmenorrhea.

7. A patient presents the following prescription at the pharmacy:
Lantus Solostar Pens #3
Inject 25 units q AM

How many days will the prescription last?
a. 12 days
b. 25 days
c. 36 days
d. 50 days

8. The following information appears on a prescription presented at the pharmacy:
Tetracycline 250 mg   #60

1 cap PO BID 1 hr ac or 2 hr pc with adequate water for acne

Refill ×2

How should the directions appear on the prescription label?
a. Take 1 capsule twice a day 1 hour before meals or after meals with adequate water for acne.
b. Take 1 capsule by mouth every 12 hours 1 hour before meals or after meals with adequate water for acne.
c. Take a capsule by mouth 1 hour before meals or 2 hours after meals with adequate water for acne.
d. Take 1 capsule by mouth twice a day 1 hour before meals or 2 hours after meals with adequate water for acne.

9. The following prescription is presented at the pharmacy:
Dr. Roberta Amos
1850 Town Center Drive Suite 550
Reston, VA 2019
703-437-5977

Maureen Leib   June 26, 202X
11602 Brandon Hill Way   Reston, VA 20194

Latanoprost ophthalmic solution 2.5 mL
1 gtt in each eye at bedtime for glaucoma

Refill ×2   Dr. Roberta Amos

How many days will the prescription last?
a. 15 days
b. 25 days
c. 30 days
d. 50 days

10. A patient presents the following prescription to the pharmacy:
Stuart Sheifer
3580 Joseph Siewick Drive Suite 305
Fairfax, VA 22033

Paul Chung   July 25, 202X
43251 Parkers Ridge Drive Leesburg, VA 20176

Metoprolol tartrate 100 mg #60
1 tab PO bid

Refill ×3   Stuart Sheifer

Which of the following auxiliary labels is appropriate for a prescription of metoprolol tartrate?
a. Caution: Federal law prohibits the transfer of this drug to any person other than the patient for whom it was prescribed
b. May cause drowsiness
c. May discolor urine or feces
d. None of the above

11. The following prescription is presented at the pharmacy:
Raymond Hoare
2921 N 11th St
Arlington, VA 22204
703-979-1400

Alfredo Beltran   July 3, 202X
1530 Key Blvd   Arlington VA 22209

Ibuprofen 600 mg   #60
I tab PO TID with food

Refill ×1   Raymond Hoare

How many times a day should the patient take their medication?
a. 1
b. 2
c. 3
d. 4

12. Which person code should the pharmacy technician input for a patient who is the spouse of the cardholder of the prescription drug plan?
a. 01
b. 02
c. 03
d. 04

13. The following prescription is presented at the pharmacy:
Aleta Mizner
10635 Konneyaut Trail
Conneaut Lake, PA 16316
814-724-2345

Levothyroxine 100 mcg   #90
1 tab PO QD

Refill ×3   Aleta Mizner

Which auxiliary label is appropriate for this medication?
a. Avoid exposure to sunlight
b. May cause drowsiness
c. Take on an empty stomach
d. All the above

14. The following prescription is presented at the pharmacy to the pharmacy technician:
Lisinopril 20 mg   #90

I tab PO q8h

The pharmacy technician reviews the prescription and detects an error while inputting the prescription into the pharmacy's computer and informs the pharmacist of the situation. Which error did the technician detect?
a. Medication dosage form
b. Medication strength
c. Medication frequency of administration
d. Route of administration

15. The following prescription is presented at the pharmacy to the pharmacy technician:
John Cheung
218 Catoctin Circle SE
Leesburg, VA 20175
703-709-5424

Yosra Altahab   May 23, 202X
11602 Bromley Village Lane Reston, VA 20194

Metoprolol Succinate 200 mg #60
1 TAB PO BID for hyperlipidemia

Refill ×6   John Chung

Which error did the pharmacy technician observe?
a. Metoprolol succinate is not available as a 200 mg tablet.
b. Metoprolol succinate is not indicated for hyperlipidemia.
c. Metoprolol succinate is not taken twice a day.
d. Both b and c.

16. The following prescription is presented at the pharmacy:
William Dagit
18105 Watercraft Place
Cornelius, NC 28031
704-892-4000

Andrew Shed   July 14, 202X
1912 Hidden Knoll Apt 200   Raleigh, NC 27606

Diphenhydramine 12.5 mg/5 mL   60 mL
Nystatin Suspension   60 mL
Lidocaine Viscous 2%   60 mL
Aluminum/Magnesium/
   Simethicone 200-200-20 mg/5 mL   60 mL

Label as Magic Mouthwash.

Gargle, swish, and spit 5 mL every 6 hours as needed for sore throat.

Refill ×1   William Dagit

Which beyond-use-date should be assigned to the prescription if the prescription was filled on July 16, 202X?
a. July 23, 202X
b. July 30, 202X
c. August 6, 202X
d. August 13, 202X

17. The following prescription was presented at the pharmacy:
Jean LaPierre
170 Reynolds Avenue
Meadville, PA 16335
814-350-1056

Patty Fiely   June 18, 202X
720 North Morgan Street   Meadville, PA 16335

Montelukast 5 mg   #30
1 TAB PO q PM for bronchospasms

Refill ×2   Jean LaPierre

Which prescribing errors are present in the prescription?
a. Medication dosage form
b. Medication dose
c. Route of administration
d. There are no errors in the prescription

18. The following prescription is presented at the pharmacy:
Lee Ivory
381 Elden Street
Herndon, VA 20170
703-481-1505

John Glenn   May 15, 202X
1600 N Oak St   Arlington, VA 22209

Amoxicillin 250 mg/5 mL   150 mL
5 mL PO q8h

Refill 0 times   Lee Ivory

How many days will the prescription last the patient?
a. 5 days
b. 7 days
c. 10 days
d. 15 days

19. The following prescription is presented at the pharmacy:
Henry Chen
University of Pittsburgh Medical Center
3549 Fifth Avenue
Pittsburgh, PA 15213
412-647-2345

Kathy Vardaro   August 7, 202X
300 Craft Avenue   Pittsburgh, PA 15213

Furosemide 40 mg   #60
I TAB PO BID for hypertension

Refill ×5   Henry Chen

What error is present in the prescription?
a. Frequency of administration
b. Medication dose
c. Medication dosage form
d. There are no errors in the prescription

20. The following prescription is presented at the pharmacy:
Donald Wong
UPMC-Mercy
1400 Locust Street
Pittsburgh, PA 15219
412-232-8111

Tom Harrison   August 1, 202X
1800 Darlington Road   Pittsburgh, PA 15217

Escitalopram 20 mg   #30
1 TAB PO QD for epilepsy

Refill ×1   Donald Wong

What error(s) is (are) present on the prescription?
a. Frequency of administration
b. Medication dosage
c. Medication indication
d. Medication route of administration

21. The following prescription is presented at the pharmacy:
Dr. Michael Silverstein
381 Elden Street Suite 100
Herndon, VA 20170
703-481-1505

Ed Tarboosch   June 26, 20XX
11602 Bromley Village Lane   Reston, VA 20194

Latanoprost ophthalmic solution   2.5 mL
1 gtt in each eye at bedtime

Refill ×2   Dr. Michael Silverstein

Which DAW code should the pharmacy technician enter into the pharmacy computer system?
a. DAW 0
b. DAW 1
c. DAW 2
d. DAW 3

22. The following prescription is presented at the pharmacy:

Terry McManus N.P.
2921 N 11th St
Arlington, VA 22204
703-979-1400

Katy Ha   April 1, 222X
1121 Arlington Blvd   Arlington VA 22209

Zolpidem 10 mg   #14
1 tab PO at bedtime

Refill ×3   Terry McManus
                                 BM4525892

What is incorrect about the prescription?
a. The prescriber's DEA number is incorrect.
b. The medication's dose is incorrect.
c. The route of administration is incorrect.
d. Nothing is incorrect.

23. The following prescription is presented and filled at the pharmacy:

Safia Yousaf
Georgetown University Hospital
3800 Reservoir Road
Washington, DC 20007
202-444-3772

Moustafa Abdul   April 11, 202X
1530 Key Blvd, Arlington, VA 22209

Synthroid 100 mcg   #90
1 TAB PO q AM

Dispense as Written

Refill ×3   Safia Yousaf

Prescription Label
Your Friendly Pharmacy
1 Great Valley Drive
Wilkes Barre, PA 18708
1-800-378-0220

RX 101110231
Moustafa Abdul   Filled: April 17, 202X

Levothyroxine 100 mcg   #90
Take one tablet by mouth every morning.

Safia Yousaf
3 refills by April 10, 202Y
Use by April 16, 202Y

What dispensing error was detected?
a. Incorrect medication dispensed.
b. Medication frequency of administration is incorrect.
c. Route of administration is incorrect.
d. There is no dispensing error.

24. The following prescription is presented at the pharmacy to the pharmacy technician:

Kendall Beltran
Allegheny General Hospital
320 E. North Avenue
Pittsburgh, PA 15212
412-359-3131

Ken Arnst   February 11, 202X
408 Heights Drive   Gibsonia, PA 15044

Omeprazole 5 mg   #60
Chew one capsule three times a day for GERD.

Refill ×5   Kendall Beltran

After reviewing the prescription, which prescribing error(s) did the pharmacy technician observe?
a. Frequency of administration
b. Medication dosage
c. Route of administration
d. All the above

25. The following prescription is presented and filled at the pharmacy:

Henry Alonzo
3400 Paradise Road Suite 100
Las Vegas, NV 89169
702-784-5700

Carmen DeSoto August 8, 202X
7398 Smoke Ranch Road   Las Vegas, NV 89128

Prednisone 5 mg   #30
I TAB PO QD

Refill ×1   Henry Alonzo

Prescription Label
Your Friendly Pharmacy
1 Great Valley Drive
Wilkes Barre, PA 18708
1-800-378-0220

RX 101111112
Carmen De Soto   Filled: August 16, 202X

Prednisolone 5 mg   #30
Take one tablet by mouth every day.

Henry Alonzo
1 refill by August 7, 202Y
Use by August 15, 202Y

Which dispensing error(s) occurred?
a. Frequency of administration
b. Incorrect medication
c. Medication dosage
d. Route of administration

26. The following prescription is presented at the pharmacy counter:

Deno DiCiantis
Meadville Medical Center
751 Liberty Center
Meadville, PA 16335
814-333-5000

Sam McKnight   October 11, 202X
910 Market Street   Meadville, PA 16335

Metronidazole 500 mg   #42
I TAB PO q8hr for 14 days

Refill   Deno DiCiantis

While checking the filled prescription, the pharmacy technician observes the following auxiliary labels are affixed to the prescription bottle of metronidazole.

- Caution: Federal law prohibits the transfer of this drug to any person other than the patient for whom it was prescribed.
- Do not drink alcohol when taking medications.
- Finish all medication as prescribed.

Which auxiliary label(s) is (are) inappropriate for a prescription of metronidazole?

a. Caution: Federal law prohibits the transfer of this drug to any person other than the patient for whom it was prescribed.
b. Do not drink alcohol when taking medications.
c. Finish all medication as prescribed.
d. None of them are appropriate for a prescription of metronidazole.

27. The following prescription is presented at the pharmacy to the pharmacy technician:
Rich Kunze
22087 Colonial Acres Court
Virginia Beach, VA 23456
757-270-1345

Joey Manno   September 13, 202X
9395 Rivershore Drive   Crittendon, VA 23433

Naproxen 500 mg   #60
I TAB PO Q12hr prn moderate pain

Refills ×2   Rich Kunze

While reviewing the prescription, what error(s) did the pharmacy technician observe?
a. Incorrect dosage form
b. Incorrrect frequency of administering the medication
c. Incorrect medication strength
d. There are no errors on the prescription

28. The following prescription is presented at the pharmacy:
Hector Gonzalez
313 Park Avenue
Falls Church, VA 22041
703-571-4899

Antonio Cabrerra   April 15, 202X
5400 Leesburg Pike   Falls Church, VA 22041

Metformin ER 1000 mg #90
I Tab PO BID

Refill ×3   Hector Gonzalez

The pharmacy technician reviews the prescription and detects an error while inputting the prescription into the pharmacy's computer and informs the pharmacist of the situation. Which error did the technician detect?
a. Medication dosage form
b. Medication strength
c. Medication frequency of administration
d. Route of administration

29. The following prescription is presented at the pharmacy counter to the pharmacy technician. The pharmacy technician is reviewing the prescription for completeness.
Elizabeth Rosales
4230 North Fairfax Drive
Arlington, VA 22201
703-637-7000

Hector Gutierrez   August 7, 202X
2100 Columbia Pike   Arlington VA 22204

Losartan 200 mg   #90
1 CAP PO QD prn diabetes mellitus

Refill ×3   Elizabeth Rosales

What error(s) is (are) identified on the prescription by the pharmacy technician?
a. Medication dosage form
b. Medication indication
c. Medication strength
d. All the above

30. The following prescription is presented at the pharmacy to the pharmacy technician:
Robert Shore
11800 Sunrise Valley Drive Suite 500
Reston, VA 20191
703-621-4501

Clark Andersen   February 27, 202X
441 Springvale Rd   Great Falls, VA 22066

Atorvastatin 20 mg   #30
I TAB PO QD after evening meal for dyslipidemia

Refill ×3   Robert Shore

While reviewing the prescription, what issue(s) is (are) observed by the pharmacy technician?
a. Medication frequency
b. Medication strength
c. Route of administration
d. No issues were observed

31. The following prescription is presented and reviewed at the pharmacy counter for completeness and accuracy:
Tre Landry
11800 Sunrise Valley Drive South Suite 500
Reston, VA 20191
703-627-4501

Herschel Williams   March 3, 202X
1215 Newport Cove   Reston, VA 20194

Simvastatin 60 mg   #90
I TAB PO BID for diabetes mellitus

Refill ×3   Tre Landry

Which error(s) was (were) observed and reported to the pharmacist?
a. Medication frequency
b. Medication indication
c. Medication strength
d. All the above

32. A patient presents the following prescription to be filled at the community pharmacy:
Joan Ritter
2921 N 11th St
Arlington, VA 22204
703-979-1400

Horace Wilson   October 11, 202X
1600 N Oak Apt 405   Arlington, VA 22209

Amlodipine 10 mg   #90
I TAB PO QD

Refills ×2   Joan Ritter

Prescription Label
Your Friendly Pharmacy
1 Great Valley Drive
Wilkes Barre, PA 18708
1-800-378-0220

RX 101111345
Horace Wilson   Filled: October 18, 202X

Amlodipine 5 mg   #90
Take one tablet by mouth every day for hyperlipidemia.

Joan Ritter
2 refills by October 10, 202Y
Use by October 17, 202Y

What error(s) are present on the filled prescription?
a. Medication dosage
b. Medication frequency
c. Medication Indication
d. Both a and c

33. The following prescription is presented at the pharmacy:
Andrew Shedlock
2610 Cates Avenue
Raleigh, NC 27606
919-470-3130

Tonya Coleman   December 14, 202X
403 West Creek Circle   Raleigh, VA 27606

Gabapentin 300 mg   #270
I CAP PO TID for seizures

Refills 2   Andrew Shedlock

Prescription Label
Your Friendly Pharmacy
1 Great Valley Drive
Wilkes Barre, PA 18708
1-800-378-0220

RX 10111789
Tonya Coleman   Filled: December 18, 202X

Gabapentin 300 mg   #270
Take one capsule by mouth three times a day for
  seizures.

Andrew Shedlock
2 refills by December 13, 202Y
Use by December 17, 202Y

Which dispensing error(s) occurred?
a. Frequency of administration
b. Medication dosage
c. Medication indication
d. No errors

34. The following prescription is presented at the pharmacy and is reviewed by the pharmacy for completeness and accuracy:
Dr. Michael Silverstein
381 Elden Street Suite 100
Herndon, VA 20170
703-481-1505

Terrence Frye   December 21, 202X
11400 South Lakes Drive   Reston, VA 20191

Seroquel SR 400 mg   #60
1 TAB PO BID for bipolar disorder

Refill ×1   Michael Silverstein

Which prescribing error was discovered?
a. Frequency of administration
b. Medication dosage
c. Route of administration
d. No prescribing errors were observed

35. The following prescription is presented and filled at the pharmacy:
Henry Alonzo
3400 Paradise Road Suite 100
Las Vegas, NV 89169
702-784-5700

Tom Roach   August 8, 202X
318 MaGee Place   Pittsburgh, PA 15213

Tobrex Ophthalmic Solution 0.3%
I-2 gtt ou q 4h

Refill ×1   Henry Alonzo

How should the signa appear on the prescription label?
a. Instill 1–2 drops in each ear every 4 hours.
b. Instill 1–2 drops in each eye every 4 hours.
c. Instill 1–2 drops in right ear every 4 hours.
d. Instill 1–2 drops in right eye every 4 hours.

36. The pharmacy technician is reviewing the following prescription label:
Ibuprofen 600 mg   #60

Take one tablet by mouth every 6 hours as needed for pain.
The following auxiliary labels were affixed to the patient's prescription bottle of ibuprofen 600 mg:
• Do not drink alcohol when taking this medication.
• May cause dizziness.
• Take with food or milk.
Which auxiliary label(s) is (are) inappropriate for ibuprofen?
a. Do not drink alcohol when taking this medication.
b. May cause dizziness.
c. Take with food or milk.
d. None of the auxiliary labels are inappropriate for ibuprofen.

37. The following prescription was presented at the pharmacy:
Henrietta Wilson
713 Washington Road
Mt Lebanon, PA 15228
412-344-9466

Aloysius Demetrious   November 13, 202X
904 Maplewood Drive   Pittsburgh, PA 15234

Glyburide 5 mg   #90
I tab PO QD for diabetes mellitus

Refill ×3

Prescription Label
Your Friendly Pharmacy
1 Great Valley Drive
Wilkes Barre, PA 18708
1-800-378-0220

RX 10101098
Aloysius Demetrious Filled: November 17, 202X

Glipizide 5 mg   #90

Take one tablet by mouth four times daily for diabetes
   mellitus.
Henrietta Wilson
3 refills by November 12, 202Y
Use by November 16, 202Y
What dispensing error(s) was (were) detected?
a. Incorrect medication
b. Incorrect frequency
c. Incorrect medication strength
d. Both a and b

38. The following prescription is presented and reviewed at
the pharmacy counter for completeness and accuracy:
Tre Landry
11800 Sunrise Valley Drive South Suite 500
Reston, VA 20191
703-627-4501
Gabriel Watson   March 3, 202X

Hydrocodone/acetaminophen 300 mg/15 mg   #30
1 TAB PO q 4–6 hours as needed

Refill ×1   Tre Landry

Which prescription omissions/errors were observed by
   the pharmacy technician?
a. DEA number is missing.
b. Patient address is missing.
c. Refills are not permitted.
d. All the above.

39. The following prescription is presented at the pharmacy
counter to the pharmacy technician:
Elizabeth Rosales
4230 North Fairfax Drive
Arlington, VA 22201
703-637-7000

Roberta Harrison   March 3, 202X
224 Maple Avenue   Vienna, VA 22180

Prozac 20 mg   #60
I CAP PO QD

Dispense as Written

Refill 1   Elizabeth Rosales

Prescription Label
Your Friendly Pharmacy
1 Great Valley Drive
Wilkes Barre, PA 18708
1-800-378-0220

RX 101110231
Roberta Harrison   Filled: March 10, 202X

Prilosec 20 mg   #60
Take one capsule by mouth four times a day.

Elizabeth Rosales
1 refill by March 2, 202Y
Use by March 9, 202Y

Which error(s) was (were) observed by the pharmacy
   technician?

a. Incorrect frequency of administration
b. Incorrect medication
c. Incorrect route of administration
d. Both a and b

40. The following prescription is presented and filled at the
pharmacy:
Safia Yousaf
Georgetown University Hospital
3800 Reservoir Road
Washington, DC 20007
202-444-3772

Bobby Wilson   April 11, 202X
1530 Key Blvd   Arlington, VA 22209

Timolol Ophthalmic Solution 0.25%   10 mL
I gtt od qd for glaucoma

Refill ×3   Safia Yousaf

Prescription Label
Your Friendly Pharmacy
1 Great Valley Drive
Wilkes Barre, PA 18708
1-800-378-0220

RX 101110231
Bobby Wilson   Filled: April 17, 202X

Timolol Ophthalmic Solution 0.25%   10 mL
Instill one drop in left eye daily for glaucoma.

Safia Yousaf
3 refills by April 10, 202Y
Use by April 16, 202Y

What dispensing error was detected?
a. Incorrect medication is dispensed.
b. Medication frequency of administration is incorrect.
c. Route of administration is incorrect.
d. There is no dispensing error.

41. The following prescription is presented at the pharmacy:
Andrew Shedlock
2610 Cates Avenue
Raleigh, NC 27606
919-470-3130

Martha Wells   July 6, 202X
1000 Main Street   Raleigh, NC 27695

Venlafaxine ER 75 mg   #30
I CAP PO QD

Refill 1   Andrew Shedlock

Prescription Label
Your Friendly Pharmacy
1 Great Valley Drive
Wilkes Barre, PA 18708
1-800-378-0220

RX 101110235
Martha Wells   Filled: July 9, 202X

Venlafaxine ER 75 mg   #30
Take one capsule once a day.

Refill 1   Andrew Shedlock

Andrew Shedlock
1 refill by July 5, 202Y
Use by August 15, 202Y

What error(s) was (were) observed by the technician?
a. Route of administration not indicated
b. Incorrect dosage form
c. Incorrect frequency of administration
d. All of the above

42. The following prescription is presented at the pharmacy:
Dr. Michael Silverstein
381 Elden Street Suite 100
Herndon, VA 20170
703-481-1505

Davey Horne   August 8, 202X
23050 Autumnwood Drive   Reston, VA 20194

Amoxicillin/clavulanate 500 mg/125 mg   #30
I TAB PO q 8 h for sinus infection

Refill 1   Michael Silverstein

Prescription Label
Your Friendly Pharmacy
1 Great Valley Drive
Wilkes Barre, PA 18708
1-800-378-0220

RX 101110532
David Johns   Filled: August 16, 202X

Amoxicillin/clavulanate 250 mg/125 mg   #30
Take one tablet by mouth every 8 hours for sinus
    infection.

Michael Silverstein
1 refill by August 7, 202Y
Use by August 15, 202Y

Which error(s) was (were) observed by the pharmacy
    technician?
a. Incorrect frequency of administration
b. Incorrect medication strength
c. Incorrect patient
d. Both b and c

43. The pharmacy technician is reviewing the following
prescription label for an adult patient:
Nitroglycerin 0.4 mg   #100

Take one tablet sublingually every 5 minutes with a maxi-
    mum of 3 doses within 15 minutes as needed for angina.
What error(s) did the pharmacy technician observe?
a. Frequency of doses
b. Medication strength
c. Route of administration
d. No errors observed

44. The pharmacy technician is reviewing the following
prescription label:
Glyburide 5 mg   #90
Take one tablet by mouth once a day for diabetes
    mellitus.

The following auxiliary labels were affixed to the pre-
    scription bottle of glyburide:
• Caution: Federal law prohibits the transfer of this
    drug to any person other than the patient for whom it
    was prescribed.

• Discolor urine or feces.
• Do not drink alcohol when taking medications.

Which auxiliary label(s) should is (are) inappropriate to
    be affixed to the prescription bottle of glyburide?
a. Caution: Federal law prohibits the transfer of this
    drug to any person other than the patient for whom it
    was prescribed.
b. Discolor urine or feces.
c. Do not drink alcohol when taking medications.
d. a and b are inappropriate auxiliary labels to be affixed
    to a prescription bottle of glyburide.

45. The following prescription is presented at the pharmacy
to the pharmacy technician:
Subash Bazaz
11800 Sunrise Valley Drive Suite 500
Reston, VA 20191
703-621-4501

Babak Mohassel   December 3, 202X
11604 Brandon Hill Way   Reston, VA 20194-1215

Doxycycline 100 mg   #28
I CAP PO QD for pneumonia.

Refill ×1   Subash Bazaz

Which issue was observed by the pharmacy technician
    when reviewing the prescription?
a. Frequency of dose
b. Medication indication
c. Medication strength
d. No issues are present

46. The following prescription was presented to the
pharmacy technician:
Dennis Finton
390 Park Avenue
Meadville, PA 16335
814-724-2280

Jocelyn Mizner   August 9, 202X
10635 Konneyaut Trail   Conneaut Lake, PA 16316

Amoxicillin 500 mg   #21
I CAP PO Q8hr for 10 days for sinus infection

Refill ×0   Dennis Finton

What prescribing error was observed?
a. Medication frequency
b. Medication strength
c. Medication dosage form
d. No prescribing errors are present

47. The following prescription was presented at the
pharmacy:
Haroon Rashid
2901 Telestar Court Suite 100
Falls Church, VA 22042
703-208-9798

Carrie Clark   March 1, 202X
441 Springvale Road, Great Falls, VA 22066

Warfarin 2 mg   #90
I TAB PO QD as directed by physician.

Refill ×3   Haroon Rashid

Prescription Label
Your Friendly Pharmacy
1 Great Valley Drive
Wilkes Barre, PA 18708
1-800-378-0220

RX 10101011
Carrie Clark   Filled: March 10, 202X

Warfarin 5 mg   #90
Take one tablet by mouth every day as directed by physician.

Haroon Rashid
3 refills by February 28, 202Y
Use by March 9, 202Y

What dispensing error was detected?
a. Dispensing date
b. Medication strength
c. Route of administration
d. No dispensing error detected

48. The pharmacy technician is reviewing the following prescription label:
Tetracycline 250 mg   #60

Take one capsule twice a day for acne vulgaris.

The following auxiliary labels were affixed to the patient's prescription bottle of tetracycline 250 mg:
• Avoid exposure to sun.
• Do not take if pregnant, nursing, or trying to conceive.
• Do not take dairy products, antacids, or iron preparations.

Which auxiliary label(s) is (are) inappropriate for tetracycline?
a. Avoid exposure to sun.
b. Do not take if pregnant, nursing, or trying to conceive.
c. Do not take dairy products, antacids, or iron preparations.
d. None of the auxiliary labels is inappropriate for a tetracycline prescription.

49. The following prescription is presented and filled at the pharmacy:
Nancy Alonzo
3400 Paradise Road Suite 100
Las Vegas, NV 89169
702-784-5700

Alphonzo Ruiz   August 20, 202X
7398 Smoke Ranch Road   Las Vegas, NV 89128

Carvedilol 12.5 mg   #60
I TAB PO BID for hypertension

Refill ×1   Nancy Alonzo

Prescription Label
Your Friendly Pharmacy
1 Great Valley Drive
Wilkes Barre, PA 18708
1-800-378-0220

RX 101111112
Carmen De Soto   Filled: August 30, 202X

Captopril 12.5 mg   #60
Take one tablet by mouth twice a day for hypertension.

Nancy Alonzo
1 refill by August 19, 202Y
Use by August 29, 202Y

Which dispensing error(s) occurred?
a. Incorrect frequency of administration
b. Incorrect medication
c. Incorrect medication dosage
d. Incorrect route of administration

50. The pharmacy technician is reviewing the following prescription label for an adult patient:
Fluticasone propionate nasal 50 mcg/actuation   #1
2–4 actuations inhaled TID

Which error was observed by the technician?
a. Dosage is incorrect.
b. Frequency of inhalations is incorrect.
c. Number of actuations/dose is incorrect.
d. Route of administration is incorrect.

51. The pharmacy technician is reviewing the following prescription label for an adult:
Amitriptyline 5 mg   #90
Take one tablet by mouth every 12 hours for bipolar disease.

Which error(s) was (were) observed by the technician?
a. Dosage is incorrect.
b. Frequency of dosages is incorrect.
c. Medication indication is incorrect.
d. All are incorrect.

52. The following prescription was presented at the pharmacy:
Henrietta Wilson
713 Washington Road
Mt Lebanon, PA 15228
412-344-9466

Alba Solar   February 15, 202X
Bower Hill Road   Mt Lebanon, PA 15228

Symbicort 160 mcg/4.5 mcg   120 actuations
2 puffs inhaled BID

Prescription Label
Your Friendly Pharmacy
1 Great Valley Drive
Wilkes Barre, PA 18708
1-800-378-0220

RX 101117231
Alba Solar   Filled: February 20, 202X

Symbicort 80 mcg/4.5 mcg   60 actuations
Two puffs inhaled once a day

Henrietta Wilson
1 refill by February 14, 202Y
Use by February 19, 202Y

Which error(s) was (were) observed by the pharmacy technician while verifying the completed prescription?
a. Incorrect frequency of administration
b. Incorrect medication strength
c. Incorrect quantity dispensed
d. All the above

53. The following prescription is presented and filled at the pharmacy:
Kim Tran
Georgetown University Hospital
3800 Reservoir Road
Washington, DC 20007
202-444-3772

Alicia Nieve   April 11, 202X
1530 Key Blvd   Arlington, VA 22209

Beconase AQ 25 g   180 metered sprays
2 sprays in each nostril BID

Refill ×3   Kim Tran

How many days' supply should be indicated by the pharmacy technician when inputting the prescription in the computer?
a. 22 days
b. 30 days
c. 45 days
d. 90 days

54. The following prescription is presented at the pharmacy:
Kim Curi
381 Elden Street Suite 100
Herndon, VA 20170
703-481-1505

Anna Bailes January 12, 202X
12001 Sunrise Valley Drive   Reston, VA 20191

Hydrocortisone 25 mg Suppositories   #12
I Supp PR BID prn hemorrhoids

Refill 1   Kim Curi

Prescription Label
Your Friendly Pharmacy
1 Great Valley Drive
Wilkes Barre, PA 18708
1-800-378-0220

RX 101160231   Filled: January 19, 202X
Ana Bailes

Hydrocortisone 25 mg Suppositories   #12
Insert one suppository orally twice a day as needed for hemorrhoids.

Kim Curi
1 refill by January 11, 202Y
Use by January 18, 202Y

Which error was observed by the pharmacy technician while verifying the filled prescription?
a. Incorrect dosage
b. Incorrect frequency of administration
c. Incorrect route of administration
d. All the above

55. The following prescription is presented at the pharmacy to the pharmacy technician:
Kendall Beltran
Allegheny General Hospital
320 E. North Avenue
Pittsburgh, PA 15212
412-359-3131

Aurora Bissiris   April 15, 202X
342 Friendship Blvd   Bloomfield, PA 15224

Hydrocortisone Cream 2.5%   30 g
Apply BID-QID TOP prn itching aa

Refill 1   Kendall Beltran

Prescription Label
Your Friendly Pharmacy
1 Great Valley Drive
Wilkes Barre, PA 18708
1-800-378-0220

RX 101210231   Filled: April 21, 202X
Aurora Bissiris

Hydrocortisone Ointment 2.5%   30 g
Apply 2–4 times a day topically as needed for itching to affected area.

Kendall Beltran
1 refill by April 14, 202Y
Use by August 20, 202Y

Which error was discovered by the pharmacy technician while conducting prescription verification?
a. Incorrect dosage form
b. Incorrect dosage strength
c. Incorrrect frequency of administration
d. Incorrect route of administration

56. The following prescription is presented at the pharmacy counter and reviewed by the pharmacy technician for completeness and accuracy:
Deno DiCiantis
Meadville Medical Center
751 Liberty Center
Meadville, PA 16335
814-333-5000

Carol Jonesy   May 13, 202X
520 N Main Street   Meadville, PA 16335

Trazodone 50 mg   #60
I TAB PO BID for depression

Refill 1   Deno DiCiantis

Which omission was observed by the pharmacy technician while receiving the patient's prescription?
a. Medication frequency of administration
b. Medication route of administration
c. Medication strength
d. No omissions were observed

57. The following prescription is presented at the pharmacy to the pharmacy technician:
Subash Bazaz
11800 Sunrise Valley Drive Suite 500
Reston, VA 20191
703-621-4501

Avi Agrawal   March 9, 202X
1514 Coat Ridge Court   Herndon, VA 20170

Sulfamethoxazole/Trimethoprim 200 mg/40 mg/5 mL
   Suspension   30 days' supply
5 mL PO BID

Refill   Subash Bazaz

What volume of sulfamethoxazole/trimethoprim 200 mg/40 mg/5 mL suspension should be dispensed?
a. 30 mL
b. 120 mL
c. 240 mL
d. 300 mL

58. The following prescription is presented and filled at the pharmacy:
Henry Alonzo
3400 Paradise Road Suite 100
Las Vegas, NV 89169
702-784-5700

Clarice Tse   August 8, 202X
7398 Smoke Ranch Road   Las Vegas, NV 89128

Miconazole 2% Cream   30 g
Apply BID TOP for fungal infection

Refill ×1   Henry Alonzo

Prescription Label
Your Friendly Pharmacy
1 Great Valley Drive
Wilkes Barre, PA 18708
1-800-378-0220

RX 101111112
Clarice Tse   Filled: August 16, 202X

Miconazole 7 Vaginal Cream 45 g
Insert one applicatorful in vagina at bedtime for 7 days.

Henry Alonzo
1 refill by August 7, 202Y
Use by August 15, 202Y

What error(s) was (were) observed in the filled prescription by the pharmacy technician?
a. Incorrect frequency of administration
b. Incorrect medication dispensed
c. Incorrect route of administration
d. All the above

59. The pharmacy technician is reviewing the following prescription label:
Amoxicillin 500 mg   #30
Take one capsule every 8 hours for infection.

The following auxiliary labels were affixed to the patient's prescription bottle of amoxicillin 500 mg:
• Do not take with dairy products, antacids, or iron preparations.
• Finish all medication as prescribed.
• Do not take if pregnant, nursing, trying to conceive.
Which auxiliary label(s) is (are) inappropriate to be affixed to the patient's prescription bottle of amoxicillin 500 mg?
a. Do not take with dairy products, antacids, or iron preparations.
b. Finish all medication as prescribed.
c. Do not take if pregnant, nursing, trying to conceive.
d. Both a and c.

60. The pharmacy technician is reviewing the following filled prescription label:
Xarelto   20 mg   #60

Take one tablet twice a day for deep vein thromboembolism.

What error is detected in the label?
a. Medication dosage form
b. Medication strength
c. Medication frequency
d. There are no errors in the label

61. The following prescription is presented at the pharmacy and reviewed by the pharmacy technician for accuracy and completeness:
Elizabeth Kline
2921 Columbia Pike
Arlington, VA 22204
703-979-1425

Mary Shedlock   March 10, 202X
11608 Brandon Hill Way   Reston, VA 20194-1215

Methylprednisolone 4 mg   #20
Day 1: 2 tab po before breakfast, 1 tab after lunch and after dinner, and 2 tabs at bedtime
Day 2: 1 tab po before breakfast, after lunch, and after dinner and 2 tabs at bedtime
Day 3: 1 tab po before breakfast, after lunch, after dinner, and at bedtime
Day 4: 1 tab po before breakfast, after lunch, and at bedtime
Day 5: 1 tab po before breakfast and at bedtime
Day 6: 1 tab po before breakfast

Refill ×0

What prescribing error(s) was (were) observed by the pharmacy technician?
a. Medication quantity
b. Medication strength
c. Route of administration
d. All the above

62. The following prescription is presented at the pharmacy:
Andrew Shedlock
2610 Cates Avenue
Raleigh, NC 27606
919-470-3130

Claudia Romero   June 11, 202X
5701 Hillsborough St Raleigh, NC 27606

Rosuvastatin 20 mg   #90
I TAB PO QD

Refill 3   Andrew Shedlock

How many days will the prescription last?
a. 15 days
b. 30 days
c. 60 days
d. 90 days

63. The following prescription is presented at the pharmacy to the pharmacy technician:
Kendall Beltran
Allegheny General Hospital
320 E. North Avenue
Pittsburgh, PA 15212
412-359-3131

Dan Dyke   August 17, 202X
1001 N Negley Avenue   Pittsburgh, PA 15206

Cyclobenzaprine 5 mg   #30
I TAB PO QD prn muscle spasms

Refill 2   Kendall Bertran

Prescription Label
Your Friendly Pharmacy
1 Great Valley Drive
Wilkes Barre, PA 18708
1-800-378-0220

RX 101111412
Dan Dyke   Filled: August 25, 202X

Cyclobenzaprine 10 mg   #60
Take one tablet by mouth four times a day.

Kendall Bertran
2 refill by August 16, 202Y
Use by August 24, 202Y

Which error(s) was (were) detected by the pharmacy
   technician while verifying the completed prescription?
a. Incorrect frequency of administration
b. Incorrect medication strength
c. Incorrect quantity dispensed
d. All the above

64. The following prescription is presented at the pharmacy
to the pharmacy technician:
Rich Kunze
22087 Colonial Acres Court
Virginia Beach, VA 23456
757-270-1345

Cora Miller   July 10, 202X
3100 Hunters Chase Drive   Virginia Beach 23452

Atenolol 50 mg   #90
I TAB PO QD for hypertension

Refill 2   Rich Kunze

Prescription Label
Your Friendly Pharmacy
1 Great Valley Drive
Wilkes Barre, PA 18708 tablets
1-800-378-0220

RX 101111122
Cora Miller   Filled: July 16, 202X

Atenolol 50 mg   #90
Place one tablet under the tongue each day for hypertension.

Rich Kunze
0 refill by July 9, 202Y
Use by July 15, 202Y

Which error(s) was (were) detected by the pharmacy
   technician while performing prescription verification?
a. Incorrect medication strength
b. Incorrect refills indicated
c. Incorrect route of administration
d. Both b and c

65. The following prescription is presented and filled at the
pharmacy:
Daphne Edwin
Georgetown University Hospital
3800 Reservoir Road

Washington, DC 20007
202-444-3772

Amos Jenkins   April 15, 202X
1530 Key Blvd   Arlington, VA 22209

Pravastatin 20 mg   #30
1 TAB PO QD for dyslipidemia

Refill ×3   Daphne Edwin

Prescription Label
Your Friendly Pharmacy
1 Great Valley Drive
Wilkes Barre, PA 18708
1-800-378-0220

RX 101110231
Amos Jenkins   Filled: April 24, 202X

Pravastatin 40 mg   #30
Take one tablet by mouth daily for dyslipidemia.

Daphne Edwin
3 refills by April 14, 202Y
Use by April 13, 202Y

Which dispensing error was detected by the technician?
a. Incorrect frequency of administration
b. Incorrect medication
c. Incorrect medication strength
d. Incorrect route of administration

66. The following prescription is presented and filled at the
pharmacy:
Roberto Benitez
201 State Street
Erie, PA 16550
814-877-6000
BB1234563

Melissa Major   September 30, 202X
7812 Hamot Road   Erie, PA 16507

Lorazepam 0.5 mg   #60
1 TAB PO TID for anxiety

Refill ×1   Roberto Benitez

Prescription Label
Your Friendly Pharmacy
1 Great Valley Drive
Wilkes Barre, PA 18708
1-800-378-0220

RX 111112222
Melissa Major   Filled: October 5, 202X

Alprazolam 0.5 mg   #60
Take one tablet by mouth three times a day as needed
   for anxiety.

Roberto Benitez
1 refill by September 29, 202Y
Use by October 4, 202Y

Which dispensing error(s) occurred?
a. Frequency of administration
b. Incorrect medication
c. Medication dosage
d. Route of administration

67. The pharmacy technician is reviewing the following prescription label:

Dr. Michael Silverstein
381 Elden Street Suite 100
Herndon, VA 20170
703-481-1505

Helena Wilson   December 15, 202X
6592 Williamsburg Blvd   Falls Church, VA 22041

Lo Loestrin FE   1 month
I TAB PO QD

Refill 6   Michael Silverstein

The following auxiliary labels were affixed to the patient's prescription package:
- Do not smoke when taking medications.
- May cause dizziness.
- May cause drowsiness.

Which auxiliary label(s) is (are) inappropriate to be affixed to the patient's package of Lo Loestrin FE?
a. Do not smoke when taking medications.
b. May cause dizziness.
c. May cause drowsiness.
d. Both b and c.

68. The following prescription is presented and filled at the pharmacy:

Cristina Alonzo
3400 Paradise Road Suite 100
Las Vegas, NV 89169
702-784-5700

Deborah Guardado   September 8, 202X
7398 Smoke Ranch Road   Las Vegas, NV 89128

Ibuprofen 600 mg   #120
I TAB PO QID PRN moderate pain

How many days will the prescription last?
a. 30 days
b. 40 days
c. 60 days
d. 120 days

69. The pharmacy technician is reviewing the following prescription label:

Acetaminophen/codeine 300 mg/30 mg   #30
Take one tablet by mouth every 4–6 hours as needed for pain.

The following auxiliary labels were affixed to the patient's prescription bottle of acetaminophen/codeine 300 mg/30 mg:
- Caution: Federal law prohibits the transfer of this drug to any person other than the patient for whom it was prescribed.
- Do not drink alcohol when taking medications.
- Do not take with grapefruit.
- May cause drowsiness.

Which auxiliary label is inappropriate to be affixed to the patient's prescription bottle of acetaminophen/codeine 300 mg/30 mg?
a. Caution: Federal law prohibits the transfer of this drug to any person other than the patient for whom it was prescribed.

b. Do not drink alcohol when taking medications.
c. Do not take with grapefruit.
d. May cause drowsiness.

70. The pharmacy receives the following prescription:

Tony Vardaro
209 Lilly Ridge Drive
Canonsburg, PA 15317
814-333-3600

Augustus Bennett   March 10, 202X
408 Heights Drive   Gibsonia, PA 15044

Albuterol 90 mcg/actuation   200 actuations
2 puffs inhaled every 4–6 h prn asthma

Refill ×3

How many days will the prescription last the patient?
a. 16 days
b. 25 days
c. 33 days
d. 50 days

71. The pharmacy receives the following prescription:

Guiseppe Catalano
Georgetown University Hospital
3800 Reservoir Road
Washington, DC 20007
202-444-3772

Devri Langhelm   April 10, 202X
1530 Key Blvd   Arlington, VA 22209

Dilantin 100 mg   #90
1 CAP PO TID for epilepsy

Dispense as Written

Refill ×3   Guiseppe Catalano

Prescription Label
Your Friendly Pharmacy
1 Great Valley Drive
Wilkes Barre, PA 18708
1-800-378-0220

RX 101110230
Devri Langhelm   Filled: April 17, 202X

Phenytoin 100 mcg   #90
Take one capsule by mouth three times a day for epilepsy.

Guiseppe Catalano
3 refills by April 9, 202Y
Use by April 16, 202Y

Which error was observed by the pharmacy technician on the completed prescription?
a. Incorrect dosage form
b. Incorrect medication dispensed
c. Incorrect route of administration
d. No errors were observed

72. The following prescription is presented at the pharmacy:
Andrew Shedlock
2610 Cates Avenue
Raleigh, NC 27606
919-470-3130

Diana Namugenyi   August 21, 202X
1301 Hillsborough St   Raleigh, NC 27605

Ofloxacin Otic Solution 0.3% 5 mL
10 gtt ad QD × 7 days

Refill 1   Andrew Shedlock

Prescription Label
Your Friendly Pharmacy
1 Great Valley Drive
Wilkes Barre, PA 18708
1-800-378-0220

RX 101117230
Diana Namugenyi   Filled: August 25, 202X

Ofloxacin Otic Solution 0.3% 5 mL
Instill 10 drops in left ear four times a day for 7 days.

Andrew Shedlock
1 refill by August 20, 202Y
Use by August 15, 202Y

Which error(s) was (were) observed by the pharmacy technician when verifying the filled prescription?
a. Incorrect duration of therapy
b. Incorrect frequency of administration
c. Incorrect route of administration
d. Both b and c

73. The following prescription is presented at the pharmacy:
Dr. Michelle Lee
381 Elden Street Suite 100
Herndon, VA 20170
703-481-1505

Emily Marchena   February 7, 202X
8666 Bruton Parish Ct   Manassas, VA 20110

Sumatriptan 25 mg   #12
25 mg PO initially after signs of headache; may repeat dose once after 2 hours

Refill 1   Michelle Lee

Prescription Label
Your Friendly Pharmacy
1 Great Valley Drive
Wilkes Barre, PA 18708
1-800-378-0220

RX 101617230
Emily Marchena   Filled: February 11, 202X

Sumatriptan 25 mg   #12
Place one tablet (25 mg) under the tongue initially after the first signs of headache. May repeat dose once after 2 hours.

Michelle Lee
1 refill by February 6, 202Y
Use by February 10, 202Y

Which error was observed by the pharmacy technician when verifying the filled prescription?
a. Incorrect frequency of administering medication
b. Incorrect medication strength dispensed
c. Incorrect patient receiving the prescription
d. Incorrect route of administration

74. The following prescription is presented at the pharmacy counter:
Deno DiCiantis
Meadville Medical Center
751 Liberty Center
Meadville, PA 16335
814-333-5000

Joe Alfier   June 11, 202X
726 Morgan Street   Meadville, PA 16335

Flovent HFA 110 mcg/actuations   #1 canister
2–4 puffs inhaled twice a day as needed for asthma

Refill 2   Deno DiCiantis

Prescription Label
Your Friendly Pharmacy
1 Great Valley Drive
Wilkes Barre, PA 18708
1-800-378-0220

RX 101117237
Joe Alfier   Filled June 15, 202X

Flovent HFA 220 mcg/actuation   #1 cannister
2–4 inhalations inhaled once a day as needed for asthma

Deno DiCiantis
2 refills by June 10, 202Y
Use by June 14, 202Y

Which error(s) was (were) observed by the pharmacy technician while reviewing the filled prescription?
a. Incorrect frequency of administration
b. Incorrect medication strength
c. Incorrect number of inhalations per dose
d. Both a and b

75. The following prescription is presented at the pharmacy to the pharmacy technician:
Subash Bazaz
11800 Sunrise Valley Drive Suite 500
Reston, VA 20191
703-621-4501

Gail Romans   March 9, 202X
11240 Colts Neck   Reston, VA 20191

Protonix 20 mg   #30
I TAB PO QD

Refill 1

Prescription Label
Your Friendly Pharmacy
1 Great Valley Drive
Wilkes Barre, PA 18708
1-800-378-0220

RX 101417230   Filled March 14, 202X

Pantoprazole 20 mg   #30
Take one tablet by mouth each day.

Subash Bazaz
1 refill by March 8, 202Y
Use by March 13, 202Y

Which error was observed by the pharmacy technician while reviewing the completed prescription?
a. Incorrect frequency of administration
b. Incorrect medication dispensed
c. Incorrect route of administration
d. No error observed

76. The following prescription is presented at the pharmacy to the pharmacy technician:
Kendall Beltran
Allegheny General Hospital
320 E. North Avenue
Pittsburgh, PA 15212
412-359-3131

Esther Gonzalez   February 2, 202X
2782 Bigelow Blvd   Pittsburgh, PA 15213

Tegretol 200 mg   #180
2 TAB PO TID

Refill 3   Kendall Beltran

Prescription Label
Your Friendly Pharmacy
1 Great Valley Drive
Wilkes Barre, PA 18708
1-800-378-0220

RX 141117230
Esther Gonzalez   Filled February 5, 202X

Tegretol XR 200 mg   #180
Take two tablets by mouth three times a day.

Kendall Beltran
3 refills by February 1, 202Y
Use by February 4, 202Y

Which dispensing error(s) was (were) observed by the pharmacy technician?
a. Incorrect dosage form
b. Incorrect dosage strength
c. Incorrect frequency of administration
d. Incorrect route of administration

77. The following prescription is presented and filled at the pharmacy:
Roberto Benitez
201 State Street
Erie, PA 16550
814-877-6000

Roberto Fuentes   September 30, 202X
7812 Hamot Road   Erie, PA 16507

Lantus Solostar Pen #1
25 units SQ q am

Refill ×1   Roberto Benitez

Prescription Label
Your Friendly Pharmacy
1 Great Valley Drive
Wilkes Barre, PA 18708
1-800-378-0220

RX 111122222
Roberto Fuentes   Filled: October 1, 202X

Lantus SoloStar Pen #1
Inject 25 units under the skin each morning.

Roberto Benitez

If the Lantus SoloStar insulin is opened on October 2, 202X, which beyond-use date should be assigned?
a. October 16, 202X
b. October 30, 202X
c. November 14, 202X
d. November 28, 202X

78. The pharmacy technician is reviewing the following prescription label:
sulfamethoxazole/trimethoprim 800 mg/160 mg #28
1 Tab PO BID for UTI

The following auxiliary labels were affixed to the patient's prescription bottle of sulfamethoxazole/trimethoprim 800 mg/160:
• Avoid exposure to sunlight.
• Finish all medication as prescribed.
• Take with water.
Which auxiliary label(s) is (are) inappropriate to be affixed to the patient's prescription bottle of sulfamethoxazole/trimethoprim 800 mg/160?
a. Avoid exposure to sunlight.
b. Finish all medication as prescribed.
c. Take with water.
d. None of the auxiliary labels are inappropriate for a prescription of sulfamethoxazole/trimethoprim 800 mg/160.

79. The following prescription is presented at the pharmacy to the pharmacy technician:
Antonio Gutierrez
170 Reynolds Avenue
Meadville, PA 16335
814-724-2347

Bruce Fisher   May 28, 202X
404 Chestnut Street Meadville, PA 16335

Alprazolam 0.5 mg #90
1 tab PO TID prn anxiety

Refill ×1   Dr. Antonio Gutierrez

What omission was observed by the pharmacy technician?
a. DEA number
b. Inscription
c. Signa
d. Subscription

80. The following prescription is presented at the pharmacy:
Henry Liu
381 Elden Street Suite 100
Herndon, VA 20170
703-481-1505

Truc Tran   April 1, 202X
106 Spring Street   Herndon, VA 20170

Janumet 50/1000 mg #180
I TAB PO BID for diabetes mellitus

Refill 1   Henry Liu

Prescription Label
Your Friendly Pharmacy
1 Great Valley Drive
Wilkes Barre, PA 18708
1-800-378-0220

RX 101117630
Truc Tran   Filled: April 5, 202X

Janumet XR 50/1000 mg   #180
Take one tablet by mouth twice a day for diabetes mellitus.

Henry Liu
1 refill by March 31, 202Y
Use by April 4, 202Y

Which error was observed by the pharmacy technician
   on the filled prescription?
a. Incorrect frequency of administration
b. Incorrect medication
c. Incorrect route of administration
d. No error observed

81. The following prescription is presented at the pharmacy:
Young Kim
Georgetown University Hospital
3800 Reservoir Road
Washington, DC 20007
202-444-3772

Fatima Koroma   April 11, 202X
1530 Key Blvd   Arlington, VA 22209

Diphenhydramine 12.5 mg/5 mL   80 mL
Viscous Lidocaine 2%   80 mL
Dexamethasone 0.5 mg/5 mL   80 mL

Label as Magic Mouthwash.
Gargle, swish, and spit 5 mL every 6 hours as needed for
   sore throat.

Refill ×1   Young Kim

Prescription Label
Your Friendly Pharmacy
3400 M Street
Washington, DC 22209
202-444-3854

RX 101110244
Fatima Koroma   Filled: April 12, 202X

Magic Mouthwash 240 mL
Gargle, swish, and spit 5 mL every 6 hours as needed for
   sore throat.

Young Kim
3 refills by April 10, 202Y

Which beyond-use date should be assigned to the finished compounded prescription?
a. April 18, 202X
b. April 26, 202X
c. May 3, 202X
d. May 10, 202X

82. The following prescription is presented at the pharmacy:
Nicholas Trucco
2610 Cates Avenue
Raleigh, NC 27606
919-470-3130

Otis McClure   September 26, 202X
235 S Capital St   Raleigh, NC 27609

Sildenafil 25 mg   #8
I TAB PO 30 min prior to anticipated sexual activity

Refill 3   Nicholas Trucco

Prescription Label
Your Friendly Pharmacy
1 Great Valley Drive
Wilkes Barre, PA 18708
1-800-378-0220

RX 101117255
Otis McClure   Filled October 1, 202X

Sildenafil 50 mg   #8
Place one tablet between the cheek 30 minutes prior to
   anticipated sexual activity.

Nicholas Trucco
3 refills by September 25, 202Y
Use by September 30, 202Y

Which error(s) was (were) observed by the pharmacy technician while verifying the completed
   prescription?
a. Incorrrect medication
b. Incorrect medication strength
c. Incorrect route of administration
d. Both b and c

83. The following prescription is presented at the pharmacy
to the pharmacy technician:
Rich Kunze
22087 Colonial Acres Court
Virginia Beach, VA 23456
757-270-1345

Randy Shope   October 13, 202X
852 Atlantic Avenue   Virginia Beach, 23456

Diclofenac Gel 1%   100 g
Apply to aa QID as needed for pain

Refill 1   Rich Kunze

Prescription Label
Your Friendly Pharmacy
1 Great Valley Drive
Wilkes Barre, PA 18708
1-800-378-0220

RX 101117279
Randy Shope   Filled: October 15, 202X

Diclofenac Gel 1%   100 g
Apply to affected area four times a day as needed for pain.

Rich Kunze
1 refill by October 12, 202Y
Use by October 14, 202Y

Which error(s) was (were) observed by the pharmacy
   technician while verifying the filled prescription?
a. Incorrect frequency of administration
b. Incorrect medication
c. Incorrect route of administration
d. No errors were observed

84. The pharmacy technician is conducting a final verification of a compounded solution and observes instability in the preparation. Which is a sign of instability in a solution?
   a. Creaming
   b. Difficulty in resuspending
   c. Discoloration
   d. Emulsion breakage

85. The pharmacy technician is checking the pharmacy for out-of-date medications in the pharmacy stock observes that a 45-gram tube of cream with lot number AbC2489712 with expiration date of 0131202X on the tube, but the box containing the cream has lot number DeF52348761 with an expiration of 0331202X. The pharmacy technician suspects the medication may have been tampered and informs the pharmacist of the situation. What action(s) should be taken?
   a. Report it to FDA Office of Criminal Investigations.
   b. Report it to law enforcement.
   c. Report it to the state board of pharmacy.
   d. All the above.

86. The following prescription is presented and filled at the pharmacy:
Jocelyn Itraheta
3400 Paradise Road Suite 100
Las Vegas, NV 89169
702-784-5700

David Hollander   August 8, 202X
7398 Smoke Ranch Road   Las Vegas. NV 89128

Humalog KwikPen Insulin   #6
20 units SC BID for diabetes mellitus.

Refill ×1   Jocelyn Iraheta

Prescription Label
Your Friendly Pharmacy
1 Great Valley Drive
Wilkes Barre, PA 18708
1-800-378-0220

RX 101114212
David Hollander   Filled: August 16, 202X

Humulin N KwikPen Insulin #6
Inject 20 units subcutaneously twice a day for diabetes mellitus.

Jocelyn Iraheta
1 refill by August 7, 202Y
Use by August 15, 202Y

Which error(s) was (were) observed by the pharmacy technician while checking the filled prescription?
   a. Incorrect dosage
   b. Incorrect route of administration
   c. Incorrect medication
   d. No errors were observed

87. A physician prescribes the following prescription:
Metformin 500 mg   3 months' supply
1 TAB PO BID

How many tablets should be dispensed?
   a. 30 tablets
   b. 60 tablets
   c. 90 tablets
   d. 180 tablets

88. The following prescription is presented at the pharmacy:
Althea Massie
3800 Reservoir Road
Washington, DC 20007
202-444-3772

Bessie Williams   August 15, 202X
1415 1st ST NW, Washington, DC 20001

Alendronate 70 mg   #12
One TAB PO once a week for osteoarthritis

Refill ×3   Althea Massie

How many days will the prescription last?
   a. 7 days
   b. 12 days
   c. 84 days
   d. 90 days

89. The following prescription is presented at the pharmacy counter:
Deno DiCiantis
Meadville Medical Center
751 Liberty Center
Meadville, PA 16335
814-333-5000

Heidi Loper   October 15, 202X
230 Allegheny Street Meadville, PA 16335

Sertraline 50 mg   #30
I TAB PO QD for depression

Refill   Deno DiCiantis

Prescription Label
Your Friendly Pharmacy
1 Great Valley Drive
Wilkes Barre, PA 18708
1-800-378-0220

RX 101427230
Heidi Loper   Filled: October 18, 202X

Sertraline 50 mg   #30
Take one tablet by mouth daily for depression.

Deno DeCiantis
0 refill by October 14, 202Y
Use by October 17, 202Y

Which error was observed by the pharmacy technician?
   a. Incorrect indication
   b. Incorrect medication strength
   c. Incorrect route of administration
   d. None of the above

90. The following prescription is presented at the pharmacy to the pharmacy technician:
Jennifer Escoto
Allegheny General Hospital
320 E. North Avenue
Pittsburgh, PA 15212
412-359-3131

Veronica Richardson September 9, 202X
101 Bradford Road   Wexford, PA 15090

Zestril 10 mg   #90
I TAB PO QD for hypertension

Refill ×3   Jennifer Escoto

Prescription Label
Your Friendly Pharmacy
1 Great Valley Drive
Wilkes Barre, PA 18708
1-800-378-0220

RX 101547230
Veronica Richardson Filled: September 16, 202X

Zetia 10 mg   #90
Take one tablet by mouth four times a day.

Jennifer Escoto
3 refills by September 8, 202Y
Use by September 15, 202Y

Which error(s) was (were) observed by the pharmacy technician while verifying the filled prescription?
a. Incorrect frequency
b. Incorrect medication
c. Incorrect route of administration
d. Both a and b

91. The pharmacy technician is reviewing the following prescription label:
Amiodarone 200 mg #60
I TAB PO BID × 2 weeks then 1 TAB PO QD × 2 weeks then ½ TAB PO QD

Which auxiliary label(s) should the pharmacy technician affix to prescription bottle?
a. Do not take with grapefruit.
b. May cause drowsiness.
c. Take at bedtime.
d. All the above.

92. The following prescription is presented and filled at the pharmacy:
Roberto Benitez
201 State Street
Erie, PA 16550
814-877-6000

David Major   September 30, 202X
7814 Hamot Road   Erie, PA 16507

Trulicity 1.5 mg/0.5 mL   6 mL
1.5 mg SC weekly for diabetes mellitus

Refill ×2   Roberto Benitez

How many days will the prescription last?
a. 12 days
b. 28 days
c. 30 days
d. 84 days

93. The following prescription is presented at the pharmacy and the pharmacy technician is reviewing for completeness:
Andrew Shedlock
2610 Cates Avenue
Raleigh, NC 27606
919-470-3130

Catie Jones   November 3, 1997
4285 Trinity Road   Raleigh, NC 27607

Meloxicam 7.5 mg   #30
I CAP PO TID

Which concern(s) are observed by the pharmacy technician and must be corrected prior to filling the prescription?
a. Medication dosage form
b. Medication frequency
c. Medication strength
d. All the above

94. The following prescription is presented at the pharmacy:
Luisa Aburito
381 Elden Street Suite 100
Herndon, VA 20170
703-481-1505

Ileana Mendez Espinoza   August 16, 202X
3334 Woodburn Village Drive Annandale, VA 22030

Clopidogrel 75 mg   #90
I TAB PO QD for thrombosis

Refill ×3   Luisa Aburito

Prescription Label
Your Friendly Pharmacy
1 Great Valley Drive
Wilkes Barre, PA 18708
1-800-378-0220

RX 11114552   Filled: August 20, 202X
Clopidogrel 75 mg   #90
Take one tablet by mouth twice a day for thrombosis.

Refill ×3   Luisa Aburito

3 refills by August 15, 202Y
Use by August 19, 202Y

What error(s) was (were) observed by the pharmacy technician?
a. Medication frequency
b. Medication indication
c. Medication strength
d. All the above

95. The following prescription is presented at the pharmacy to the pharmacy technician:
Rich Kunze
22087 Colonial Acres Court
Virginia Beach, VA 23456
757-270-1345

Natalie Bonomo   September 13, 202X
9300 Rivershore Drive Crittendon, VA 23433

Coreg CR 20 mg   #60
Chew 1 TAB q AM prn anxiety

Refill ×1   Rich Kunze

Prescription Label
Your Friendly Pharmacy
1 Great Valley Drive
Wilkes Barre, PA 18708
1-800-378-0220

RX 111115532
Natalie Bonomo   Filled: September 20, 202X

Coreg CR 20 mg   #60
Chew 1 tablet every morning as needed for anxiety.

Rich Kunze
1 refill by September 12, 202Y
Use by September 19, 202Y

Which error(s) was (were) observed by the pharmacy
   technician while verifying the filled prescription?
a. Incorrect frequency
b. Incorrect indication
c. Incorrect route of administration
d. Both b and c

96. The following prescription is presented at the pharmacy
   to the pharmacy technician:
   Subash Bazaz
   11800 Sunrise Valley Drive Suite 500
   Reston, VA 20191
   703-621-4501

   Yosra Altahan   March 17, 202X
   1257 Waynewood Dr   Alexandria, VA

   Potassium Chloride 10 mEq   #90
   1 CAP PO BID for low potassium

   Prescription Label
   Your Friendly Pharmacy
   1 Great Valley Drive
   Wilkes Barre, PA 18708
   1-800-378-0220

   RX 111125532
   Yosra Altahan   Filled: March 23, 202X

   Potassium Chloride 10 mEq   #90
   Take one capsule by mouth twice a day for low potassium.

   Subash Bazaz
   1 refill by March 16, 202Y
   Use by March 22, 202Y

   Which error(s) was (were) observed by the pharmacy
      technician while verifying the filled prescription?
   a. Incorrect frequency
   b. Incorrect indication
   c. Incorrect route of administration
   d. No errors were observed

97. The following prescription is presented at the pharmacy
   counter on August 12, 2023 and is being reviewed by the
   pharmacy technician for completeness and accuracy:
   Marielle Levy
   Meadville Medical Center
   751 Liberty Center
   Meadville, PA 16335
   814-333-5000

   Larry Esposito   September 9, 2016
   639 Terrace Street   Meadville, PA 16335

   Citalopram 20 mg   #30
   I TAB PO qd for obsessive compulsive disorder.

   Refill ×1   Marielle Levy

Which error(s) was (were) observed by the pharmacy
   technician?
a. Medication dose
b. Medication frequency
c. Prescription date
d. All the above

98. The following prescription is presented and filled at
   the pharmacy:
   Madeline Martin
   3400 Paradise Road Suite 100
   Las Vegas, NV 89169
   702-784-5700

   Janeen Asfour   August 8, 202X
   7398 Smoke Ranch Road Las Vegas, NV 89128

   Chlorhexidine osopharyngeal 480 mL
   15 mL swish and spit twice a day

   Refill ×1   Madeline Martin

   How many days will the prescription last?
   a. 7 days
   b. 12 days
   c. 16 days
   d. 30 days

99. The pharmacy receives the following prescription:
   Marietha Mayem
   Georgetown University Hospital
   3800 Reservoir Road
   Washington, DC 20007
   202-444-3772

   Chuck Najjoum   April 11, 202X
   1530 Key Blvd   Arlington, VA 22209

   Tamsulosin 0.4 mg   #90
   1 CAP PO QD for BPH

   Refill ×3   Marietha Mayem

   Prescription Label
   Your Friendly Pharmacy
   1 Great Valley Drive
   Wilkes Barre, PA 18708
   1-800-378-0220

   RX 10567231
   Chuck Najjoum   Filled: April 17, 202X

   Tamsulosin 0.4 mg   #90
   Take one capsule by mouth four times a day for benign
      prostatic hyperplasia.

   Marietha Mayem
   3 refills by April 10, 202Y
   Use by April 16, 202Y

   What error(s) was (were) observed by the pharmacy
      technician while verifying the filled prescription?
   a. Incorrect frequency
   b. Incorrect indication
   c. Incorrect route of administration
   d. All the above

100. The pharmacy technician is reviewing the following
   prescription label:
   Amlodipine 10 mg   #90
   I TAB PO QD

The following auxiliary labels were affixed to the patient's prescription bottle of amlodipine 10 mg.
* Caution: Federal law prohibits the transfer of this drug to any person other than the patient for whom it was prescribed.
* May cause drowsiness.
* May cause dizziness.

Which auxiliary label(s) is (are) inappropriate to be affixed to the patient's prescription bottle of amlodipine 10 mg?
a. Caution: Federal law prohibits the transfer of this drug to any person other than the patient for whom it was prescribed.
b. May cause drowsiness.
c. May cause dizziness.
d. Both b and c are inappropriate to be affixed to a prescription bottle of amlodipine 10 mg.

101. The following prescription is presented at the pharmacy:
Martina Donayre
2610 Cates Avenue
Raleigh, NC 27606
919-470-3130

Mary Ann Pannich June 14, 202X
11607 Bromley Village Lane Reston, VA 20194

Simvastatin 40 mg #60
I TAB PO PM

Refill ×2   Martina Donayre

Prescription Label
Your Friendly Pharmacy
1 Great Valley Drive
Wilkes Barre, PA 18708
1-800-378-0220

RX 101117456
Mary Ann Pannich Filled June 19, 202X

Simvastatin 40 mg #60
Take one tablet by mouth in the morning.

Martina Donayre
2 refills by June 13, 202Y
Use by June 18, 202Y

Which error(s) was (were) discovered by the pharmacy technician while verifying the filled prescription?
a. Incorrect dosage form
b. Incorrect medication strength
c. Incorrect time of administration
d. Both a and c

102. The following prescription is presented at the pharmacy to the pharmacy technician:
Maryuri Avilla
16364 115th Avenue
Jupiter, FL 33478
561-747-4882

Vincente Barlowe   February 13, 202X
7654 Grand Blvd Unit 4   Port Richey, FL 34668

Neomycin/Polymyxin B/Hydrocortisone Otic
   Suspension   1 bottle
IV gtt as TID

Refill   Maryuri Avilla

Prescription Label
Your Friendly Pharmacy
1 Great Valley Drive
Wilkes Barre, PA 18708
1-800-378-0220

RX 101117987
Vincente Barlowe   Filled: February 20, 202X

Neomycin/Polymyxin B/Hydrocortisone Ophthalmic
   Suspension
Instill five drops in the left eye three times a day.

Maryuri Avilla
0 refill by February 12, 202Y
Use by February 19, 202Y

Which error(s) did the pharmacy technician observe while verifying the filled prescription?
a. Incorrect amount of medication to administer
b. Incorrect medication selected
c. Incorrect route of administration
d. All the above

103. The following prescription is presented at the pharmacy to the pharmacy technician:
Subash Bazaz
11800 Sunrise Valley Drive Suite 500
Reston, VA 20191
703-621-4501

Laura Elsberg   September 1, 202X
1548 Deer Point Way   Reston, VA 20194

Advair Diskus 250 mcg/50 mcg #1
One puff inhaled every 12 hours for COPD

Refill ×2   Subash Bazaz

Prescription Label
Your Friendly Pharmacy
1 Great Valley Drive
Wilkes Barre, PA 18708
1-800-378-0220

RX 101117652
Laura Elsberg   Filled: September 6, 202X

Advair Diskus 100 mcg/50 mcg   #1
One puff inhaled every 12 hours for chronic obstructive pulmonary disease

Subash Bazaz
1 refill by August 31, 202Y
Use by September 5, 202Y

Which error was observed by the pharmacy technician?
a. Incorrect frequency
b. Incorrect indication
c. Incorrect strength
d. None of the above

104. The pharmacy technician is checking a suspension the pharmacy technician has compounded and observes instability in the preparation. Which is a sign of instability in a suspension?
a. Creaming
b. Difficulty in resuspending
c. Emulsion breakage
d. Nonuniform appearance

105. The following prescription was presented at the pharmacy:

Haroon Rashid
2901 Telestar Court Suite 100
Falls Church, VA 22042
703-208-9798

Robert Klein	April 15, 202X
3800 Woodburn Village Drive	Annandale, VA 22003

Atenolol 50 mg   #90
I TAB PO QD for hypertension

Refill 3   Haroon Rashid

Prescription Label
Your Friendly Pharmacy
1 Great Valley Drive
Wilkes Barre, PA 18708
1-800-378-0220

RX 101117666
Robert Klein   Filled: April 20, 202X

Atenolol 25 mg   #90
Take one tablet four times a day.

Haroon Rashid
3 refills by April 14, 202Y
Use by April 19, 202Y

Which error(s) was (were) observed by the pharmacy technician during medication verification?
a. Incorrect frequency of administration
b. Incorrect medication strength
c. Missing route of administration
d. All the above

106. The following prescription is presented at the pharmacy:

Althea Massie
3800 Reservoir Road
Washington, DC 20007
202-444-3772

G.E. Branche	May 18, 202X
218 Catoctin Circle SE	Leesburg, VA 20176

Propranolol ER 80 mg   #60
1 CAP PO QD for hypertension

Refill 2   Althea Massie

Prescription Label
Your Friendly Pharmacy
1 Great Valley Drive
Wilkes Barre, PA 18708
1-800-378-0220

RX 101168930
G. E. Branche   Filled: May 24, 202X

Propranolol ER 80 mg #60
Take one capsule by mouth once a day for hypertension.

Althea Massie
1 refill by May 17, 202Y
Use by May 23, 202Y

Which error was observed by the pharmacy technician while verifying the filled prescription?
a. Incorrect frequency of administration
b. Incorrect medication
c. Incorrect patient
d. No errors observed

107. The following prescription is presented to the pharmacy:

Antonio Gutierrez
170 Reynolds Avenue
Meadville, PA 16335
814-724-2347

Anita Consuelo	October 12, 202X
170 Spring Street	Meadville, PA

Duloxetine 60 mg   #30
1 CAP PO QD for neuropathic pain

Refill 1   Antonio Gutierrez

Prescription Label
Your Friendly Pharmacy
1 Great Valley Drive
Wilkes Barre, PA 18708
1-800-378-0220

RX 101117888
Anita Consuelo   Filled October 18, 202X

Duloxetine 60 mg   #30
Take one capsule by mouth once daily for neuropathic pain.

Antonio Gutierrez
1 refill by October 11, 202Y
Use by October 17, 202Y

Which error was observed by the pharmacy technician while verifying the filled prescription?
a. Incorrect strength
b. Incorrect frequency of administration
c. Incorrect route of administration
d. No error was observed

108. The pharmacy receives the following prescription:

Tony Vardaro
209 Lilly Ridge Drive
Canonsburg, PA 15317
814-333-3600

Freddie Moon	January 11, 202X
280 Walnut Street	Pittsburgh, PA 15232

Allopurinol 100 mg #90
I TAB PO QD for gout

Refill 1   Tony Vardaro

Prescription Label
Your Friendly Pharmacy
1 Great Valley Drive
Wilkes Barre, PA 18708
1-800-378-0220

RX 101117626
Freddie Moon   Filled by January 14, 202X

Alopurinol 100 mg   #90
Take one tablet by mouth four times a day for gout.

Tony Vardaro
1 refill by January 10, 202Y
Use by January 13, 202Y

Which error(s) was (were) observed by the pharmacy
    technician while verifying the filled prescription?
a. Incorrect frequency of administration
b. Incorrect medication strength
c. Incorrect patient
d. All the above

109. The following prescription is presented at the
    pharmacy to the pharmacy technician:
    Solomon Habte
    Allegheny General Hospital
    320 E. North Avenue
    Pittsburgh, PA 15212
    412-359-3131

    Kennya Alvarado   March 9, 202X
    5859 Wilkins Avenue   Pittsburgh, PA 15217

    Ondansetron 8 mg   #30
    I TAB PO q 8h prn n/v

    Refill 1   Solomon Habte

    How many days will the prescription last?
    a. 5 days
    b. 10 days
    c. 15 days
    d. 30 day

110. The following prescription is presented and filled at
    the pharmacy:
    Joel Burke
    3400 Paradise Road Suite 100
    Las Vegas, NV 89169
    702-784-5700

    Leigh-Ann Carter Sinclair   August 8, 202X
    3400 Paradise Road   Las Vegas, NV 89169

    Lisinopril/Hydrochlorothiazide 10/12.5 mg   #90
    I TAB PO QD for hypertension

    Refill ×1   Joel Burke

    Prescription Label
    Your Friendly Pharmacy
    1 Great Valley Drive
    Wilkes Barre, PA 18708
    1-800-378-0220

    RX 101118759
    Leigh-Ann Carter Sinclair   Filled: August 16, 202X

    Lisinopril/Hydrochlorothiazide 20/12.5 mg   #90
    Take one tablet by mouth each day for hypertension

    Joel Burke
    1 refill by August 7, 202Y
    Use by August 15, 202 V

    Which error(s) was (were) observed by the pharmacy
        technician on the filled prescription?
    a. Incorrect frequency of administration
    b. Incorrect medication strength
    c. Incorrect route of administration
    d. No errors were observed

111. The pharmacy technician is reviewing the following
    prescription label:
    Celecoxib 200 mg   #90
    Take one capsule by mouth daily for rheumatoid
        arthritis.

    The following auxiliary labels were affixed to
        the patient's prescription bottle of celecoxib
        200 mg:
    • Avoid exposure to sunlight.
    • Do not drink alcohol when taking medications.
    • Take with food.
    Which auxiliary label(s) is (are) inappropriate to be
        affixed to the patient's prescription bottle of cel-
        ecoxib 200 mg?
    a. Avoid exposure to sunlight.
    b. Do not drink alcohol when taking medications.
    c. Take with food.
    d. All the above are appropriate auxiliary labels for
        celecoxib 200 mg.

112. The following prescription is presented to the
    pharmacy:
    Surekha Cohen
    1530 Key Blvd Suite 101
    Rosslyn, VA 22209
    703-571-2222
    AC1234563

    Liz Rosales   June 15th, 202X
    1121 Arlington Blvd   Rosslyn, VA 22209

    Clonazepam 0.5 mg   #90
    I TAB PO TID prn anxiety

    Refill 1   Surekha Cohen

    Prescription Label
    Your Friendly Pharmacy
    1 Great Valley Drive
    Wilkes Barre, PA 18708
    1-800-378-0220

    RX 101117352
    Liz Rosales   Filled June 20, 202X

    Lorazepam 0.5 mg   #90
    Take one tablet by mouth three times a day as needed
        for anxiety.

    Surekha Cohen
    1 refill by December 14, 202Y
    Use by June 19, 202Y

    Which error was observed by the pharmacy technician
        while verifying the completed prescription?
    a. Incorrect medication
    b. Incorrect frequency of administration
    c. Incorrect route of administration
    d. No error was observed

113. The following prescription is presented to the
    pharmacy:
    Tristan Tran
    3300 Gallows Road
    Falls Church, VA 22042
    703-776-4001
    BT1234563

Howard Chou   January 7, 202X
3301 Woodburn Road   Annandale, VA 22003

Tramadol 50 mg   #30
I tab PO q 4–6 h prn moderate pain

Refill   Tristan Tran

Prescription Label
Your Friendly Pharmacy
8124 Arlington Blvd
Falls Church, VA 22042
703-560-7280

RX 101117288
Howard Chou   Filled: January 7, 202X

Tramadol 50 mg   #30
Take one tablet by mouth every 6 hours as needed for
    moderate pain.

Tristan Tran
0 refill by July 6, 202X
Use by January 6, 202Y

What error was observed by the pharmacy technician
    while verifying the filled prescription?

a. Incorrect medication dosage
b. Incorrect frequency of administration
c. Incorrect route of administration
d. No error was observed

114. The following prescription is presented to the
    pharmacy:
    Sheila Ryan
    Virginia Hospital Center
    1701 N. George Mason Dr.
    Arlington, VA 22205
    703-558-5000

Robert Boderman   June 30, 202X
9608 Barroll Lane   Kensington, MD 20895

Zocor 40 mg   #90
I TAB PO QD

Refill 1   Sheila Ryan

Prescription Label
Your Friendly Pharmacy
1 Great Valley Drive
Wilkes Barre, PA 18708
1-800-378-0220

RX 101117832
Robert Boderman   Filled: July 5, 202X

Simvastatin 40 mg #90
Take one tablet by mouth once a day.

Sheila Ryan
1 refill by June 29, 202Y
Use by July 4, 202Y

Which error was observed by the pharmacy technician
    while checking the filled prescription?
a. Incorrect frequency of administration
b. Incorrect medication

c. Incorrect route of administration
d. No error was observed

115. The following prescription is presented at the
    pharmacy to the pharmacy technician:
    Elizabeth Kline
    2921 Columbia Pike
    Arlington, VA 22204
    703-979-1425

John E. Smith   May 15, 202X
2921 11th St S   Arlington, VA 22204

Bupropion 100 mg #90
I TAB PO TID

Refill 1   Elizabeth Kline

Prescription Label
Your Friendly Pharmacy
1 Great Valley Drive
Wilkes Barre, PA 18708
1-800-378-0220

RX 101151730   Filled: May 20, 202X

John R. Smith
Bupropion 100 mg #90

Take one tablet by mouth three times a day.

Elizabeth Kline
1 refill by May 14, 202Y
Use by August 19, 202Y

Which error was observed by the pharmacy technician
    while verifying the filled prescription?
a. Incorrect frequency of administration
b. Incorrect medication
c. Incorrect medication strength
d. Incorrect patient

116. The following prescription was presented at the
    pharmacy:
    Haroon Rashid
    2901 Telestar Court Suite 100
    Falls Church, VA 22042
    703-208-9798

Mary Ludden   August 8, 202X
3840 North Fairfax Drive Arlington, VA 22015

Eliquis 5 mg   #120
I TAB PO BID for thromboembolism prophylaxis

Refill 2   Haroon Rashid

Prescription Label
Your Friendly Pharmacy
1 Great Valley Drive
Wilkes Barre, PA 18708
1-800-378-0220

RX 101158627
Mary Ludden   Filled: August 12, 202X

Eliquis 2.5 mg   #120
Take one tablet by mouth three times a day for throm-
    boembolism prophylaxis.

Haroon Rashid
2 refills by August 7, 202Y
Use by August 11, 202Y

Which error(s) was (were) observed by the pharmacy technician?
a. Incorrect frequency of administration
b. Incorrect medication strength
c. Incorrect route of administration
d. Both a and b

117. The following prescription is presented at the pharmacy counter:
Betya Yarhi
Meadville Medical Center
751 Liberty Center
Meadville, PA 16335
814-333-5000

Martin Feldman   November 3, 202X
232 Church Street   Meadville, PA 16335
Lisinopril 20 mg   #90
I TAB PO QD for hypertension
Refill 1   Betya Yarhi

Prescription Label
Your Friendly Pharmacy
1 Great Valley Drive
Wilkes Barre, PA 18708
1-800-378-0220

RX 101158630
Martin Feldman   Filled: November 6, 202X

Lisinopril/hydrochlorothiazide 20/12.5 mg   #90
Take one tablet by mouth daily for hypertension.

Betya Yarhi
1 refill by November 2, 202Y
Use by November 5, 202Y

Which error(s) was (were) observed by the pharmacy technician while verifying the filled prescription?
a. Incorrect frequency of administration
b. Incorrect medication
c. Incorrect medication strength
d. Both b and c

118. The following prescription is presented at the pharmacy:
Matthew Kennedy
381 Elden Street Suite 100
Herndon, VA 20170
703-481-1505

Maryori Espinalo   May 12, 202X
2416 Wanda Way   Reston, VA 20190

Celecoxib 200 mg   #90
I CAP PO BID prn rheumatoid arthritis

Refill 1   Matthew Kennedy

How many days will the prescription last?
a. 30 days
b. 45 days
c. 60 days
d. 90 days

119. The following prescription is presented at the pharmacy:
Henry Chen
11800 Sunrise Valley Drive Suite 500
Reston, VA 20191
703-621-4501

Ginger Clevinger   November 12, 202X
13630 Bent Tree Circle   Centreville, VA

Lantus Insulin 10 mL vial
Inject 20 Units SC BID

Refill 2   Henry Chen

How many days will one vial of Lantus Insulin last the patient?
a. 7 days
b. 10 days
c. 25 days
d. 50 days

120. The following prescription is presented and filled at the pharmacy:
Minji Kwon
3400 Paradise Road Suite 100
Las Vegas, NV 89169
702-784-5700

Mateo Cardinale   August 8, 202X
7398 Smoke Ranch Road   Las Vegas, NV 89128

Sertraline 50 mg   #30
I TAB PO QD for OCD

Refill ×1   Minji Kwon

Prescription Label
Your Friendly Pharmacy
1 Great Valley Drive
Wilkes Barre, PA 18708
1-800-378-0220

RX 101721112
Mateo Cardinale   Filled: August 16, 202X

Sertraline 50 mg   #30
Place one tablet under the tongue for obsessive compulsive disorder.

Minji Kwon
1 refill by August 7, 202Y
Use by August 15, 202Y

Which error(s) are (were) detected by the pharmacy technician when verifying the prescription?
a. Medication dosage
b. Medication indication
c. Route of administration
d. All the above

121. The pharmacy technician is reviewing the following prescription label:
Hydrochlorothiazide 50 mg #90

Take one tablet by mouth once a day in the morning for hypertension.

The following auxiliary labels were affixed to the patient's prescription bottle of hydrochlorothiazide 50 mg:

- Caution: Federal law prohibits the transfer of this drug to any person other than the patient for whom it was prescribed.
- May cause dizziness.
- Take with a full glass of orange juice or eat a banana.

Which auxiliary label(s) is (are) inappropriate for a prescription of hydrochlorothiazide 50 mg?

a. Caution: Federal law prohibits the transfer of this drug to any person other than the patient for whom it was prescribed.

b. May cause dizziness.

c. Take with a full glass of orange juice or eat a banana.

d. Both a and b.

APPENDIX D

Chapter Review Question Answers

Chapter 1

1. a. Adalimimab is the generic name for Humira. Enoxaparin is the generic name for Lovenox. Rituximab is the generic name for Rituxan. Tacrolimus is the generic name for Prograf.
2. d. Taxotere is the brand name for docetaxel. Cubicin is the brand name for docetaxel. Retavase is the brand name for reteplase recombinant injection. Sandimmune is the brand name for cyclosporine.
3. b. Lantus is the brand name for insulin glargine. Apidra is the brand name for insulin glulisine. NovoLog is the brand name for insulin aspart. Tresiba is the brand name for insulin degludec.
4. b. Amphotericin B liposome is an antifungal agent. Amiodarone is indicated for ventricular arrhythmias. Argatroban is indicated as an anticoagulant. Paclitaxel is indicated for ovarian and breast cancer.
5. d. Docetaxel is classified as a mitosis inhibitor. Acyclovir is classified as an antiviral agent. Azathioprine is classified as an immunosuppressant. Carboplatin is a classified as an alkylating agent.
6. a. Amiodarone has a narrow therapeutic index. Ampicillin, azithromycin, and calcium gluconate do not have a narrow therapeutic index.
7. a. Compounded sterile products are assigned to one of two risk levels depending on the batch size, complexity of the compounding process, the length of time between the start of the compounding, and administration of the drug to the patient and the preparation site.
8. d. Enoxaparin is administered subcutaneously. Alteplase is administered intravenously. Bivalirudin is administered intravenously. Cefazolin may be administered intramuscularly or intravenously.
9. c. The minimum inflow velocity for a Type A 2 biological safety cabinet is 100 feet/minute.

10. b. The ante room must be classified as an ISO Class 6. The IV hood must be classified as an ISO Class 5. The clean room must be classified as an ISO Class 7. The nonhazardous room must be an ISO Class 8.
11. b. ISO Class 5 and 6 areas must be tested for sterility every 6 months. ISO 7 and 8 areas must be tested every for sterility every 12 months.
12. a. A buffer area is an example of a secondary engineering control. A Class II biological cabinet is an example of a primary engineering control. Environmental monitoring is used to evaluate a primary engineering control. Viable air sampling is an example of environmental monitoring.
13. b. Fluconazole is an antifungal agent indicated for candidiasis. Chlorpromazine is an antipsychotic indicated for psychosis. Fluorouracil is am antimetabolite indicated for various cancers. Heparin is an anticoagulant indicated for thromboembolism.
14. c. Normal saline solution is indicated for providing extracellular fluid replacement to the body. D5W is used to hydrate and provide calories to the body. Hartman's and lactated Ringer's solution are used for fluid and electrolyte replacement.
15. d. Water for injection USP not sterile. It cannot be used in aseptic compounding of sterile products. Bacteriostatic water for injection USP is sterile water with antimicrobial agents that can be used for injection. Purified water USP is not intended for parenteral administration; it is used in the reconstitution of oral products. Sterile water for injection USP has been sterilized but has no antimicrobial agents; it can be used in parenteral solutions.
16. a. Amiodarone is an example of a high-alert parenteral medication used in an acute care setting. Glyburide, rivaroxaban, and warfarin are classified as high-alert medications in an acute care setting, but they are orally not parenterally.

339

17. d. A multidose container used in an ISO 5 or better environment has an in-use time of 28 days unless otherwise specified by the manufacturer. A single-dose container has an used in an ISO an ISO 5 or better environment has an in-use time of 6 hours.

18. c. The maximum number of particles per cubic meter for a Class 7 environment is 352,000. The maximum number of particles per cubic meter for a Class 5 environment is 3520. The maximum number of particles per cubic meter for a Class 6 environment is 35,200. The maximum number of particles per cubic meter for a Class 8 environment is 3,520,000.

19. a. USP <797> requires temperature to be monitored and documented at least once daily.

20. d. USP <797> requires viable particles to be monitored by a qualified certifier every 6 months.

21. d. All personnel who compound sterile preparations must be evaluated for gloved finger tip testing every 12 months (annually).

22. d. The BUD for a compounded sterile preparation where sterility testing was performed and passed and stored in a refrigerator is 45 days. A compounded sterile preparation where sterility testing was not performed and passed and is stored at controlled room temperature would be assigned a BUD of 14 days. A BUD of 28 days would be assigned to a compounded sterile preparation where sterility testing was not performed and passed and is stored in the refrigerator. A BUD of 30 days would be assigned to a compounded sterile preparation where sterility testing was performed and passed and is stored at controlled room temperature.

23. c. The in-use time assigned to a single-dose container in an ISO-5 environment or better environment is 6 hours. An ampule must be used immediately after opening in an ISO-5 environment or better environment. Pharmacy bulk is assigned an in-use time as specified by the manufacturer after opening in an ISO-5 environment or better environment. An in-use time of 28 days is assigned to a multidose container after opening in an ISO-5 environment or better environment.

24. a. When an additive contains acetate or a lactate salt is added to a CSP, it will increase the buffer capacity of the compound. An additive containing calcium, magnesium, or phosphate added to a CSP may cause the drug to precipitate.

25. a. A Class II biological cabinet must be on a minimum of 10 minutes before beginning to compound. A vertical laminar airflow system must be on at least 30 minutes before beginning to compound.

26. a. An IV hood is found in ISO Class 5 environment. The ante area is an ISO Class 6 environment, the clean room is an ISO Class 7 area, and the nonhazardous room is a ISO Class 8 environment.

27. d. The clean room must be tested every 12 months to comply with USP <797> air standards. The IV hood and the ante area must be tested every 6 months to comply with USP <797> air standards.

28. a. The differential airflow shall be a minimum of 40 feet/minute between buffer area and ante area when compounding Category 1 and Category 2 compounds.

29. a. The ante area must maintain a minimum of 20 ACPHs.

30. c. Viable air samples be collected from ISO Class 5, 7, and 8 environments every 6 months.

31. a. USP <797> requires the pressure differential (velocity across line of demarcation) be completed a minimum of once a day by the compounding. It is recommended that be done during each shift.

32. c. Time of infusion = volume of fluid (or amount of drug)/rate of infusion. Time of infusion = 500 mL/125 mL/hour = 4 hours.

33. b. An individual should wash their hands, under the fingernails, on the wrists, and up to the elbow for 30 seconds with a facility-approved agent.

34. a. The sequence to remove personal protective equipment is gloves, goggles/face shield, gown, and mask/respirator.

35. d. The sequence of cleaning a laminar flow workbench is the top of the hood, the horizontal IV pole to include all the hooks and brackets, each side of the hood, rear wall of the hood, and then the flat work surface.

36. a. The sequence to remove air bubbles from a syringe are (1) Draw back on the plunger, allowing fluid into the syringe. (2) Turn the large air bubbles around the syringe to pick up smaller air bubbles. If smaller air bubbles continue to exist, tap the syringe to displace them. (3) Hold the syringe upright and pull the plunger back to clear the hub. (4) Slowly push the plunger to remove any remaining air.

37. b. A compounding record must be maintained a minimum of 3 years from the date the medication was prepared.

38. d. Sodium is responsible for establishing total body water volume. Calcium, magnesium, and phosphate are necessary for good bone growth. Chloride controls water balance inside and outside of the cells. Phosphate aids in fighting infection.

39. c. An ophthalmic medication should have a pH of 7.4.

40. b. Cracking occurs when there is a separation of oil and water in an emulsion. Aggregation occurs when triglycerides clump together in an emulsion. Creaming results when an accumulation of a triglyceride forms at the top of an emulsion. Separation may occur when one of the ingredients separates out in a mixture.

41. b. An 80-bag batch would require testing of 10% of the batch size or 8 bags. A batch of 40 bags would require 10% of the batch size or 4 bags. A batch size of 101–500 would require 10 bags to be tested. A batch of 600 bags would require 2% of the batch size or 12 bags to be tested.

42. b. American Society of Testing and Materials–tested chemotherapy gloves may be worn when transporting intact supplies or compounded hazardous drugs or receiving or stocking hazardous drugs.

43. d. Gloves, gowns, and hair, face, beard, and shoe covers and eye/face protection and respiratory protection must be worn when collecting and disposing of waste and spills. Also, gloves, gowns, and hair, face, beard, and shoe covers and eye/face protection and respiratory protection must be worn when receiving damaged or broken hazardous drugs. Gloves, gowns, and hair, face, beard, and shoe covers must be worn when compounding sterile and nonsterile hazardous drugs and routine cleanup of hazardous drugs.

44. d. A hazardous drug label must read: "Caution Hazardous Drug: Observe Special Handling, Administration, and Disposal Requirements"
45. a. Acetic acid is an example of a hazardous waste that is corrosive. Lead and mercury are hazardous wastes that are toxic. Nitroglycerin is an example of a hazardous waste that is reactive.
46. d. A spill kit contains a NIOSH-approved respirator mask. A spill kit contains an absorbent chemotherapy pad and towel. A spill kit contains a disposable chemotherapy-resistant gown with cover, not a disposable gown with back covers. A spill kit contains chemotherapy gloves, not latex gloves.
47. a. Counting or repackaging tablets and/or capsules is an unintentional exposure risk associated with dispensing a hazardous medication. Expelling air or diluting injectable HDs from syringes, reconstituting an HD, and weighing or mixing components are examples of an unintentional exposure risk associated with dispensing a hazardous medication when compounding or manipulating a hazardous drug.
48. d. Methotrexate is an example of an HD. Ampicillin, insulin glargine, and levothyroxine are not classified as HDs.
49. a. Enoxaparin is indicated for deep vein thrombosis. Epoetin alpha recombinant is used to treat anemia. Famotidine is used to treat duodenal and gastric ulcers. Fluorouracil is indicated in various cancers such as breast or colorectal and pancreatic acid.
50. d. Chlorpromazine is classified as an antipsychotic. Amiodarone is an antiarrhythmic, amphotericin B is an antifungal agent, and carboplatin is an alkylating agent.

Chapter 2

1. c. Refrigerated antineoplastic HDs must be stored in a dedicated refrigerator in a negative pressure area with at least 12 ACPH (e.g., storage room, buffer room, or containment segregated compounding area).
2. a. Antineoplastic HDs and all HD APIs must be unpacked (i.e., removed from external shipping containers) in an area that is neutral/normal or negative pressure relative to the surrounding areas. HDs must not be unpacked from their external shipping containers in sterile compounding areas or in positive pressure areas.
3. a. A Class II Type A1 must maintain a minimum inflow velocity of 75 feet/minute. A Class II Type A2, Class Type B1, and Class II B1 must maintain a minimum inflow velocity of 100 feet/minute.
4. d. Disinfecting is the process of inhibiting or destroying microorganisms. Cleaning refers to the process of removing contaminants from objects and surfaces, normally accomplished by manually or mechanically using water with germicidal detergents or enzymatic products. Deactivation refers to the treatment of an HD contaminant on surfaces with a chemical, heat ultraviolet light, or another agent to change the HD to a less hazardous agent. Decontamination is the process of inactivating, neutralizing, or removing of HD contaminants from nondisposable surfaces and transferring it to absorbent, disposable materials such as wipes, pads, or towels.

5. c. USP <800> states that a C-PEC must be deactivated, decontaminated, and cleaned at least monthly.
6. b. USP <800> states that a gown must be changed according to manufacturer's information for permeation of the gown. If no permeation information is provided, the gown should be changed every 2–3 hours or immediately after a spill or splash.
7. c. Decontamination is the process of inactivating, neutralizing, or removing HD contaminants from nondisposable surfaces and transferring it to absorbent, disposable materials such as wipes, pads, or towels. Cleaning is the process of removing contaminants (e.g., organic and inorganic material) from objects and surfaces, normally accomplished by manually or mechanically using water with germicidal detergents or enzymatic products. Deactivation refers to the treatment of an HD contaminant on surfaces with a chemical, heat ultraviolet light, or another agent to change the HD to a less hazardous agent. Disinfecting is the process of inhibiting or destroying microorganisms. Surfaces must be cleaned before disinfecting takes place.
8. d. NIOSH recommends an assessment of the workplace to identify and assess the hazards in the workplace to prevent the worker from being exposed to hazardous drugs.
9. b. The employee does not need to be isolated from other employees from being exposed to the hazardous medication. After an employee has been accidentally exposed to a hazardous medication, Safety Data Sheets should be referred to decontaminate as instructed, postexposure examination should be conducted, and an incident report should be completed.
10. a. After a hazardous medication spill has occurred, the first thing to be done is to assess the size and scope of the spill. Obtain a spill kit and respirator, don the PPEs to include double gloves and respirator, and contain the spill using a spill kit.
11. c. Chemotherapy gloves should be worn for handling all HDs, including non-antineoplastics, and for reproductive risk–only HDs. Gloves are required for compounding sterile and nonsterile hazardous drugs, administration of hazardous drugs, and cleanup of hazardous drug spills. Gloves must be powder-free since powder may absorb the hazardous material. Double gloves should be worn during any handling of HD shipping cartons or drug vials and handling of HD waste or waste from patients recently treated with HDs.
12. c. When cutting, crushing, or manipulating tablets or capsules, the pharmacy technician does not need to wear eye/face protection. A pharmacy technician compounding an oral liquid drug or topical drug or withdrawing a subcutaneous injection from a vial is required to wear eye/face protection.
13. c. Cyclophosphamide is an example of a medication containing a manufacturer's information (MSHI). Anastrozole, clomiphene and fluconazole are examples of drugs that meet the NIOSH definition of a hazardous drug but are not drugs that have MSHI or are classified by the National Toxicology Program as "known to be human carcinogen," or classified by the International Agency for Research on Cancer (ARC) as " carciogenic or "probably carcinogenic."

14. d. A hazardous drug is any drug identified as hazardous or potentially hazardous on the basis of at least one of six criteria, which includes teratogenicity. Corrosivity, ignitability, and reactivity are characteristics of hazardous waste.

15. b. A waste is determined to be a hazardous waste if it is specifically listed on one of four lists: F, K, P, and U lists.

16. c. After compounding a hazardous medication, the pharmacy technician should dispose of their gloves in a yellow container, which is used for chemotherapy waste. Hazardous pharmaceutical waste is placed in a black container. A red sharps container is used to dispose of hypodermic needles, syringes with attached needles (or needleless plungers), scalpels, razor blades, and broken glass.

17. d. Hazardous drugs are classified into three groups: antineoplastic drugs, non-antineoplastic drugs, or drugs that pose a reproductive risk for men or women.

18. c. Environmental sampling must be performed at least every 6 months.

19. b. The health care facility must maintain SOPs for the safe handling of HDs for all situations in which these HDs are used throughout a facility. It must be reviewed at least every 12 months by the designated person, and the review must be documented. Revisions in forms or records must be made as needed and communicated to all personnel handling HDs.

20. c. USP <800> addresses Hazardous Drugs-Handling in Healthcare Settings. USP <795> addresses Pharmaceutical Compounding-Nonsterile Preparation; USP <797> addresses Pharmaceutical Compounding-Sterile Preparations; and USP <825> addresses Radiopharmaceuticals-Preparation, Compounding, Dispensing and Repackaging.

21. d. The first thing to be done after an individual has been accidentally exposure to a hazardous drug is to remove the individual's contaminated clothes.

22. a. Carcinogenicity is the ability to cause cancer in humans, animals, or both. Genotoxicity is the ability to cause a change or mutation in genetic material. Reproductive toxicity causes fertility impairment in humans. Teratogenicity is the ability to cause defects in fetal development or fetal malformation.

23. d. Any health care worker who handles HDs should be enrolled in a medical surveillance program

24. c. The EPA is responsible for enforcing the RCRA.

25. b. Two pairs of gloves are required to be worn when compounding both sterile and nonsterile hazardous medications.

Chapter 3

1. d. The FDA is responsible for the safety, efficacy, and security of medications. The CMS is responsible for administering Medicare, Medicaid, the Children's Health Insurance Program (CHIP) and the Health Insurance Portability and Accountability Act standards. The DEA is responsible for enforcing the Controlled Substance Act, the Combat Methamphetamine Epidemic Act of 2005, and the Ryan Haight Online Pharmacy Consumer Protection Act of 2008. The EPA is responsible for regulating the handling of hazardous waste.

2. a. USP <795> addresses pharmaceutical compounding of nonsterile preparations. USP <797> addresses pharmaceutical compounding of sterile preparations. USP <800> covers hazardous drug handling in health care settings. USP <825> addresses radiopharmaceutical preparation, compounding, dispensing, and repackaging.

3. d. HIPAA was enacted to improve the portability and continuity of health coverage in the group and individual markets. The ACA requires health care entities receiving federal financial assistance (e.g., Medicaid and Medicare) to engage in practices designed to prevent discrimination on the basis of age, race, color, nationality, or gender, including gender identity. The Drug Supply Chain Security Act outlines critical steps to build an electronic, interoperable system to identify and trace certain prescription drugs as they are distributed in the United States. The FDCA clearly defines adulteration and misbranding of medications.

4. d. The Substance Abuse and Mental Health Services Administration's goal is to reduce the impact of substance abuse and mental illness in communities. The DEA enforces the Controlled Substance Act, which deals combating substance abuse of controlled substances; it does not address mental illness in communities. The EPA is responsible for regulating hazardous waste. The NRC oversees medical uses of nuclear material through licensing, inspection, and enforcement programs.

5. b. Alprazolam is classified as Schedule IV Controlled Substance. Acetaminophen with codeine is a Schedule III Controlled Substance. Methylphenidate is a Schedule II Controlled Substance. Pregabalin is a Schedule V Controlled Substance.

6. b. The Controlled Substance Act requires an inventory of all controlled substances to be conducted every 2 years.

7. d. URAC accredits specialty pharmacies. Accreditation Commission for Health Care accredits acute inspection services, compounding pharmacies, and durable medical equipment, prosthetics, orthotics, and supplies providers. The Center for Pharmacy Accreditation accredits outpatient pharmacy practices in community, hospitals, health systems, and clinics. The Joint Commission accredits and certifies hospitals and health care organizations that provide ambulatory and office-based surgery, behavioral health, home health care, laboratory, and nursing care center services.

8. d. The United States Pharmacopoeia (USP) established USP <797>, which is a pharmacy standard for compounding sterile products in the United States. Congress enacts statutes and laws. The PTCB certifies pharmacy technicians. The state board of pharmacy issues regulations that oversee the practice of pharmacy in the state.

9. a. A certification is a legal document certifying that an individual meets certain objective standards usually provided by a neutral professional organization, such as pharmacy technician being certified by either the PTCB or NHA. A code is a collection of laws, rules, or regulations that are systematically arranged. A regulation is a rule and administrative code issued by governmental agencies at all levels, municipal, county, state, and federal. For example, state boards of

pharmacy issue regulations that affect the practice of pharmacy within the state. A statute is a written law passed by a legislature on the state or federal level.

10. b. The Drug Listing Act of 1972 required every medication to be assigned an 11-digit number known as a National Drug Code.

11. d. DEA Form 222 is used to order Schedule II Controlled Substances for a pharmacy. DEA Form 41 is used to by pharmacy or a reverse distributor to document destruction of controlled substances. DEA Form 106 is used to document the theft or loss of controlled substances from a pharmacy. DEA Form 107 is used to document the theft or loss of listed chemicals.

12. d. A pharmacy should refer to federal, state and local regulations prior to the disposal of hazardous drug waste.

13. d. A medication guide must be provided to the patient or the patient's agent when a drug is dispensed in an outpatient setting (e.g., retail pharmacy, hospital ambulatory care pharmacy), and the product will then be used by the patient without direct supervision by a health care professional; when a drug is subject to a REMS that includes specific requirements for reviewing or providing a medication guide as part of an element to assure safe use (possibly in conjunction with distribution); and when a patient or the patient's agent requests a medication guide.

14. b. A medication guide is required to be provided to a patient when receiving a prescription for celecoxib. Medication guides do not need to be provided to a patient when they are receiving amoxicillin, cetirizine, or famotidine.

15. b. The Combat Methamphetamine Epidemic Act of 2005 permits a maximum amount of 3.6 g of pseudoephedrine per day to be purchased by an individual.

16. c. Under the Combat Methamphetamine Epidemic Act of 2005 an individual must be at least 18 years of age to purchase pseudoephedrine.

17. a. A pharmacy is required to provide patient package inserts to all patients receiving metered-dose inhalers (e.g., albuterol), oral contraceptives, estrogen, and progesterone.

18. d. During an administrative inspection, the DEA will review the following documents: the initial inventory, biennial inventory, closing inventory, receiving records (DEA Form 222 and CSOS), distribution records, DEA Form 106, DEA Form 41, reverse distributor, and return to manufacturer documentation and dispensing records.

19. c. Under the Poison Prevention Packaging Act of 1970, nitroglycerin is exempted from being dispensed in a child-resistant container. Furosemide, levothyroxine, and warfarin are required to be dispensed in a child-resistant container.

20. c. Pharmacists and pharmacy technicians must demonstrate competency and undergo written/electronic testing at least every 12 months.

21. b. Pharmacists and pharmacy technicians who compound nonsterile preparations must demonstrate competency in hand hygiene, garbing, cleaning and sanitizing, handling and transporting components and CNSPs, measuring and mixing, proper use of equipment

and devices to compound CNSPs and documentation of compounding processes to include Master Formulation and Compounding Records.

22. b. A Category 2 CSP may be assigned a BUD of greater than 12 hours at controlled room temperature or more than 24 hours if refrigerated. A Category 1 CSP may be assigned a BUD of 12 hours or less at controlled room temperature or 24 hours or less when refrigerated. A Category 3 CSP is assigned a BUD longer than Category 2 CSPs. There is no such thing as a Category 4 CSP.

23. b. Hand hygiene is required before beginning any compounding, which includes washing hands and forearms up to the elbows with soap and water for at least 30 seconds.

24. b. A compounded cream with preservatives would be assigned a BUD of 35 days. Nonpreserved aqueous dosage forms (e.g., emulsions, gels, creams, solutions, sprays, or suspensions) are assigned a BUD of 14 days. Nonaqueous dosage forms (e.g., suppositories and ointments) are assigned a BUD of 90 days. Compounded solid dosage forms (e.g., capsules tablets, granules, powders) are assigned a BUD of 180 days.

25. d. Medication errors may be caused human, organizational, technical, and manufacturing errors.

26. d. A medication education error is one where proper education material is not provided to the patient. An example is the failure of the pharmacist or pharmacy technician to provide a medication guide to the patient. An adverse drug error occurs when a drug utilization review warning is missed or ignored, such as the pharmacy technician overrides a warning for warfarin in a 75-year-old patient and does not inform the pharmacist of the situation. A compliance error occurs when a patient fails to adhere to the directions provide by their physician and pharmacist regarding taking their medication—an example would be a patient the completing their 30-day therapy in 10 days, and the pharmacist fails to address the issue with the patient. A documentation error occurs when essential information is missing or incorrect. An example of this is when the medication list in the pharmacy information system is not updated with current information

27. b. A cold environment should not exceed 8°C (46°F). The temperature in a freezer is maintained thermostatically between −25°C and −10°C (−13°F and 14°F). A cool environment is any temperature between 8°C and 15°C (46°F and 59°F). Room temperature is any temperature between 15°C and 30°C (59°F and 86°F).

28. d. If specific disposal instructions are not listed on a medication guide or package insert, then mix medicines (liquid or pills; do not crush tablets or capsules) with an unappealing substance such as dirt, cat litter, or used coffee grounds.

29. a. CarBAMazepine is identified as a high-alert medication in a community pharmacy. Insulin U-100 and sacubitril/valsartan are identified as high-alert medications in a long-term care pharmacy. Insulin U-500 insulin is identified as a high-alert medication in an acute care setting.

30. c. The ISMP has identified limiting the variety of medications that can be removed from an ADC using the override function as a best practice. Other best practices include dispensing vinCRIStine and other vinca alkaloids in a mini bag of a compatible solution and not in a syringe; eliminating the prescribing of fentaNYL patches for opioid-naive patients and/or patients with acute pain, and weighing each patient as soon as possible on admission and during each appropriate outpatient or emergency department encounter.

31. b. Both the FDA and ISMP have issued lists of look-alike/sound-alike medications.

32. d. Strategies used to reduce the risk of potential errors involving look-alike and sound-alike medications include using both the brand and generic names on prescriptions and labels; including the purpose of the medication on prescriptions; configuring computer selection screens to prevent look-alike names from appearing consecutively; and changing the appearance of look-alike product names to draw attention to their dissimilarities.

33. d. Three behaviors are found in a Just Culture and include human error, at-risk behavior, and reckless behavior.

34. d. Medicare Part D requires participating pharmacies to implement a continuous quality improvement program.

Chapter 4

1. d. Drug diversion may result in an individual becoming addicted to the substance and losing their professional license or certification. Drug diversion may result in an individual experiencing an increased risk of developing an infection such as hepatitis C, not a decreased risk of infection.

2. d. An example of a behavioral sign of an impaired health care worker is their unreliability in meeting deadlines. Bloodshot eyes, hand tremors, and significant weight loss are examples of physical signs of an impaired health care worker.

3. b. Replacing controlled substances by a product of similar appearance during prepackaging is an example diversion during dispensing. Altering a written prescription is an example diversion during prescribing. Removing expired controlled substances from the holding area is an example of diversion of waste and removal. Ordering controlled substances on a stolen DEA Form 222 is an example of diversion during procurement.

4. d. The DEA recognizes five classes of drugs that are frequently abused: opioids, depressants, hallucinogens, stimulants, and anabolic steroids.

5. a. Automation and technology is an example of a system-level control. Chain of custody is an example of a provider-level control. Legal and regulatory requirements are an example of core administrative element. Prescribing and administration is an example of a provider-level control.

6. a. The container of a drug product being compromised would occur during the procurement of the medication.

The container of a drug product being compromised would not occur during the preparation and dispensing, the prescribing, or the administration of the medication.

7. d. During the monitoring and surveillance of controlled substances, appropriate processes and practices would be implemented to address the purchasing, inventory management, administration, waste and disposal, and documentation of controlled substances. Automation and technology controls would address automated dispensing and prepackaging devices and diversion monitoring software. Human resource management controls policies and procedures that would address employee and provider policies. Investigation and reporting practices address what should be done when a suspected diversion of a controlled substance occurs.

8. d. High-risk areas include surgery centers, operating rooms, and procedural and anesthesia areas and emergency departments.

9. b. Organizational oversight refers to establishing best practices that ensure the chain of custody and the health care worker being responsible for handling-controlled substances at all times. Federal and state laws and regulations govern the procurement, prescribing, administration, and waste or removal of controlled substances.

10. b. Removing a health care worker's access to controlled substances immediately upon termination from the institution is an example ensuring the chain of custody of controlled substances. Completing a DEA Form 41 (Registrant Record of Controlled Substances Destroyed) is used to request permission from the DEA to destroy controlled substances. External diversion is diversion performed by an individual not employed by the health care organization or pharmacy.

11. d. DEA Form 224a is used to renew a pharmacy's registration with the DEA every 3 years. DEA Form 222 is used to order Schedule I and II Controlled Substances. DEA Form 223 is a DEA Certificate of Registration. DEA Form 224 is the Application for New Registration.

12. b. The letter M indicates the prescriber is a midlevel practitioner (physician assistant or nurse practitioner). The letter A indicates the practitioner received their DEA number prior to 1985. The letter G is assigned to prescribers under the Department of Defense. The letter X is assigned to prescribers employed by a Drug Addiction Treatment facility.

13. d. Interns, residents, staff physicians, and midlevel practitioner may use a hospital's DEA number to prescribe controlled substances.

14. d. Schedule I and II Controlled Substances can be ordered using DEA Form 222.

15. d. Advantages of the Controlled Substance Ordering System (CSOS) includes eliminating the maximum number of line items per order; permitting the electronic ordering of schedule I, II, III, and IV controlled substances; and resulting in lower transaction costs to the pharmacy.

16. b. DEA Form 41 must be retained by the pharmacy for at least 2 years.

17. c. DEA Form 107 is used is used to report the theft or loss of listed chemicals I and II. DEA Form 41 is used to request the destruction of controlled substances.

DEA Form 106 is used the theft or loss of controlled substances. DEA Form 224 is used to register a pharmacy to be able to dispense controlled substances.

18. a. Schedule I Controlled Substances have no currently accepted medical use in the United States. Schedules II, III, IV, and V have accepted medical uses in the United States.

19. a. Acetaminophen with codeine is a classified as a Schedule III Controlled Substance. Alprazolam is a Schedule IV Controlled Substance, codeine/guaifenesin is a Schedule V Controlled Substance, and hydrocodone with acetaminophen is a Schedule II Controlled Substance.

20. a. A biennial inventory must be conducted at least every 2 years. An initial inventory must be performed when a DEA registration is issued for a pharmacy. An inventory for damaged substance is conducted when a controlled substance is either damaged, defective, or impure. A perpetual inventory indicates the actual quantity of a specific medication on hand at a specific time.

21. d. After a pharmacy has been burglarized for controlled substances, the local DEA must be notified within 1 business day. A completed DEA Form 41, Report of Theft or Loss of Controlled Substance, must be submitted as soon as possible. A report must be filed with State Board of Pharmacy.

22. c. The Combat Methamphetamine Epidemic Act of 2005 requires an individual be at least 18 years of age to purchase an SLCP.

23. c. A drug dispensing machines showing discrepancies and overrides may indicate drug diversion. A physician self-prescribing controlled substance may indicate drug diversion *not* a prescriber receiving a written prescription for controlled substances from another physician. Controlled substance waste not being documented may indicate drug diversion; controlled substance waste being documented would not indicate diversion.

24. b. According to the Combat Methamphetamine Epidemic Act of 2005, a maximum of 3.6 g of the chemical can be sold in 1 day. The maximum amount that can be purchased in 30 days is 9 g, of which no more than 7.5 g can be imported by private or commercial carrier or US Postal service.

25. d. Controlled substance diversion may be identified by comparing controlled substance purchase invoices to controlled substance purchase orders and receipt into the pharmacy's perpetual inventory; identifying unusual peaks in quantity or frequency of controlled substance purchases; and reconciling invoices to statements or wholesale purchase history reports to detect missing invoices.

Chapter 5

1. a. A contraindication is a specific situation in which a medication, procedure, or surgery should not be used because it may have adverse effects on an individual. A drug allergy is an abnormal reaction of the immune system to a drug (medication). A drug intolerance refers to an inability to tolerate the adverse effects of a medication, generally at therapeutic or subtherapeutic doses. An idiosyncratic reaction is a drug reaction that occurs rarely and unpredictably among the population.

2. d. A social history is a summary of lifestyle practices and habits that may have a direct or indirect effect on their health. Lifestyle practices includes diet, exercise, sexual orientation, level of sexual activity, and occupation. Habits take into consideration use of tobacco, alcohol, and other substances. A family medical history is a record of the relationships among family members along with their medical histories. This includes current and past illnesses. A family history may show a pattern of certain diseases in a family. A medical history consists of past surgical history, family medical history, social history, allergies, and medications the patient is taking or may have recently stopped taking. A medication history is a compilation of filled prescription information to include medication name, dosage, quantity, and date filled.

3. c. Hypertension is high blood pressure. Hyperglycemia refers to high blood sugar levels. Hyperlipidemia is high blood cholesterol. Hyperthyroidism refers to elevated thyroid levels.

4. c. Dermatitis is inflammation of the skin. Endocarditis is inflammation of the heart muscle. Colitis is inflammation of the colon. Phlebitis is inflammation of the vein.

5. b. Fibromyalgia is chronic muscle pain. Ostealgia refers to bone pain. Nephralgia is kidney pain. Neuralgia is nerve pain.

6. b. Primary nonadherence occurs when a new medication is prescribed for a patient, but the patient fails to obtain the medication (or its appropriate alternative) within an acceptable period of time after it was initially prescribed. Intentional medication nonadherence is an active process whereby the patient chooses to deviate from the treatment regimen. Secondary nonadherence refers to a patient taking insufficient doses required to experience a therapeutic effect, missing doses, or discontinuing their therapy early. Unintentional medication nonadherence is a passive process in which the patient may be careless or forgetful about adhering to treatment regimen.

7. b. A patient is considered adherent if they take 80% of their prescribed medication doses.

8. d. The minimum age for a pediatric patient to be immunized against for measles, mumps, and rubella is 12 months.

9. d. A pediatric patient receiving Prevnar 13 should receive a four-dose series at 2, 4, 6, and 12 to 15 months.

10. b. A patient receiving Comirnaty may receive the second dose no earlier than 21 days after the first dose.

11. d. Gardasil is recommended for all individuals through age 26 years.

12. b. Shingrix is the brand name for Zoster (recombinant). Gardasil is the brand name for the human papillomavirus vaccine. Trumenba is the brand name for the meningococcal serogroup B vaccine. Varivax is the brand name for varicella vaccine.

13. c. Meningococcal serogroups A, C, W, Y vaccine is indicated for first-year college students who live in residential housing (if not previously vaccinated at age 16 years or older) or military recruits. Hepatitis A

vaccine is indicated for not at-risk individuals who want protection from hepatitis A. Human papillomavirus vaccine is recommended for all individuals through the age of 26. mRNA-1273 (Spikevax) vaccine is indicated for COVID-19.

14. c. The use of abbreviations found on the ISMP's Do Not Use or ISMP's error-prone abbreviations, symbols, and dose designations is an example of prescribing error. According to the ISMP these abbreviations, symbols, and dose designations should *never* be used when communicating medical information verbally, electronically, and/or in handwritten applications. This includes internal communications; verbal, handwritten, or electronic prescriptions.

15. d. A root cause classification considered technical is one whereby the equipment used in processing or compounding a prescription is not working properly. A root cause classification considered human is an error caused by an individual by not following procedures, missing or ignoring a step, or lack of training. A root cause classification considered to be manufacturing is error caused during manufacturing in which the medication is not manufactured according to specifications, or the packaging or educational materials provided are incorrect. A root cause classified as organizational is one whereby the health care organization's policy and procedures lack appropriate directions for the staff to perform their jobs properly, including training.

16. c. A medication education error is one where proper education material is not provided to the patient. An example is the failure of the pharmacist or pharmacy technician to provide a medication guide to the patient is classified as medication education error. A compliance error indicates inappropriate patient behavior regarding adherence to a prescribed medication regimen. Documentation error occurs when essential information is missing or incorrect such as the pharmacy's information system is not current. A wrong drug error occurs when a drug was dispensed that is different than the drug prescribed.

17. a. An adverse drug error occurs when a drug utilization review warning is missed or ignored. An example occurs when a pharmacy technician overrides a drug utilization review warning and fails to inform the pharmacist. A deteriorated drug error is one where a drug dispensed has expired or for which the physical or chemical dosage-form integrity has been compromised. Wrong label/mislabeling error occurs when incorrect information in entered on the label. This type of error could involve wrong directions on the label to include the route of administration, frequency of administration, and timing of administration. A wrong formulation error occurs when a different dosage form or salt is dispensed without the prescriber's permission.

18. b. A category B medication error is one that occurred but did not reach the patient. A Category A medication error is one where circumstances exist that have potential for causing errors. A category C medication error is one where the error reached patient but did not cause harm. A category D medication error is one where the error reached patient and did not cause harm but needed monitoring or intervention to prove no harm resulted.

19. d. The physician should write *right eye* instead of using OD. *Left ear* should be written out instead of using the abbreviation AS. *Left eye* should be written out instead of using the abbreviation OS. *Right ear* should be written out instead of using the abbreviation AD.

20. d. The metric system is the approved system of measurement for the practice of pharmacy in the United States.

21. b. The drugs buPROPion and busPIRone are drugs bearing confused drug names. The drugs buPROPion and busPIRone are not controlled substances. The drugs buPROPion and busPIRone may be crushed. The drugs buPROPion and busPIRone are not proprietary drug names but are nonproprietary drug names.

22. b. Primary nonadherence occurs when a new medication is prescribed for a patient, but the patient fails to obtain the medication (or its appropriate alternative) within an acceptable period of time after it was initially prescribed. Intentional medication nonadherence occurs when the patient chooses to deviate from their treatment regimen. Secondary nonadherence occurs when a patient fills a prescription but does not take the medication as it was intended and/or prescribed. Unintentional medication nonadherence occurs when the patient may be careless or forgetful about adhering to treatment regimen.

23. c. Excessive polypharmacy occurs when the patient is concurrently using 10 or more medications. Polypharmacy occurs when a patient is taking 5 to 9 medications. The term *no polypharmacy* is used when a patient is taking 4 or fewer medications.

24. d. A patient's ability to pay for their medication is not a component of their health literacy. It is a factor that may affect their adherence to their medication therapy. Health literacy requires a patient to be able to read, listen, communicate, and comprehend to follow a medication regimen.

25. b. The Joint Commission requires two identifiers be provided by a patient prior to point of care testing.

Chapter 6

1. a. Angiotensin-converting enzyme inhibitors are indicated for conditions affecting the cardiovascular. Angiotensin-converting enzyme inhibitors are not indicated for conditions affecting the circulatory, endocrine, or respiratory systems.

2. c. A syrup is a concentrated solution of sugar in water or other aqueous liquid. An emulsion is a two-phase system in which one liquid is dispersed in the form of small globules throughout another liquid. The dispersed liquid is known as the internal phase, whereas the dispersion medium as the external or continuous phase. Emulsions may be oil in water or water in oil. A suspension is a coarse dispersion containing finely divided insoluble material suspended in a liquid medium. A tincture is a dilute solution consisting of a medicinal substance in alcohol or in alcohol and water, usually 10% to 20% by volume

3. b. An ophthalmic solution is a parenteral dosage form. Bulk powders, rectal suppositories, and sublingual tablets are examples of enteral dosage forms.

4. c. Room temperature is 20°C to 25°C. Cool is 8°C to 15°C. A cold temperature does not exceed 8°C. Excessive heat is any temperature greater than 40°C.

5. a. Enbrel must be refrigerated. Spikevax must be stored in an ultracold freezer. Synthroid should be stored at room temperature. Zostavax should be stored in the freezer.

6. c. An opened vial of insulin be stored at room temperature for no more than 28 days.

7. c. Insulin should be administered subcutaneously at a 45° to 90° angle. An intradermal injection should be administered at a 5° to 15° angle. An intravenous injection should be injected at 15° to 35° angle. An intradermal injection should be administered at 90° angle.

8. b. Pruritis means intense itching. Otalgia refers to an earache. Rhinitis is a runny nose. Erythema refers to skin redness.

9. d. Tachycardia refers to a rapid heart rate. Ostealgia means bone pain. Glycosuria refers to glucose in the urine. Dysuria means painful urination.

10. d. A medication (drug) allergy is an abnormal reaction of the immune system to a medication (drug). An adverse drug event is the harm experienced by a patient as a result of exposure to a medication. Drug intolerance is the inability of an individual to tolerate the adverse effects of a medication, generally at therapeutic or subtherapeutic doses. Idiosyncratic drug reaction is an adverse effect that cannot be explained by the known mechanisms of action by a medication.

11. b. Family history is a component of an individual's medical history. Exercise, religion, and substance use are parts of an individual's social history.

12. b. Primary nonadherence adherence occurs when a new medication is prescribed for a patient, but the patient fails to obtain the medication. Intentional medication nonadherence is an active process whereby the patient chooses to deviate from the treatment regimen. Secondary nonadherence occurs when a patient fills a prescription but does not take the medication as it was intended and/or prescribed. Unintentional medication nonadherence is a passive process in which the patient may be careless or forgetful about adhering to treatment regimen.

13. c. A patient with a blood pressure of 115/70 is classified as normal. Normal blood pressure is <120/≤80. Hypertensive crisis occurs when an individual's blood pressure is >180/>120. Elevated blood pressure occurs when an individual's blood pressure is 120 to 129/<80. An individual is classified as having stage 1 hypertension has blood pressure being 130 to 139/80 to 89.

14. b. Cholesterol is a non-water-soluble lipid, which is transported in lipoprotein particles, which are water soluble. Apolipoprotein B is the primary protein contained within low-density lipoprotein and very low-density lipoprotein. Triglycerides are the dominant form of body-stored fat consisting of three fatty molecules and a molecule of the alcohol glycerol. Very low-density lipoprotein cholesterol particles carry triglycerides in the blood.

15. c. A demonstrated outcome associated with MTM is increasing a patient's understanding and self-management skills of their medication. Goals of MTM include cutting health care costs due to duplicate or unnecessary prescriptions, decreasing medication-related morbidity and mortality, and reducing preventable adverse events.

16. d. A pharmacy technician can schedule eligible patents for medication therapy review. Only a pharmacist can assess, identify, and prioritize medication-related problems; design a plan to address each identified medication-related problem; and provide suggestions to address a patient's identified medication problems to the physician.

17. d. Herbal products, nonprescription medications, prescription medications, and dietary supplements are listed on a patient's personal medication record.

18. d. A pharmacy technician may remind patients of follow-up physician appointments and scheduled laboratory tests. In addition, a pharmacy technician may review a patient's refill history.

19. a. A pharmacy technician may assist the pharmacist in developing written communication to a physician when intervening or referring a patient during medication therapy management. Only the pharmacist may consult the physician on the selection medications for a patient. Only the pharmacist may develop a collaborative agreement with a physician. The pharmacist may provide suggestions to the physician to address medication problems.

20. d. Each state determines what is permitted under a CPA. The magnitude of services that can be performed by pharmacists within the CPA also differs from state to state. Some states have strict limitations, and others leave more of the decision-making up to the discretion of the provider. Once a state has allowed CPA and has defined the specific terms, individual organizations can decide what they will permit pharmacists to do. Services performed by pharmacists under CPAs are not limited to modification of drug therapy and monitoring of laboratory tests. States may require credentialing for pharmacists to participate in CPAs, and other states may stipulate specific continuing education or completion of a certificate training program.

21. b. Chronic conditions covered under Medicare Part D include hypertension, Alzheimer disease, bone disease/arthritis (e.g., osteoporosis, osteoarthritis, rheumatoid arthritis), chronic heart failure, diabetes, dyslipidemia, end-stage renal disease, mental health disorders (e.g., depression, schizophrenia, bipolar disorder), respiratory disease (e.g., asthma, chronic obstructive pulmonary disease, or chronic lung disorder).

22. b. CPT 99605 is used in billing for medication therapy management service(s) for a pharmacist who provides face-to-face services with a new patient, to include an assessment and intervention for the initial visit of 15 minutes. CPT 99064 is not used in billing for MTM services. CPT 99606 is used in billing for medication therapy management service(s) for a pharmacist who provides face-to-face services with an established patient, to include an assessment and intervention for a visit of 15 minutes. CPT 99607 is used in billing for medication therapy management service(s) for a pharmacist who provides face-to-face services to a patient for an additional 15 minutes and is used in conjunction with CPT 99605 or CPT 99607.

23. d. Proton pump inhibitors are used to treat conditions affecting the gastrointestinal system.
24. b. An enteric-coated tablet is a tablet coated with a material that permits transit through the stomach to the small intestine before the medication is released. A capsule is a solid dosage form in which the drug is enclosed in a hard or soft soluble container, usually in the form of gelatin. The gelatin shell dissolves in the stomach and releases the medication from the capsule. A sublingual tablet dissolves when placed beneath the tongue and absorbs into the blood through tissue there. A troche is administered buccally between the gums and the inner lining of the mouth cheek.
25. a. Asthma is a chronic (long-term) condition that affects the airways in the lungs. A dysrhythmia is an abnormal rhythm of the heart. Edema is a build-up of fluid in the body tissues. Pneumonia is a severe inflammation of the lungs in which the alveoli (tiny air sacs) are filled with fluid.

Chapter 7

1. c. A pharmacy technician documents the patient's immunization. Only a pharmacist may counsel the patient, determine the appropriateness of the vaccine for the patient, and verify the vaccine order.
2. d. A vaccine is a preparation that is used to stimulate the body's immune response against diseases. An antibody is a complex molecules (immunoglobulins) made in response to an antigen's presence. An antigen is a substance that causes antibody production, resulting in an immune response. A cytokine is a protein that signals cells of the immune system.
3. b. Hepatitis B vaccine may be administered at birth to a newborn. Hepatitis A and measles, mumps, and rubella and varicella vaccines may be administered when the patient is 12 months old.
4. d. There are five doses administered in a series for DTaP. They are administered at 2, 4, 6, 15 to 18 months, and 4 to 6 years.
5. c. Gardasil 9 is the brand name for the human papillomavirus vaccine. Bexsero is the brand name for the meningococcal serotype B vaccine. Engerix-B is the brand name for the hepatitis B vaccine. Prevnar 13 is the brand name for the pneumococcal 13-valent conjugate vaccine.
6. c. Human papillomavirus vaccination is recommended for all persons through the age of 26 years.
7. d. After receiving their first dose of Tdap vaccine, the patient should receive subsequent doses every 10 years.
8. b. A reconstituted vaccine that is not used immediately or comes in a multidose vial should be maintained at 2°C to 8°C (36°–46°F); it should not be frozen.
9. d. VAR vaccine must be used within 30 minutes of being reconstituted. Hib vaccine must be used within 24 hours of being reconstituted. MMR vaccine must be use within 8 hours of being reconstituted. RZV vaccine must be within 6 hours of being reconstituted.
10. a. The varicella vaccine is administered subcutaneously and uses a ⅝″ needle to patients regardless of their age.

Vaccines administered intramuscularly may use a ⅝″, 1″, 1¼″, or 1½″ needle length depending on the age of the patient and the location site.
11. a. The RZV vaccine requires to be reconstituted with AS01B§ adjuvant suspension. ActHIB vaccine is reconstituted with 0.4% sodium chloride. Hib vaccine is reconstituted with 0.9% sodium chloride. iImovax, M-M-R II, ProQuad (MMRV), and RabAvert vaccines are reconstituted with sterile water.
12. a. HPV vaccine is administered intramuscularly. MMR, VAR, and ZVL vaccines are administered subcutaneously.
13. d. To administer a vaccine IM into an infant, toddler, child, or adult, the needle should be inserted at a 90° angle. To administer a subcutaneous vaccine into an infant, child, or adult, the needle should be inserted at 45° angle.
14. a. FluMist Quadrivalent is administered intranasally. Prevnar 13 and Trumenba are administered intramuscularly. Rotarix is administered orally.
15. c. A sharps container should be replaced when it is three-quarters filled.
16. d. A needlestick injury should be washed with soap and water. Eyes that have been exposed to patient blood or bodily fluids should be irrigated with clean water or saline or sterile irrigants.
17. a. An alcohol swab is used to clean the skin prior to administering a vaccine subcutaneously or IM. Hydrogen peroxide, merthiolate, and sterile water are not used to clean the skin prior to administering a vaccine subcutaneously or intramuscularly.
18. d. The diluent for Varivax may be stored at either room temperature or in the refrigerator. The diluent for Menveo, RabAvert, and Shingrix must be stored in the refrigerator.
19. d. Rotarix is administered as an oral drop. Gardasil and Prevnar 13 are administered intramuscularly. Measles, mumps, and rubella are administered subcutaneously.
20. c. The deltoid muscle is the site of injection for an adult receiving an intramuscular injection. The anterolateral thigh muscle is the primary site of administration for an intramuscular injection for a newborn, infant, or toddler and is an alternate site children and adults. Injections are not administered into the bicep muscles. A child older than 1 year of age and adults may receive a subcutaneous injection into the fatty tissue covering the triceps muscle.
21. b. The office address and the individual's name and title who administered the vaccine must appear on the patient's medical record. Other information required to be recorded on a patient's medical record the date of when the dose of the vaccine was administered, *not* the date when the next dose is to be administered. The edition date of the VIS and the date the VIS is provided must appear on the patient's medical record, *not* the original date of the VIS. The vaccine manufacturer and lot number of the vaccine need to be recorded on the patient's medical record; the expiration date of the vaccine does *not* need to be recorded on the patient's medical record.

22. a. Prior to storing vaccines in the storage unit, the unit must demonstrate 2 consecutive days of temperatures have been recorded within the recommended range.

23. b. Freezers should maintain temperatures between −50°C and −15°C (−58°F and +5°F).

24. d. The vaccine coordinator should be notified immediately upon discovery of temperature excursion. Contacting the vaccine manufacturer, documenting the details of the incident, and labeling exposed vaccines "Do Not Use" and segregating them from other vaccine in the storage unit should be done after notifying the vaccine coordinator.

25. b. VAERS is used to report an adverse event associated with the administration of a vaccine. MERP is used to report a medication error. VERP is used to report an error associated with a vaccine. A VIS is a vaccine information sheet that explains the benefits and risks associated with a vaccine.

Chapter 8

1. c. Only the pharmacist can interpret point-of-care test results. Both the pharmacist and pharmacy technician may be responsible for collecting demographic, social, and clinical data and consent forms, insurance, and payments from the patient. ensuring the test and reagents are stored properly, identify and recording the test results in a log.

2. a. An institution's exposure control plan must be reviewed and updated every year.

3. b. An institution must offer free hepatitis B vaccinations to all employees with occupational exposure to blood or other potentially infectious materials.

4. b. The OSHA Bloodborne Pathogen Standard requires that employees be trained annually.

5. d. Amniotic fluids, saliva and serum may contain biohazardous waste.

6. b. A red container indicates it contains biohazardous waste. A black indicates it contains Resource Conservation Recovery Act (RCRA) hazardous waste; a white container with a blue lid indicates it contains pharmaceutical waste, and a yellow container indicates it contains chemotherapy waste.

7. b. The Joint Commission requires at least two identifiers be provided by the patient prior to administering the point-of-care testing.

8. c. Stage 1 hypertension has a reading of 130 to 139/80 to 89. Normal blood pressure is <120/≤80; elevated blood pressure is 120 to 129/<80; and hypertensive crisis is >180/>120.

9. d. 3-Hydroxy-3-methylglutaryl coenzyme A reductase inhibitors are not indicated for hypertension. Angiotensin converting enzyme inhibitors, beta-adrenergic antagonists, diuretics, and calcium channel blockers are indicated for hypertension.

10. a. A1C is used to diagnose diabetes. Dyslipidemia is diagnosed using by measuring plasma levels of total cholesterol, triglycerides, and individual lipoproteins. Hypertension is diagnosed through a blood pressure monitor. Hypothyroidism is diagnosed through blood plasma test measuring thyroid-stimulating hormone.

11. b. COVID-19 is caused by the SARS-CoV-2 virus. Acute pharyngitis is caused by group A Streptococcus; influenza is caused by influenza virus; and syphilis is caused by *Treponema pallidium*.

12. d. A symptom is a physical or mental problem that a person experiences that may indicate a disease or condition. The chief complaint is a statement from the patient indicating the reason they are seeking medical attention. A medication allergy is the abnormal reaction of the immune system to as a result of a medication. A family history is a RECORD OF THE RELATIONSHIPS AMONG FAMILY MEMBERS ALONG WITH THEIR MEDICAL HISTORIES and may reveal potential indicators of genetic predisposition to disease.

13. c. The Centor Score may be used as a screening tool to identify GAS pharyngitis. The Centor Score is not used as a screening tool for chlamydia, gonorrhea, or influenza-like illness.

14. b. The CMS conducts laboratory inspections for facilities providing point-of-care testing. The CDC, DEA, and FDA do not conduct laboratory inspections for facilities providing point-of-care testing.

15. b. A facility wishing to participate in a the CLIA Waiver Process must follow the manufacturer's instructions for the waived tests the pharmacy is performing; enrolling the laboratory in the CLIA program by completing an application (Form CMS-116); pay the certificate fee every 2 years; and submit the application process to your local state agency.

16. c. A Certificate of Waiver permits a laboratory to administer tests the FDA categorizes as waived tests. They are required to enroll in the CLIA program. Laboratories with Certificate of Waiver are only surveyed if a complaint has been made; the testing is beyond the scope of the certificate; there's a risk of harm due to incorrect testing or to collect waived test information.

17. d. An INR analyzer measures blood-clotting time (PT) for people who are taking anticoagulation medications such as warfarin. Blood glucose can be measured using a glucometer (blood glucose monitor). A serum chemistry analyzer is used to perform tests on whole blood, serum, plasma, or urine samples to determine concentrations of analytes such as cholesterol. An HgbA1c analyzer is used to measure glycated hemoglobin, which is a marker for diabetes mellitus.

18. c. The COVID-19 test is a qualitative test. A1C, cholesterol, and lipid panels are quantitative tests.

19. c. The summary explains what the test detects. The intended use describes the test purpose, substance detected or measured, test methodology, appropriate specimen type, and FDA-cleared conditions for use. Precautions alert the user of practices or conditions affecting the test, potential hazards, and safety precautions. The test principle describes the test methodology and technical reactions of the test and the interactions with the sample to detect or measure a specific substance.

20. c. Sensitivity is the proportion of patients who do have the disease that test positive. A false-negative result occurs when a patient with the underlying disease tests negative. A false-positive result occurs when a patient

without the underlying disease tests positive. Specificity refers to the proportion of patients that do not have the disease that test negative.

21. d. Quantitative (numerical) results should be recorded in the appropriate units of measurement. Qualitative results should be recorded using words or abbreviations rather than symbols. For example use: "Positive" or "Pos," "Reactive" or "R" instead of "+" and "Negative" or "Neg," "Nonreactive" or "NR" instead of "-".

22. b. The person performing the quantitative test should initial the results after verifying all of the information has been entered correctly.

23. b. A refrigerator used to store patient samples is kept between +2°C and +8°C.

24. d. Recording temperatures requires dating and initialing/signing the temperature log; posting a temperature log on the refrigerator and/or freezer door; and reading and recording the thermometer(s) in the refrigerator and/or freezer daily.

25. d. Some the records a point-of-care facility must maintain include daily temperature checks, test system or equipment function checks, and maintenance; quality control results; and test or product recall notices.

Chapter 9

1. a. An HMO requires a patient to use network providers only a point-of-service and a PPO may permit network providers or out-of-network providers.

2. d. A Patient assistance program is a program created by pharmaceutical and medical supply manufacturers to help financially needy patients purchase necessary medications and supplies. A drug discount card provides the patient the ability to purchase medications at a contracted provider rate. A health savings account is a type of savings account that permits the patient to set aside money on a pretax basis to pay for qualified medical expenses. Manufacturer-sponsored prescription coupons (manufacture discount programs) are provided by pharmaceutical companies to encourage use of specific medications.

3. b. Medicare Part B covers physician visits, clinical laboratory services, and outpatient and preventative care screenings. Medicare Part A covers inpatient hospital stays, inpatient stays at most skilled nursing facilities, and hospice and home health care. Medicare Part C is known as Medicare Advantage (MA) and can be combined with Medicare Part D through a Medicare Advantage Prescription Drug (MA-PD). Medicare Part D is provided by private insurers and approved by Medicare and can be purchased to work in conjunction with Medicare Part A and B or combined with Part C through an MA-PD plan.

4. a. To be eligible for Medicare Part D Assistance for Low Income Beneficiaries, an individual must be enrolled in Medicare Parts A and B.

5. c. Medicaid is a joint federal and state program.

6. a. A copayment is the portion of the prescription bill that the patient is responsible for paying. A deductible is the amount paid by a policyholder out of pocket before the insurance pays a claim. The EAC is a state Medicaid Agency's best estimate of the price paid by pharmacies for a particular drug. Usual/customary/reasonable is the amount paid for a medical service in a geographic area based on what providers in the area usually charge for the same or similar medical service.

7. a. Code 01 is assigned to the cardholder of the insurance plan for a prescription. Code 02 is assigned to the spouse of the cardholder, and code 03 is assigned to a dependent. Code 04 is not assigned.

8. c. RxBIN (bank identification number) is a six-digit number used to identify the company that will reimburse the pharmacy for the prescription being filled. Group code refers to employer that contracted the insurance company for the policy. RxPCN is a number/code identifying which company processes the prescription claim. The subscriber is the individual who purchased the insurance plan.

9. b. A DAW 1 code indicates substitution is not allowed by provider and the brand name medication must be dispensed. DAW 0 indicates no product selection was indicated on the prescription and a generic medication can be dispensed. DAW 2 indicates that substitution is allowed; however, the patient requested the product be dispensed. DAW indicates that substitution is allowed, and the pharmacist selected the product dispensed.

10. c. A patient's NPI number is not transmitted during adjudication. Patient information during adjudication includes patient name, date of birth, gender, patient's relationship to the cardholder, cardholder/member identification number, and group number.

11. c. A code 9 indicates the patient's birthdate is incorrect. If the date the prescription was filled is incorrect, the rejection code is 15. An incorrect day's supply would have a rejection code of 19. If the patient's gender is incorrect the rejection code would be 10.

12. a. A generic drug is classified as tier 1. Preferred brand drugs are tier 2. Nonpreferred brand drugs are tier 3. Preferred specialty drugs are tier 4.

13. d. A CPT code consists of six digits.

14. c. An NPI number consists of 10 digits.

15. b. If two or more plans cover dependent children of separated or divorced parents, who do not have joint custody of their children, the child's primary plan is determined in this order: the plan of the custodial parent, the plan of spouse of the custodial parent (if the parent has been remarried), and the plan of the parents without custody. The birthday rule is used in primary coverage of a married couple.

16. d. AWP is the national average of list prices charged by wholesalers to pharmacies. AAC refers to the price determined by CMS/HHS of the pharmacy providers' actual prices paid to acquire drug products marketed or sold by specific manufacturers. AMP is the average price paid to the manufacturer for the drug in the United States by wholesalers for drugs distributed to retail community pharmacies and retail community pharmacies that purchase drugs directly from the manufacturer. ASP is the weighted average of all nonfederal sales to wholesalers.

17. d. A request for an override for a medication with restricted limitations may be done based on age or sex restrictions, early refill on a medication, and the quantity

to be dispensed. Other exceptions include dispensing a brand-name medication instead of the generic medication, medication quantity limit, or a 7+-hour emergency supply of the medication.

18. c. The prescriber's office is responsible for obtaining the prior authorization. The pharmacy can request the process to be started. The patient is not involved in the prior authorization process.

19. c. A CPT code of 99605 should be used for a new patient, face to face visit of 15 minutes. A CPT G0108 is used for Individual diabetes training. A DAW 0 indicates no product selection was indicated.

20. a. The CMS oversees CHIP, Medicare, and Medicaid. HRSA is responsible for the oversight of the 340B program. The Joint Commission (TJC) accredits and certifies hospitals and health care organizations that provide ambulatory and office-based surgery, behavioral health, home health care, laboratory and nursing care center services. URAC accredits specialty pharmacies, specialty pharmacy services, mail order services pharmacies, infusion pharmacies, Medicare home infusion therapy supplier accreditation, and pharmacy benefit accreditation.

21. c. The Joint Commission organization established national patent safety goals for ambulatory care, assisted living communities, behavioral health care and human services, critical access hospital, home care, laboratory, nursing care centers, and office-based surgery.

22. d. URAC developed the Opioid Stewardship designation.

23. d. The CMS publishes the Medicare Advantage (Medicare Part C) and Medicare Part D Star Ratings each year to measure the quality of health and drug services received by consumers enrolled in Medicare Advantage and Prescription Drug Plans (or Part D plans).

24. b. The False Claims Act encourages submitting suspected fraud and abuse against the government by protecting and rewarding individuals in whistleblower cases. The Anti-Kickback Statute makes it illegal to knowingly offer incentives to induce referral for services that are paid by government health care programs. The Physician Self-Referral Law makes it illegal for physicians and members of their immediate family to have financial relationships with clinics to which they refer their patients. The Sarbanes-Oxley Act established a comprehensive reform of financial practices for businesses that focuses on publicly held corporations, financial reporting, audit procedures, and their internal financial controls.

25. c. For-profit hospitals are *not* eligible to participate in the 340B Program.

Chapter 10

1. c. Amlodipine is not available as 7.5 mg strength. It is available as a 2.5 mg, 5 mg, and 10 mg tablet.
2. d. The lowest available dose of atorvastatin is 10 mg.
3. c. Gabapentin is only available as a 400 mg tablet.
4. c. Duloxetine is the generic name for Cymbalta. Bupropion is the generic name for Wellbutrin XL or Wellbutrin SR; citalopram is the generic name for Celexa; and fluoxetine is the generic name for Prozac.

5. c. Solve by setting up the following proportion: 1 tablet/1 day = X tablets/90 days. Cross multiply and divide; 90 tablets should be dispensed.

6. c. Ferrous sulfate may discolor the urine or feces.

7. b. Coreg is not taken twice a day; it is taken once a day. Coreg CR is indicated for hypertension. Coreg CR is available as a capsule. Coreg CR is a brand-name drug.

8. b. Instill one (i) drop in left eye (os) each (q) evening (pm).

9. b. Alprazolam is a controlled substance and requires the auxiliary label: Caution: Federal law prohibits the transfer of this drug to any person other than the patient for whom it was prescribed to be affixed to the prescription bottle

10. d Acetaminophen with codeine is a Schedule III controlled substance and must be filled within 6 months of being written and can have a maximum of five refills.

11. b. 200 inhalations/8 inhalations per day = 25 days.

12. a. Losartan is a generic drug name. The physician indicated on the prescription that no product selection was indicated and therefore a DAW code 0 should be inputted. A DAW 1 indicates substitution is not allowed by the provider.

13. c. (5 mL/1 teaspoon) (3 tsp/1 tbsp) (2 tbsp/1 fl oz) (16 fl oz/1 pt) = 480 mL

14. d. The formula makes 100 g of psoriasis ointment. One pound is equal to 454 g. Calculate the factor needed to enlarge the formula by dividing the weight to be compounded by the total weight of the formula (454 g/100 g) = 4.54. Multiply the quantity of each ingredient by 4.54. Coal tar 2 g × 4.54 = 9.08 g of coal tar.

15. d. Solve by: Volume (mL) × % (expressed as a decimal) = milliliters of active ingredient; 240 mL × (2.5 mL/100 mL) = 6 mL.

16. b. Solve by: 1 mL/20 drops = 5 mL/x drops where x = 100 drops in the bottle; (100 drops)/(2 drop/dose)/2 doses per day) = 25 days.

17. c. The spouse of the cardholder is assigned 02 as a relationship code.

18. d. Furosemide is a diuretic and as a result loses potassium during enuresis. Orange juice and potassium are a source of potassium and can help replenish the lost potassium.

19. d. A medication guide must be provided to the patient or the patient's agent when the patient or the patient's agent requests a medication guide; when a drug is dispensed in an outpatient setting (e.g., retail pharmacy, hospital ambulatory care pharmacy), and the product will then be used by the patient without direct supervision by a health care professional; the first time a drug is dispensed to a health care professional for administration to a patient in an outpatient setting, such as in a clinic or dialysis or infusion center; the first time a drug is dispensed in an outpatient setting of any kind, after a medication guide is materially changed (e.g., after addition of a new indication, new safety information), and when a drug is subject to a REMS that includes specific requirements for reviewing or providing a medication guide as part of an element to assure safe use (possibly in conjunction with distribution, the medication guide must be provided in accordance with the terms of the REMS.

20. b. The FDA requires a medication guide be distributed to the patient when they receive a prescription of ciprofloxacin. Medication guides do not need to be distributed to patients receiving a prescription for amoxicillin or tetracycline.

21. d. QOD appears on the TJC's "Do Not Use" List. AC, BID, and PO do not appear on the TJC's "Do Not Use" List.

22. d. Medication tampering should be reported to the FDA Office of Criminal Investigations, professional and pharmacy boards, law enforcement, and local public health officials upon confirmation of the tampering incident.

23. c. Signs of instability of solution includes discoloration, precipitates, haziness, gas formation, and microbial growth and unclear and inappropriate color and/or odor.

24. a. USP <797> states a Category 3 sterile preparation that has been aseptically processed, tested for sterility, and passed all applicable tests for a Category 3 CSP should be assigned a BUD of 60 days.

25. Amoxicillin suspension is considered a nonpreserved aqueous dosage form and USP <795> assigns it a BUD of 14 days.

Index

Page numbers followed by "*b*" indicate boxes, "*f*" indicate figures, "*t*" indicate tables.

G

Gabapentin, 237t–247t
Garbing and gloving competency evaluation, 29
Gastroesophageal reflux disease, 156
Gel, 150, 248
Gestational diabetes mellitus, 158
Glaucoma, 156
Glimepiride, 237t–247t
Glipizide, 237t–247t
Gloved fingertip sampling, 29–30
Gloves, PPE, 52
Gonorrhea, 197–198
Gowns, PPE, 52–53
Graves' disease, 156
Gravimetric analysis, weighing and measuring components, 37
Group health plans, 209

H

Hair covers, PPE, 53
Handbook on Injectable Drugs (Trissel), 22
Hand hygiene
    compounded sterile preparation, 31–32, 31f
    and personal protective equipment, 59, 193
Handling of hazardous drugs, 77
Hazard Communication Program, 57–58
Hazardous drug management
    accidental exposure of, 51–52
    antineoplastic, 48
    ASHP's recommendation procedure
        general spill procedure, 60–61
        spills in containment primary engineering control, 61
    biological safety cabinets, 49–50
    containment supplemental engineering controls, 55–56
    dispensing final dosage forms, 55–56
    disposal of, 77
    domains, 47b
    eligibility requirements, 47b
    engineering controls, 47–50
        nonsterile hazardous drugs manipulation, 50
        receiving and storing hazardous, 47–48
        sterile hazardous drugs manipulation, 48–50
    environmental monitoring, 60
    facility cleaning
        cleaning, 50–51
        deactivating, 50–51
        decontaminating, 50–51
        disinfecting areas, 50–51
    federal regulations, disposal of hazardous drugs, 56–57
    handling of, 77
    ISO Class 7 anteroom, 49
    ISO Class 7 buffer room, 49
    personal protective equipment
        disposal process, 54
        requirements, 52–54
    refrigerated antineoplastic, 48
    spill control of, 60

Hazardous drug management *(Continued)*
    sterile and nonsterile, 48
    transport and receiving, 54–55
Hazardous waste management, in pharmacy, 68
Head covers, PPE, 53
Health care
    reimbursement systems, 210–214
    services reimbursement, 223
Health history collection, 198
Health Insurance Portability and Accountability Act (HIPAA) standards, 65–66, 145
    administrative simplification provisions, 67
    electronic health care transactions and code sets standard, 67
    privacy rule, 67
    purpose of, 67
    security rule, 67
Health literacy, 144–145, 157
Health savings account, third party reimbursement types, 210
Heart rate, 194
Hepatitis B vaccination, 192
Hepatitis C, screening tests, 201
Herbal supplements (botanical), 129, 155
HgbA1c analyzers, 201
High-alert drug classifications
    in acute care settings, 20–21
    narrow therapeutic index medications, 21
High-deductible health plan, 209
High-density lipoprotein cholesterol, 158
High-efficiency particulate air (HEPA)-filtered supply air, 49
HIV screening tests, 201
HMO, health insurance, 209
Home pregnancy, screening tests, 201
Hospital's number, DEA, 69
Household system of measurement, pharmacy conversions, 259
HRSA 340B audit data requests, 231
Human blood and blood products, point-of-care testing, 193
Human body fluids, point-of-care testing, 193
Human, medication error, 135
Humoral immunity, 171
Hydralazine, 237t–247t
Hydrochlorothiazide, 237t–247t
Hydrocodone/acetaminophen, 237t–247t
Hydroxyzine, 237t–247t
Hypercholesterolemia. *See* Hyperlipidemia
Hyperlipidemia, 156, 158–159
    laboratory values, 159t
    lipid levels, 159t
    types of, 158t
Hypertension, 156
    category of, 196t
    classifications, 158t
    laboratory measures, 158
    signs and symptoms, 195–196
    treatments, 196
Hypotension, 156
Hypothyroidism, 156

I

Ibuprofen, 237t–247t
Ideal body weight (IBW), 31

Idiopathic medication, 129
Idiosyncratic drug reaction, 155
Idiosyncratic reaction, 129
Ignitability, RCRA, 56
Illegible prescriptions, medication error, 135
Immediate-use compounded sterile preparations, 22
Immunity, 171
Immunization (vaccination/inoculation), 129, 155, 171
    active immunity, 171
    adjuvants, 171
    adult immunization schedule recommendations, 173t–175t
    anaphylaxis, 171
    antibodies, 171
    antigen, 171
    antigen-presenting cell, 171
    attenuated, 171
    child and adolescent immunization schedule recommendations, 172t–173t
    cold chain, 171
    combination vaccinations, 173t
    cytokine, 171
    documentation, 180–181, 180t–181t
    domains, 170b
    eligibility requirements, 170b
    emergency medical protocol, 185, 185t
    handling of vaccines, 181
    history, 155
    humoral immunity, 171
    immunity, 171
    immunization, 171
    inactivated vaccine, 171
    innate immunity, 171
    live attenuated vaccine, 171
    lyophilization, 171
    natural immunity, 171
    passive immunity, 171
    pharmacy technician role, 170–171
    preservative, 171
    receiving of vaccines, 182
    requirements, 170t–171t
    schedule
        adult, 133ta–134ta
        child and adolescent, 131–135, 131ta–133ta
    stabilizers, 171
    storing of vaccines, 182–183
    terminology, 171–172
    toxoid, 171
    vaccination, 171
    and vaccination schedules, 172–175
    vaccine, 172
    vaccine administration preparation, 175–177
        with diluents, 175t–176t
        infection control, 175
        intramuscular injections, 176–177, 177t
        reconstituting vaccines, 175–176
        subcutaneous injection, 176, 176t
    vaccine administration procedures
        inhalation for live attenuated influenza vaccine, 179
        intramuscular, 178–179, 178f
        multiple vaccinations, 179
        oral drop, 179
        rotateq, 179
        rotavirus vaccine, 179
        subcutaneous, 177–178, 177f

J

K

L

M